Memorable Psychiatry

Second Edition

Jonathan Heldt, M.D.

Also available from the same author:
Memorable Psychopharmacology
Memorable Neurology

The content of this book is not intended to be a replacement for proper medical training, nor is it intended to substitute for professional medical advice, diagnosis, or treatment. Always seek the advice of your physician or other qualified health provider with any questions you may have regarding a medical condition.

Editing and behavioral consultation provided by **Juliane Heldt, BCBA (Board Certified Behavior Analyst)**.

Copyright © 2018, 2021 Jonathan Heldt.

All rights reserved.

Revision 2.1. Last revised September 1, 2021.

ISBN: 1737210818
ISBN-13: 978-1737210818

DEDICATION

To **my grandparents Steve and Young-cha Pai** who crossed more oceans, worked longer hours, and endured greater hardships than anyone should have to so they could provide for their family. Thank you for giving us the life we have today.

CONTENTS

	Acknowledgments	i
1	Introduction	1
2	Diagnosis	3
3	Evaluation	17
4	Psychiatric Emergencies	33
5	Depression	59
6	Bipolar Disorder	81
7	Schizophrenia	101
8	Addiction	129
9	Anxiety	155
10	OCD	175
11	PTSD	197
12	Dissociation	215

13	Somatization	233
14	Personality	251
15	Borderline	271
16	Antisocial	291
17	Psychopathy	309
18	Eating Disorders	321
19	Development	335
20	Autism	357
21	ADHD	373
22	Dementia	389
23	Sleep	413
24	Final Review	429

ACKNOWLEDGMENTS

A world of thanks to **Juliane Heldt, BCBA (Board Certified Behavior Analyst)** for putting my books into the hands of so many people who would not otherwise have seen them. Thank you for being the best editor, publicist, supporter, interdisciplinary consultant, and sister I could ask for.

1 INTRODUCTION

Welcome to the most fascinating field in medicine. Psychiatry deals with the most complex organ in the human body—the **brain**—and the way in which it works not only with the other parts of the body but also with other people and society as a whole. More than any other discipline of medicine, psychiatry requires a meaningful understanding of the world and its complexities. However, too often psychiatry is experienced not as fascinating but as bewildering, mystifying, or illogical. The central tension of psychiatry—how little we know about the brain and its inner workings—is viewed not as a target for curiosity but instead as a barrier to entry. Attempts to make sense of the mind's workings (such as the algorithmic diagnoses that form the basis for most textbooks on psychiatry) often risk going too far in the opposite direction, trading in the dynamic intricacies of the human mind for a simplified "cookbook" of what can go wrong with the brain. This makes psychiatry less bewildering, but it also risks turning it into something boring, tedious, and rote.

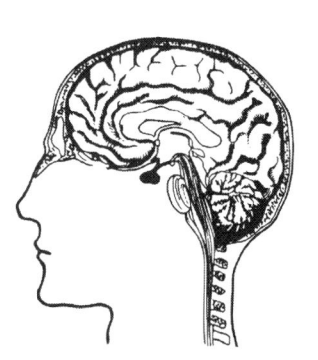

There is a middle ground. This book aims to make the disorders we treat understandable through the use of clear explanations, analogies, and mnemonics. A good understanding of these disorders is essential for allowing **clarity in diagnosis** and avoiding the pitfalls of overdiagnosis, including use of ineffective or even harmful treatments. In addition, this book also aims to provide **practical clinical tools** that you can use when working with patients in the real world.

By design, some of the mnemonics and analogies included may be silly, shocking, or amusing. This is done to the information more accessible, as provoking an emotional response is one of the best ways of getting information to stick. Nothing in this book is intended to stigmatize, trivialize, or humiliate anyone struggling with any of the disorders mentioned.

We'll begin our study of mental disorders with an overview of the line between normalcy and illness. From there, we will learn how to perform a clinical evaluation of someone with a psychiatric problem as well as how to respond to psychiatric emergencies. After that, the book begins in earnest as we learn about all of the major disorders in psychiatry, including depression, mania, psychosis, anxiety, addiction, personality disorders, and many more.

Through each chapter, we will not only learn about each disorder in isolation but also discover out how to differentiate between different psychiatric disorders, many of which have similar or overlapping symptoms. Unfortunately, this means that the going will be a little rough at the beginning, as there is no way to compare diagnoses across categories without bringing up disorders that we have not covered yet. However, rest assured that **it will get easier as time goes on**! In addition, don't be afraid to skip ahead if you need more information on any given subject. Frequent references between chapters will also be made to facilitate understanding. A general understanding of physiology (including the autonomic nervous system) and pathology will be helpful for understanding all of the concepts, but it is not required.

Finally, pay attention to any information presented in boxes! These concepts are particularly high-yield. The most high-yield information has been collected together in a double-sided page at the end of this book. Feel free to reference this as you progress through the book, or you may even consider snapping a photo to take with you as a handy on-the-go memory aid!

> **Concepts in boxes** are particularly **high-yield**!
>
> *An **easy way** to remember them will be in **italics** below.*

Now, let's begin…

2 DIAGNOSIS

In medicine, **diagnosis** is the process of determining what condition best explains a patient's illness. Accurate diagnosis is the basis upon which clinicians make decisions about how best to relieve suffering, and without a diagnosis, appropriate treatment remains out of reach. Diagnosis is accomplished through a careful evaluation of a patient's **signs** (*objective* findings that you can observe directly, such as redness of the eyes) and **symptoms** (*subjective* concerns that the patient tells you about, such as a headache). Signs and symptoms in psychiatry are collectively referred to as **phenomenology**.

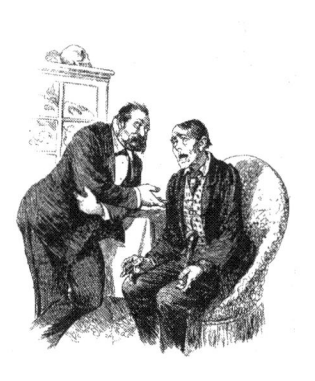

Within psychiatry, many of the conditions we treat are **syndromes** rather than specific disease processes. A syndrome is a set of signs and symptoms that tend to occur together. For example, when someone says that they have a "cold," they are saying that they have a set of signs and symptoms (such as cough, runny nose, sore throat, fatigue, muscle aches, and loss of appetite) that tend to mean something when they cluster together.

Diagnosing a syndrome is not the same as identifying the underlying cause. Using the same example, saying you have a cold is not the same thing as identifying a rhinoviral infection. However, even if it doesn't identify the exact cause of the problem, diagnosing a syndrome is still helpful because it suggests a certain **prognosis** and **treatment response**. For example, identifying that someone has a cold suggests that the signs and symptoms will probably go away on their own in a few days or weeks (its prognosis) and that antibiotics are unlikely to help (its treatment response).

The process of diagnosing a syndrome applies to the majority of conditions that are seen in psychiatry. By saying that someone has depression, we are not saying that we have identified the specific anatomic, physiologic, or cellular processes associated with that disorder. Rather, we are saying that we have recognized a consistent set of signs and symptoms (in the case of depression, things like sadness, fatigue, insomnia, and an inability to enjoy activities) that tend to occur together and predict a certain prognosis (6 to 12 months before recovery in most cases) and treatment response (a beneficial effect from serotonin-boosting medications and psychotherapy). It is possible that, with future research, we will eventually discover more of the mechanisms underlying these syndromes. However, at least at this time, the precise pathology of most mental disorders remains out of our grasp.

Because of this, psychiatric syndromes are referred to as **disorders** rather than diseases. This is because the biological, psychological, and social impairment that they create in peoples' lives (the "disorder") can often be observed objectively, even if there is less agreement on what is causing the impairment (the "disease"). However, the lack of clear objective findings that definitively rule in or out a certain disease makes psychiatric diagnosis an inherently **subjective process**.

> Most **psychiatric disorders** are **syndromes** and not specific pathologies, making psychiatric diagnosis an inherently **subjective** process.
>
> *Syndromes are subjective, pathologies are provable.*

As with any subjective process, not everyone is going to agree. This is made especially difficult because a diagnosis implies a distinction between what is **normal and abnormal**. For example, a boy who is worried about a test at school may believe that having a sore throat is "abnormal enough" to be able to stay home from school. For his mother, however, the lack of a fever suggests that his condition is "normal enough" that he still needs to go to school. The mother may ask a doctor to come by to provide a more formal evaluation. However, even a doctor's professional opinion remains a subjective determination as long as objective markers of a specific disease process are missing.

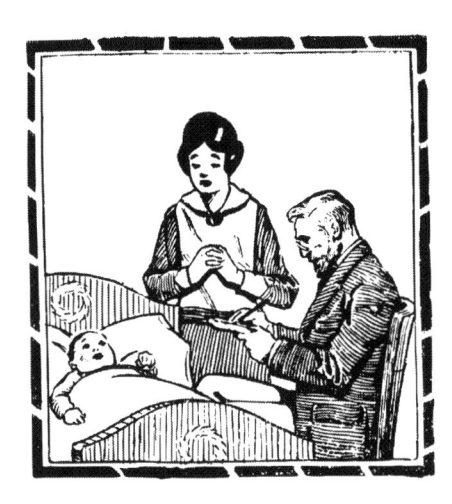

NORMAL VERSUS ABNORMAL

A central tenet of psychiatry is the notion that there are people whose ability to function has been compromised by emotional, cognitive, and/or behavioral problems. These individuals are said to be suffering from **mental disorders** that are distinct enough from "normal" life to warrant medical attention. There is general agreement in the medical community that mental disorders exist. However, there is much less agreement on where to draw the line between normalcy and illness.

At the center of this disagreement is the idea that words like "normal" and "abnormal" are **binary descriptions of dimensional concepts**. Most psychiatric syndromes are not binary "yes-or-no" conditions that are either there or not. Rather, the majority of psychiatric disorders occur on a **spectrum** where some people are severely impaired, others have only mild symptoms, and still others have no symptoms at all. However, the act of diagnosis *is* a binary decision where you either say that someone has the diagnosis or they don't. This attempt to shoehorn non-binary disorders into a binary diagnostic system is inherently problematic, and disagreements are bound to arise.

To understand this better, imagine that you have been given an assignment to define what "abnormally tall" is. On the surface, this seems like a simple task. You initially think, "6 foot 5 inches seems pretty tall." However, you realize that most people will have their own equally arbitrary definition of the height over which someone becomes "too tall," so you decide to be scientific about it. Given that height falls on a normal distribution, you decide that everyone above the 95th percentile should be considered "abnormally tall." You find that in the United States this corresponds to approximately 6'2" for men and 5'8" for women. Upon further reflection, you realize that this distribution varies widely from country to country, making it feel less standardized than you first thought. You then decide to normalize this by only comparing someone's height to their own personal growth trajectory. However, this wouldn't capture someone who has always been abnormally tall even from a young age, so you throw out this idea.

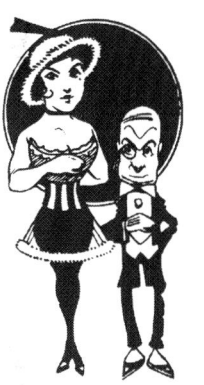

You then decide to go the other way and define "abnormally tall" as being whenever someone *feels* that they are too tall. No, wait, that's too loose and open to various interpretations. Let's try to be scientific again but take a different approach. Maybe there are some biological traits associated with height that you can use to define it rather than everyone having their own arbitrary definitions? For example, certain brain tumors cause an excess of growth hormone which can result in people being really tall. However, you realize that these specific abnormalities won't account for everyone, as there are some really tall people who *don't* have pituitary tumors and other people *with* pituitary tumors who are average height.

Instead, you consider defining "abnormally tall" in terms of how functionally impairing it is, such as needing to special-order clothing that will fit or frequently stooping down to avoid hitting one's head on doorways. However, that also seems very culturally dependent. Getting frustrated, you begin to wonder: why even *have* a definition of "abnormally tall" in the first place? These are all just extremes of normalcy, and it's not good to hold people to any particular standard. Maybe we should be focusing on challenging the obsession that we as a society have with height and appearance rather than making people feel bad for thinking they are too tall or too short. However, then you realize that—like it or not—everyone still has an idea of what "abnormally tall" looks like, even if they don't agree.

Increasingly tired of this assignment, you decide to combine several approaches by saying that if someone is over 95th percentile for height given their country of origin *or* there is a known biological abnormality, then you will say that they are "abnormally tall" provided that this is associated with functional difficulties, personal distress, or medical problems.

ADVANTAGES AND DISADVANTAGES OF DIAGNOSIS

This story illustrates the challenges of trying to define the line between normal and abnormal, even for a concept as simple, objective, and easily measured as height. When you make the concepts involved more abstract (such as the "invisible" concepts in mental health), reaching consensus becomes even more difficult. Indeed, this complexity underlies the reasons why agreeing on diagnostic schemes for mental disorders has been (and will likely remain) such a contentious process. Everyone has their own internal sense of what "abnormal" is, which makes consensus difficult to achieve. Given the trouble of coming up with a diagnostic scheme for even one "disorder," you might be tempted to conclude that there is no point in even having diagnoses at all. However, there are several reasons why diagnosis remains important:

It predicts prognosis and treatment response. Diagnosis predicts prognosis and treatment response, even for conditions that are syndromes rather than clearly defined pathological processes.

It facilitates communication. Diagnosis provides an efficient shorthand for people to communicate quickly with others. For example, rather than saying, "This young lady has grandiose thoughts that she is going to colonize the moon, is displaying erratic behavior, is talking incredibly fast, and hasn't felt the need to sleep for over 2 weeks," someone could simply say, "She is experiencing a manic episode."

It allows research to be coordinated. By standardizing definitions of what constitutes a specific condition, researchers in different places are able to work together to study the causes of and treatments for these disorders. Without this standardization, one group could not be sure that they are studying the same condition as another group, and research efforts would become uncoordinated and ineffective.

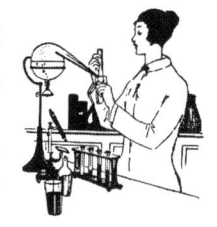

It validates distress. Diagnosis by a qualified professional provides validation of the distress that people with mental disorders experience. This does more than merely offer emotional support. Professional validation of distress carries weight in many areas of life, such as engaging the support of family and friends, satisfying employers (as in a doctor's off-work letter), explaining behavior to authorities, and justifying reimbursement from health insurance companies, among many other things.

It supports community building. A diagnosis can serve as a rallying point for groups of people affected by similar conditions to support one another and work towards positive change, both for themselves (as in Alcoholics Anonymous) and for society as a whole (such as advocacy groups like the National Alliance on Mental Illness).

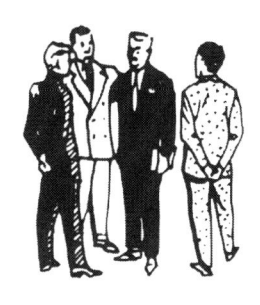

Nevertheless, there are also some downsides associated with diagnosis that cannot be ignored. Despite the benefits of diagnosis, it is not an entirely benign process, for these reasons:

It can lead to overdiagnosis and overtreatment. By making a set of signs and symptoms into a recognizable "disorder," providers are encouraged to actively look for these patterns. This can lead to the overdiagnosis and overtreatment of things that are not necessarily pathological. For example, someone who feels emotions strongly but remains functional still risks being diagnosed with a mood disorder by an overzealous clinician.

It can be stigmatizing. Especially in the realm of mental health, diagnosis can be a highly stigmatizing experience. People often feel "labeled" with a diagnosis and may be treated differently by others as a result. Receiving a diagnosis may also change someone's self-image, leading to decreased self-esteem or lack of belief in their own abilities. Like labels, psychiatric diagnoses and the stigma associated with them can be hard to peel off, and people often find that the negative effects of diagnosis persist even after the initial problem has gone away.

It can lead to a sense of premature closure. Providing a psychiatric diagnosis can "medicalize" normal problems in living and give both the patient and their provider a sense of premature closure. This is especially problematic in psychiatry, as all mental disorders have not only a biological component but psychological and environmental causes as well. For example, someone who has been diagnosed with depression may start believing that they have found the explanation for their distress ("I have a chemical imbalance") and then stop looking for other things they can do to potentially improve their mood, such as strengthening the relationships in their life or doing more activities that they enjoy. A doctor may similarly be convinced that they have figured the situation out and neglect to look for other possible explanations, such as thyroid abnormalities, that could account for changes in mood.

THE ALGORITHMIC APPROACH TO DIAGNOSIS

Despite these disadvantages, psychiatric diagnosis seems here to stay, as the potential advantages are too great to ignore. In modern psychiatry, the most common diagnostic system is the **algorithmic** approach to diagnosis, meaning that each disorder is presented as a set of criteria which are either met or not, resulting in a diagnosis. If we continue with the concept of "abnormally tall" from before, the criteria could be presented algorithmically as:

Excessive Height Disorder:
    A.   The patient meets criteria for at least one of the following:
           a.   Height above the 95th percentile adjusted for country of origin
           b.   Evidence of an underlying biological abnormality (e.g., elevated levels of insulin-like growth factor-1)
    B.   The person has functional difficulties, personal distress, and/or medical problems as a result of Criterion A

Using this algorithmic approach, we can say that someone definitely does or does not qualify for a diagnosis of "Excessive Height Disorder." This decreases ambiguity and ensures that two people who use the same term are in fact talking about the same diagnosis, greatly increasing the **reliability** of psychiatric diagnosis. However, this may have come at the expense of their **validity** or the extent to which the diagnostic criteria actually correspond to the real-life syndrome that they are trying to describe. To use an analogy, someone trying to come up with diagnostic criteria for a mental disorder is akin to an archer trying to hit a target. A *reliable* archer would have all of their arrows hit at approximately the same place. However, this does not mean that they are on target. A *valid* archer would hit the target but would not necessarily do this consistently. Only an archer who is *both reliable and valid* would consistently hit the target.

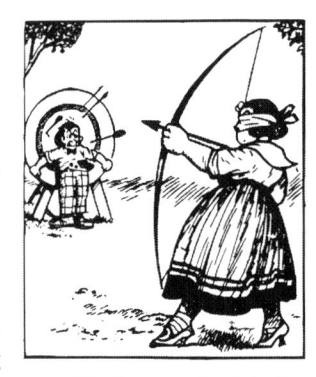

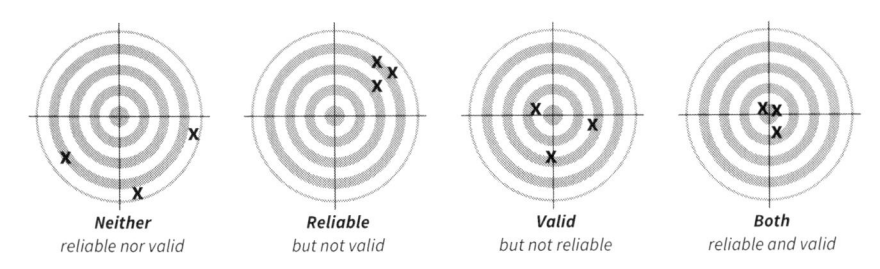

Neither	**Reliable**	**Valid**	**Both**
reliable nor valid	but not valid	but not reliable	reliable and valid

In the same way, using an algorithmic approach to diagnosis makes it so that specific terms are more *reliable*, but it is no guarantee of the *validity* of this diagnosis (it does not necessarily capture the real-life clinical syndrome that they are referring to). We'll talk a few times in this book about times when the validity of a diagnosis has been sacrificed for reliability (I'm looking at you, antisocial personality disorder).

Despite concerns about validity, the increased reliability of algorithmic diagnosis has proven to be popular and enduring. For proof of this, look no further than the Diagnostic and Statistical Manual of Mental Disorders (DSM) published by the American Psychiatric Association and the International Classification of Diseases (ICD) developed by the World Health Organization. Both the DSM and the ICD contain specific algorithmic diagnostic criteria for hundreds of mental disorders and are the dominant classification systems in the United States and across the world.

Throughout this book, we will make reference to diagnostic criteria in the DSM and in particular the fifth edition (DSM-5) which was published in 2013. This is done when the diagnostic criteria have proven helpful for understanding a disorder (such as the SIGECAPS symptoms seen in depression). In addition, we will make reference to the official names for each disorder as listed in the DSM but will not use them exclusively. For example, Alzheimer's disease will be discussed as a form of "dementia" rather than a subtype of "major neurocognitive disorder." This is done to help prepare you for actual clinical experiences where these non-technical terms continue to be used frequently by both professionals and patients. However, keep in mind that the names of disorders found in the DSM are often carefully chosen with the goal of decreasing stigma and increasing scientific accuracy, so in your own practice you should consider what the most appropriate term should be.

THE DIATHESIS-STRESS MODEL

The beginning of this chapter introduced two fundamental dilemmas: how to separate normal from abnormal, and the nature of mental disorders. As a field, we have tried to address the first question using an algorithmic approach to diagnosis. For the second question, a number of models have been proposed to explain the possible origins of mental disorders. One model known as the **diathesis-stress model** states that the majority of psychiatric syndromes can be conceptualized as the result of a complex interaction between each individual's inherent vulnerability to that syndrome (their **diathesis**) and the environmental influences that are present (the **stress**).

For example, let's say that someone is slicing bread for dinner and accidentally makes a deep cut in their finger. This person will likely begin bleeding and require immediate medical attention. However, is this bleeding a *disorder*? No. Cuts and scrapes happen all the time, and bleeding is a normal and physiologic response to this form of injury. This person's bleeding is more accurately conceptualized as a medical **condition**: a state that is not necessarily *pathological* but may still need medical attention. (Another example of a medical condition is pregnancy: not pathological, but may still need medical care!) However, let's say that this person also had hemophilia, which is a genetic deficiency in one of their clotting factors. In this case, even an accidental cut from a kitchen knife can be a potentially deadly event if the bleeding is not be controlled. In this way, when an environmental stress (an accidental cut from a knife) meets a pre-existing diathesis (a deficiency in clotting factors), a disorder is formed.

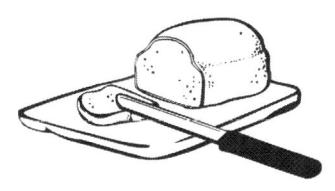

Like the concept of a disorder itself, the concepts of stress and diathesis are not binary but instead occur on a spectrum. There are big stressors and little stressors, just as there are severe diatheses and minor diatheses. It is the combination of the stressor and the diathesis that ultimately determines the severity of a disorder. Continuing the same example from earlier, someone with hemophilia (a severe diathesis) may live their entire lives without ever having a problem as long as they never run into an injury of any kind (no stressors). However, if they have so much as a nosebleed (a little stressor), that may still create a major disorder. On the other hand, someone with an intact clotting system (no diathesis) is not likely to have too many problems from just a small cut (a little stressor) but may still end up bleeding to death if they are injured in a major car crash (a big stressor).

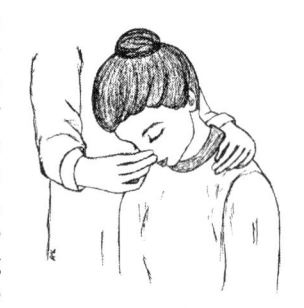

The diathesis-stress model explains much of what we see in psychiatry. Post-traumatic stress disorder (PTSD) is a helpful example. Not everyone who experiences trauma (a stressor) will go on to develop symptoms of PTSD. In fact, the majority of those who exposed to trauma do not go on to develop PTSD. However, people with a particular set of vulnerabilities (including certain genes, personality traits, coping styles, and social supports) can experience PTSD even after what most would consider to be a minor trauma:

Large diathesis + Small stressor = Disorder

Similarly, someone with only a minor diathesis for PTSD may still develop symptoms if they experience a severe enough trauma:

Small diathesis + **Large stressor** = Disorder

In contrast, someone with a significant vulnerability to trauma who experiences a major trauma may end up with an incredibly severe disorder, while another person who experiences the same trauma but has no vulnerability may not end up with a disorder at all:

Large diathesis + **Large stressor** = **Severe disorder**

~~No diathesis~~ + **Large stressor** = ~~No disorder~~

The concept of both diatheses and stressors contributing to mental disorders is well validated, and you should be incredibly skeptical of anyone who offers a singular explanation for any mental disorder. In the end, it's never just one thing.

PUTTING IT ALL TOGETHER

Diagnosis is one of the most powerful tools that psychiatrists and other healthcare providers use in their daily practice. Like any tool, diagnosis is not inherently good or bad. Rather, whether the process of psychiatric diagnosis is used in a constructive or destructive way depends largely on the skills and intentions of the person using it. To maximize your chances of making a helpful diagnosis, consider using the following Principles of Psychodiagnostics which can serve as guidelines for how to maximize the benefits of diagnosis while minimizing the drawbacks:

1. Normalcy is always on the differential. Normalcy should always be considered as a possible explanation for any patient presenting with a psychiatric complaint. Many mental disorders resemble normal aspects of everyday life (such as depression resembling sadness), making it essential to consider normalcy as an explanation before applying a diagnosis. Occasionally the line between normalcy and illness is clear, but most of the time it is not. In these cases, carefully considering both the advantages and disadvantages of diagnosis can help in making an informed decision.

2. At extremes, the quantitative becomes qualitative. The process of diagnosis is inherently problematic because it involves shoehorning **quantitative** (non-binary) concepts into **qualitative** (binary) diagnoses. Using the same example from earlier, someone's height is a *quantitative* measure that can be counted in centimeters or inches. However, we also have *qualitative* terms like "short" and "tall." For those in the middle (say, someone of around average height), there is generally poor agreement for who qualifies for these terms. However, at **extremes** (say, someone who is 7 feet tall), there is no disagreement: this person is tall by any standard you would use. In this way, you can see that at extremes, a quantitative measure (being 7 feet tall) becomes a qualitative measure (this person is "tall"). Mental disorders are the same way. Milder presentations of certain conditions can result in disagreement between different providers, but for severe cases there is often little doubt that a particular patient is suffering from a mental disorder. Therefore, it seems reasonable to reserve use of diagnosis for those cases that are impairing enough to be considered severely disruptive to someone's life.

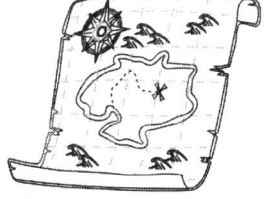

3. The diagnosis is not the disease. Please keep in mind that the diagnostic criteria we are about to review are *not* the diseases themselves! They are, at best, a starting point for arriving at a true understanding of the conditions that we treat. These lists and algorithms should never take the place of a thorough clinical evaluation and will not bring you any closer to truly understanding a patient's experience. This distinction is frequently confused in psychiatry, and it's not uncommon to hear a clinician say something like, "He seems really depressed, but he technically doesn't meet DSM criteria for major depressive disorder." This is absolutely the wrong way to use the DSM, as it confuses a *representation* of a disorder with the disorder itself. To use an analogy, diagnostic criteria are like maps: they are helpful for understanding a territory, but they should never be confused for the territory itself! Trying to understand these disorders by memorizing the criteria is like traveling to Yosemite and then staring at your map the whole time. In the same way, the diagnostic criteria outlined in the DSM act like a map of mental disorders: they provide guidelines and boundaries, but ultimately they are stand-ins for the disorders rather than being the disorders themselves.

4. Context over content. Psychiatry is filled with lots of bizarre and exotic-sounding symptoms, including hallucinations, shady impostors, government conspiracies, and multiple personalities. Because of this, it is easy to get swept up in the **content** of what you're hearing. However, the content of a patient's symptoms is far less important than the **context** of how these symptoms have come about. As one example, when most people hear the term "auditory hallucinations," they immediately think of schizophrenia. After all, hearing voices has to be pathological, right? However, research has revealed that around 5% of people hear voices and are not in any way troubled or impaired by them. If you focused solely on the *content* of the case, it would be easy to jump to a diagnosis of schizophrenia. However, by focusing on the *context*, you would notice that these people still lead lives free of distress and remain functional both at home and in the community. In contrast, you should be more inclined to diagnose someone with schizophrenia when they are presenting with auditory hallucinations in the context of worsening performance at work, difficulty communicating with others, and a sudden lack of self-care. This is just one of many examples, and we will return to the idea of prioritizing context over content many times throughout this book.

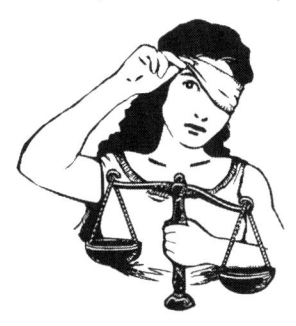

5. Taking someone seriously does not mean always taking them literally. The language of medicine is not always used in the same way by every person. For example, a patient may tell their therapist that they are "very depressed" after having a single stressful day at work. To take this statement at its literal face value and diagnose clinical depression would be an example of gross overdiagnosis. However, to ignore the distress at the heart of what the patient is saying would also not be the right thing to do. The middle ground is to always take what your patient tells you *seriously*, even if you do not always take it *literally*.

This distinction is necessary because the language of psychiatry is often used as an **idiom of distress**. Idioms of distress are a culturally understood way of expressing that you are suffering and require assistance. For example, you can probably think of at least one movie where a character on-screen immediately downs an entire glass of wine in response to an awkward or stressful situation. In our culture, drinking an entire glass of wine at once is a culturally-accepted expression of distress. In the medical field, similar idioms of distress can include saying you have a particular mental or physical disorder ("Work's been really stressful, I've been having panic attacks all week"), using medical terminology to demonstrate the seriousness of your situation ("I'm a danger to myself, a danger to others, and I'm gravely disabled"), or asking for diagnostic tests ("I need to get my brain scanned").

Complicating the matter further is the complex relationship between distress and disease. Too often, someone coming into a doctor's office saying that they are in distress is immediately treated as though they have a disease. This is reasonable, as distress is often caused by disease, so the presence of distress should prompt a search for an underlying cause. However, it is wrong to assume that distress *is* itself a disease, as there are many cases where someone can be in distress in the absence of any biological disease process (such as difficult situations at work or in the home). The simplest way to capture the relationship between distress and disease is to remember that **distress is not disease but can be caused by a lot of things, including disease**.

Making a distinction between taking someone seriously and taking them literally should not be seen as an encouragement to *never* take someone literally. The majority of the time, taking someone's statements at face value is the best approach, both for diagnostic accuracy and for preserving the provider-patient relationship (after all, who likes having everything they say doubted all the time?). But you also should not completely ignore the downsides of overliteralizing expressions of distress, and the best way to do this is to always take your patient seriously, even if your clinical intuition and expertise tells you that what they're saying shouldn't be taken literally at this moment.

6. It's never just one thing. Finally, keep the diathesis-stress model in mind! When you are feeling overworked, it's easy to assume that your patients' difficulties are their own fault or that they have brought it on themselves. The diathesis-stress model can help to remind you that patients are often under extremely stressful circumstances that are not always under their control. In addition, discussing the diathesis-stress model with patients can help them to have a balanced view of their disorder, which can reduce not only the stigma associated with mental disorders ("I always thought that my depression was something I brought upon myself") but also help to prevent the premature sense of closure that can occur with receiving a medical diagnosis ("I knew I was vulnerable to depression, but I never realized how much the little things I was doing each day contributed to feeling the way I did"). By understanding that every disorder involves both a stress and a diathesis, our profession and our patients can both maintain a more balanced view of these conditions.

> **Psychiatric diagnosis** is a powerful tool with many **advantages and disadvantages** that must be taken into account.
>
> Remember the **Principles of Psychodiagnostics**:
> 1. *Normalcy is always on the differential.*
> 2. *At extremes, the quantitative becomes qualitative.*
> 3. *The diagnosis is not the disease.*
> 4. *Context over content.*
> 5. *Taking someone seriously does not mean always taking them literally.*
> 6. *It's never just one thing.*

And with those principles in mind, we are now ready to learn about the process of psychiatric evaluation!

REVIEW QUESTIONS

1. A 23 y/o M is referred for psychiatric evaluation for evaluation of obsessive-compulsive disorder. He reports repetitive thoughts that he is unclean and is covered in bugs. In order to relieve the distress caused by these thoughts, he has taken to picking at his skin to the extent that he breaks the skin and causes bleeding. Physical examination of the patient is shown below:

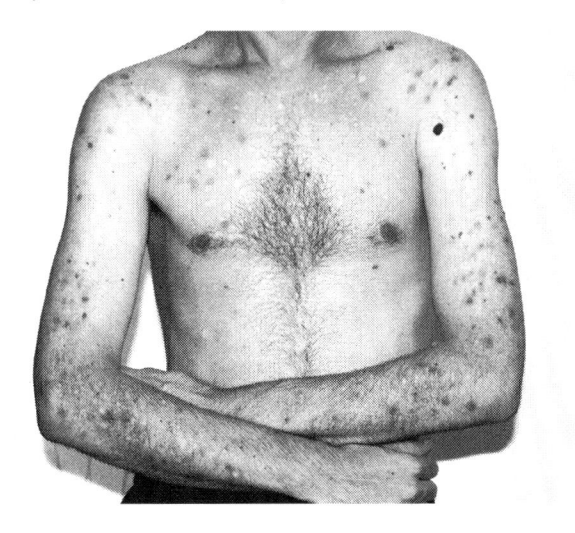

   How would this patient's visible physical injuries best be classified?
   A. Symptom
   B. Sign
   C. Behavior
   D. Disorder
   E. Syndrome

2. A research team is developing a set of 3 screening questions for heroin addiction that takes only one minute to complete. Answering "Yes" to at least 2 of these questions is considered a positive screen for heroin use. To make sure that these questions are helpful, they compare patients' responses to these questions to the results of their urine toxicology tests. The team finds that 100% of patients who answered "Yes" to at least 2 of the questions have use of heroin confirmed on urine testing. However, 52% of patients who have a positive urine test do not screen positive using the questions. What is the best description of this screening test?
   A. It is reliable but not valid
   B. It is valid but not reliable
   C. It is both reliable and valid
   D. It is neither reliable nor valid
   E. None of the above

1. **The best answer is B.** Physical findings that can be observed objectively are considered signs. His subjectively reported feelings, such as a sensation of distress that precedes skin picking, would be considered symptoms (answer A), while his skin picking itself would be the behavior (answer C). Finally, it is the combination of his reported symptoms, signs, and behaviors that would comprise a disorder or syndrome (answers D and E).

2. **The best answer is B.** Because the screening questions accurately capture what they are hoping to (with use of heroin being confirmed by urine testing in 100% of cases), it would be considered a highly valid test (ruling out answers D and E). However, because it only identifies patients with disordered use of heroin less than half of the time, it would not be considered a reliable test (answers A and C).

3 EVALUATION

A **psychiatric evaluation** is the process by which clinicians gather information about a patient with the goal of establishing an accurate diagnosis. The primary tools used for this process are the **psychiatric interview** and the **mental status exam**. The importance of learning how to correctly perform these two assessments cannot be overstated! Unlike in other fields of medicine (where physical exam findings, lab tests, and imaging can help to diagnose a disease even in the absence of a well-taken history), in psychiatry the clinical interview will often be your primary or even only source of diagnostic data.

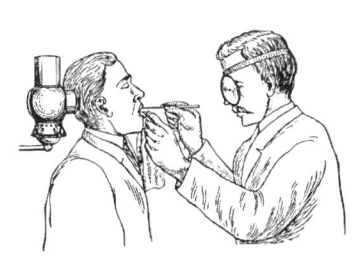

Being able to evaluate a patient with a psychiatric concern is a critical skill for all healthcare providers regardless of their specialty, as mental disorders are often comorbid with physical ailments. In fact, it is estimated that up to a quarter of all primary care patients have a psychiatric condition. In addition, many psychiatric syndromes can interact with or closely mimic diseases in nearly every other field of medicine (including body dysmorphic disorder in plastic surgery, panic attacks in emergency medicine, post-partum depression in obstetrics and gynecology, conversion disorder in neurology, or Munchausen syndrome by proxy in pediatrics, all of which we will discuss in more detail in later chapters). Despite a high prevalence of psychiatric conditions in nearly all fields of medicine, less than half of patients actually end up receiving adequate mental health care. Much of this has to do with clinicians feeling ill-informed or unprepared about what to do when presented with a psychiatric concern. To help yourself feel more comfortable in these situations, spend some time learning how to do a good psychiatric interview and mental status exam.

THE PSYCHIATRIC INTERVIEW

The psychiatric interview is a **structured clinical assessment** that focuses on matters related to mental health. It is similar to the history and physical performed when seeing a patient in any medical setting but includes a greater focus on **psychological and social aspects of health**. The primary goal of conducting a psychiatric interview is to obtain information that will lead to an accurate diagnosis and a solid treatment plan. However, a psychiatric interview should also be used as an opportunity to build rapport and create a **therapeutic alliance** with your patient.

There are many elements of the psychiatric interview to remember, so let's use the mnemonic **CHAMPION'S PSYCH EVAL** to list them all out. By mentally running through this mnemonic during the interview, you can make sure that you're not forgetting any major parts of the evaluation before you leave the room. We'll go over each of these elements one by one:

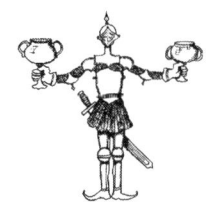

Chief Complaint
How Can We Help?
Additional Information
Medical History
Psychiatric History
Ideation
Orientation
Navigation
'Social Support

Prescriptions
Substances
Youth and Development
Collateral
Housing

Employment
Victimization
Ancestry
Legal Issues

CHIEF COMPLAINT
First, introduce yourself, then begin the interview by asking about the patient's reason for coming to medical attention. Try to keep the conversation **open-ended** at first by asking questions that cannot be answered with a simple yes or no (such as asking, "Tell me about what brought you in" rather than, "Are you depressed?"). Providing at least a few minutes of "free" speech at the beginning of the interview can help to focus the rest of the conversation, as the patient will often bring up whatever is concerning them the most at this time.

HOW CAN WE HELP?
After framing the nature of the problem, ask the patient how they think that you can be of help. After all, the patient came to medical attention for a specific reason, and it can be helpful to make their desires known from the beginning of the interview. Common reasons for coming to psychiatric attention include wanting to know the origin of specific symptoms, obtaining a prescription for medication, or desiring to begin therapy. In emergency settings, patients may ask to be admitted to the hospital (or, in cases where they were brought involuntarily, may want to leave). By knowing the patient's preferences from the very beginning of the interview, you can focus the rest of the interview on gathering the information necessary to determine whether their request is appropriate or not.

ADDITIONAL INFORMATION
Once you have a sense of the patient's main concern, gather some additional information on the problem by taking a **history of present illness** (HPI). You can use the mnemonic **OLD CARTS** to remind yourself of the key components of an HPI, including **O**nset (when the problem began), **L**ocation (where the problem is, which may or may not be germane to a psychiatric complaint), **D**uration (how long it has lasted), **C**haracter (what it feels like), **A**ggravating factors (what makes it worse), **R**elieving factors (what makes it better), **T**iming (when it occurs), and **S**everity (how intense or disabling it is).

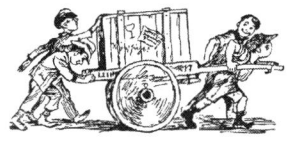

A structured **history of present illness** can help to clarify the chief complaint.

OLD CARTS:
***O**nset*
***L**ocation*
***D**uration*
***C**haracter*
***A**ggravating factors*
***R**elieving factors*
***T**iming*
***S**everity*

MEDICAL HISTORY
While a psychiatric interview is mostly focused on mental health, make sure to inquire about physical health as well by taking a **past medical history**! This will help you screen for current threats to health as well as determine which psychiatric treatments would be appropriate given their conditions (for example, you wouldn't prescribe lithium to a patient with chronic kidney disease).

PSYCHIATRIC HISTORY
Asking about a patient's **past psychiatric history** (including hospitalizations, therapy, medications, and history of suicide attempts or self-harm) can help clue you into the nature and severity of their problem. Consider doing a **psychiatric review of systems** where you ask screening questions about some of the most common disorders such as mood disorders, anxiety, and schizophrenia to help rules these diagnoses out.

IDEATION
The next three elements are all words that end in "-ation" which should help to clue you in when using the mnemonic. The first is ideation. There are two types of ideation that you will be asked about in psychiatry: **suicidal ideation** and **homicidal ideation**. Because most psychiatric conditions increase the risk of suicide, screening for suicidal ideation should be done for **every patient** presenting with a mental health concern. In contrast, assessment of homicidal ideation can be done only in cases where it is relevant. Because suicide and violence are two of the most tragic outcomes of mental disorders, we'll spend more time going over these in greater detail in Chapter 4.

ORIENTATION
The next "-ation" is orientation. This can be assessed by asking about **person** ("What is your name?"), **place** ("Where are we at this moment?"), **time** ("Do you know what the date is?"), and **situation** ("Why are you here right now?"). If your patient has been answering all other questions coherently, it can be disruptive (and even a bit insulting) to ask the orientation questions. However, for anyone who appears confused or has had recent changes in cognition, assessing orientation can provide valuable insights into their current mental status. Decreased levels of orientation are most often related to delirium or dementia (discussed in Chapters 4 and 22, respectively).

NAVIGATION
The final "-ation" is often overlooked, but asking about a patient's ability to safely navigate their environment can at times be crucial for coming up with a plan, especially in emergency settings when the patient's **disposition** is in question. For example, when working with a patient who would like to return home but was brought in by ambulance, ask yourself, "How would they get there? Do they have a family member willing to pick them up? If not, are they too impaired to take a cab or a bus?"

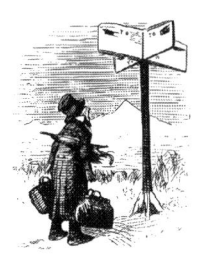

SOCIAL SUPPORT
Friends and family play a key role in mental health, so knowing your patient's level of **social support** can often directly impact management. For example, you should be much more hesitant to discharge a suicidal patient who is socially isolated and lives alone compared to someone who will return home to a large supportive family who has volunteered to keep a close eye on them over the next few days.

PRESCRIPTIONS
It is important to know the **names, dosages, schedules, and indications** for all medications that a patient is taking. Remember to ask about **over-the-counter drugs** and **supplements** as well. For patients you will be treating, asking about past psychiatric medication trials can help to direct future treatment. Try to outline exactly when each of these trials occurred as well as the outcome (was the medicine stopped due to side effects or was it simply ineffective?). Asking about past **allergic reactions** is important as well, especially in acute situations where emergency medications may be needed.

SUBSTANCES
Mental health and **substance use** are intricately linked. Not only can specific drugs produce clinical signs and symptoms that mimic a variety of mental disorders, but many mental disorders can also be triggered or exacerbated by use of substances. At a minimum, ask patients if they drink alcohol, smoke cigarettes, or use any recreational drugs. In cases where substance use appears to play a large role, consider taking a full substance history, including specific substances used, age of first use, amount and frequency of use, time of last use, positive or negative effects of use, and any history of treatment efforts. (We'll introduce a mnemonic for this in Chapter 8!)

YOUTH AND DEVELOPMENT
Assessing **developmental history** can provide important diagnostic clues, especially when working with children and adolescents. A developmental history should begin with an assessment of prenatal development and continue on to developmental milestones such as speech and motor abilities (which will be discussed further in this book in Chapter 19).

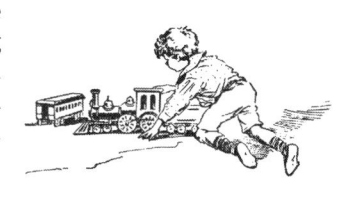

COLLATERAL
A key aspect of evaluating the patient's support network is to identify someone from whom you can obtain **collateral information**. Collateral should be sought from the people who know the patient best, such as family members, roommates, friends, or their healthcare providers. Collateral contacts can be crucial in determining the diagnosis and making a treatment plan, as they can provide additional information from an outside perspective that the patient is not able to give. In addition, collateral can help you to determine how **culturally normative** certain beliefs or behaviors are.

HOUSING
From here, we are going to shift our focus to a few of the highest yield social determinants of mental health, staring with **housing**. Many of your patients won't live in traditional houses but rather in group homes, nursing facilities, rehabilitation programs, or out on the street. This can be important diagnostically (as certain disorders, such as addiction or schizophrenia, are more likely to result in chronic homeless than others). However, it can and should factor into your clinical decision making as well, such as providing referrals to social resources as appropriate.

EMPLOYMENT
Knowing about a patient's **employment status** and **financial situation** can both help to provide important insights into the patient's functional status and overall level of support (including whether the patient is working or if they are supported by family or disability payments). Financial topics can be sensitive, so avoid asking specifically how much money the patient makes. Instead, ask how they support themselves on a day-to-day basis.

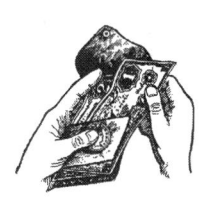

VICTIMIZATION
Inquiring about **abuse, neglect, and domestic violence** may give your patients a rare opportunity to speak with someone about their experience and take steps to either manage or remove themselves from a dangerous situation. While screening for abuse is important for all patients, it is particularly crucial when working with **dependents** (people who rely on others for their safety and survival, including children, the elderly, and the disabled). In many places, healthcare providers are **mandated reporters** who are required to report cases of suspected abuse to local agencies. Be familiar with the laws in your area of practice!

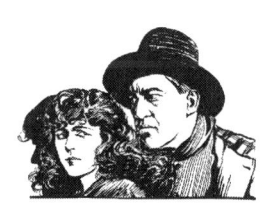

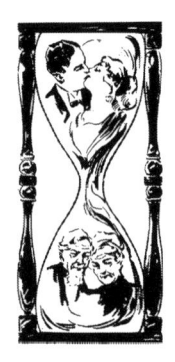

ANCESTRY
Nearly all psychiatric syndromes are **heritable** to a certain degree, and knowing how mental disorders have affected other people in the patient's family can inform current diagnosis and treatment decisions. For example, certain forms of dementia are strongly heritable, so knowing that multiple first-degree relatives have been affected by early-onset Alzheimer's disease increases the probability of this diagnosis significantly in someone presenting with memory loss. Importantly, suicides also seem to run in families, so knowing if there is a history of suicide attempts can help to determine the patient's level of risk.

LEGAL
Legal issues are another frequently forgotten part of the interview. However, knowing about your patient's past and present intersections with the legal system may reveal important information. For example, a past arrest for driving under the influence of alcohol may suggest a substance use disorder, impulsivity due to mania, or reckless disregard for the rights of others related to antisocial personality disorder. However, it should never be assumed that any interaction with the legal system is automatically reflective of psychiatric pathology, as by definition legal situations often involve more than one side to the story.

A **psychiatric interview** is a **structured evaluation** of the patient's **present circumstances** and **past history**.

CHAMPION'S PSYCH EVAL:

Chief Complaint	**P**rescriptions
How Can We Help?	**S**ubstances
Additional Information	**Y**outh/Development
Medical History	**C**ollateral
Psychiatric History	**H**ousing
Ideation	**E**mployment
Orientation	**V**ictimization
Navigation	**A**ncestry
'Social Support	**L**egal Issues

Finally, while diagnosis in psychiatry is highly reliant upon subjective symptoms rather than objective signs, the **physical exam** remains a core part of evaluation, as certain psychiatric conditions or treatments can have physical signs (such as swollen salivary glands due to recurrent vomiting in someone with bulimia nervosa or a tremor from lithium toxicity). In addition, a thorough **review of systems** can help to identify other medical conditions that need to be taken into consideration when deciding upon treatment. The review of systems can be as comprehensive or brief as the situation allows. Young otherwise healthy adults may not need a full review, but you may decide to be more thorough when working with elderly patients or those with multiple medical conditions.

THE MENTAL STATUS EXAM

The mental status exam (abbreviated MSE) is **psychiatry's equivalent of the physical exam**. Just as you would use findings from the physical exam to argue for or against the presence of a specific disease (such as a heart murmur suggesting a valve problem), you can use findings from the mental status exam to rule specific diagnoses in or out. Unlike a physical exam, however, a mental status exam does not need to be performed separately, as conducting a full psychiatric interview will often allow you to comment on all aspects of the mental status exam.

When reviewing findings from the mental status exam, it's important to keep in mind that a single finding rarely, if ever, proves definitive for diagnosing a specific mental disorder. For example, speaking very rapidly can be a sign of a manic episode. However, much often than not, differences in rates of speech are entirely within the realm of normalcy, as some people simply talk faster than others. In contrast, for someone who not only speaks rapidly but also wears excessive make-up, cannot complete a single sentence without changing their train of thought, and plans to save the world by reuniting the members of the Beatles, it is more likely to be a sign of a specific mental process. As always, focus on *context over content*, and avoid reading too much into any single finding without first putting the overall picture together.

The mental status exam can be broken down into the following domains: **A**ppearance, **B**ehavior, **M**otor, **S**peech, **A**ffect and mood, thought **P**rocess, thought **C**ontent, **P**erception, **O**rientation, **C**ognition, **I**nsight, and **J**udgment. You can remember these using the phrase "**A B**eautiful **M**ental **S**tatus **A**lways **P**leases **C**ustomers, **P**rovided **O**f **C**ourse **I**t's **J**ustified!" We'll go over each of these one by one:

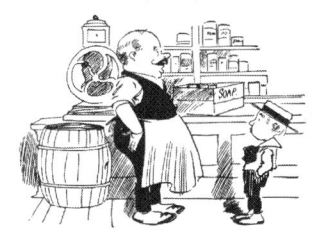

APPEARANCE
A patient's **appearance** can contain important diagnostic clues. Someone's **apparent age** can increase the likelihood of certain diagnoses (such as ADHD in children or dementia in older adults). Specific **facial features** can suggest certain diagnoses as well (such as a masked facies suggesting Parkinson's disease or a flat nasal bridge suggesting Down syndrome). Someone's level of **grooming** can also be telling, with patients who appear disheveled or unkempt possibly reflecting a lack of self-care which can be found in a variety of psychiatric syndromes including schizophrenia and severe depression. **Weight** can provide diagnostic clues as well, especially when it comes to eating disorders.

BEHAVIOR
The domain of **behavior** encompasses many aspects. First, evaluate the patient's level of **alertness** (ranging from awake and alert to drowsy, stuporous, or comatose). Next, **cooperativeness**, **rapport**, and **eye contact** all provide information about the quality of the relationship you have with the patient. One's overall **level of activity** can also provide important clues. Decreased activity can occur in severe states of depression (**psychomotor retardation**), while increased activity (**psychomotor agitation**) can be a sign of anxiety or mania. Most of these can be observed spontaneously without the need to be specifically elicited.

MOTOR

A basic neurological examination of **movement** and **gait** is often performed as part of the mental status exam, as motor abnormalities can be observed either due to specific mental conditions (such as motor tics in Tourette syndrome or waxy flexibility in catatonia) or as a side effect of the medications used to treat them (such as extrapyramidal symptoms caused by antipsychotic drugs).

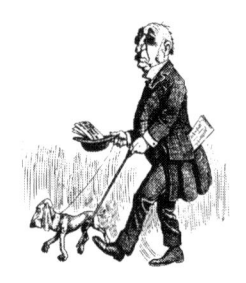

SPEECH

When evaluating **speech**, listening to *how* words are being said can be just as informative as the words themselves. Take a note of the patient's level of **verbality**. Are they talking much more than normal (hyperverbal), or are they barely talking at all (hypoverbal)? Are they talking unusually quickly or slowly (**rate of speech**)? Does their speech contain the melodic quality that normal speech has (known as **prosody**)? Does their speech feel pressured, like they can barely contain the words they have inside of them, or are they having difficulty getting words out (halting speech)? Are their words slurred or hard to understand (articulation), or are they completely unable to speak (aphasia)? Abnormalities in speech can be a sign of a variety of mental conditions (such as absent prosody suggesting depression or poor articulation suggesting alcohol intoxication).

AFFECT AND MOOD

Affect and mood refer to a patient's current **emotional state**. A patient's **mood** reflects their *internal* emotional experience. As such, mood is assessed primarily by asking, "How are you feeling right now?" You can report the patient's response verbatim (such as "good," "okay," "frustrated," "angry," and so on). In contrast, **affect** is the patient's *external* emotional expression which can be evaluated semi-objectively by the interviewer. Affect is most often described by the words euthymic (a normal, well-balanced mood), dysthymic (a sullen mood), and euphoric (an intensely elated mood). However, there are other affective states as well (including irritable, angry, playful, or suspicious). You can also note the **range of affect**. Someone with a full range of affect will show a variety of facial expressions throughout the interview, whereas someone with a restricted range would show only a narrow range of emotion. A labile affect involves rapid shifts from extremes of emotions (such as going from laughing to crying in a matter of seconds) and can be seen in certain syndromes such as borderline personality disorder, whereas a blunted or flat affect refers to a lack of emotional expression and can be suggestive of schizophrenia or advanced dementia. Finally, you can comment on the **appropriateness** of one's affect. For example, someone in a manic state may appear ecstatic even when talking about the recent death of a family member while someone who is depressed may seem sad even when talking about a joyous occasional, both of which would be examples of an inappropriate affect.

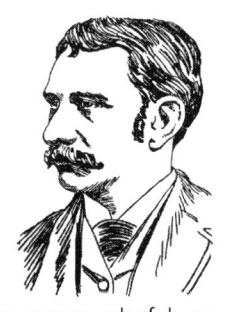

THOUGHT PROCESS
Thought process refers to the nature of the connections between one's thoughts. The majority of people have a **linear and logical** thought process, meaning that they proceed from one topic to another in a natural and straightforward way that is easy for a listener to follow. This is not always the case in psychiatry, however, as some mental disorders involve a degree of thought disorganization that makes it difficult to follow one's train of thought. When asked a question, a patient may veer off into unrelated topics before eventually answering the question (**circumstantiality**) or may never answer the original question at all (**tangentiality**). The rate and amount of thoughts matters as well: someone in a manic state may have so many thoughts that they cannot keep track of them (**flight of ideas**), whereas someone who is depressed or psychotic may appear to have a complete lack of spontaneous thinking (**poverty of thought**). At other times, thoughts can become so disorganized that the words coming out of someone's mouth make absolutely no sense (**word salad**). We will discuss this and other ways in which thought process can become derailed more fully in later chapters.

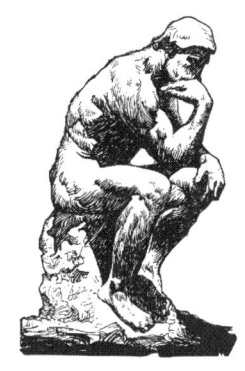

THOUGHT CONTENT
Thought content involves the specific ideas and beliefs that a patient has in mind. Specific areas of thought content which are relevant to psychiatry include **suicidal ideation**, **homicidal ideation**, **preoccupations** (thoughts that command the entirety of the person's attention to the point where they cannot focus on anything else), and **delusions** (false beliefs that are inconsistent with the patient's background and cannot be corrected by reasoning). Given that no one has the ability to read minds, thought content can only be assessed through what the patient tells you directly.

PERCEPTION
Perception refers to one's ability to accurately take in information about the world. Common impairments in perceptions include **illusions** (misperceptions of genuine stimuli, such as seeing a drape moving in a dark room and assuming it is a person) and **hallucinations** (false perceptions in the absence of any external stimuli, such as hearing someone's voice saying mean things about you even when no one else is in the room). The specific form that the hallucination takes on matters, with **auditory hallucinations** (hearing voices) being common in psychiatric syndromes like schizophrenia and **visual hallucinations** (seeing things) being more often related to non-psychiatric medical conditions.

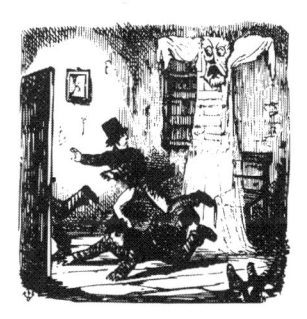

ORIENTATION
You may remember orientation (assessing person, place, time, and purpose) as one of the elements of the psychiatric interview! Some sources consider it to be part of the mental status exam as well.

COGNITION
Cognition refers to the patient's general level of intellectual ability. A variety of questions can be used to assess these domains, including **memory** ("I'm going to tell you 5 words then ask you to repeat them to me in 10 minutes"), **attention** ("Can you spell the word 'world' backwards?"), **general knowledge** ("Who is the current president?") and **executive functioning** ("Can you draw a clock for me?"). There are also standardized cognitive tests, such as the Montreal Cognitive Assessment (MoCA) or Mini-Mental State Examination (MMSE), that can provide an even greater level of detail on the patient's current cognitive level. Impairments in cognition can be either temporary (as in delirium) or chronic (as in dementia or intellectual disability).

INSIGHT AND JUDGMENT
Finally, insight and judgment are two related domains that involve the patient's ability to accurately understand their situation (**insight**) as well as to know how to act appropriately within it (**judgment**). Many mental disorders can directly impair insight, including conditions like schizophrenia where delusions and hallucinations can lead one to believe things that are not consistent with reality. Insight and judgment are closely linked, as it can be hard to make appropriate decisions if your understanding of the situation is lacking. For example, a drunk person who decides to drive is doing so as a result of alcohol impairing not only their insight but also their judgment ("I'm thfine to drife!").

When assessing these domains, it's important to remember that evaluations of insight and judgment are inherently subjective. A multitude of factors, including culture, religion, and worldview, influence every patient's experience of illness and may make them disagree with your diagnosis or with what you believe to be the best course of action. Be very mindful not to use "poor insight and judgment" as a synonym for "the patient disagrees with me." Instead, keep in mind the subjectivity inherent to any patient-provider interaction.

> A **mental status exam** consists of a **structured evaluation** of multiple domains and is the **psychiatric equivalent of a physical exam**.
>
> *A Beautiful Mental Status Always Pleases Customers,*
> *Provided Of Course It's Justified:*
> *Appearance*
> *Behavior*
> *Motor*
> *Speech*
> *Affect and mood*
> *Thought Process*
> *Thought Content*
> *Perception*
> *Orientation*
> *Cognition*
> *Insight*
> *Judgment*

A STATISTICAL FRAMEWORK FOR EVALUATION

The psychiatric interview and mental status exam are both intended to help guide the interviewer towards or away from particular diagnoses. In this way, every step of the interview can be seen as a **medical test**, the result of which either increases or decreases the likelihood of a particular diagnosis. For example, asking someone, "Over the past 2 weeks, have you had little interest or pleasure in doing things that you normally enjoy?" will help to rule in or out a diagnosis of major depressive disorder, with a response of "Yes" suggesting depression and "No" arguing against it. During a mental status exam, specific signs can similarly help to support or argue against a specific diagnosis. When assessing an adult patient, for example, a complete lack of any eye contact argues *for* a diagnosis of autism while sustained eye contact strongly argues *against* it.

It can be strange to think of the psychiatric interview and mental status exam as essentially a series of dozens (if not hundreds) of consecutive medical tests, but viewing them within that framework opens up a deeper understanding of the process. As with any medical test, steps within the psychiatric interview and mental status exam are prone to error. The two types of error are **false positives** (also known as type I errors) and **false negatives** (or errors). A false positive occurs when a test suggests the presence of a diagnosis that is *not* actually there, while a false negative occurs when a test suggests the absence of something that *is* actually there, as seen in the following example:

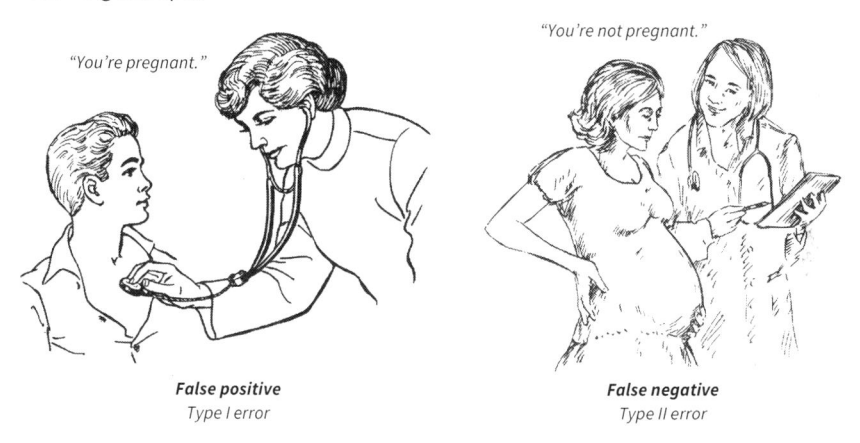

"You're pregnant."

"You're not pregnant."

False positive
Type I error

False negative
Type II error

No test is perfect 100% of the time, and there will always be false positives and false negatives associated with any medical examination. The concept of **sensitivity** and **specificity** can help us to better understand exactly what each step of the evaluation process is telling us. Sensitivity and specificity both describe the *ways* in which you can trust (or not trust) what a test is telling you.

The se**n**sitivity of a test tells you how good it is at avoiding false **n**egatives. If a highly sensitive test is **n**egative, then you can be relatively certain that that diagnosis is **ruled out**. Using the same example as earlier, if someone answers "No" to the question of "Over the past 2 weeks, have you had little interest or pleasure in doing things that you normally enjoy?" you can be almost certain that this person is not currently suffering from a major depressive episode, as this question is highly sensitive. For this reason, highly sensitive tests are often used for screening as they can rapidly and efficiently rule out a diagnosis. Use the mnemonic **Sn-N-out** to remember that if a **Sen**sitive test is **N**egative then the diagnosis is **Out**.

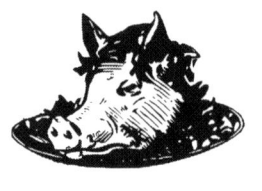

Sensitivity is a statistical measure of the **true positive rate** and is helpful for **ruling out** a diagnosis.

Sn-N-out = If a Sensitive test is Negative then the diagnosis is Out.

Conversely, specificity tells you how good a test is at avoiding false positives. If a highly specific test is positive, then you can be relatively certain that that diagnosis is **ruled in**. For example, the presence of certain types of delusions (such as believing that one's thoughts are being broadcasted to the world or that one's movements are under someone else's control) are highly specific for schizophrenia and can reliably be used to differentiate schizophrenia from other syndromes that also involve psychotic experiences. For this reason, if someone says that they have these beliefs, you can be relatively certain that they are suffering from schizophrenia. Use the word **Sp-P-in** to remember that if a **Sp**ecific test is **P**ositive then the diagnosis is **In**. Tests with perfect specificity (meaning that if they are positive then the diagnosis can be ruled in 100% of the time) are called **pathognomonic** signs. For example, someone with an asymmetric pill-rolling resting tremor is almost certain to have Parkinson's disease. While pathognomonic signs are incredibly helpful, they are basically non-existent in psychiatry due to the complexities of the nervous system and human behavior.

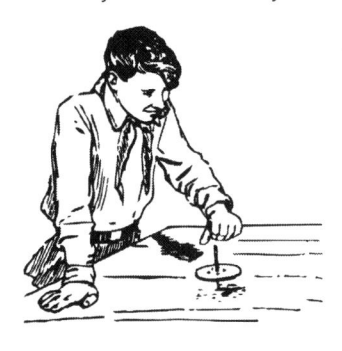

Specificity is a statistical measure of the **true negative rate** and is helpful for **ruling in** a diagnosis.

Sp-P-in = If a Specific test is Positive then the diagnosis is In.

It is worthwhile to keep in mind that Sp-P-In and Sn-N-Out are **rules of thumb**, and the actual reality is not as simple as these mnemonics make them out to be. Very few tests are both 100% sensitive and 100% specific, and any improvements in a test's sensitivity often lowers its specificity (and vice versa). Because of the limitations of sensitivity and specificity, it may be more helpful to consider using **likelihood ratios** which combine sensitivity and specificity into a single metric. Likelihood ratios tell us in very practical terms how much more certain we can be after doing a test. Likelihood ratios are highly dependent upon the **pre-test probability**. In the absence of any information about a particular patient, the pre-test probability is equivalent to the **base rate** of a given condition in the general population. For example, the base rate of Alzheimer's disease in the general population is less than 1%. However, in particular circumstances, the pre-test probability can be either higher or lower. Let's say that we are evaluating a 75-year-old for Alzheimer's disease. Using the general base rate of Alzheimer's disease (less than 1%) would be unwise, as age is a major risk factor for this form of dementia, with the base rate for a 75-year-old being roughly 10%. However, if this same patient has also had recent onset of memory loss and confusion while driving, the pre-test probability of him having Alzheimer's disease goes up even further (to, say, 50%). To help gain further diagnostic clarity, we order brain imaging. The MRI has a positive likelihood ratio of 19 for diagnosing Alzheimer's disease, meaning that if the scan is positive (if there are signs of brain degeneration) then we can be *19 times more certain* that this patient has Alzheimer's disease (equivalent to a post-test probability of over 95%). In contrast, if this same test were positive for a 75-year-old with no memory difficulties, the post-test probability would only be 70% (still significant, but not nearly as definitive). In this way, likelihood ratios help to guide the clinician towards or away from particular diagnoses provided that they are based on an accurate pre-test probability.

EFFECT SIZES

While this book will be primarily focused on diagnosis, we will also discuss treatment strategies for most of the disorders we will talk about. When discussing treatment, a different set of biostatistics will be used. We will primarily use **effect size** to describe the effectiveness of a treatment. Effect sizes are superior to other statistics about treatment (such as p-values, which measure statistical significance) because they answer not only the question, "Is this treatment effective for this condition?" but also the arguably more important question, "How effective is it?"

To understand the benefits of using effect sizes, consider the question, "Is food effective at treating hunger?" On the surface, it seems that we can answer that question with a definitive yes. However, the answer depends largely on the amount and type of food, as a sandwich is going to be significantly more satisfying than a stick of celery. To answer the question, "How effective is each type of food at treating hunger?" we would need to use effect size. In statistical terms, the effect size of a sandwich is going to be larger than the effect size of a celery stick even though we would say that both are effective anti-hunger treatments.

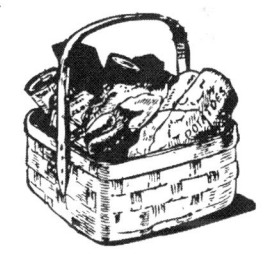

To use a more clinically relevant example, consider the question, "Are antidepressants effective at treating depression?" The majority of studies show that approximately 60% of all patients get better after starting an antidepressant. This would seem to suggest that antidepressants are, in fact, effective. However, these same studies also show that around 40% of people taking placebos *also* get better. This 20% difference cannot be ignored (meaning that antidepressants are likely effective). However, we can get a much clearer picture by asking, "*How* effective are they?" There are many different ways to calculate effect size, but one of the most common is known as **Cohen's d**. The significance of this number is arbitrarily defined, but generally a score of **0.2** shows a **small** effect size, **0.5** shows a **medium** effect size, and **0.8** and above is a **large** effect size. So where do antidepressants fall on this scale? Published studies show that antidepressants have an effect size of between 0.2 to 0.4, which is considered a small effect size. This may seem like a damning indictment of antidepressants. However, a small effect size does not mean no effect size, and many other medications commonly used in modern medicine also have a small effect size, including treatments for osteoporosis, high cholesterol, and stroke prevention. (For what it's worth, the use of mnemonics in teaching new material has an effect size of 1.6, which is considered between "very large" and "huge." So you've made the right choice in picking up this book!)

PUTTING IT ALL TOGETHER

Accurate diagnosis is the foundation upon which we are able to provide effective treatments for people suffering from psychiatric disorders. However, we cannot formulate accurate diagnoses without a firm foundation in the process of psychiatric evaluation. This chapter has hopefully given you the tools necessary to do so (the psychiatric interview and the mental status exam) as well as provided a statistical framework for interpreting specific findings from these exams. This framework will set the stage not only for understanding information in subsequent chapters but also for evaluating patients in clinical settings.

As a final note, when approaching the differential diagnosis for a patient presenting with psychiatric concerns, it can be helpful to have a list of all major categories of mental disorders prepared. Use the mnemonic **A MAP TO MIND SPACE** to keep these handy for rapid recall. You can use this mnemonic to make sure you are not forgetting any potential explanations for the signs and symptoms you are seeing!

Keeping a framework of the **major categories of psychiatric disorders** in mind while evaluating a patient can help to structure your clinical decision making.

A MAP TO MIND SPACE:

Addiction

Mood
Anxiety
Psychosis

Trauma-related
OCD and related

Medical conditions
Intoxicants
Normalcy
Delirium

Somatoform
Personality
ADHD/autism
Cognitive (dementia)
Eating disorders

REVIEW QUESTIONS

1. A 46 y/o F is brought into the emergency department by her wife who is concerned because the patient has stopped eating or responding to questions for the past week. On exam, the patient's facial expression shows a furrowed brow. She rocks continuously back and forth in her chair while wringing her hands. When interviewed, she looks up in response to questions but does not answer them verbally, instead looking down at the floor. Which of the following aspects of the mental status exam *cannot* be evaluated at this time?
   A. Appearance
   B. Behavior
   C. Alertness
   D. Mood
   E. Affect

2. A nurse practitioner is about to see a new patient in her clinic. She reviews the patient's packet of information prior to the visit and sees that the PHQ-9 (a self-report questionnaire for depression) is positive, with the patient scoring 12 points. Scores of 10 or greater on the PHQ-9 have a sensitivity of 88%, a specificity of 88%, and a positive likelihood ratio of 7.1 for major depressive disorder. Which of the following conclusions can the nurse practitioner make with certainty?
   A. This patient has major depressive disorder
   B. This patient does not have major depressive disorder
   C. This patient is more likely than not to have major depressive disorder
   D. This patient is more likely than not to *not* have major depressive disorder
   E. None of the above

3. A 26 y/o F who recently gave birth is discussing the risks and benefits of starting an antidepressant with her doctor. The doctor knows that this particular antidepressant has an effect size of 0.3 for post-partum depression. Which of the following statements can be made to the patient?
   A. "This medication has a 30% chance of working."
   B. "You are likely to feel around 30% better after starting this medication."
   C. "It is more likely than not that this medication will be effective."
   D. "It is more likely than not that this medication will be ineffective."
   E. None of the above

1. **The best answer is D.** Because mood is a self-reported item that reflects a patient's subjective experience of their internal emotions, it cannot be evaluated in a patient who is non-verbal. One could try to infer this patient's mood by their behaviors and facial expressions (such as her hand wringing), but this would be classified as their affect rather than their mood (answer E). The other aspects of the mental status exam can be evaluated by an observer even for patients who do not respond to questions.

2. **The best answer is E.** While sensitivity and specificity are very helpful measures of a medical test's performance, they rarely tell us anything with certainty. Only in cases of 100% sensitivity or specificity can a diagnosis be ruled in or out with certainty (answers A and B). In addition, while it may be tempting to conclude that a positive screen on a test with 88% specificity can make us certain that a diagnosis of major depressive disorder is at least more likely than not, this is not the case either. Instead, we would need to know the pre-test probability (that is, what percentage of people coming into the clinic are likely to have major depressive disorder) and then use that to calculate the chance that this patient has major depressive disorder based on the positive likelihood ratio. Without knowing the pre-test probability, we cannot make any of these conclusions with certainty.

3. **The best answer is C.** In medicine, effect sizes tell us the strength of an association between two items. In this case, an effect size of 0.3 between antidepressants and post-partum depression tells us that there is likely to be an effect as the effect size is greater than 0 (answer D). Effect sizes do not tell us the chance of a medication working (answer A) or the precise amount that a medication will work (answer B). Instead, interpreting effect sizes is largely based on arbitrarily defined cut-offs (such as above 0.2 being a small effect size, above 0.5 being a medium effect size, and above 0.80 being a large effect size).

4 PSYCHIATRIC EMERGENCIES

The term **psychiatric emergency** refers to any dangerous or life-threatening situation that occurs as a consequence of a mental disorder, including **suicide**, **violence**, **abuse**, **delirium**, **catatonia**, and **homelessness**. Each of these states must be recognized and addressed **independently of the diagnosis**. For example, someone coming to the emergency room with a plan to commit suicide should be triaged and evaluated immediately regardless of whether their suicidal thoughts are coming from an underlying diagnosis of depression, bipolar disorder, schizophrenia, borderline personality disorder, or any other condition. That's not to say that finding the underlying diagnosis is not important! However, in an emergency situation, coming up with the right diagnosis is a secondary priority to **making sure that the patient and others are safe**.

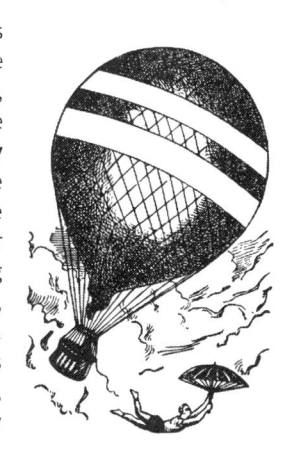

Psychiatric emergencies can be difficult to recognize. When most people think of emergencies, they tend to picture medical conditions like heart attacks, strokes, or car accidents. In contrast, when most people think of psychiatry, they tend to think of chronic conditions such as depression or anxiety that are usually seen in less acute settings. Nevertheless, certain circumstances related to mental disorders absolutely require rapid evaluation and treatment, as they can result in immediate harm if left unaddressed.

Unlike the conditions we will cover for the rest of the book, psychiatric emergencies are *not* disorders in and of themselves (there is no "suicide disorder," for example). Because of this, recognizing the presence of a psychiatric emergency is merely the **starting point** for a full evaluation in search of an underlying cause. Once the situation has been stabilized, use the tools we learned in the last chapter (the psychiatric interview and mental status exam) to do a more thorough evaluation.

SUICIDE

Suicide is by far the **most common psychiatric emergency**, with over 50% of all urgent psychiatric consults being related to suicidal thoughts or attempts. Suicide is a major public health concern and is the tenth most common cause of death worldwide. While adults between the age of 45 and 65 are at the highest risk, suicide is a leading cause of death among teenagers and young adults due to the fact that most people in this group are otherwise healthy. For every death by suicide, there are as many as 25 suicide attempts. Women *attempt* suicide more often, while men *die* by suicide more often due to use of more lethal methods such as firearms. With the exception of dementia and intellectual disability, **all mental disorders** increase the lifetime risk of suicide. Because of this, screening for suicidal ideation should be done on **every patient** presenting with a mental health concern.

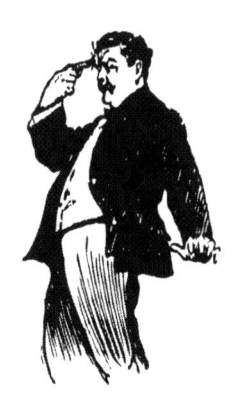

People with suicidal ideation may recognize the dangerousness of their situation and bring themselves in for medical attention, or they may be brought in by others. As with any psychiatric emergency, first make sure that the patient is safe. There are several steps to take when assessing a patient with thoughts of suicide. This involves doing the same things that you would for any patient presenting with any psychiatric complaint, including conducting an interview, performing an exam, and ordering labs and imaging if appropriate. However, for a patient with thoughts of suicide or a high likelihood of future attempts, a few additional considerations must be taken. You can remember these steps using the mnemonic **DIOS MIO**:

D is for Detainment. All states allow involuntary detainment of people who are determined to be a **danger to themselves** as a consequence of a mental disorder. You should consider detaining a patient at high risk for suicide to prevent them from leaving the hospital and carrying out their plans to harm themselves.

I is for Inpatient. For suicidal patients who have a mental disorder that could benefit from treatment, inpatient hospitalization may be an appropriate option for intensive monitoring and treatment.

O is for Observation. You should consider what level of observation is needed, including arranging for a one-to-one sitter if necessary to ensure safety.

S is for Sharps. You should be careful that patients thinking of suicide do not have access to any means by which to harm themselves while in the hospital such as access to glass or other potentially sharp items.

M is for Medical clearance. Patients with suicidal ideation can have medical problems as well, which should be assessed to determine whether the patient would be best served by medical or psychiatric hospitalization.

I is for Injuries. This involves conducting a careful and thorough physical exam for signs that a patient has already tried to harm themselves, such as cuts from a knife or injuries from jumping off a building.

O is for Occult overdoses. People coming into the hospital with thoughts of suicide may have already ingested certain drugs in an attempt to overdose. While the effects of some drugs are immediately noticeable, for others the signs and symptoms of an overdose are not apparent for several hours. Because of this, you should consider ordering labs (like an acetaminophen and acetylsalicylic acid level) for patients with suicidal ideation.

> When evaluating a patient with **suicidal ideation**, consider what steps you need to take to **assure their immediate safety**.
>
> ***DIOS MIO*:**
> **D**etainment
> **I**npatient
> **O**bservation
> **S**harps
> **M**edical clearance
> **I**njuries
> **O**ccult overdoses

While there are many considerations to make, the ultimate question often comes down to whether someone having thoughts of suicide is safe to go home or whether they will need inpatient hospitalization (the **I** in DIOS MIO). This is a complicated question, as not every patient with suicidal ideation will require hospitalization. In the majority of cases, the decision is based on whether or not this person will try to commit suicide in the **near future**, in which case the 24/7 monitoring and treatment offered by a hospital should be sought. However, it is necessary to keep in mind that **hospitalization does not inherently prevent suicide**. People can and do commit suicide while hospitalized, even with the closest observation. At best, being in the hospital can *delay* suicide, but it does not inherently prevent it. Why then do we consider hospitalizing someone presenting with suicidal ideation? The key is that hospitalization can be helpful in treating the **underlying mental disorder** that is contributing to the risk of suicide. For example, for someone in a severe episode of depression, treatment in the hospital can help to rapidly reduce the feelings of hopelessness and isolation that make them feel that suicide is the only option.

When assessing someone's immediate risk for suicide, consider factors with **high likelihood ratios** for suicide attempts in the near future, including access to **g**uns, **R**ecent suicide attempts in the past few weeks, **O**ngoing thoughts of suicide, recent **S**elf-harm, and use of **E**thanol or other disinhibiting **S**ubstances that may increase impulsivity. You can remember these factors using the mnemonic **Guns & ROSES**.

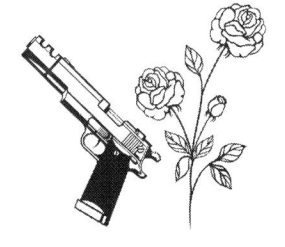

> A number of factors raise the **likelihood of a suicide attempt** in the **near future**.
>
> **Guns & ROSES:**
> **G**uns
> **R**ecent attempts
> **O**ngoing thoughts
> **S**elf-harm
> **E**thanol
> Other **S**ubstances

However, even considering these factors, accurate prediction of suicide remains out of our grasp. This is because suicide has an overall **low base rate** in the general population (around 0.01%). This means that, even if likelihood ratios predicted that someone was *100 times* more likely to attempt suicide, their chance of doing so would still only be around 1%, leaving a 99% chance of a false positive. Therefore, at the end of the day, your **clinical judgment and intuition** remain the best tools available for predicting which patients are at the highest risk and most in need of inpatient hospitalization.

Just as important as knowing which factors increase the foreseeability of suicide is knowing what has *not* been found to reduce the risk. One of these factors is the idea of "**contracting for safety**," or the notion that if a patient promises a clinician that they will not harm themselves then they are at lower risk of suicide. However, there is no evidence that safety contracts are protective against suicide or accurately identify patients at a lower risk of suicide, so don't use them for this purpose. In addition, there is a tendency to see "**passive**" suicidal ideation (where someone expresses a wish to end their life but has not developed a specific plan to do so) as being lower risk compared to "**active**" suicidal ideation (where they have developed a plan). However, this idea is not supported by data. It can still be helpful clinically to stratify suicidality as "active" or "passive," but do not let this sway you too much. If the foreseeability of someone committing suicide is high, you should still consider admitting them even if they have "only" passive suicidal ideation.

Once safety is assured, the task then becomes determining what is contributing to the desire to commit suicide. In the United States, the vast majority of people who die by suicide (up to 98% by some estimates) show evidence of having had a mental disorder. **Mood disorders** like depression and bipolar disorder are most frequently found, with around one-third of all fatal suicide attempts involving a mood disorder. However, they are not the only causes, with addiction, schizophrenia, and personality disorders each accounting for around 15% of the total.

Consistent with the idea that *it's never just one thing*, suicide is rarely the result of any single cause or stressor. Rather, suicide often stems from a combination of a **desire** to end one's own life as well as the **means** to do so. A desire to commit suicide is related to a number of different factors, including life experiences, personality traits, cultural influences, and religious beliefs. Two thought patterns are frequently reported by people planning a suicide attempt: a feeling that one is a **burden** on others as well as a lack of any sense of **belonging** to a group. Once these thought patterns are present, the risk of suicide increases significantly.

While thinking of suicide can represent a psychiatric emergency in and of itself, it is not until one has acquired the means to lethally self-harm that the possibility of committing suicide becomes imminent. The means of committing suicide has a large impact on the dangerousness of the situation, with certain suicide methods being significantly more lethal than others (for example, firearms are associated with a mortality rate of over 90%, while the mortality rate from overdosing on medications is less than 5%). In most cases, suicides are **planned** and involve preparatory thoughts and actions for several weeks or months leading up to the attempt (such as acquiring a firearm or storing up medications for an overdose). However, up to a quarter of all suicides appear to be **impulsive** in response to a specific situation or circumstance.

While there are moral and philosophical issues surrounding suicide (such as whether someone has the right to take their own life and whether it is ethical to involuntarily commit someone), the fact remains that only around 20% of people who survive a suicide attempt report feeling that they wish the attempt had succeeded. This suggest that taking steps to prevent suicide, including hospitalization, may be warranted to help someone get through a particularly difficult time of their lives and survive until the underlying mental disorder or environmental stressor is addressed.

NON-SUICIDAL SELF-HARM

Some people actively hurt or harm themselves *without* any intention of dying. Most often, this involves making non-lethal cuts on their body (although other methods such as burning are used as well). This behavior is not uncommon, with around 10% of adults having self-harmed at some point in their life. There is some overlap between non-suicidal self-injurious behavior and suicide, as people who self-harm often have thoughts of suicide. However, as a general rule, most people who self-harm are not necessarily suicidal. In fact, only 5% of patients who self-harm commit suicide within 10 years of the self-harm incident. For this reason, self-harm differs enough from suicide that it warrants separate discussion.

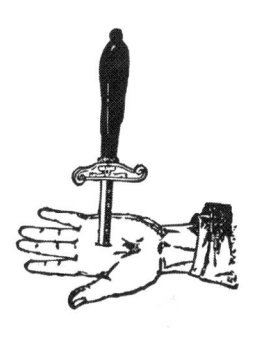

The question that most people have when learning about self-harm is: *why*? For the majority of people, the idea of self-harm (and the pain that this would naturally involve) makes little sense. Yet people who engage in self-harm report that, paradoxically, self-harm helps them to feel *better*. It is believed that many people who self-harm have a profoundly unbalanced emotional state that turns an act which causes most people pain into one that actually brings relief from an inner sense of emotional turmoil. (There are other reasons why people self-harm as well, which we will talk about in subsequent chapters.) While self-harm is associated with a number of mental disorders, it is most associated with **borderline personality disorder**, with over 90% of people with this condition having engaged in self-harm. In addition, a diagnosis of borderline personality disorder increases the risk of self-harm by over 5 times, and dialectical behavior therapy (a treatment for this disorder) is one of the few interventions that appears to reliably reduce this behavior. While self-harm is not a perfectly sensitive or specific marker of this disorder, it is correlated enough that the presence of self-harm should at least put borderline personality disorder on your differential.

VIOLENCE

Violence or threats against others can be a psychiatric emergency. However, in contrast to suicide (which is related to a mental disorder in the vast majority of cases), violence should *not* automatically be assumed to be psychiatric in origin. In fact, the idea that people with mental disorders are more likely to be violent is a myth, as individuals with a mental disorder are much more often the *victims* of violence rather than its perpetrators. Nevertheless, in some cases, certain mental disorders can increase the risk of violence, and mental health providers must be ready to evaluate violence and respond to the situation. When discussing violence, it can be helpful to make a distinction between **agitation** and **aggression**. Both agitation and aggression can result in violence, but the underlying causes are distinct and require a different treatment approach.

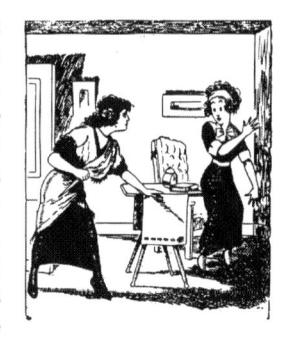

AGGRESSION

When most people think of violence, they tend to think of aggression, which is more common in non-medical settings. Aggression is often **organized** and involves a specific target. It can be premeditated (such as someone who has been planning to attack someone else for weeks) or impulsive (such as someone suddenly striking another person during an argument). While aggressive acts can sometimes have their roots in a mental disorder, it is more often the result of **conflict between ordinary people**. This is not to say that it *never* occurs as a consequence of a mental disorder. For example, someone with schizophrenia may develop a delusional belief that the Catholic church is trying to kill them and may spend months planning an attack on a neighbor who wears a crucifix around their neck. In addition, several categories of mental disorders are defined by the presence of aggressive acts (including antisocial personality disorder which will be discussed in more detail in Chapter 16). However, aggression originating from a psychiatric condition in this way is the exception rather than the rule, and most cases of aggression do not involve mental disorders.

Because aggression is not always psychiatric in origin, you need to make a distinction between threats requiring **legal intervention** (such as calling the police) and those stemming from a mental disorder (in which case psychiatric treatment and hospitalization would be more appropriate). Use the psychiatric interview to screen for signs of a mental illness that could be underlying threats of violence. Using the earlier example of someone with schizophrenia who has a delusional belief revolving around the Catholic church, this sort of delusional belief is likely psychiatric in origin, making inpatient hospitalization a good option in this case. In contrast, someone who was brought in after stabbing their partner during a fight is more likely to require legal, rather than psychiatric, attention. In addition, unless there is a primary psychiatric disorder driving the risk of violence, use of medications like antipsychotics or mood stabilizers do little to alter the risk of violence.

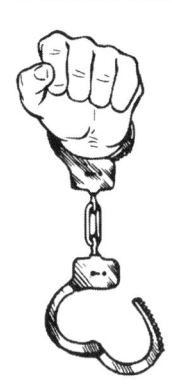

Psychiatrists and other health care providers have a **duty to protect** potential victims of violence in most states. This means that, if a patient expresses a desire to inflict violence upon an identifiable target, you have a legal duty to make a reasonable attempt at protecting the identified victim. This often involves notifying the victim and/or law enforcement. (The details vary by state, so be familiar with the laws governing your local area of practice.) The duty to protect was based upon some tragic cases when a potential victim was not warned of the threat on their life and ended up being killed.

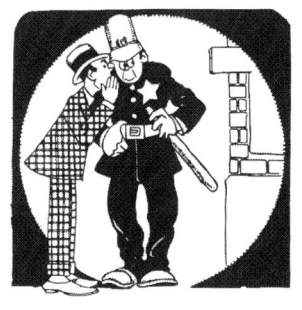

AGITATION
In contrast to the purposeful and organized violence seen in aggression, agitation is a state of psychological and physiologic tension, excitement, or restlessness that can result in **purposeless** and **disorganized** acts of violence. Unlike aggression, agitation *is* associated with **medical or psychiatric conditions** more often than not. In particular, any psychiatric conditions that present with confusion or fear (including psychosis, mania, anxiety, delirium, dementia, and substance intoxication) should be on the differential for someone in a state of agitation.

When working with an agitated patient, the primary goal is rapid **de-escalation**. Verbal de-escalation should always be attempted first provided it is safe to do so and involves establishing rapport with the patient and setting firm limits on behavior ("You will not harm or attack yourself or anyone else"). In addition, because agitation results from a sense of confusion, using simple and concrete statements can help to provide a sense of orientation ("My name is Dr. Cruz. I'm a doctor here in the hospital. It is 11:00 on Saturday night. Your family brought you here because they are concerned about you.") which can be quite calming. If verbal de-escalation is not working, medications (including benzodiazepines and/or antipsychotics) can be offered. These medications can help to rapidly reduce the inner tension driving the state of agitation.

When both verbal and pharmacologic de-escalation have failed to make the situation safe, physical restraints (such as arm or leg straps) may be needed. Restraints are *not* treatment, but they may be needed to prevent further harm from being inflicted by the patient (either to themselves or those around them). Restraints are associated with both physical and mental harm, including a high risk of physical injury, organ damage, psychological trauma, and even death from strangulation. Because of this, **restraints should be avoided whenever possible**. However, for highly agitated patients, it is not always possible to avoid use of restraints. Therefore, try to find a balance by minimizing the use of restraints whenever possible while still allowing for their use in extreme circumstances when someone's safety is at risk.

VIOLENCE RISK ASSESSMENT
Psychiatrists are often asked to assess the risk of violence in a given situation, as many states allow for people who are a **danger to others** to be detained against their will provided that this danger stems directly from a mental disorder that could potentially be treated during psychiatric hospitalization. As with suicide, there is no way to accurately predict who will go on commit a violent act. Nevertheless, several factors

do appear to increase the foreseeability of a violent act. To remember these, use the mnemonic **PV'd MALES** which stands for **P**revious **V**iolence, **M**ale, **A**dult (as opposed to children or the elderly), **L**ow intelligence, **E**stranged from others, and **S**ubstance use. Of these, previous violence is *by far* the most important risk factor, as it is associated with the highest likelihood ratio.

A number of factors significantly raise the **likelihood of violence** in the near future.

PV'd MALES:
Previous **V**iolence
Male
Adult
Low intelligence
Estranged
Substance use

While substance use is listed as a risk factor for violence, this does not necessarily apply to all drugs. The specific substances that have been associated with an increased risk of violence include **P**hencyclidine (PCP), **I**nhalants, **S**teroids, **S**timulants such as methamphetamine or cocaine, and **E**thanol. You can remember these specific substances using the mnemonic **PISS-E**.

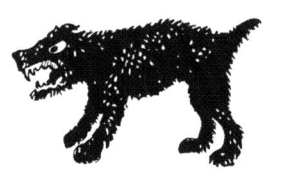

Specific substances increase the **likelihood of violence** during **intoxication**.

PISS-E:
Phencyclidine (PCP)
Inhalants
Steroids
Stimulants
Ethanol

Once the risk of violence has been determined, attention can then turn to diagnosing and treating the underlying mental disorder (if any) that is driving this risk. Whether it involves agitation or aggression, in cases where there is a treatable psychiatric condition, inpatient hospitalization may be needed for close monitoring and immediate treatment. In some cases, violent acts may have already been committed, in which case the patient may instead be seen in legal (rather than medical) settings. These intersections between mental health and the legal system form the basis for the field of **forensic psychiatry**.

ABUSE AND NEGLECT

Abuse is a form of violence that involves physical, sexual, verbal, emotional, or other forms of cruelty inflicted upon others. Unlike agitation or aggression (states that are diagnosed in *perpetrators* of violence), abuse is more often diagnosed in *victims* of violence, making it necessary to have a separate discussion of how to evaluate these patients. While all forms of abuse can constitute an emergency, recognizing the presence of abuse is particularly urgent when it involves vulnerable groups who are not able to defend themselves such as children, the elderly, or the disabled. Child abuse is unfortunately **common**, with around 25% of people reporting a history of verbal abuse, 15% reporting physical abuse, and 10% reporting sexual abuse during childhood. Child abuse is associated with both immediate harms to the child (including a risk of permanent injury or death) as well as increasing the risk of a multitude of mental and physical disorders later in life. For this reason, quick and accurate recognition of the signs of child abuse is crucial.

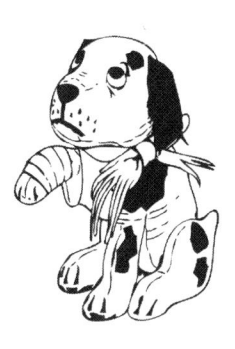

Diagnosing abuse is based on unusual details from the patient's **history** as well as certain objectively observable **signs**. Use the phrase **Fuzzy DETAIL** to remember aspects of a reported history that are suggestive of abuse:

Fuzzy is for Fuzzy or vague. Parents or other caregivers who are abusing their child may try to provide an alternative explanation for any observed injuries in an attempt to deflect attention. These fabricated histories are often vague so as to provider fewer opportunities for doctors and other healthcare providers to find inconsistencies.

D is for Denied. In some cases, parents or other caregivers will outright deny injuries that are objectively observable. This is highly suggestive of abuse.

E is for Evolving. Be wary of stories that are constantly evolving and changing, especially if these changes seem to conveniently fit any new details that emerge.

T/A are for Tardy or Absent. For serious injuries, parents and other caregivers have a responsibility to bring their child to medical attention as soon as possible. Any delay in seeking treatment (or especially a complete failure to bring their child to medical attention) should be looked into.

I is for Inconsistent. Any form of inconsistency should be a red flag for abuse (for example, if the caregiver's explanation of the injuries is inconsistent with the observed physical exam or if various caregivers provide differing explanations).

L is for Lacking. Sometimes, caregivers will try to provide no explanation or give an explanation that is clearly insufficient (such as saying that widespread bruises are the result of the child bumping their knee during sports).

> **Explanations for injuries** that are **inconsistent** or **lacking** should raise a red flag for **child abuse**.
>
> *Fuzzy DETAIL:*
> *Fuzzy or vague*
> *Denied*
> *Evolving*
> *Tardy*
> *Absent*
> *Inconsistent*
> *Lacking*

In addition to the presence of fuzzy details while taking a history, specific objective findings on physical examination can also suggest intentional injury. Use the mnemonic **TEN-4 Over & OUT** to remember these features:

TEN is for Torso, Ears, or Neck. The vast majority of "normal" injuries during childhood (those that are unrelated to abuse) occur on the knees, shins, forehead, and other parts of the body that sit over bony prominences. In contrast, bruises on other areas of the body should warrant investigation, with the torso, ears, and neck being among the most common sites of intentional injury to children.

4 is for Four months. Infants below the age of four months are largely sedentary, as they cannot yet move around. Because of this, any injuries in infants younger than 4 months or who cannot yet move around are highly suggestive of abuse ("those who cannot cruise cannot bruise").

Over is for Over the body. A pattern of injuries occurring in multiple areas of the body or involving multiple organ systems is incredibly unusual and suggests abuse.

O is for Obvious patterns. Sometimes, abuse-related injuries will follow an obvious pattern, such as an elliptical pattern signaling a bite wound or multiple punctate scars being related to cigarette burns as seen in the following image:

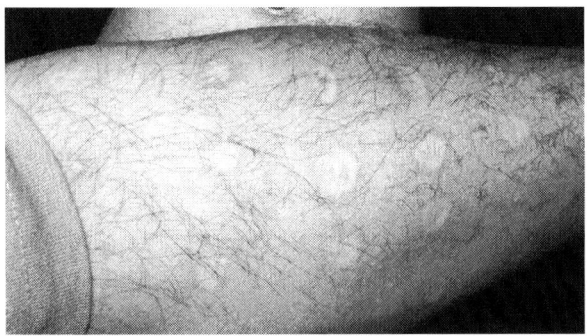

Multiple punctate scars suggestive of intentional injury.

U is for Unexposed. Any cuts, bruises, or other injuries to areas that are not commonly exposed (such as the genitals or anus) are essentially pathognomonic for sexual abuse. The presence of sexually transmitted infections in children is also suggestive of sexual abuse, although this is not necessarily pathognomonic depending on the specific infections involved (for example, gonorrhea and syphilis are almost always associated with abuse while human papillomavirus and chlamydia can be passed from mother to child during childbirth and may have long incubation periods before overt symptoms appear).

T is for Timing. Injuries that appear to be in different stages of healing suggest that they were incurred at various times, raising the possibility of abuse.

> Specific patterns seen on **physical exam**, including injuries to **unusual** or **unexposed** parts of the body, are strongly **suggestive of abuse**.
>
> *TEN-4 Over & OUT:*
> *Torso, Ears, and Neck*
> *Less than 4 months old*
> ***Over** the body*
> ***Ob**vious patterns*
> ***U**nexposed body parts*
> ***T**iming*

Not all abuse is physical. **Psychological abuse** can include shaming, ridiculing, terrorizing, threatening, isolating, or exploiting a child (or someone that the child loves) for various reasons and can be equally damaging. Psychological abuse can be incredibly difficult to diagnose, as it does not always leave objective evidence in the same way that physical and sexual abuse can (although abnormal weight loss or failure to meet milestones can sometimes occur).

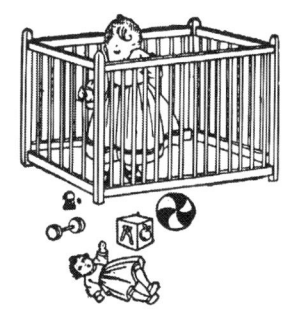

While abuse specifically refers to acts of *commission* (meaning that a harmful act was done), **neglect** involves the *omission* of specific acts that are necessary to provide for a child's basic needs, resulting in harm. While neglect is often more subtle than abuse, it can be equally damaging both physically and mentally. Indeed, neglect is actually *more* common than abuse yet remains underrecognized and underreported. Neglect can take various forms, including **physical** neglect (failure to provide basic food, clothing, hygiene, and shelter), **medical** neglect (failure to provide access to health care), **educational** neglect (failure to provide access to school or other educational opportunities), **social** neglect (failure to provide social opportunities), and **emotional** neglect (lack of affection, nurturing, and positive interactions). Neglect is not always intentional, as some families are unable to meet the needs of their dependents due to poverty or other factors. However, that does not necessarily mean that the damaging effects of neglect are any less, and a variety of disorders related to antisocial behavior appear to have direct links to a history of childhood neglect. For this reason, rapid recognition of neglect is essential, even though the lack of objective signs in many cases can make this challenging.

While none of these features on their own are diagnostic of abuse or neglect with any degree of certainty, the more that are present the more troubling the picture becomes. In some cases, hospitalization of the victim may be necessary to treat injuries and/or protect them from further harm. In cases of sexual assault, additional measures (such as preventing pregnancy, providing prophylaxis against sexually transmitted infections, and collecting forensic evidence) must be taken as well. If abuse is suspected, examining siblings or other dependents in the home may reveal additional injuries. As a reminder from the previous chapter, healthcare providers across the United States are mandated reporters of child abuse, meaning that all cases of suspected child abuse must be reported to appropriate agencies.

DELIRIUM

Delirium is an acute state of **cognitive impairment** in someone who is **medically unwell**. Delirium is common in **hospitalized patients**, with anywhere from 10 to 30% of all hospitalized patients experiencing some form of delirium. It is even more common in those parts of the hospital with the sickest patients, such as the intensive care unit where rates of delirium approach 50 to 75%. While the diseases which cause delirium are not necessarily psychiatric in origin, psychiatrists are often consulted on delirium given their specialty in evaluating mental status.

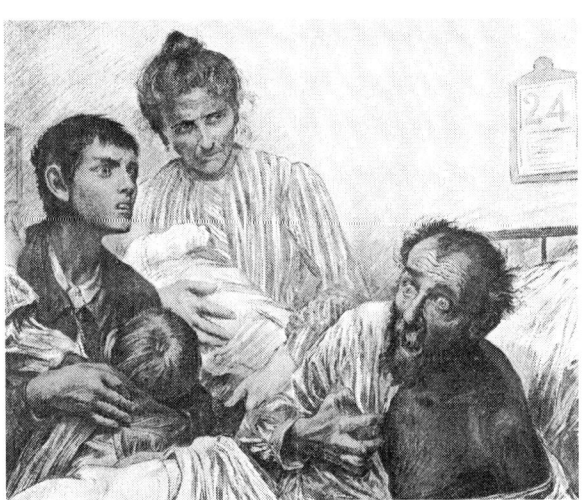

Patient in a state of delirium.

Delirium has been found to be an independent predictor of multiple negative outcomes, including worse recovery from illness and a higher rate of death. Because of this, assessing and treating delirium promptly is crucial. You can remember the key features of delirium using the phrase **Where THE F AM I?**:

Where is for Disorientation. The "Where?" in this mnemonic should remind you of the disorientation that occurs in delirium. Asking orientation questions (person, place, time, and situation) can help to clarify the severity of a patient's confusion, as their ability to answer these questions will be lost in reverse order.

T is for Thought disorganization. Confusion in delirium manifests in various ways, including rapid changes in consciousness, lack of awareness, inattention, and an inability to speak or comprehend language. Emotional lability and sleep disturbances are not uncommon as well.

H is for Hallucinations. Delirium can cause major disruptions in one's perception, with hallucinations being common. These hallucinations are generally **visual** in nature (as opposed to auditory hallucinations, which are more likely to be psychiatric as we will discover in Chapter 7). Paranoia and combativeness are not uncommon as well.

> **Visual hallucinations** generally have a **medical** than psychiatric cause.
>
> *Vis*ual hallucinations come from diseases of the **vis**cera.

E is for Energy changes. Delirium can have varying effects on a patient's energy and activity levels. Some people become *hyper*active with restlessness, babbling, and even agitation, all of which tends to get the treatment team's attention. In contrast, *hypo*active forms of delirium, in which a patient simply shuts down and becomes slow, sleepy, and apathetic, are much more likely to be underdiagnosed.

F is for Fluctuating. Delirium typically has a **waxing-and-waning** course, with moments of lucidity alternating with moments of confusion. Someone with delirium may be fully oriented and lucid at lunch, then be actively hallucinating and unable to remember their own name by dinnertime.

A is for Acute. Delirium is specifically an **acute** rather than chronic condition, meaning that it both comes on quickly (often over only a few hours or days) and that it tends to be **transient**, with most patients getting better over time provided that the underlying causes are addressed. While delirium is **reversible** in most cases, in cases of prolonged illness, neuronal injury can result in persistent cognitive deficits.

M is for Medical causes. By definition, delirium is caused by an **underlying medical condition**, with common causes being infections (such as respiratory or urinary tract infections), metabolic derangements (such as hyperglycemia or hyponatremia), blunt force trauma (especially involving the head or spine), and states of shock and hypoperfusion (such as severe blood loss).

I is for Intoxicants. Aside from medical conditions, delirium can also be caused or exacerbated by various **medications** and **recreational substances**. Recognition of delirium should always prompt a close review of the patient's medication list to look for and remove any potentially deliriogenic drugs.

Delirium is an acute state of **changes in awareness, attention, and cognition** in someone who is **medically unwell**.

Where THE F AM I?
Where (disorientation)
Thought disorganization
Hallucinations
Energy changes
Fluctuating
Acute
Medical causes
Intoxicants

Treatment of delirium should be **multimodal**, including medical, psychiatric, social, and environmental interventions. Use the mnemonic **U R SAFE** to remember the various strategies for treating delirium (think of "U R SAFE" as being your response when a delirious patient asks "Where THE F AM I?"):

U is for Underlying cause. Like all psychiatric emergencies, delirium is not a disease in and of itself but rather is a syndrome that is *caused* by a disease. Therefore, the presence of delirium should initiate an **immediate work-up** to determine the primary cause. Once a cause is found, immediate treatment should be rendered (such as using antibiotics to treat an underlying infection or stopping any deliriogenic medications).

R is for Reorientation. Gently reorienting the patient when they become confused can be helpful as long as it is not done excessively or in a way that provokes agitation.

S is for Sleep. The normal sleep-wake cycle is often impaired during delirium, with patients sleeping during the day and then up all night. This sleep disturbance may itself hinder immune system function and the body's ability to heal. For that reason, efforts to promote healthy sleep patterns (such as turning off the lights at night and minimizing unnecessary beeping or other disruptive noises) can promote recovery.

A is for Antipsychotics. Medications known as antipsychotics can reduce the severity and duration of delirium, with a **small effect size** of around 0.4. Some antipsychotics are also sedating which, if timed properly, can help to promote sleep as well.

F is for Family and friends. Involving important people in the patient's life can help them to remain engaged and cognitively stimulated. When they can't be around, placing pictures of family and friends in the room can help to create a comforting environment for the patient.

E is for Environment. Frequent room changes and visits from staff members can create a disorienting environment that is not conducive to healing. Instead, focus keeping a calm, quiet, and consistent environment that is comfortable and easy for the patient to understand.

> **Treatment of delirium** is inherently **multimodal**, including medical, psychiatric, social, and environmental interventions.
>
> *U R SAFE*:
> **U**nderlying cause
> **R**eorientation
> **S**leep
> **A**ntipsychotics
> **F**amily and friends
> **E**nvironment

CAPACITY

Capacity is the determination of whether a patient has the cognitive ability to make their own medical decisions. Most people at a baseline mental state should be able to thoughtfully consider whether they want specific medical or surgical interventions. However, patients who are delirious may not be able to make these decisions. A capacity evaluation provides a structured framework for determining whether or not a patient is able to provide their own consent. Psychiatrists may be asked to evaluate capacity in difficult cases. However, **all medical providers** should be able to perform a capacity evaluation. You can use the mnemonic **CURBSIDE** to remember the elements of a capacity evaluation. If a patient meets all of these criteria, they are deemed to have capacity. However, if they are missing *even one* of these elements, they do not have capacity for that decision.

C is for Communicate. Is the patient able to communicate meaningfully with others? If this basic criterion is not met, then assessment of capacity is impossible to perform. For example, if someone is comatose or unresponsive to questions, then by definition they do not have capacity.

URB is for Understanding Risks and Benefits. Is the patient able to understand both the risks and benefits of the decision they are making? For example, a patient with gas gangrene (a severe infection that is uniformly fatal without treatment) may be told that limb amputation is necessary. This procedure obviously carries risks, including lifelong deformity and disability, yet given the 100% mortality rate without treatment, the benefits outweigh the risks in nearly all cases. A patient with capacity must be able to understand and compare these risks and benefits when making a decision.

S is for Situation. Is the patient able to fully appreciate the situation that they are in, or does it seem like they are minimizing or exaggerating the gravity of their condition? Continuing the same example, the patient with gas gangrene must be able to comprehend that their life is at risk if they decline treatment.

I is for Impact. Does the patient appreciate the likely impact that their decision will have on their situation? For example, if the patient with gas gangrene wants to decline treatment and leave the hospital, they need to be able to state that they will likely continue to become sick and potentially die.

D is for Decide. Is the patient able to clearly express a preference for a particular choice given their situation, such as deciding to undergo or forego surgery?

E is for Explain. Finally, the patient must be able to explain their decision taking into account all of the above! Put another way, the patient must be able to synthesize their understanding of their situation, the risks and benefits of the proposed intervention, and the impact of their choice into a coherent decision.

A **capacity evaluation** involves a **structured evaluation** of a patient's ability to **make medical decisions** in a reasonable way.

CURBSIDE:
*C*ommunicate
*U*nderstand *R*isks and *B*enefits
*S*ituation
*I*mpact
*D*ecide
*E*xplain

Capacity provides a **clear standard** for allowing patients to have autonomy over treatment decisions without putting severely ill patients at risk of not receiving appropriate treatment. It's important to know that making bad decisions is *not* the same as lacking capacity! For example, if the patient with gas gangrene is able to communicate an understanding of the risks and benefits of amputation, the situation they are in, the impact of their decision, and an ultimate decision to discontinue care, they are protected in doing so even if the majority of doctors would think that they are "crazy" for making this decision. It's also important to note that capacity applies to a specific *decision*, not to a specific *patient*. Someone may have the capacity to make one decision (such as disagreeing with the specific antibiotic being proposed) while lacking the capacity to make another (such as wanting to leave the hospital) at the same time. For this reason, capacity should be evaluated on an ongoing basis with each new major decision rather than being applied as a blanket "label" to the patient.

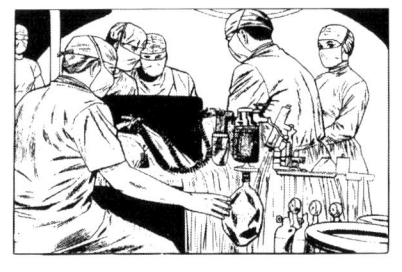

In situations where a patient has capacity, their decision on the matter should be respected, even if it is in disagreement with what the treatment team would like to do. In cases where a patient *lacks* capacity, a surrogate decision maker should be sought (often a spouse, family member, or close friend). The surrogate decision maker should be encouraged to make decisions **as the patient would have** to the best of their knowledge, rather than basing the decision on the surrogate's own values and beliefs. In cases where the patient lacks capacity but a surrogate decision maker cannot be found, the treating team may be required to make decisions on the patient's behalf.

CATATONIA

Catatonia is an abnormal mental state characterized by **changes in consciousness and behavior** where the patient acts in a way that appears senseless or purposeless to an outside observer. Unlike delirium which has an underlying *medical* cause, catatonia is related to an underlying **psychiatric condition** in most cases. In the modern day, catatonia most often occurs with **mood disorders**, with over half of all cases being related to bipolar disorder and an additional third being related to depression. However, it can be seen in schizophrenia as well, with up to 15% of cases being associated with psychosis.

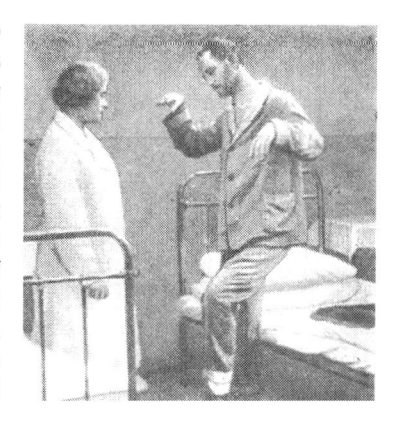

People in a state of catatonia act in very specific ways that can help you to recognize when this state is occurring. Use the mnemonic **LIMP MEN** to remember these core features of catatonia:

L is for Lethargy. The lethargic **stupor** that is characteristic of catatonia involves an apparent lack of mental activity. Patients with catatonia can appear sedated or even comatose despite being awake.

I is for Immobility. The stupor seen in catatonia can extend from mental lethargy to a state of physical **immobility** or a complete paucity of movement. Left untreated, immobility can have severe consequences, including malnutrition, dehydration, and muscle breakdown.

M is for Mutism. Catatonia often renders patients **mute**, resulting in minimal or absent verbal communication.

P is for Positioning. Catatonia involves various abnormalities of positioning which are some of the most characteristic signs of this condition. **Catalepsy** is a state of severe muscular rigidity resulting in difficulty changing position. This can lead to **posturing** or the maintenance of odd or uncomfortable-seeming positions, sometimes for hours on end. A patient with catatonia may even allow someone else to move them into different positions and then continue to hold those positions, a phenomenon known as **waxy flexibility**.

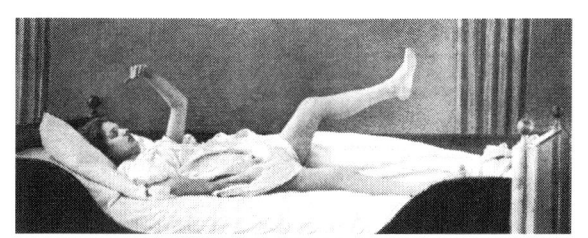

Catalepsy with posturing.

M is for Motor abnormalities. While most of the signs in catatonia involve *decreased* activity due to mental stupor and physical rigidity, people in a state of catatonia can show *increases* in specific behaviors as well. **Grimacing** involves the patient making various facial expressions or holding them for prolonged periods of time. Patients may also engage in **mannerisms** which are odd-appearing caricatures of normal actions such as waving their hand back and forth repeatedly. **Stereotypy** involves frequent, repetitive, and purposeless movements such as attempting to walk into a wall over and over. Finally, catatonia can at times lead to **agitation** involving restlessness and impulsivity, which can be dangerous and requires immediate attention.

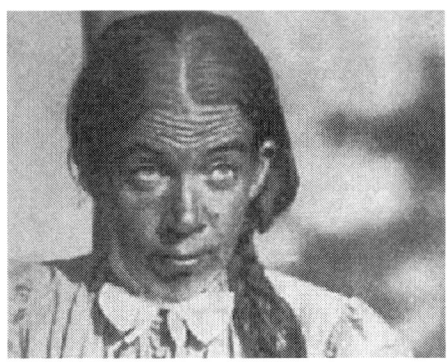

Grimacing.

E is for Echolalia and echopraxia. The "echos" in catatonia involve mimicry of people around the patient. This can manifest as **echolalia**, or repeating specific words or phrases over and over, and **echopraxia**, or mimicking the movements of others in a reflexive or purposeless way.

N is for Negativism. Finally, **negativism** involves a complete lack of response to any external stimuli such as greetings or instructions. Negativism can even extend to situations where most people would react involuntarily, like a patient standing motionless when a ball is thrown at them on accident.

Catatonia is a state of **stupor** related to a **psychiatric disorder** resulting in abnormalities in **movement, speech**, and **positioning**.

LIMP MEN:
Lethargy (stupor)
Immobility
Mutism
Positioning
Motor abnormalities
Echolalia/echopraxia
Negativism

A particularly severe form of catatonia known as **malignant catatonia** involves not only the core features of catatonia but also significant **autonomic nervous system instability**, including sweating, fever, and changes in blood pressure, heart rate, and respiration. The presence of autonomic instability in a patient with catatonia is ominous, as over half of all patients with malignant catatonia will die without treatment (and even with treatment the mortality rate can be up to 10%).

Benzodiazepines are the mainstay of treatment for all cases of catatonia and are effective up to 80% of the time. Benzodiazepines will often produce dramatic improvements in behavior and cognition within minutes of administration, which can be helpful not only therapeutically but also diagnostically for confirming suspected cases. In cases of malignant catatonia or severe cases where benzodiazepines have not worked, **electroconvulsive therapy** (ECT) should be considered. Notably, you should **avoid antipsychotics** as they tend to worsen catatonia! You can remember the strategies for treating **CAT**-atonia by embedding them into the word itself: **C**onvulsive therapy (ECT), **A**voiding antipsychotics, and minor **T**ranquilizers (benzodiazepines).

> **Benzodiazepines** are the **first-line treatment for catatonia**. ECT should be used in malignant or treatment-refractory cases. **Antipsychotics** should be **avoided**.
>
> To treat **CAT**-atonia:
> **C**onvulsive therapy (ECT)
> **A**void antipsychotics
> Minor **T**ranquilizers (benzodiazepines)

HOMELESSNESS

Access to shelter is a basic human necessity. However, many people struggle with **homelessness** and lack a consistent place to sleep. It is common to encounter homelessness in emergency settings, as around a third of homeless patients have visited a hospital due to a lack of food or shelter. While some view homelessness as being outside the purview of medicine and psychiatry, the fact remains that homelessness is as **dangerous** as many of the other conditions that we treat, with homeless people being 3 times as likely to die than people with homes, with the median age of death being in one's 40s. For this reason, it is important both to understand the nature of homelessness and to have a structured approach for providing the best quality of care for these patients.

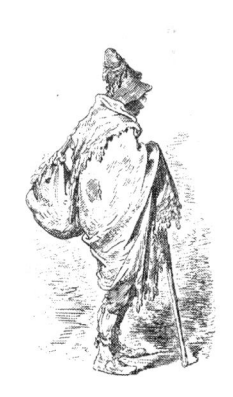

Like violence, homelessness is not *inherently* medical or psychiatric in origin. Studies have shown that most cases of homelessness can be attributed to **economic factors** such as housing supply and unemployment. However, for some patients, psychiatric disorders, substance abuse, and serious medical conditions have played a large role in their inability to secure housing.

While people often refer to "the homeless" as a single group, in reality people struggling with homelessness are a **heterogenous** population. While some homeless people do sleep on the streets, in parks, or out in the open, this is not the norm. Two-thirds of homeless people reside in shelters, while the rest either temporarily stay with family and friends or live in makeshift housing like cars, tents, or boxes. While many people picture the average homeless person as a single adult male, the reality is that 40% of homeless people are women and 20% are children. **Minority groups** are disproportionately represented in homeless populations due to the systemic barriers to employment and housing that they face.

The majority of people seeking shelter are **transitionally homeless** (80%), meaning that they are temporarily without a home but are able to eventually secure a new residence. The remaining 20% is split between the **episodically homeless**, who repeatedly drift in and out of homelessness, and the **chronically homeless**, who are consistently unable to find shelter. Many chronically homeless people started off their lives in similar circumstances, with many having been **institutionalized** or placed in foster care as children. A criminal history can also make it hard for patients to get back on their feet, with many housing options being closed to them.

Hospitals, and emergency departments in particular, tend to be ill-equipped to respond to homelessness. One study found that less than 5% of homeless patients were discharged from the emergency department with a plan that specifically addressed their homelessness. With this in mind, having a structured framework for meeting the needs of homeless patients is invaluable. Use the mnemonic **A TRIP HOME** to remember the core aspects of caring for homeless patients, including things to screen for, referrals to make, and interventions to offer.

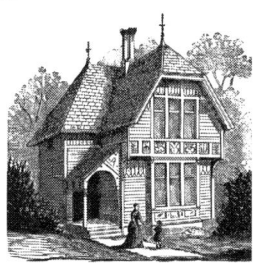

A is for Addiction. Substance use is common in the homeless population, with up to 50% having a history of alcohol use disorder and around 40% having struggled with other substance use disorders. Make sure to screen for substance use and offer referrals to detox and rehab programs as needed.

T is for Traumatization. A history of trauma, abuse, or violence is very common in homeless patients, with a third of women, 25% of men, and 40% of transgender people without homes having been physically or sexually assaulted in the past year. It is important to engage in **trauma-informed care** that includes screening for trauma, taking time to approach sensitive issues in a nuanced way, and being mindful of the patient's boundaries during an exam (such as asking for permission when asking potentially sensitive questions such as screening for sexually transmitted infections).

R is for Rehabilitation. Cognitive impairments such as such as learning disabilities or memory deficits are common in homeless patients, especially those who are elderly, have a severe mental disorder, or have experienced severe head trauma. This can contribute to an inability to care for oneself, with a third of patients having difficulty doing at least one **activity of daily living** (ADL) such as dressing, bathing, or eating.

Make sure to assess for cognitive and functional abilities, and offer referrals to services such as occupational therapy as appropriate.

I is for Immunization. Infectious diseases are widespread in homeless populations, so consider offering **immunizations** against influenza and other diseases as appropriate as well as ordering **labs** to screen for infections like HIV and hepatitis C.

P is for Psychiatric services. Between a quarter and a third of all homeless people have a severe mental disorder such as schizophrenia, depression, or bipolar disorder. This is especially true for those who are episodically or chronically homeless. For this reason, it is important to screen for a variety of psychiatric diagnoses and to offer treatment as needed. Some patients with severe forms of psychiatric pathology may need either temporary **hospitalization** or long-term **institutionalization** to regain stability. However, these steps should be taken rarely, as it is estimated that only 5% of homeless people with serious mental disorders need to be institutionalized, with the other 95% being able to live in the community with appropriate support.

H is for Housing. Naturally, for patients who lack a home, trying to secure housing should be among your top priorities. **Shelters** can provide a temporary solution, although many patients are reluctant to go due to concerns about shelters being loud, unclean, crowded, lacking in privacy, or dangerous. Longer-term placements in **supportive housing** (placements with medical care and other services embedded within them) have been shown to significantly reduce subsequent shelter use, hospitalization, incarceration, and even risk of death. It's important to note that not all supportive housing is the same! Some placements can insist upon abstinence from drugs as a condition for continued housing, although evidence of long-term success from this approach is mixed. Instead, placements that take a **Housing First** mentality (which views housing, not sobriety, as the primary goal) seem to have the best outcomes, with patients in these programs spending over twice as much time in stable housing with no difference in substance use or psychiatric symptoms.

O is for Outreach. Homeless patients can struggle with navigating traditional clinical settings. Instead, refer patients to **outreach programs** that embed clinical services in the places where homeless people often go as part of their daily life, such as shelters and soup kitchens. Outreach programs significantly improve access to care, with 90% of patients in these programs getting consistent medical care compared to less than 40% in traditional clinics.

M is for Multidisciplinary. Care for the homeless is necessarily **multidisciplinary**, as no one profession can address all of the issues that homeless people face. Doctors, nurses, social workers, therapists, and other disciplines should all be involved whenever possible. In particular, **case managers** can help the patient coordinate various aspects of their care and help to advocate on the patient's behalf. Studies have shown that case management can improve housing stability, alleviate psychiatric symptoms, reduce substance use, and increase employment, all while minimizing costs.

E is for Essentials. Finally, one of the best ways to help homeless patients is to focus on practical, tangible solutions to the problems they face. Giving out shoes, warm clothes, blankets, bus tokens, and food vouchers can go a long way towards addressing the basic needs of these patients and helping to build trust and rapport. When prescribing medications, try to simplify the medication regimen as much as possible by choosing medications that are inexpensive, have once-daily dosing (rather than needing to be taken multiple times per day), and/or that don't need to be taken with food. In addition, make sure to update contact information such as phone numbers, as these can change often for homeless patients. Using a pragmatic approach, you can help to address your patients' needs and get them back on track.

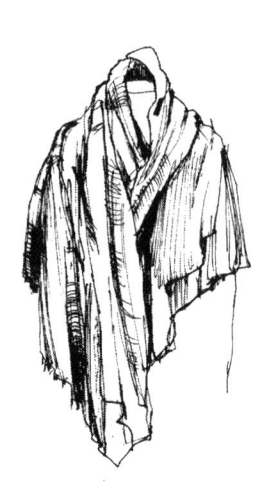

While it won't always be possible to accomplish each of these steps (especially in emergency settings), try to keep each of them in mind as the standard of care for homeless patients!

Homelessness is **dangerous** for patients and should be addressed promptly using **evidence-based strategies**.

A TRIP HOME:
Addiction
Traumatization
Rehabilitation
Immunization
Psychiatric services
Housing
Outreach
Multidisciplinary
Essentials

PUTTING IT ALL TOGETHER

Psychiatric emergencies are among the most tragic outcomes of mental illness. While suicide, violence, abuse, delirium, catatonia, and homelessness do not represent a comprehensive list of psychiatric problems you may encounter in emergency settings, they each warrant separate consideration and treatment in addition to any associated disorders. Because psychiatric emergencies are a hodgepodge of different situations, there aren't very many unifying themes to bring them all together. Instead, take some time to review what we've learned as well as the associated mnemonics for each before moving on!

REVIEW QUESTIONS

1. A 51 y/o M calls a suicide hotline saying that he is having thoughts of shooting himself with a handgun. He says that he is out of his medications and has not seen his psychiatrist in over 10 months. What is the most appropriate next question for the counselor to ask?
    A. "What medications do you take?"
    B. "Who is your psychiatrist?"
    C. "Where are you right now?"
    D. "Have you ever had a manic episode?"
    E. "Do you have a history of non-suicidal self-harm like cutting?"

2. A 22 y/o M is brought into the Emergency Department by police who found him running in a busy city square waving a gun around and yelling nonsensically. The gun has been confiscated. In the hospital, he is uncooperative with a psychiatric interview and instead yells and swings his fists wildly, nearly hitting a nearby staff member. What is the best next step?
    A. Determine any potential targets of violence and contact them
    B. Speak to the patient loudly and firmly
    C. Determine whether the gun was loaded or not
    D. Obtain a urine sample for a toxicology test
    E. Administer medications

3. (Continued from previous question.) Serum and urine samples are collected. Toxicology testing shows the presence of a single substance. Which of these substances is *least* likely to have been identified?
    A. Alcohol
    B. Steroids
    C. Heroin
    D. Phencyclidine
    E. Methamphetamine

4. An 81 y/o F is admitted to the hospital for intravenous antibiotic treatment of a urinary tract infection. During the second night of hospitalization, she awakens at 2:30 in the morning and attempts to climb out of bed, pulling an IV out of her arm in the process. She continues to repeat, "I'm going home, I'm going home, I'm going home." On interview, she knows her name but not where she is or why she is in the hospital. What is the best next step?
    A. Restrain the patient
    B. Initiate an immediate work-up for causes of delirium
    C. Administer antipsychotic medications
    D. Arrange for a sitter
    E. Increase the dose of antibiotics

5. (Continued from previous question.) After several minutes, the patient calms and agrees to return to her hospital bed. However, when the nurse attempts to replace the IV, the patient begins yelling, "I don't want it! I don't want it!" What is the best next step?
    A. Perform a capacity evaluation
    B. Attempt to find a surrogate decision maker
    C. Consult psychiatry
    D. Consult ethics
    E. Restrain the patient and place the IV

6. A 19 y/o M is brought to the hospital by his mother who says that the patient has been acting "like a zombie" for the past three days. He has a history of a single manic episode one year ago which was successfully treated. Due to the patient's stability, his medications were discontinued one month ago. Initial vital signs are HR 126, BP 142/90, RR 10, and T 101.1°F. The patient is unable to participate in an interview and does not respond to any questions asked, instead staring motionlessly at the ground throughout the entire interview. Neurologic exam is notable for muscular rigidity. The doctor accidentally drops her pen on the ground which makes a sharp noise, but the patient does not flinch or even move at all in response to this. An attempt to conduct a neurologic exam shows that the patient will leave his arms in any position that they are put in, even against gravity. Which of the following aspects of the patient's presentation predicts the worst prognosis?
    A. Mutism
    B. Negativism
    C. Waxy flexibility
    D. Catalepsy
    E. Hyperthermia

7. (Continued from previous question.) Which of the following is the best next step?
    A. Admitting to the hospital for observation
    B. Administering lorazepam
    C. Arranging for electroconvulsive therapy
    D. Restarting previous medications for bipolar disorder
    E. Starting an antipsychotic

1. **The best answer is C.** The most important first step in responding to a psychiatric emergency like suicidal ideation is to immediately assess for the patient's safety. Asking the patient's location will permit the hotline counselor to intervene by calling emergency medical services. Other questions may be helpful in fleshing out the patient's history or determining a diagnosis but ultimately are less important than securing the patient's safety.

2. **The best answer is B.** This patient is exhibiting signs of severe agitation. In these cases, the best approach is to attempt rapid behavioral de-escalation. Verbal de-escalation should be attempted first, with other measures such as restraints and/or medications (answer E) being performed only after verbal de-escalation has failed. Other steps to obtain additional history (answers C and D) or fulfilling one's duty to protect (answer B) are important but take secondary priority after managing the acute behavioral emergency.

3. **The best answer is C.** All of the substances listed are associated with an increased risk of violence except for opioids, which tend to cause sedation rather than agitation.

4. **The best answer is D.** This patient is suffering from delirium, a psychiatric emergency that requires prompt assessment and intervention. In the majority of cases, the presence of delirium should initiate an immediate work-up for causes; however, in this case the presence of a urinary tract infection provides a reasonable explanation for delirium, and a further work-up may not be necessary and is, at the very least, not an immediate priority (answer B). Antipsychotic medications are helpful at reducing the duration of delirium, so using them in this patient is not unreasonable (answer C); however, arranging for a sitter who can provide verbal reassurance is more likely to result in immediate behavioral de-escalation. Restraining the patient (answer A) may be necessary in cases of severe delirium where verbal de-escalation and administration of antipsychotics have not been effective, but it should be used as rarely as possible owing to the significant medical and psychological risks associated with restraint. Finally, changing the dose of antibiotics should only be done as clinically necessary for treatment of her infection and is irrelevant to the discussion of treatment of delirium (answer E).

5. **The best answer is B.** As mentioned in the previous question, this patient lacks an understanding of where she is or why she is in the hospital. Because of this, it is already clear that she lacks capacity to make this decision as she is unable to appreciate her situation (answer A). In cases where the patient lacks capacity, a surrogate decision maker should be sought. Consulting psychiatry (answer C) may help to provide clarity on cases where the presence or absence of capacity is not clear cut, but would not provide much helpful information in cases like these where the lack of capacity is immediately evident. Ethics consultation (answer D) may be required in the future if a surrogate decision maker is unable to be found, but this must be confirmed first. Finally, administering non-voluntary treatment should not be done unless if the situation is immediately life-threatening. In this case, an infection is unlikely to be immediately life-threatening, giving the provider time to search for a surrogate decision maker.

6. **The best answer is E.** This patient is exhibiting clear signs of catatonia, including mutism (not speaking), negativism (not reacting to loud sounds), waxy flexibility (maintaining his arms in any position they are placed in), and catalepsy (muscular rigidity) (answers A, B, C, and D, respectively). However, only hyperthermia (the presence of a fever) is suggestive of malignant catatonia, a life-threatening form of catatonia with a high mortality rate.

7. **The best answer is C.** While administering a benzodiazepine such as lorazepam (answer B) is indicated as a first-line treatment for most cases of catatonia, for cases of malignant catatonia electroconvulsive therapy is the first-line treatment, as evidence suggests that early use of ECT for malignant catatonia results in better outcomes and lowered mortality rates. Observation (answer A) is inappropriate for a potentially life-threatening condition. Using medications to treat the underlying bipolar disorder (answers D and E) may be helpful for long-term treatment but would not be expected to result in immediate treatment of catatonia.

5 DEPRESSION

Let's begin our whirlwind tour of psychiatric pathology with **depression**. Depression has the highest lifetime prevalence of any single psychiatric disorder, with 20% of all people experiencing a depressive episode during their lifetime. Because of this, depression has been called the "common cold" of psychiatry. Despite how widespread it is, depression is not easy to diagnose. What we currently call "depression" is, in fact, an **illness with many faces**, and it is likely that the various disorders that we currently lump together under this term are in fact many separate conditions, each with their own unique causes and treatment considerations. It is this mix of **ubiquity** and **heterogeneity** that makes diagnosing depression such a challenge: most people have a preconceived idea of what "depression" means based on their own personal experiences, but this notion will differ drastically from one person to the next.

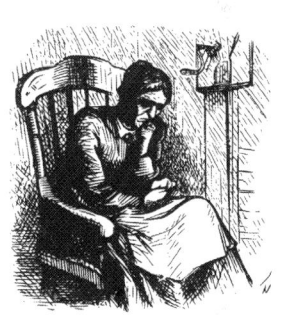

To help you make sense of this, we will first learn about depression in its most prototypical form: specifically, **episodic unipolar major depressive disorder** and its various subtypes. From there, we'll go over all the misdiagnoses and missed diagnoses that patients and medical professionals alike often lump together under the term depression. Because the approach to treatment can vary so widely for all the different clinical entities that are often called depression, it is imperative to accurately diagnose the situation as soon as possible. If you were to treat every person who walks through your door complaining of "depression" as if they have episodic unipolar major depressive disorder, you are likely to enter your patients into a cycle of failed treatments and dashed expectations. For this reason, knowing the patterns of "textbook" depression is essential.

SIGNS AND SYMPTOMS OF DEPRESSION

The specific signs and symptoms of depression are captured in the mnemonic **SIGECAPS**. Legend has it that SIGECAPS refers to an outdated practice where a doctor making a prescription would write "SIG" for directions and then "E-CAPS" for energy capsules, an older term for antidepressants. Use this memory device to remember:

S is for Sleep. Disturbances in sleep are a core symptom of depression and are experienced by more than 90% of people during an episode. Depression causes not only difficulty in falling asleep but also early morning awakenings, disrupting both the **amount** and **quality** of sleep that people are able to get. Research shows that depression is even able to alter someone's circadian rhythm, making them feel perpetually jetlagged. Due to this, people with depression classically complain of severe symptoms of depression in the mornings which partially lift by the afternoon.

I is for Interest or enjoyment. A hallmark symptom of depression is an inability to feel pleasure, known as **anhedonia**. Anhedonia is evidenced by decreased interest in activities that are normally pleasurable such as participating in hobbies or socializing with others. Anhedonia is what makes depression a **non-reactive** state, meaning that someone's mood will remain the same no matter what is going on around them. For example, someone in a state of depression would feel no joy even in situations that would normally inspire mirth, such as celebrating a birthday, getting a promotion at work, being with family and friends, or riding a giant chicken. Out of all the symptoms of depression, anhedonia is the **most sensitive** marker, and the absence of anhedonia reliably rules out major depressive disorder.

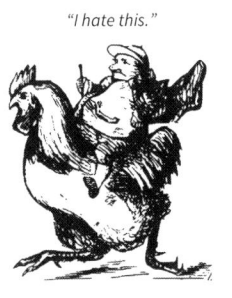

"I hate this."

G is for Guilt or hopelessness. People in a state of depression often find that their thoughts become narrowed and, after a while, they are only able to focus on negative thoughts. The thought content in depression often revolves around feelings of **guilt** ("I deserve this"), **worthlessness** ("All I am is a burden on people"), or **hopelessness** ("There's no way out of this hole I am in"). Thought patterns of depression are often **ruminative**, as certain thoughts are "chewed over" repeatedly in the mind.

E is for Energy. Levels of energy and activity are often severely decreased in depression, sometimes to the point where even getting out of bed in the morning is a major challenge. The **fatigue** seen in depression exceeds what would be expected just from the sleep disturbances present in this disorder, suggesting that fatigue is a core feature of the disorder rather than merely a side effect of other symptoms.

C is for Concentration. The rumination, poor sleep, and low energy experienced during a depressive episode often make it difficult to concentrate, leading to impairments in work, school, and relationships. In contrast to syndromes like attention deficit hyperactivity disorder where concentration deficits are chronic, in depression the ability to concentrate improves when the mood episode ends.

A is for Appetite. The majority of people with depression find that their appetite and food intake are significantly decreased, which can result in noticeable weight loss or even malnutrition over time. People in a state of depression often describe food as unappetizing or flavorless ("It's like I'm eating cardboard").

P is for Psychomotor retardation. While many features of depression are symptoms that can only be *subjectively* reported, in some cases depression involves signs that can be *objectively* observed by others. Psychomotor retardation refers to a general **slowing of speech and physical movements** which together suggest an inner slowing of cognition as well. It is generally considered to be a sign of severe depression.

S is for Suicidal thoughts. For people in the depths of depression who are unable to find any pleasure in life and are constantly haunted by feelings of guilt, worthlessness, and hopelessness, suicide can seem like the only way out. Over half of all people who die by suicide were in a depressive episode at the time of their death, making the link between depression and suicide incredibly robust.

> A **major depressive episode** involves **depressed mood, anhedonia**, and a variety of **other signs and symptoms**.
>
> *Depressed mood + SIGECAPS:*
> *Sleep disturbance*
> *Interest or enjoyment (decreased)*
> *Guilt or hopelessness*
> *Energy (decreased)*
> *Concentration (impaired)*
> *Appetite (decreased)*
> *Psychomotor retardation*
> *Suicidal thoughts*

Having **at least 5** of these 9 symptoms for **2 or more weeks** is diagnostic of a major depressive episode per DSM-5 criteria. However, it's important to note that the DSM criteria do not capture the entirety of depression. There are a variety of additional signs and symptoms that are clinically seen in depression, including a slouched posture, monotone speech that lacks prosody, severe anxiety, a high rate of unexplained medical symptoms like headaches and stomach pain, feelings of depersonalization and derealization ("It's like I'm seeing the world through a fog"), and a general lack of motivation. While not officially recognized in the diagnostic criteria, these signs and symptoms can be helpful for diagnosing depression as well.

> Per the DSM-5, patients must have **5 out of 9** symptoms for a period of **2 weeks** or more to qualify for **major depressive episode**.
>
> *The timeframe for depression is **two blue weeks**.*

DEPRESSION ACROSS THE LIFESPAN

The signs and symptoms of depression are important to understand, but ultimately they are only the first step in being able to diagnose depression. This is because evaluating signs and symptoms can only give you a cross-sectional snapshot of a patient at a single moment in time. However, diagnosis should be based on **longitudinal** information and take into account the patient's history across their entire lifespan as much as possible. Because of this, we will spend some time discussing the epidemiology, prognosis, and treatment response associated with depression to provide you with additional tools for getting the diagnosis right.

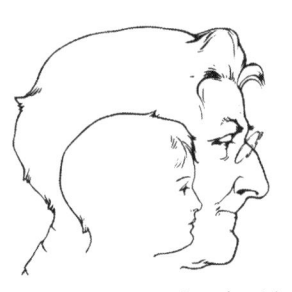

EPIDEMIOLOGY

As mentioned previously, depression is the single most common psychiatric disorder, with over 20% of all people experiencing at least one depressive episode during their lifetime. This gives depression a **high base rate** in the population, putting it high on your differential for *all* patients presenting with any psychiatric concern (even if you know nothing else about them). For patients specifically presenting with any kind of mood-related concerns, it should be at or near the top of your differential.

Depression can develop at any age, although it begins most often in **early adulthood** with a median age of 32. However, up to a quarter of people with depression do not have their first episode until after the age of 50, so a lack of prior episodes (even in an elderly patient) does not automatically rule out a major depressive episode. **Women** are diagnosed with depression twice as often as men.

PROGNOSIS

Evaluated longitudinally, the signs and symptoms of major depressive disorder tend to occur in discrete **episodes**. Untreated, an episode of depression usually lasts between **6 to 12 months**. After this time, most patients will spontaneously recover and enter a period of normal reactive mood known as **euthymia** (although many will have some residual depressive symptoms even between episodes). Functioning is often significantly impaired *during* an episode of depression but **preserved between episodes**. (This is in contrast to other disorders, such as schizophrenia or personality disorders, where functioning is continuously impaired.)

After a single episode of depression, the risk for developing another episode is approximately 50%. This means that as many as half of all people diagnosed with depression will only have a single **isolated** episode during their lifetime. For the other half, depression becomes a **recurrent** disorder, with the risk of recurrence increasing to 80% after a second lifetime episode and getting even higher with each additional episode after that.

The relationship between depression and life events is complex. Although exact numbers are hard to come by, depressive episodes are *sometimes but not always* precipitated by stressful life events. Generally, these life events involve some form of a major disruption to one's **social circumstances**, with the most common being conflict with one's partner, moving geographically, being forced to change jobs, receiving a diagnosis of a major medical illness, having a family member leave home, or experiencing the death of a relative or close friend. Interestingly, the relationship between major life events is most clearly established for one's first lifetime episode of depression. After that, depression seems to take on "a life of its own," with episodes happening more and more often without a clear link to life events.

Depression carries a significant **mortality rate**. Mood disorders are found in the majority of people who die by suicide, and up to 5% of people with depression will eventually take their own lives. Depression also worsens outcomes for a variety of medical illnesses including cancer, heart disease, and stroke, leading to decreases in life expectancy of up to 10 years even after removing suicide from the equation.

TREATMENT

With treatment, the average length of a major depressive episode is reduced from 6 months to less than **3 months**. Treatment for depression consists of **psychotherapy**, **medications**, or a **combination** of the two. While psychotherapy and antidepressants are both effective, the combination of the two is better than either one alone.

Several types of psychotherapy have been shown to be helpful. The most well-studied is **cognitive behavioral therapy** (CBT) which focuses on the connections between thoughts, feelings, and behavior and teaches specific skills for breaking out of the cycle of depression. CBT is associated with a **medium effect size** (around 0.5) for treating depression. Other types of therapy, including behavioral activation, acceptance and commitment therapy (ACT), interpersonal therapy (IPT), and psychoanalytic therapy, have evidence supporting their use as well.

Medications used to treat depression are known as **antidepressants**, although this is a marketing term more than a scientific one. Most of these drugs work by increasing the amount of various neurotransmitters, including **serotonin**, **dopamine**, and **norepinephrine**, that is active and available in the brain. The most common class of antidepressant is **serotonin reuptake inhibitors** (SRIs) that boost levels of serotonin in the brain, although other neurotransmitters like norepinephrine and dopamine can play a role as well. Antidepressants are helpful for treating depression, with a **small-to-moderate effect size** of around 0.4. Antidepressants also take some time to work, with a full effect often not being seen for up to 2 months after beginning the medication.

Treatment response in depression appears to follow a "Rule of Thirds," as about one-third of patients who receive treatment experience complete recovery from their symptoms (known as **remission**), one-third notice the improvement of some but not all symptoms (known as **response**), and one-third do not get any better with the first treatment tried (known as **treatment resistance**). Patients who have not received any benefit even after multiple trials of therapy and medications are considered to have **treatment-resistant depression**. In these cases, treatments such as electroconvulsive therapy (ECT) may be considered. While ECT is an invasive and complicated procedure, it is highly effective, with a **large effect size** around 0.8 even for people who have not received any benefit from other treatments tried.

MECHANISMS OF DEPRESSION

Throughout this book, we will explore what is known about the underlying pathophysiology of the disorders that we are studying with the goal of using this information both to improve diagnostic accuracy as well as to identify those people who are most likely to benefit from specific treatments. However, it is worth keeping in mind that the brain is a complicated organ, and given how little we know about it, these mechanisms should be seen as **likely hypotheses** rather than established facts.

Looking at the pathophysiology of this condition, it is worth stating right off the bat that there is **no evidence that depression results from an inherent "chemical imbalance"** of any kind. While medications that increase serotonin are effective at reducing the symptoms of depression in the majority of people who take them, that does *not* mean that depressed people lack serotonin, and decades of research have yet to provide much evidence for the "chemical imbalance theory" of depression.

Instead, depression appears to involve specific changes in the way that people process information. To put it simply, depressed people see the world differently. Depression involves a tendency to focus on negative, rather than positive, stimuli. When presented with a list of words, for example, people with depression are more likely to focus on words like "hate" or "pain" rather than "love" or "comfort." When shown a variety of faces, a depressed person will fixate on people with negative facial expressions (like anger or disgust) while blocking out those with positive expressions (like smiling or laughter). Like an invisible magnet, depression draws one's mind preferentially towards negative stimuli, not only in terms of what occupies attention in the current moment but also what information is remembered weeks or months down the line.

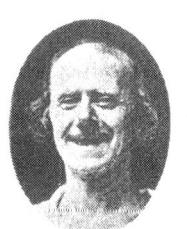

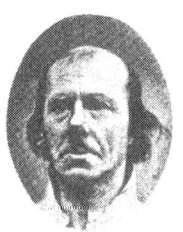

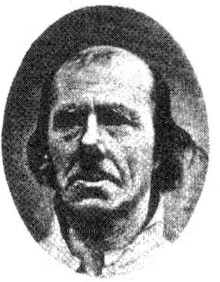

*Perspective of a **non-depressed** person.* *Perspective of a **depressed** person.*

On a neurobiological level, these differences in emotional processing are reflected in the amygdala and other parts of the **limbic system**. In someone who is depressed, these brain regions are *hyper*active when shown a sad or angry face and *hypo*active when shown happy or smiling faces. This phenomenon is referred to as a **negative affective bias**: *negative* for sad or pessimistic, *affective* for one's current emotional state, and *bias* for being drawn to certain stimuli over others. Negative affective biases tend to accumulate, trapping people in a vicious cycle where the negative thought patterns of depression are constantly reinforced.

Negative affective biases explain much of what is seen in the phenomenology of depression. For one, each person at their baseline has an intrinsic tendency to focus on either positive or negative stimuli and, like many things in psychiatry, this occurs on a spectrum. Research has found that people who have a greater tendency towards negative emotional processing (even when not in an episode of depression) are at higher risk for developing depression compared to people with a greater tendency towards positive stimuli, suggesting that this represents an **inherent vulnerability** towards depression regardless of one's current mood state. In addition, negative affective biases tend to accumulate in a **snowball-like effect**, explaining the "slide" into depression that people experience (rather than depression being a state that comes on all at once like a flu). Finally, negative affective biases lead people with depression to consistently **underestimate their chances of success** at various activities, leading to the specific cognitive and behavioral patterns seen in depression such as feelings of hopelessness ("I never do anything right"), isolating oneself socially ("I'm not going to see people, they will all just laugh at me"), and a lack of desire to engage in pleasurable or rewarding activities ("Maybe it works for other people, but it won't work for me"). (This tendency towards *under*estimation of success will form the basis of a crucial distinction between depression and mania in the next chapter.)

The involvement of negative affective biases also explains much of what we see during treatment of depression. In particular, negative affective biases provides a mechanism for why antidepressants take so long to work. As mentioned previously, antidepressants often take up to 2 months to have a full effect, which makes them different from other drugs (like stimulants or alcohol) that exert psychological effects almost immediately after taking them. However, studies have demonstrated that antidepressants *do* in fact have immediate effects—just not the ones you might expect. Within minutes of taking an antidepressant, a significant lessening of negative affective biases is observed, with people becoming more able to focus on positive stimuli, less reactive to negative facial expressions, and more accurate at estimating their chances of success at various activities. It is believed that this change in emotional processing sets the stage for a *gradual* unlearning of depressive thought patterns and behaviors. In fact, studies have found that the extent to which an antidepressant will ultimately improve mood for a particular person can be predicted by how much it changes their affective processing within the first few days of treatment. Negative affective biases also explain why antidepressants do not elevate mood in non-depressed people (they are not "happy pills"), as they won't work if there are no negative affective biases to lift. They also explain why drugs and CBT are both effective in treating depression and in roughly the same amount of time, as both types of treatments reduce negative affective biases and allow someone with depression to establish new thoughts patterns and different ways of interpreting the world.

No one theory is going to explain a condition as complex as depression, and additional mechanisms are likely at work (including prominent dysregulation of the **hypothalamic–pituitary–adrenal axis**, discussed further in Chapter 9). Nevertheless, negative affective biases serve a practical purpose by helping to confirm a diagnosis of depression and to provide a specific neurobiological target for treatment.

HOW TO DIAGNOSE DEPRESSIVE DISORDERS

Like most mental disorders, a diagnosis of depression is determined primarily using the psychiatric interview and the mental status exam. Specific symptoms of depression, as well as their timing across the lifespan, should be directly assessed. Certain findings on the mental status exam (including slowed movements, absent prosody, dysthymic affect, a ruminative thought process, and suicidal ideation) may also argue for the diagnosis.

Even once you have diagnosed major depressive disorder, however, your job is not yet done. There are various **subtypes** of major depressive disorder that should be considered as well, all of which fit the phenomenology and life course of "textbook" depression to some extent. The presence of any of these subtypes can carry implications for treatment, so make sure to keep them on your differential. Unlike the misdiagnoses and missed diagnoses we will talk about in the next section, all of these entities would accurately be considered to be unipolar major depressive disorder.

MAJOR DEPRESSIVE DISORDER
Major depressive disorder is the prototypical depressive disorder and can be diagnosed when the SIGECAPS symptoms are present for at least two blue weeks. Notably, these episodes of depression occur *without* accompanying episodes of mania (making it a *uni*polar, rather than a *bi*polar, disorder). Even a *single* major depressive episode is sufficient to diagnose major depressive disorder per DSM-5 standards despite the fact that only 50% of people will go on to have another episode. For clarity, people with multiple episodes of depression are said to have **recurrent** major depressive disorder.

MELANCHOLIC DEPRESSION
Historically, the "melancholic" specifier was used to describe **severe** episodes of depression that seemed to come "out of the blue" (as opposed to being brought on by life events) and were completely **non-reactive** to external circumstances. **Neurovegetative symptoms** such as psychomotor retardation, severe loss of appetite, weight loss, fatigue, inattention, and disrupted sleep are particularly pronounced. It is unclear if melancholic depression represents a distinct subtype of major depressive disorder as opposed to simply a very severe form. In any case, treatment is largely the same as for "textbook" depression, although more intensive forms of treatment such as ECT may be considered earlier.

ATYPICAL DEPRESSION
Atypical depression has some unique features compared to "textbook" depression. Most notably, mood remains **reactive** in atypical depression, and many people with atypical depression will experience a lifting of depressive symptoms during happy life events or a worsening of symptoms when things don't go their way. Patients with atypical depression often display a long-standing pattern of **interpersonal rejection sensitivity**, even when not in an episode of depression. Other unique features of atypical depression are an *increase* in appetite (rather than a decrease) which can result in weight gain, sleeping too much (rather than too little), and a

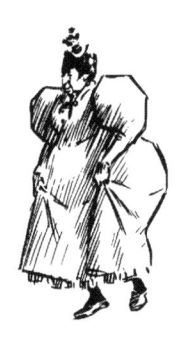

sensation that one's limbs feel too heavy to lift (known as **leaden paralysis**). In terms of treatment, a specific class of antidepressants known as **monoamine oxidase inhibitors** (MAOIs) is particularly effective for atypical depression. You can remember the features of atypical depression by thinking of it as **ate-typical depression**: a depressed person who had mood reactivity and became happy when they **ate** food would probably start to gain weight, causing their limbs to feel heavy, and may become sensitive to people rejecting them because of their weight.

> **Atypical depression** involves **increased appetite**, **hypersomnia**, **leaden paralysis**, and **interpersonal rejection sensitivity**.
>
> *Ate*-typical depression involves **eating**, leading to **heaviness** and **rejection sensitivity**.

POSTPARTUM DEPRESSION

Around 15% women develop clinical depression within a few weeks of delivering their child. It is unclear why the postnatal state increases the risk of depression, but many factors (including hormonal changes, sleep deprivation, and childcare stress) are believed to play a role. Postpartum depression is not considered to be a separate syndrome from major depressive disorder and is treated like "textbook" depression with the exception of taking some additional considerations into account when choosing medications if the mother is breastfeeding.

Postpartum depression should be differentiated from "**baby blues**," a transient state of mild depressive symptoms that resolves within a few weeks. Baby blues occur in 80% of mothers following delivery and are considered to be a normal part of the human experience. Severe symptoms lasting more than a few weeks should raise the consideration for a diagnosis of postpartum depression (remember "two blue weeks"). Postpartum depression should also be carefully separated from **postpartum psychosis**, another psychiatric syndrome that occurs in the period following childbirth. In contrast to baby blues or postpartum depression, postpartum psychosis is characterized by symptoms of psychosis or mania, including rapid swings in mood, hallucinations, bizarre beliefs, and paranoia. Postpartum psychosis is one of the leading causes of infanticide and is considered to be a medical emergency necessitating immediate psychiatric hospitalization and treatment.

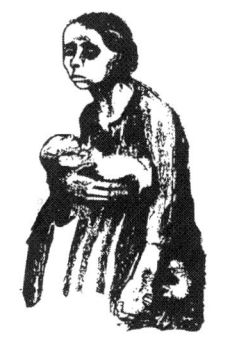

PSYCHOTIC DEPRESSION

Psychotic depression is characterized by the presence of **paranoia**, **delusions**, or **hallucinations** in addition to all of the usual symptoms of major depressive disorder. Psychotic symptoms do not occur in all cases of severe depression, but nearly all cases of psychotic depression involve severe depressive symptoms. Treatment involves a combination of both **antidepressants** and **antipsychotics**. In many cases, hospitalization and/or ECT should be considered. (Differentiating psychotic depression from other disorders where mood and psychotic symptoms co-occur, including bipolar disorder with psychotic features, schizoaffective disorder, and even schizophrenia itself, can be challenging. We will defer discussion of this until Chapter 7, as it requires a greater understanding of both mania and psychosis.)

CATATONIC DEPRESSION
Catatonia can occur in severe cases of major depressive disorder. It manifests in the specific signs and symptoms described in Chapter 4 and often requires intensive treatment in a hospital setting. As with all forms of catatonia, **benzodiazepines** should be used liberally, as they are often very effective at rapidly reversing the state of catatonia. If medications are not effective or if there are signs suggestive of malignant catatonia, ECT should be considered.

SEASONAL DEPRESSION
Seasonal depression (also known as seasonal affective disorder) is a subtype of major depressive disorder where depressive episodes have a clearly established link with the changing of the seasons. Most often, depression develops during the **winter months**. This is likely related to lower levels of sunlight during the winter, as the rate of seasonal depression increases the farther away from the equator you go. Treatment for seasonal depression involves **bright light therapy** for at least 30 minutes each day to help offset the loss of sunlight. Most houselights do not produce the full spectrum of light (as sunlight does), so specialized "light boxes" should be used. Standard treatments for major depressive disorder, including conventional antidepressants and psychotherapy, can be used as well and are equally effective.

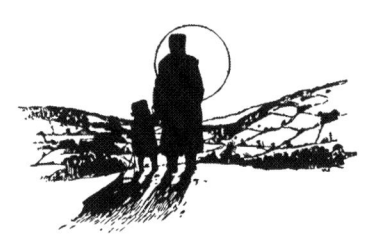

DIFFERENTIAL DIAGNOSIS OF DEPRESSIVE DISORDERS

Now that we have a good understanding of depression and its various subtypes, let's explore what actually happens when patients walk into the door complaining of "depression." Even the most well-read students can have difficulty adjusting to real-world clinical settings where cases of "textbook" depression are the **exception rather than the rule**. Even in cases where someone *technically* meets diagnostic criteria for major depressive disorder, a different diagnosis (such as bipolar disorder or borderline personality disorder) may do a much better job of explaining the patient's distress and pointing towards a helpful treatment strategy. This reflects a major shortcoming of the DSM and other algorithmic approaches to diagnosis: they have increased the *reliability* of diagnosis at the expense of sacrificing the *validity* of what the diagnostic criteria are supposed to represent.

For this reason, when evaluating a patient complaining of depression, it can be helpful to approach the psychiatric evaluation with an eye towards **misdiagnoses** and **missed diagnoses**. Misdiagnoses are fundamentally incorrect diagnoses. For example, if someone with a history of both depression and mania was diagnosed with unipolar (rather than bipolar) depression, this would simply be a wrong diagnosis. In contrast, missed diagnoses are those that are frequently encountered with depression (such as anxiety or substance abuse) and can interact with or mimic many of its symptoms. Understanding the most common misdiagnoses and missed diagnoses of depression can be exceptionally challenging, even for experienced clinicians. It will be even more challenging early in this book, as we will not have discussed many of the conditions we will be comparing with depression. Rest assured that it will get easier as you progress in knowledge. In the meantime, feel free to jump ahead to other chapters of the book to gain additional insight into these disorders.

Both when answering test questions as well as when evaluating patients in clinical settings, having a framework for evaluating mood concerns can give you a structured process for picking up on clinically important features. You can use the mnemonic **Reactive PLANETS** to remember the specific high-yield factors that commonly differentiate depression from alternative diagnoses:

R is for Reactivity. The presence or absence of mood reactivity is an important diagnostic clue. Non-reactivity suggests a mood disorder such as unipolar or bipolar depression, while a reactive mood may suggest atypical depression, borderline personality disorder, or even just plain old normalcy.

P is for Polarity. A history of both depression and mania is the diagnostic hallmark of bipolar disorder. Make sure to inquire about any history of manic or hypomanic episodes, as bipolar depression requires a fundamentally different treatment approach compared to unipolar depression.

L is for Lability. Mood symptoms can either be stable or labile. Mood symptoms from major depressive disorder or bipolar disorder are often quite stable and endure for weeks, months, or years at a time. In contrast, a labile affect (changing within minutes or hours) is often more characteristic of personality disorders or substance use.

A is for Attributability. In some cases, depression can be attributable to specific causative factors, including medical conditions (like hypothyroidism), substances (alcohol), external circumstances (postpartum depression), and timing (seasonal depression or premenstrual dysphoric disorder) among many others.

N is for Normality. Normalcy should *always* be on the differential. Take some time to consider whether the patient's reported symptoms are within the realm of normal human emotion.

E is for Episodicity. Depressive symptoms often occur in discrete episodes, which is characteristic of both unipolar major depressive disorder as well as bipolar disorder. Chronic non-episodic depression should raise your suspicion for other diagnoses, including dysthymia and personality disorders.

T is for Treatment responsivity. How well a person has responded to treatments for depression can offer a helpful clue as well. A history of failing multiple trials of conventional antidepressants should have you searching for alternate explanations, including misdiagnoses (bipolar disorder), missed diagnoses (anxiety disorders), or other attributable factors (alcohol-induced depression). However, poor treatment response in and of itself is not sufficient to rule out major depressive disorder (they may just have treatment-resistant depression). The best way of conceptualizing the effect of treatment response is to think that poor treatment response *can be but is not always* a marker of a misdiagnosis or missed diagnosis.

S is for Severity. Finally, the severity of depressive symptoms can help to differentiate between "full blown" and subsyndromal symptoms of depression as well as to differentiate between normalcy and pathology.

Diagnosing depression is more than just using **SIGECAPS**! Try to focus on the patient's pattern of symptoms **across the lifespan**.

Use **Reactive PLANETS** to systematically assess mood complaints:
*R*eactivity
*P*olarity
*L*ability
*A*ttributability
*N*ormality
*E*pisodicity
*T*reatment responsivity
*S*everity

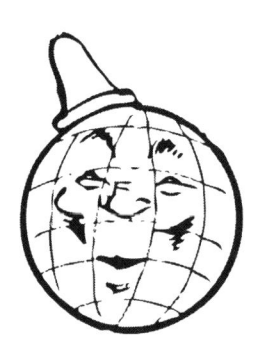

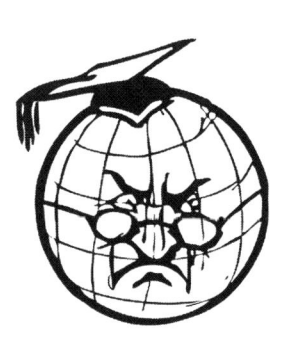

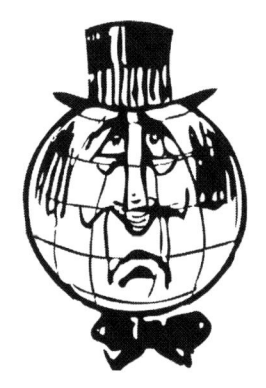

NORMALCY
Sadness, grief, misery, distress, and heartache are painful, and it's not uncommon for people to seek psychiatric care when they experience these emotions. However, to label these experiences as a mental disorder risks unnecessarily pathologizing normal human emotion. When deciding where to draw the line between illness and pathology, consider both **reactivity** and **severity**. For example, someone who recently lost a spouse after a long battle with cancer is likely to experience grief. The symptoms of grief overlap significantly with those of depression, including an intense and protracted state of poor mood, difficulty enjoying activities, trouble

concentrating, poor appetite, and difficulty sleeping. However, most people agree that grief should ultimately be considered a normal part of the human experience and not be diagnosed as a mental disorder. Focusing on reactivity and severity can help to identify those cases where distress and dysfunction are clearly in excess of what most people would experience during grief. While many people experience intense sadness while grieving, it is a minority of people who have a completely non-reactive mood, who are unable to focus on any positive stimuli, who feel completely hopeless about the future, who begin to feel worthless or lack self-esteem, or who begin having persistent thoughts of suicide following bereavement. In these cases, the line between normalcy and pathology has been crossed, and a discussion of treatment options may be helpful. While bereavement is only one example, it provides a good case study for demonstrating the challenges of separating normalcy from depression.

It's also not uncommon for people to use the language of depression as an **idiom of distress**. For example, someone who is upset because they did not get a promotion at work may tell others "I'm depressed" as a way of communicating and seeking validation for their emotions. Distress is not inherently pathological, so always make sure to ask further questions before giving a clinical diagnosis.

ADJUSTMENT DISORDER

Adjustment disorder is defined as depressive and/or anxious symptoms that occur soon after a major life stressor such as going through a divorce or losing a job. Given that we have already established that depressive episodes can also occur after major life events, how can we differentiate between depressive episodes and adjustment disorder? The key here is that the symptoms are **not so severe** that the patient would meet criteria for clinical depression. In effect, adjustment disorder is a "**diagnosis of normalcy**" that recognizes that some degree of distress is normal and expected following a major life change. The continued existence of adjustment disorder as a diagnosable "mental disorder" likely reflects the fact that it ultimately serves a practical purpose by allowing clinicians to provide treatment for grieving or suffering patients in a way that is normalizing, non-stigmatizing, and permits reimbursement for medical services. Treatment for adjustment disorder involves a specific type of psychotherapy known as **supportive therapy** that allows the patient to discuss their psychological reactions in a setting that is empathic and compassionate.

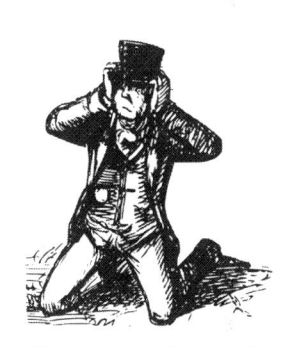

DYSTHYMIA

Dysthymia (referred to as "persistent depressive disorder" in the DSM-5) is on the spectrum of depression but differs from major depressive disorder in two crucial ways. First, it is **chronic** rather than episodic, with symptoms being present most of the time without a break for **at least two years**. Second, it is **subsyndromal** in that the patient does not quite meet full criteria for a major depressive episode but still suffers from depressed mood. Mood symptoms in dysthymia tend to avoid those symptoms of depression that are generally found more often in severe cases of depression (such as psychomotor retardation or thoughts of suicide). This suggests that dysthymia can be conceptualized as a milder but more chronic form of major depressive disorder, and this idea is supported by the fact that treatment for dysthymia is largely the same as for "textbook" depression. You can remember the common symptoms and time course of dysthymia using the mnemonic **HE'S 2 SAD** to remind you of the **H**opelessness, decreased **E**nergy, low **S**elf-esteem, abnormal **S**leep, **A**ppetite changes, and impaired **D**ecision-making that are seen, all for a minimum of **2** years.

> **Dysthymia** (also known as persistent depressive disorder) is a state of **chronic depressive symptoms** that are less severe than "textbook" depression.
>
> *HE'S 2 SAD:*
> *Hopelessness*
> *Energy (decreased)*
> *Self-esteem (decreased)*
> *2 years minimum*
> *Sleep (abnormal)*
> *Appetite (abnormal)*
> *Decision-making (impaired)*

Up to a quarter of all patients with depression have both dysthymia and major depressive disorder, a clinical situation known as "**double depression**." In these cases, the patient spends large portions of their life in a chronic subsyndromal state of depression punctuated with discrete episodes of more severe depression. People with double depression also tend to relapse much more quickly than those with "textbook" major depressive disorder. Double depression is notoriously difficult to treat, but the approach to treatment remains the same: therapy and/or medications.

BIPOLAR DEPRESSION

Depression that occurs in someone with a history of mania or hypomania should be diagnosed as bipolar (rather than unipolar) depression. Clinically, bipolar depression is often **indistinguishable from unipolar depression**. However, major differences in prognosis and treatment response between unipolar and bipolar depression suggest that these two conditions should be conceptualized as **entirely separate disorders** despite the significant overlap in symptoms. A patient presenting with current depressive symptoms can be diagnosed with bipolar I disorder if there is a clear history of even a single manic episode, while a history of even a single hypomanic episode is sufficient to diagnose bipolar II disorder. (Both mania and hypomania will be discussed further in Chapter 6.)

What complicates the process significantly is the fact that patients who have bipolar disorder will often have several depressive episodes *before* their first manic episode. How can we be certain that a patient having their first major depressive episode is not, in fact, presenting with bipolar depression? After all, around 15% of all people seeking treatment for depression will ultimately be diagnosed as having bipolar disorder, and 40 to 70% of people with bipolar disorder are initially diagnosed with unipolar depression. There are some clues that can point us in the right direction. Compared to people with unipolar depression, people with bipolar depression tend to have their first episode earlier in life, to spend more of their time impaired by mood symptoms, to have more psychomotor retardation, to display melancholic, atypical, or psychotic features, and to have a family history of mania. Treatment response can be helpful as well, as conventional antidepressants are likely to be ineffective and may actually increase the rate at which the patient alternates between mania and depression (known as "rapid cycling"). Pay close attention to the presence of any of these during the initial evaluation as well as subsequent treatment. However, at the end of the day, none of these clues are sufficient to definitively diagnose bipolar depression, and **you can never be certain** that a patient has bipolar disorder until they have "declared themselves" by having their first manic or hypomanic episode. While operating within this kind of ambiguity can be frustrating, it is worthwhile to be cautious before diagnosing bipolar depression, especially considering that the treatments for bipolar disorder (including mood stabilizers and antipsychotics) are significantly more harmful than those for unipolar depression.

CYCLOTHYMIA
Just as dysthymia can be conceptualized as a milder but more chronic form of depression, so too cyclothymia can be seen as a milder but more chronic form of bipolar disorder. Cyclothymia can be differentiated from unipolar depression by its **lower severity** and **bipolarity**. In cyclothymia, someone has periods of mild depression (that never quite meet criteria for a major depressive episode) alternating with episodes of hypomania (that never quite meet criteria for a manic episode). While conceptually cyclothymia makes sense, in practice it is rarely diagnosed as most people who have either manic or hypomanic episodes tend to have "full blown" major depressive episodes at some point during their lives.

SUBSTANCE INDUCED MOOD DISORDER
The relationship between depression and substance use is often a two-way street. The effects of certain drugs (such as alcohol or benzodiazepines) can resemble depression during intoxication, while others (including stimulants like methamphetamine) can resemble depression during withdrawal. Other substances may induce depression to the extent that someone may be depressed even when they are not actively intoxicated. The most common substance associated with depression is **alcohol**, but even prescription drugs (such as benzodiazepines or steroids) can impact mood. The key for diagnosing a substance-induced mood disorder is **attributability** and **timing**, as use of the substance will often correlate with increases in depressive symptoms while abstaining from the substance will tend to resolve the symptoms. In cases where symptoms persist even after substance use is stopped for some period of time, a diagnosis of a primary depressive disorder should be considered.

MOOD DISORDER DUE TO A GENERAL MEDICAL CONDITION
Certain medical conditions can "masquerade" as depression and remain undiagnosed for long periods of time. A classic example is **hypothyroidism**, a condition whose symptoms (such as fatigue and poor appetite) overlap significantly with and are often mistaken for clinical depression. Other examples include cardiac disease, chronic hypotension, infections, certain forms of cancer, and neurologic disorders such as multiple sclerosis. The key is for the clinician to have a **high index of suspicion** for any

physical signs or symptoms that may suggest a medical etiology. Additional clues can be found in the **attributability** and **timing** of symptom onset. As a word of caution, be mindful to not confuse a normal grief reaction to being diagnosed with an illness like cancer (which would be considered in the realm of normalcy or adjustment disorder) with the **severe** and **non-reactive** symptoms of major depressive disorder.

PREMENSTRUAL DYSPHORIC DISORDER

Premenstrual dysphoric disorder (sometimes abbreviated PMDD) is a cluster of physiological and psychological symptoms, including low mood, irritability, anxiety, fatigue, and various somatic symptoms, that occurs in some women. The symptoms of premenstrual dysphoric disorder overlap with those of clinical depression quite a bit, but the diagnostic key is the **menstrual pattern** to symptoms. Specifically, mood symptoms often begin in the luteal phase and end soon after menstruation begins. On average, symptoms last six days but can last up to two weeks. Premenstrual dysphoric disorder is not mutually exclusive with depression, as some people will have both discrete episodes of depression in addition to premenstrual dysphoria (in which case the existing symptoms of depression often get significantly worse prior to menses). Asking your patients to complete a mood chart for at least a month can help to confirm the diagnosis (although often patients will know on their own that their symptoms have a clear relationship with their menstrual cycle). Once the diagnosis is reached, treatment options can include antidepressant medications and/or psychotherapies like CBT, which have both been found to be effective.

BORDERLINE PERSONALITY DISORDER

Borderline personality disorder is a complex syndrome defined by unstable emotions, a poor sense of self, and volatile interpersonal relationships. It is the most commonly encountered personality disorder in clinical settings, and we will discuss it at length in Chapter 15. Despite how common it is, borderline personality disorder is frequently overlooked as an explanation for mood symptoms.

Mood symptoms in borderline personality disorder are characterized primarily by two features: **affective lability** and **chronic dysphoria**. Affective lability refers to rapid changes in emotional expression. In contrast to the mood episodes seen in clinical depression or bipolar disorder which often last for weeks or months, affective instability results in emotional changes within a matter of **minutes or hours**. For example, someone with borderline personality disorder may switch from joyous laughing to furious screaming within the span of 60 seconds. These changes in affect are often precipitated by external events (such as threats of abandonment), making mood notably **reactive** (rather than non-reactive as in major depressive disorder).

In addition to affective instability, people with borderline personality disorder often experience chronic dysphoria that can be mistaken for depression. The key difference is that clinical depression occurs in discrete episodes lasting months or even up to a year, whereas chronic dysphoria often persists for **years or decades**. Chronic dysphoria also needs to be distinguished from the chronic low-level depressive symptoms seen in dysthymia, which are similarly non-episodic in nature. The key lies in the difference between **dysthymia** and **dysphoria**. Dysthymia is a low-grade depression, whereas dysphoria is a state of profound dissatisfaction and disappointment with one's self and one's life. This is admittedly a difficult distinction to make, but the easiest way to keep it straight is to think that dysthymia is how you feel after someone *dies* (as in the grieving process) while dysphoria is how you feel after someone *breaks up* with you. Both are painful and difficult to experience, but dysphoria involves feelings of rejection and questioning of self-worth that typically aren't present during grief. Pay attention to the "flavor" of sadness that your patient is reporting to help distinguish between dysthymia and dysphoria.

Recognizing the presence of borderline personality disorder when assessing a patient with depression is important, as it drastically changes the approach required for successful treatment options. Attempting to treat depression in a patient with borderline personality disorder is an exercise in futility, as traditional antidepressant medications do little to help. Instead, treatment of borderline personality disorder itself must take first priority. Treatment involves specific forms of therapy such as **dialectical behavior therapy** (DBT) that specifically address the unique symptom patterns of the disorder. Because of this, **poor treatment responsivity** can be diagnostically helpful (as can **lability** and **lack of episodicity**).

SCHIZOPHRENIA

Schizophrenia is a disorder characterized by a mixture of dramatic positive symptoms (including paranoid delusions, auditory hallucinations, and thought disorganization) as well as more subtle negative symptoms (such as lack of motivation, flat affect, poor energy, social isolation, and poverty of thought). At first, the bizarre symptoms of psychosis can seem a world away from the more recognizable syndrome of depression. However, it's not uncommon for schizophrenia to be mistakenly diagnosed as depression, as the negative symptoms of schizophrenia can strongly resemble the neurovegetative symptoms found in depression (especially in early stages of the disorder before the more dramatic positive symptoms emerge).

The relationship between depression and psychosis is complicated further by the fact that depression, bipolar disorder, schizophrenia, schizoaffective disorder, and even borderline personality disorder can all feature a mixture of mood and psychotic symptoms, yet each is a distinct disorder with separate treatment considerations. We will discuss the relationship between mood and psychotic disorders at some length in Chapter 7, but in the meantime, try to focus on *process over content* when trying to differentiate depression from schizophrenia. People with psychotic depression often have relatively preserved functioning between mood episodes, whereas people with schizophrenia often have **progressive deterioration** of functioning even during periods when symptoms are not active.

ATTENTION DEFICIT HYPERACTIVITY DISORDER

Attention deficit hyperactivity disorder (ADHD) is a neurodevelopmental disorder characterized by chronic inattention and hyperactivity. It often begins in childhood, but for some it persists into adult life as well. For some, the social difficulties and low occupational attainment that often occur in untreated ADHD can lead to a sense of frustration, dissatisfaction, and helplessness which can often be misdiagnosed as depression. In these cases, the mood symptoms should improve with adequate treatment of ADHD. In cases where it does not, consideration of a separate diagnosis of depression may be warranted (as it is absolutely possible to have both depression and ADHD at the same time).

In other cases, the inattention seen in depression can be misdiagnosed as ADHD, although the episodic nature of depression should help to separate it from the **chronic** inattention seen in ADHD. In these cases, treatment of depression should naturally improve concentration.

POST-TRAUMATIC STRESS DISORDER

Post-traumatic stress disorder (PTSD) is a syndrome of cognitive and behavioral symptoms that begins following exposure to a life-threatening or violent event. There is significant overlap in symptoms between depression and PTSD, as both feature **anhedonia**, **sleep disturbance**, and **difficulty concentrating**. However, despite this overlap, depression and PTSD should be conceptualized as two distinct conditions. Depression is not a "natural effect" of experiencing trauma, and people who meet criteria for both PTSD and depression experience more distress and have worse functional outcomes than people with either diagnosis alone. In addition, there are distinct biological profiles associated with each, suggesting two separate processes (even if they do overlap in some ways). While psychotherapy and/or antidepressants can be helpful for both depression and PTSD, a more trauma-focused therapy is often necessary for successful treatment of PTSD.

ANXIETY DISORDERS

Anxiety disorders are characterized by excessive worrying. They are often comorbid with depression, with up to 60% of people with depression also having an anxiety disorder. Ignoring the presence of anxiety in a person with depression is more of a *missed* diagnosis than a *mis*diagnosis. Luckily, the same treatments are helpful in both disorders, including antidepressant medications and psychotherapies like CBT.

DEMENTIA

The term "dementia" refers to a group of neurocognitive disorders that all involve a **progressive decline in cognitive abilities** such as memory and complex thinking. In the elderly, severe depression can be mistaken for dementia, and people with depression may even score poorly on objective tests used to diagnose dementia. The term "pseudodementia" has been coined to describe patients who appear to have dementia. A prior history of depressive episodes, the presence of other symptoms of depression, and a *lack of effort* on cognitive tests (as opposed to an *inability* to engage) can all point towards a diagnosis of pseudodementia. In addition, patients with pseudodementia often have insight into their cognitive problems ("I'm losing my memory") while those with dementia do not. Identification of pseudodementia is critical, as depression is a highly treatable condition (dementia much less so).

DISSOCIATION

As mentioned previously, feelings of depersonalization and/or derealization are seen commonly in depression even though they aren't formally included in the DSM criteria for diagnosis. Dissociative disorders and depression are highly comorbid, and it is possible to have both at the same time. When dissociative symptoms are present, they tend to predict a worse response to conventional treatments. However, dissociative symptoms that occur *only* in the context of a depressive episode should not necessarily warrant a separate diagnosis of a dissociative disorder.

PUTTING IT ALL TOGETHER

If depression is an illness with many faces, you will need to be able to recognize each one to be able to arrive at the correct diagnosis. The differences in signs and symptoms between the various syndromes that can all present as "depression" can be slight, yet the prognosis and treatment response associated with each can be worlds apart. Because of this, a diagnosis of depression should be given cautiously and only after careful consideration of alternative explanations. Use the mnemonic **SIGECAPS** to remember the core signs and symptoms of depression at a single moment in time. The phrase "**two blue weeks**" can help you to recall the diagnostic timeframe. Major depressive disorder is notably a **non-reactive** and **episodic** disorder, with episodes typically lasting 6-12 months without treatment and 3-6 months with treatment. Treatment consists of therapy and/or antidepressant medications, either alone or in combination.

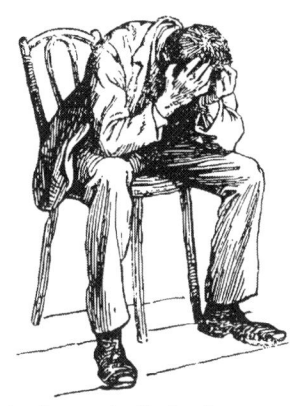

A variety of distinct clinical entities, including atypical, melancholic, postpartum, psychotic, catatonic, and seasonal depression, all should be considered various subtypes of depression but must still be recognized due to the implications they carry for treatment. In contrast, there are many misdiagnoses and missed diagnoses that may present with similar symptoms but ultimately should *not* be considered as a form of major depressive disorder. Use the **Reactive PLANETS** framework to guide your clinical judgment whenever you encounter someone presenting with problems related to mood. These questions can help you to spot when the patient's presentation differs significantly enough from "textbook" depression for consideration of an alternative explanation.

REVIEW QUESTIONS

1. A 23 y/o F comes to a psychiatrist's office for evaluation of performance anxiety. She is a graduate student in piano performance and has heard that propranolol can be a helpful medication for this. Wanting to be thorough, her psychiatrist conducts a psychiatric review of systems. To rule out depression, the psychiatrist asks about her mood, which she describes as "normal." What is the best next question to rule out a diagnosis of a current major depressive episode?
    A. "How is your sleep?"
    B. "Were you abused as a child?"
    C. "Do you enjoy things like you normally do?"
    D. "How is your appetite?"
    E. "Do you have thoughts that you would be better off dead?"

2. A 36 y/o M is seen for an initial psychiatric evaluation. He reports that since he was fired from his job 6 months ago, he has been spending all day in bed due to an inability to sleep at night and severe fatigue during the day. He has two children under the age of 3, and finances are becoming tight. He says, "I know I need to be looking for a job to take care of my wife and kids, but I just *can't*." His wife recently has taken to calling him "worthless," and he says, "After hearing it enough times, I find it hard to disagree." He is worried that his wife will divorce him and that his friends will leave him, saying, "Everyone just looks angry or disappointed at me all the time." When asked about his food intake, he reports that he has been eating only a bowl of cereal each day. He denies use of alcohol or any other substances. He has feelings of hopelessness but no thoughts of suicide. On exam, he moves and talks noticeably slower. Without treatment, how much longer would these symptoms be expected to continue?
    A. Less than 1 month
    B. Between 1 and 6 months
    C. Between 6 and 12 months
    D. More than 1 year
    E. These symptoms will likely continue until treatment is started

3. (Continued from previous question.) The psychiatrist recommends starting the antidepressant sertraline along with CBT. That night, the patient takes his first dose of the medication. Which of the following symptoms is likely to resolve first?
    A. Finding it hard to disagree when his wife calls him "worthless"
    B. Spending all day in bed
    C. Eating only a single bowl of cereal each day
    D. Moving and talking noticeably slower
    E. Feeling that everyone looks angry or disappointed at him
    F. All of these symptoms are equally likely to respond first

4. (Continued from previous question.) The patient returns to see his psychiatrist several times over the next few months. By the fourth month, he reports that his mood is entirely back to normal. The decision is made to continue both CBT and sertraline for another year. One year later, he is successfully tapered off of medication with no return of depressive symptoms. The patient says, "That was the worst few months of my life, but I'm glad it's over. I hope nothing like this ever happens again." What is this patient's risk of experiencing another episode in the future?
    A. 100% (it is certain that he will have another episode)
    B. Between 50 and 100% (it is more likely than not)
    C. 50% (it is equally likely and unlikely)
    D. Between 0 and 50% (it is less likely than not)
    E. 0% (it is completely unlikely)

5. A 47 y/o F who works as a business executive presents to a psychiatrist reporting worsening mood symptoms over the past four weeks, including depressed mood, irritability, feeling cold all of the time, difficulty sleeping, lack of energy, poor appetite, and constipation. She normally enjoys trail running but has not been able to exercise for more than a few minutes at a time for the past two months. Despite eating very little, she says that she has gained more than 15 lbs. over this same time period. She says, "My sister has suffered with depression as well and says that fluoxetine works really well for her. I was wondering if I could go on that too." Which of the following is the next best step?
    A. Prescribe fluoxetine
    B. Refer for CBT
    C. Prescribe fluoxetine along with a referral for CBT
    D. Order laboratory testing
    E. Reassure the patient that her symptoms are normal

6. A 72 y/o F sees her primary care doctor for the first time in over a decade. She says that her husband of over 50 years suffered a stroke two months ago that left him "basically like a vegetable." The patient now spends most of her time caring for her husband, which leaves her feeling exhausted and depressed. She thinks constantly about what it would mean if her husband were to die, although she also admits that "sometimes I think it would be good for him to go, which makes me feel like a horrible person." She denies feeling hopeless or having thoughts of suicide. Her appetite and concentration are intact. Which of the following is the next best step?
    A. Refer for therapy
    B. Reassure the patient that her symptoms are normal
    C. Discuss risks and benefits of medications
    D. Provide referrals to social resources such as caregiver support
    E. All of the above

1. **The best answer is C.** In addition to a sense of depressed mood, asking about anhedonia is a highly sensitive marker for ruling out depression. Someone who denies both a depressed mood and anhedonia is exceedingly unlikely to be currently in a major depressive episode. The other questions may be important to ask to get a better sense of the patient's current mental state (especially suicide, answer E) but are not as sensitive for ruling out a major depressive episode.

2. **The best answer is B.** This patient is likely suffering from major depressive disorder (although other causes cannot be entirely ruled out at this time). The average length of an untreated depressive episode is between 6 and 12 months. Given that he has already had symptoms for 6 months, it is most likely that his symptoms will last up to another 6 months (ruling out answers A, C, and D). As an episodic disorder, the symptoms of depression are unlikely to continue indefinitely even if treatment is not started (answer E).

3. **The best answer is E.** The core symptoms of depression, including feelings of worthlessness (answer A), fatigue (answer B), poor appetite (answer C), and psychomotor retardation (answer D) are all unlikely to respond to antidepressant treatment within a single day. In contrast, antidepressants have been shown to reduce negative affective biases even within the first day of treatment, suggesting that this patient's feelings that others look angry or disappointed will resolve first.

4. **The best answer is C.** Around 50% of people with a first episode of depression will have an isolated episode, while the other 50% will develop recurrent major depressive disorder.

5. **The best answer is D.** While the patient reports symptoms consistent with depression, there are also other symptoms that suggest a medical etiology, including cold intolerance, constipation, an inability to exercise, and significant weight gain in the absence of food intake. The most likely explanation is untreated hypothyroidism, which would need to be confirmed with laboratory testing. Treating her symptoms with antidepressants or CBT (answers A, B, and C) would not be appropriate until hypothyroidism has been ruled out. She should not be reassured that her symptoms are normal when there is evidence of likely medical pathology (answer E).

6. **The best answer is E.** This patient is likely suffering from adjustment disorder given the recent major life change and resulting symptoms of depression that do not meet criteria for a full disorder. Adjustment disorder is a "diagnosis of normalcy," so reassurance should be given (answer B). Treatment for adjustment disorder includes supportive therapy (answer A), with referrals to social support when indicated (answer D). It is reasonable to have a discussion about the risks and benefits of medications even if the risks likely outweigh the benefits in this case (answer C).

6 BIPOLAR DISORDER

Mania is an abnormal mental state characterized by excessive **elevations in mood and energy**. In many ways, mania can be thought of as the **opposite of depression**. While both are episodic and non-reactive mood states that result in dysfunction, with mania the culprit is too *high* of a mood rather than too low. With depression, people have trouble even getting out of bed in the morning; with mania, they haven't felt the need to sleep for days. With depression, people think of themselves as so worthless that they don't deserve to live; with mania, they see themselves as the greatest person to have ever walked the face of the earth. With depression, people are so fixated on hopeless thoughts that they can think about nothing else; with mania, they may have so many thoughts going on at once that others can't keep up. People in a manic state speak quickly, think quickly, move quickly, and act quickly. While it is definitely an oversimplification to say that mania is simply the opposite of depression, this rule of thumb will work most of the time.

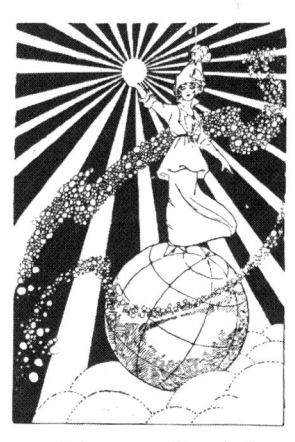

Mania is the hallmark state of **bipolar disorder**, a psychiatric condition that involves both manic highs and depressive lows. In contrast to depression, bipolar disorder is significantly more rare, with only 1% of the population experiencing a manic episode during their lifetimes. Despite this rarity, bipolar disorder can be a difficult and disabling condition due to its severity, chronicity, and onset early in life. Because of this, prompt diagnosis and treatment of bipolar disorder is essential. With this in mind, we will first learn about "textbook" mania so that you can easily recognize this syndrome when it occurs. From there, we will discuss how to diagnose bipolar disorder and its various subtypes before learning about all the misdiagnoses and missed diagnoses that frequently accompany a diagnosis of bipolar disorder.

SIGNS AND SYMPTOMS OF MANIA

While elevated (or irritable) mood and increased energy are the hallmarks of mania, they are frequently accompanied by other clinical features as well. The signs and symptoms of mania that can be seen at a particular moment in time are summarized in the mnemonic **DIG FAST**:

D is for Distractibility. People in a state of mania often describe their thoughts as "racing" and have trouble staying on any one subject. They may have difficulty finishing a conversation or even a single sentence, as their attention is quickly pulled in different directions.

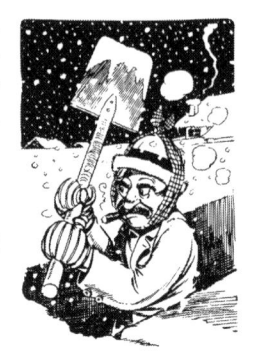

I is for Impulsivity. Impulsivity, indiscretion, and irresponsibility characterize most cases of mania, with people without having fully considered the possible consequences of their actions. Accordingly, people in a state of mania are known to engage in risky behaviors, including drug use, reckless driving, unprotected sex, and spending thousands of dollars at a time on frivolous or unnecessary purchases.

G is for Grandiosity. Thought content in mania often involves a degree of grandiosity that can border on the psychotic. People in a manic state can come to believe that they are a special or exalted figure (such as a king, president, prophet, messiah, leader, or CEO) and make plans accordingly. Often, these plans lack a clear connection to reality ("I'm going to save the world by selling microgreens right back to farmers!") and aren't very durable, changing drastically from one minute to the next.

F is for Flight of ideas. While grandiosity describes the thought *content* in mania, flight of ideas describes the thought *process*. In mania, ideas "fly" through the mind so rapidly that it is difficult for anyone to keep track of the conversation ("I have the most beautiful cat in the world. I need to pick up a dozen gallons of orange juice from the store. What is congress thinking? Is this microphone even on?"). Difficulty keeping up with a patient that you are interviewing is highly suggestive of a manic episode.

A is for Activity. More than any other sign or symptom, an increase in energy and activity (sometimes referred to as **psychomotor agitation**) is a key hallmark of mania. Specifically, the activity in a mania is **goal-directed** and involves working towards some kind of reward or outcome. The increased "busyness" of people in a manic state has been noted since the early days of psychiatric diagnosis, and it appears to be a **highly sensitive** marker of mania (analogous to anhedonia in depression). In fact, the DSM-5 changed its diagnostic criteria so that the absence of increased goal-directed activity rules out a diagnosis of mania. When this activity is blocked (such as by a well-meaning spouse or friend who is concerned about how erratically they are behaving), someone in a manic state is liable to become quite *irritable*, yelling or lashing out at the person who is getting in the way of their world-changing aspirations.

S is for Sleep. Decreased sleep is another key symptom of mania. In contrast to depression which is most often characterized by a perceived *inability* to sleep, sleep disturbance in mania is experienced as a *decreased need* for sleep (generally due to the increase in goal-directed activity). It's not uncommon for people in a manic state to keep going for days or even weeks on only a few hours of sleep per night.

T is for Talkativeness. Finally, people in a manic state are often hypersocial and exceptionally talkative, which is described on a mental status exam as *pressured speech*. They may walk around a room repeatedly shaking the hand of every single person present. Some studies have even found that specific aspects of speech, such as fluctuating pitch and high rate of speech, are highly sensitive markers of mania.

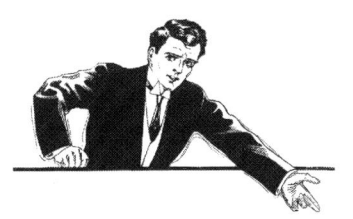

> A **manic episode** involves an **increase in psychomotor energy and activity** accompanied by other signs and symptoms.
>
> *Elevated* or *irritable* mood + **DIG FAST**:
> **D**istractibility
> **I**mpulsivity
> **G**randiosity
> **F**light of ideas
> **A**ctivity (increased)
> **S**leep (decreased need for)
> **T**alkativeness

Per DSM standards, having **at least 3** of these 7 symptoms for **1 week or more** qualifies the patient for a manic episode (think "**one fun week**" versus "two blue weeks" in depression). At least one of these symptoms must be increased goal-directed activity. Like with depression, the DSM criteria do not capture the entirety of mania, and some additional signs and symptoms can often be seen. Many people in a manic state describe a feeling of mental and physical robustness ("I've never felt better in my life!"). Friends and family will often say that there is a change in moral standards that accompanies mania (such as a trustworthy banker who suddenly begins to write bad checks). People in a state of mania are noted to be very quick witted and genuinely humorous. A variety of delusions are often seen in mania as well; they tend to be grandiose and even playful in nature and are much less stable and systematized than the complex belief systems seen in schizophrenia.

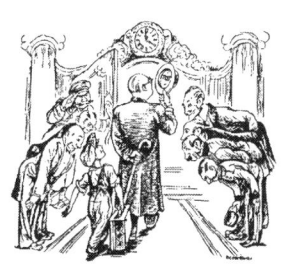

> Per the DSM-5, patients must have **3 out of 7** symptoms for a period of **1 week** or more to qualify for an **acute manic episode**.
>
> *The timeframe for mania is **one fun week**.*

BIPOLAR DISORDER ACROSS THE LIFESPAN

Some may wonder what exactly is pathological about mania. It makes sense that "too much sadness" would be a disorder; "too much happiness" less so. The key with mania lies not in the *content* of the disorder but in the *process*. Just like depression, in mania a patient's mood is notably **non-reactive**, rendering someone incapable of experiencing emotions *other* than happiness. To use an analogy, it's not a problem if a car can go fast as long as it is capable of slowing down when it needs to. However, if the car is always moving at top speed and cannot slow down for any reason, then this becomes a dangerous situation not only for the driver but also for everyone else on the road. To put it simply, mania is **life with the brakes off**.

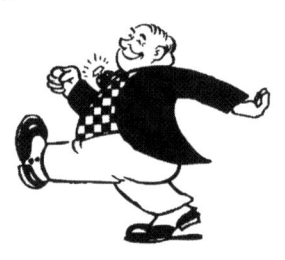

To push the car analogy even further, driving without brakes is likely to **end in a crash**. This is exactly what we see with mania, as manic episodes are frequently followed by depressive episodes. Indeed, the relationship between mania and depression is so well characterized that we don't refer to people as only having one or the other (there is no "manic disorder"). Instead, we refer to people who experience manic episodes as having **bipolar disorder** (formerly known as "manic-depressive disorder"). Let's learn more about what happens with bipolar disorder across the lifespan, including who gets it, what they can expect to happen, and what forms of treatment are effective.

EPIDEMIOLOGY
Bipolar disorder is a relatively **rare** syndrome and is found at a rate of around 1% of the population (compared to 20% for unipolar depression), making it liable to overdiagnosis rather than underdiagnosis. Compared to unipolar depression, bipolar disorder tends to begin earlier in life, with onset in **early adulthood** (the average age for a first episode is 21 years). **Men and women** are affected equally, although men with bipolar disorder have manic episodes more often than women with the disorder.

PROGNOSIS
Like major depressive disorder, functioning is often significantly impaired during a mood episode but **preserved between episodes**. However, people with bipolar disorder tend to spend more of their lives in a mood episode compared to people with unipolar depression. In fact, studies show that people with bipolar disorder spend as much as 50% of their lives in some form of abnormal mood episode, with this time divided between depression (35%), a state of milder manic symptoms known as **hypomania** (10%), and cycling between episodes (5%). It's worth pointing out that mania, while it is the hallmark state of bipolar disorder, is actually quite rare, making up only around 1% of the lives of patients with bipolar disorder! Despite this rarity, mania must be taken seriously given its potential for harm. Patients in a manic state often engage in high-risk behavior such as reckless driving or drug abuse which may cause both immediate and delayed harm to themselves, others, and their livelihood.

In contrast with depression, bipolar disorder is a **highly recurrent** syndrome. Whereas the risk of recurrence after a single depressive episode is only 50%, the risk of having another mood episode after even a single manic episode is over 90%! This has important implications, both for educating patients and families about the nature of their illness as well as deciding on how long to continue with treatments.

Bipolar disorder has an even higher **mortality rate** than unipolar depression, owing mostly to an elevated risk of suicide during depressive episodes. Up to 1% of all people with bipolar disorder will attempt suicide within a one-year span, a rate 60 times higher than the general population. In addition, people with bipolar disorder tend to use **highly lethal** means such as firearms more often, with one death for every 3 suicide attempts (versus one for every 25 attempts in the unipolar depression).

TREATMENT

Untreated, an episode of mania typically lasts around **3 to 6 months**, but with treatment a manic episode can be stopped within a matter of days or weeks. In contrast, an episode of bipolar depression can last up to a year without treatment, but this can be reduced down to 2 or 3 months with treatment. Hospitalization is often necessary for acute stabilization and ensuring safety. Given that mania is often experienced as an enjoyable state, patients may be hesitant or unwilling to consider treatment ("What do you mean you think I should be in the hospital? You must not know how amazing my life is!"). Involving family and friends to help encourage treatment can be highly effective. In cases where insight is severely impaired, a court order for involuntary treatment may be needed.

Treatment of bipolar disorder is significantly more complicated compared to unipolar depression. This is because there are not one but *two* distinct mood states, each of which requires separate treatment considerations. In addition, because of the highly recurrent nature of bipolar disorder, treatment must be focused not only on *treating* the current symptoms but also on *preventing* future episodes of both kinds. Unlike depression (where treatment generally includes either therapy, medications, or both), for bipolar disorder the standard of care is to almost always use **medications**, with psychotherapy alone not considered sufficient for treating bipolar disorder in the majority of cases.

Medications used to treat bipolar disorder are known as **mood stabilizers**. The oldest known mood stabilizer is **lithium**, which has been shown to be effective at both treating and preventing manic and depressive episodes (with a **moderate effect size** above 0.5). Interestingly, lithium appears to be most effective for patients who match "classic" mania symptomatology, with less effect noted with increasing atypical features (such as mixed features or rapid cycling, both discussed in the next section). Lithium is also one of the few medications that has been proven to **lower suicide risk**. In fact, patients taking lithium are over 80% less likely to commit suicide while taking lithium than when not.

Certain **anticonvulsant** medications can also act as mood stabilizers but tend to only treat one phase of the illness or another. For example, valproate and carbamazepine are helpful for treating mania (with a small effect size around 0.3) but do not treat depression, while lamotrigine prevents depression (with an effect size around 0.4) without having any antimanic effects. **Antipsychotics** are also effective at treating bipolar disorder with a **medium effect size** around 0.5. In fact, antipsychotics are actually *faster* at reversing a state of mania than conventional mood stabilizers and should be used as a first-line treatment in situations when urgent treatment is needed. While any antipsychotic can treat mania, only a select few can treat bipolar depression (specifically quetiapine, lurasidone, olanzapine, and cariprazine which each have effect sizes in the range of 0.2 to 0.5). While one might be tempted to use **antidepressants** like SRIs to treat bipolar depression, this would be a grave error, as conventional antidepressants are generally considered to be *ineffective* for treating bipolar depression and may actually be harmful by increasing the rate that a patient cycles between mania and depression. Finally, **electroconvulsive therapy** may be considered for patients who have not responded to less invasive treatments. ECT is effective at treating both mania and bipolar depression, with over two-thirds of patients responding well to this form of treatment.

Psychotherapy can be an incredibly helpful adjunct to medications for treating bipolar disorder. Patients receiving psychotherapy in addition to medications have less severe symptoms and a lower risk of relapse compared to people just on medications alone. In particular, CBT has been shown to have a small to medium effect size on a variety of outcomes including symptoms, treatment adherence, quality of life, and relapse prevention. Other types of therapy that also have evidence to support their use in bipolar disorder are psychoeducation, interpersonal and social rhythm therapy, family focused therapy, and integrated care management.

MECHANISMS OF BIPOLAR DISORDER

One theory suggests that bipolar disorder develops as a consequence of individual differences in processing reward-related stimuli. In particular, people with bipolar disorder tend to show an **emotional hypersensitivity to rewards**, even when not in a manic state. (In fact, reward hypersensitivity is highly predictive of developing mania even for someone who has never had a manic episode.) Someone with reward hypersensitivity shows greater behavioral, emotional, and cognitive responses to rewards, leading them to set overly ambitious goals (particularly in the area of fame, achievement, and finances) and regularly overestimate their chances of success.

To illustrate this, let's say that there is a card game that costs $20 to play. You get to flip over a single card from a full deck. If that card is an ace, you win $100; otherwise, you lose. With 4 aces in a deck of 52 cards, the odds of drawing an ace are less than 8%, making this an objectively bad deal. Someone with an average level of sensitivity to reward-related stimuli might find this interesting and decide to play. However, after losing a game or two, they would likely recognize that the odds are against them and stop playing. In contrast, someone with reward hypersensitivity might see this game and think, "If I play at least a few times, I'm sure to win! And if I win once, I can keep playing and eventually build up $1000. With this money, I can finally begin developing that smartphone app I've been thinking about." Even after losing five, ten, or twenty times, this person is likely to continue believing that they will make money off of this venture due to persistent *over*estimation of their likelihood of reward.

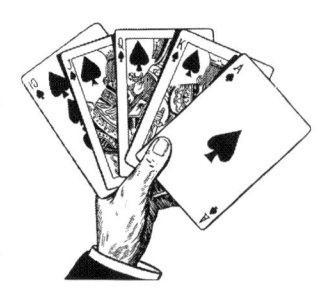

This hypersensitivity to reward-related stimuli explains why increased goal-directed activity is such a sensitive marker for mania, as many of the other symptoms of mania (including grandiosity, flight of ideas, decreased need for sleep, and talkativeness) are side effects of this core abnormality. Indeed, increased goal-directed activity is a clearly identified **prodrome** of mania and often precedes other manic symptoms by days or even weeks. This intense focus on goal-directed behavior also explains the tendency to engage in extremely pleasurable or rewarding activities such as sex, shopping, and drug use (known as **hyperhedonia**).

Reward hypersensitivity is correlated with overactivation of neural circuits in the **left lateral orbitofrontal cortex**, a region of the brain that governs the relationship between emotions and decisions. Interestingly, bipolar depression and unipolar depression are both associated with *decreased* reward sensitivity in the left lateral orbitofrontal cortex which in turn reduces motivation and the ability to gain pleasure from normally enjoyable activities. (Recall from the previous chapter that negative affective biases involve persistent underestimation of chances of success.) In this way, the left lateral orbitofrontal cortex may hold the key to both depression and mania, as it explains both the increased goal-directed activity seen in mania as well as the anhedonia that is the most sensitive marker of depression. You can remember the association of the **L**eft **l**ateral **o**rbito**f**rontal **c**ortex by thinking of it as the part of the brain that says "**L**et's **l**ive **o**utrageously! **F**orget **c**onsequences."

The **left lateral orbitofrontal cortex** is overactivated in **bipolar disorder**.

Left lateral orbitofrontal cortex = "Let's live outrageously! Forget consequences."

The involvement of reward circuits also explains what we see with treatment of mania. All of the reward-processing regions of the brain, such as the nucleus accumbens and the ventral tegmental area, involve **dopamine** signaling, so it should come as no surprise that dopamine-blocking medications have some of the strongest and most immediate effects for reversing mania.

On a clinical level, knowing about reward hypersensitivity and increased goal-directed activity serves a practical purpose by providing a highly *sensitive* marker for diagnosing mania. Asking about goal-directed activity rather than a period of "feeling happier than normal" can improve your diagnostic process and help you more accurately identify when mania is, and is not, part of the clinical picture. You can remember this by thinking that **M**ANIA involves **M**ore (goal-directed) **A**ctivity and is **N**ot **I**nherently **A**ffective in nature!

Mania involves **increased goal-directed activity** more often than elevated mood.

MANIA = More (goal-directed) Activity, Not Inherently Affective!

HOW TO DIAGNOSE BIPOLAR DISORDERS

Mania is **easy to diagnose in person**. As any experienced clinician can tell you, once you have seen someone in a state of "full blown" mania, you never forget it. This would make diagnosing bipolar disorder, of which mania is the hallmark state, a similarly simple task. However, in reality bipolar disorder is often quite challenging to diagnose. The challenge comes from the fact that, despite being the *defining* state of bipolar disorder, mania is not the most *frequent* state! So unless you happen to catch someone in the roughly 1% of their lifetime that they are manic, you must instead rely upon subjective reports from the patient or collateral. As with anything subjective, these reports are highly variable, as someone else's definition of "manic" or "bipolar" does not always align with clinical standards of diagnosis. Because of this, take any past reports of "manic" symptoms with a grain of salt, and ask patients and their families to **avoid using jargon** in favor of objective descriptions of behavior that are more likely to capture the increased goal-directed activity that defines mania.

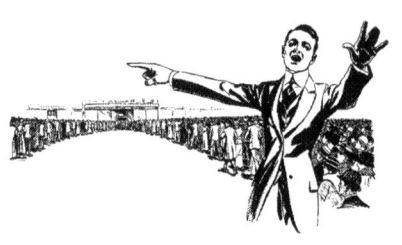

Thus far, we have limited our discussion to the state of "textbook" mania and its associated condition known as bipolar disorder. However, bipolar disorder is not a single entity, as there are a variety of different ways in which it can manifest that each carry important implications for prognosis and treatment as we'll talk about now.

BIPOLAR I DISORDER

Bipolar I disorder (also known as bipolar disorder type 1) is characterized by episodes of **mania** alternating with episodes of **depression**. The presence of even a *single* manic episode qualifies the patient for a diagnosis of bipolar I disorder regardless of how many depressive episodes they have had. (There may be rare cases of people who have only manic episodes with no episodes of depression, but the vast majority of people who have even a single manic episode will also have a major depressive episode at some point in their lifetime. Therefore, anyone presenting with mania but has no history of depressive episodes may simply have not experienced a depressive episode *yet*.)

Recognition of manic and depressive episodes is done on a clinical basis. You can use the mnemonic **DIG FAST** to remember the symptoms of mania. As discussed in Chapter 5, depressive episodes in bipolar depression are often indistinguishable from unipolar depression, so the **SIGECAPS** mnemonic applies here as well.

BIPOLAR II DISORDER

Just as mania is the hallmark state of bipolar I disorder, **hypomania** is the hallmark state of bipolar II disorder (also known as bipolar disorder type 2). Hypomania is a state of elevated mood and heightened activity that is similar to, but not quite as severe as, mania. People in a hypomanic state are productive, ecstatic, and indefatigable. These symptoms might even be noticeable by others, but by definition they are not impairing. Compared to mania, the timeframe for diagnosing an episode of hypomania is shorter, requiring only **4 days** of sustained hypomanic symptoms to be present.

Unlike mania, hypomania is not considered inherently pathological, and many people with bipolar II disorder describe being at their peak level of functioning during an episode of hypomania. So why is bipolar II disorder a problem? The problem with hypomania is that it is often, if not always, associated with episodes of severe depression, which is when most people with bipolar II will come to clinical attention. Indeed, despite the absence of "full-blown" manic episodes, bipolar II disorder should not be seen as a milder disorder compared to bipolar I. While their manic states are less pronounced, people with bipolar II disorder have **more frequent and severe depressive episodes**, leading to similar overall levels of functional impairment if not higher. In addition, people with bipolar II have higher rates of suicidal thoughts and attempts than either bipolar I disorder or unipolar depression. You can remember the predominant state of depression in bipolar II compared to I by thinking of the II as two lower-case l's in a row standing for lower lows (and lower highs as well). Treatment of bipolar II disorder has not been studied as extensively as bipolar I disorder, but it largely resembles bipolar I in that mood stabilizers and antipsychotics appear to be useful, while antidepressants are often ineffective or even harmful.

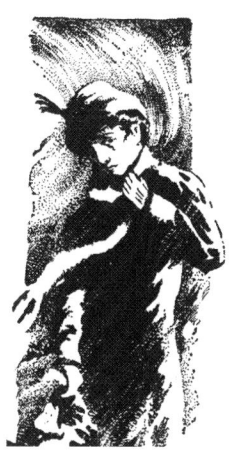

Bipolar II disorder is characterized by both **hypomanic and depressive episodes**, the latter of which are often **more frequent and severe** compared to bipolar I.

Bipolar II disorder involves lower lows than bipolar I disorder.

CYCLOTHYMIA

In theory, cyclothymia is a mild form of bipolar disorder where the patient has both **hypomanic** episodes (that do not meet criteria for a manic episode) and periods of **dysthymia** (that do not meet criteria for a major depressive episode). In a nutshell, it is bipolar disorder's version of dysthymia as it is a **more persistent but less severe** version of the prototypical disorder. As with dysthymia, patients must have the characteristic pattern of this disorder for **2 years** prior to receiving the diagnosis.

In actual clinical practice, a diagnosis of cyclothymia is incredibly **rare**. A large part of this is due to the fact that it is ultimately not that hard to meet criteria for a major depressive episode (in which case they would be diagnosed with bipolar II disorder). In addition, it is likely that someone who remains at a subsyndromal level of symptoms may never actually reach the point where they present for clinical attention. Evidence on treatment of cyclothymia is scarce, but existing data suggests that it should be treated similarly to bipolar II disorder.

To aid your understanding of the relationship between unipolar depression, dysthymia, bipolar I disorder, bipolar II disorder, and cyclothymia, schematic diagrams for these conditions are found on the next page. Take some time to study these and make sure you have a good understanding of them before moving on!

Major depressive disorder

Dysthymia

"Double depression"

Bipolar I disorder

Bipolar II disorder

Cyclothymia

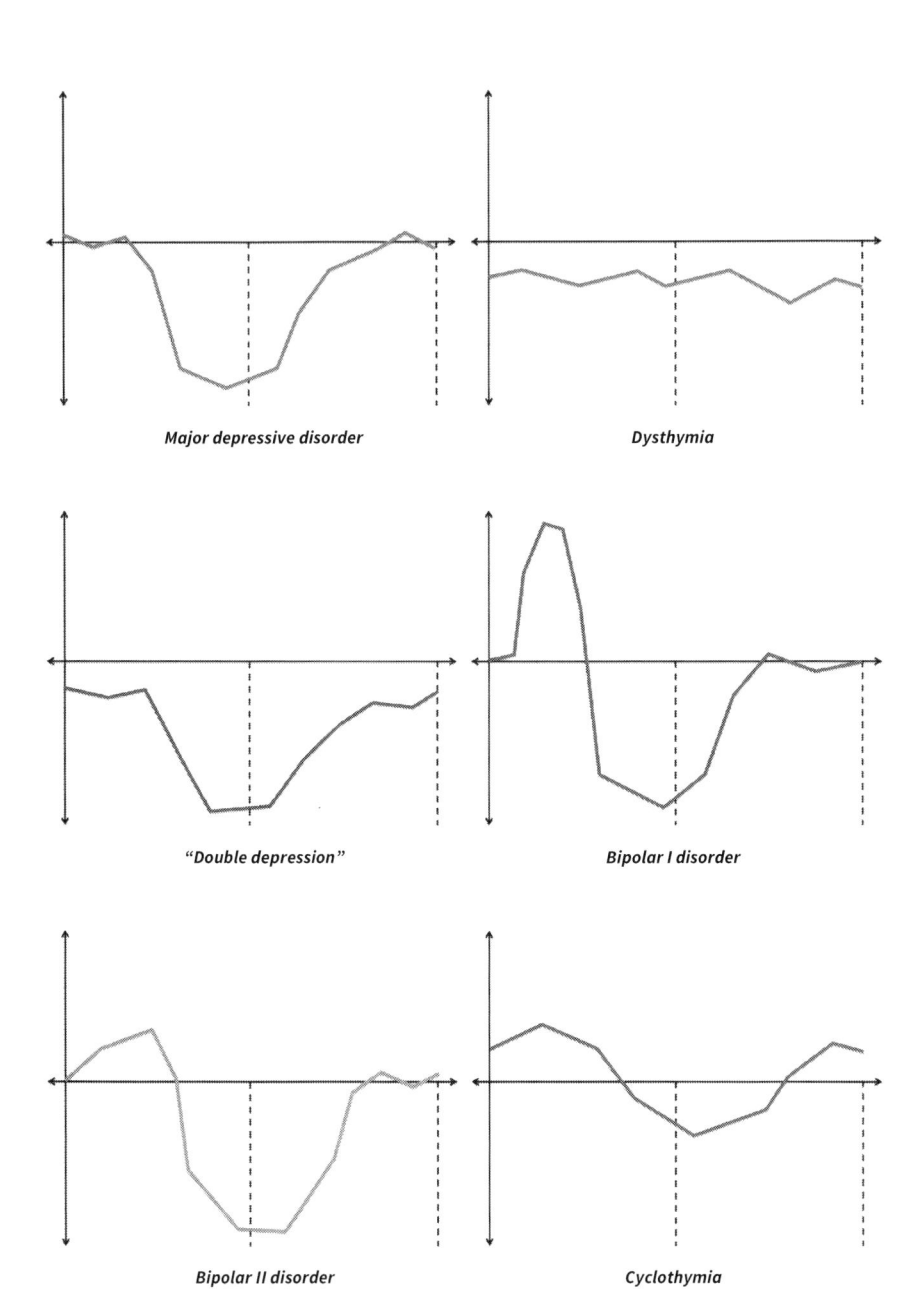

Schematic diagrams of various mood disorders. The x-axis shows time in years (with individual years marked by a dotted line), while the y-axis shows the patient's mood state (with euthymia set at the x-axis, manic symptoms above the x-axis, and depressive symptoms below the x-axis).

MIXED STATE
While classically depression and mania were considered to be mutually exclusive states, decades of clinical research have demonstrated that it is possible for someone to have **both depressive and manic symptoms at the same time**. This is known as a **mixed state** or mixed manic episode. While it may seem paradoxical to be both manic and depressed at the same time, recall that the predominant feature of **MANIA** is **M**ore **A**ctivity and that it is **N**ot **I**nherently **A**ffective. Therefore, a mixed state isn't someone who feels both happy and sad at the same time—rather, it is a combination of low mood (including thoughts of guilt, hopelessness, despair, and suicide) and increased goal-directed activity. The combination of these two states is often experienced by the patient as severe **irritability** or even outright **agitation**. The combination of profound depression and increased energy makes mixed states a **high-risk state**, with a higher chance of reckless activity or suicide compared to either depression or mania alone.

Diagnostically, mixed states are considered to be equivalent to manic episodes (so if a patient has even one mixed episode in their lifetime, they diagnosis would be bipolar I disorder). As with most bipolar disorders, treatment of a mixed state involves mood stabilizers and/or antipsychotics, with antidepressants to be avoided.

BIPOLAR DISORDER WITH PSYCHOTIC FEATURES
Just as depression can present with psychotic features, so too can bipolar disorder co-occur with symptoms resembling psychosis. This can occur during mania, depression, or a mixed state. The frequency of psychotic symptoms in bipolar disorder is even more pronounced than in unipolar depression, with more than half of all patients with bipolar disorder experiencing some degree of psychotic symptoms during their lifetime. Treatment often involves antipsychotics, either on their own or combined with a mood stabilizer like lithium or an anticonvulsant.

BIPOLAR DISORDER WITH CATATONIA
While catatonia can occur in a variety of severe psychiatric syndromes, in the modern day bipolar disorder is the **most common cause of catatonia** with more than half of all patients with catatonia meeting criteria for bipolar disorder. It can occur during mania, depression, or a mixed state. Catatonia is treated the same regardless of its etiology (using benzodiazepines or, if these are ineffective, ECT).

RAPID CYCLING BIPOLAR DISORDER
Given that most depressive episodes last 6 to 12 months and manic episodes last 3 to 6 months, the majority of people with bipolar disorder have less than one major mood episode per year. However, a small subset of patients with bipolar disorder are considered to have a **rapid cycling** variant defined as having **4 or more** distinct mood episodes within a 1 year period. Rapid cycling bipolar disorder has been associated with use of antidepressants, which may induce rapid cycling (another reason to avoid using them to treat bipolar disorder in most cases).

It's important to note that rapid cycling does *not* refer to alternations in mood episodes that happen over the course of minutes, hours, or days. As will be discussed in Chapter 15, changes in mood and affect occurring within a short period of time are more likely reflective of **affective instability** and should raise diagnostic suspicion for borderline personality disorder.

POSTPARTUM PSYCHOSIS

Postpartum psychosis is a state of disorganized restlessness and inability to distinguish reality from fantasy that occurs in the first few weeks after childbirth in around 0.1% of all deliveries. Postpartum psychosis is considered to be a **psychiatric emergency** due to the risks to both the baby and the mother, and immediate hospitalization is often required. Medication treatment generally involves mood stabilizers and antipsychotics. Despite the name postpartum "psychosis," this condition is much more strongly associated with **mania**, and women with bipolar I disorder have over a 35% chance of postpartum psychosis following delivery.

DIFFERENTIAL DIAGNOSIS OF BIPOLAR DISORDERS

Given how bipolar disorder is associated with both highs and lows, it is appropriate that the disorder itself would be affected by **both overdiagnosis and underdiagnosis**. The low base rate of the disorder in the general population ensures that overdiagnosis will remain a problem, while the rarity of mania means that underdiagnoses and misdiagnoses will continue. Nevertheless, studying the interface between bipolar disorder and many of the misdiagnoses and missed diagnoses that frequently accompany the disorder can provide clarity when approaching patients with mood symptoms. Just like with depression, you can use the mnemonic **Reactive PLANETS** (for **R**eactivity, **P**olarity, **L**ability, **A**ttributability, **N**ormality, **E**pisodicity, **T**reatment responsivity, and **S**everity) as a clinical framework for assessing any patient presenting with mood concerns.

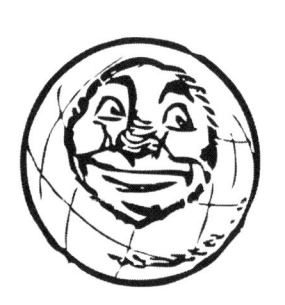

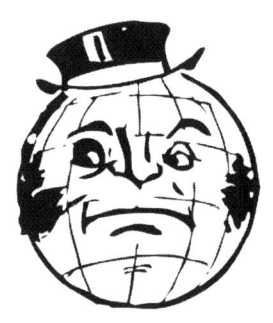

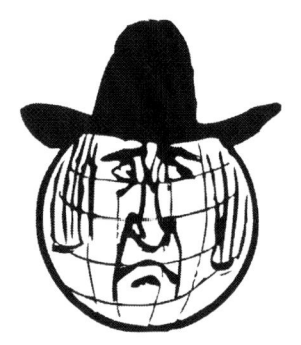

NORMALCY

There is nothing inherently pathological about having emotions or moods. However, anyone who experiences emotions strongly is at risk of being overdiagnosed as having bipolar disorder, largely due to misconceptions about what the term "bipolar" means. More than just being stigmatizing, overdiagnosis of bipolar disorder can lead to use of medications like mood stabilizers and antipsychotics that are often harmful in the long-term. The "cure" for overdiagnosis is for clinicians to understand the patterns and phenomenology of bipolar disorder well enough to consistently arrive at an accurate diagnosis. As with unipolar depression, the pathological mood states of bipolar disorder are distinguished from normal everyday swings of emotion in that they are **severe, sustained,** and **non-reactive** to external events. It is this non-reactivity that most reliably separates mood disorders from normalcy (remember that it's only a problem for a car to go fast if it is unable to brake when it needs to!).

UNIPOLAR DEPRESSION
Up to two-thirds of people with bipolar disorder are initially diagnosed as having unipolar depression. While there are certain aspects of a patient's history that can *suggest* a possible bipolar etiology (including an earlier onset in life, a family history of mania, pronounced psychomotor retardation, or the presence of melancholic, atypical, or psychotic features), you must keep in mind that until someone has declared themselves by having their first manic, hypomanic, or mixed episode, **it is impossible to accurately distinguish between unipolar and bipolar depression on the basis of clinical presentation alone**. Because of this, clinicians tend to fall into two camps: overcallers and undercallers. Overcallers cite the dangers of undertreatment and mistreatment (including a risk of inducing rapid cycling by using antidepressants) to justify a higher rate of false positives and more liberal use of mood stabilizers and antipsychotics. In contrast, undercallers are wary of the stigma of overdiagnosis as well as significant long-term toxicities associated with use of mood stabilizers and antipsychotics and prefer to err towards the side of false negatives. Given that there are risks associated with both undercalling and overcalling, try to use your best clinical judgment on the initial diagnosis while always being mindful that your diagnosis must remain flexible as new information (such as the emergence of new symptoms or a patient's response to treatment) comes to light.

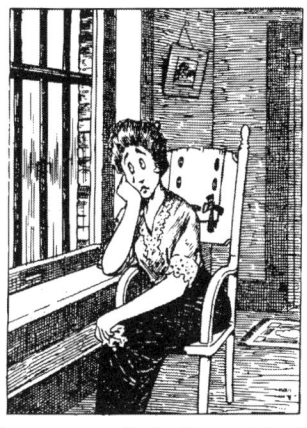

BORDERLINE PERSONALITY DISORDER
After unipolar depression, borderline personality disorder is the disorder that is most commonly confused with bipolar disorder, with as many as half of all patients with borderline personality disorder receiving a misdiagnosis of bipolar disorder at some time in their lives. This is especially common when the diagnosis is based on reported history rather personally witnessed symptoms. The reasons for this confusion stem from the fact that, at least on a superficial level, many features are shared between the two disorders. Both are characterized by extreme swings of emotion as well as a tendency towards recklessness and impulsivity. In addition, irritability can be a sign of a manic episode as easily as it can be a manifestation of the chronic anger seen in cases of borderline personality disorder.

Making the distinction between bipolar disorder and borderline personality disorder is highly dependent upon the **timing** of specific symptoms. A core feature of borderline personality disorder is affective instability resulting in rapid changes in emotional expression. However, these swings occur within the span of **seconds or minutes** in contrast to the mood episodes lasting weeks or months that are characteristic of bipolar disorder. (Even rapid cycling bipolar disorder is characterized by 4 mood shifts per year, suggesting an average of 3 months between transitions.) In addition, the affective instability and impulsivity found in borderline personality disorder tend to be **chronic** whereas the recklessness seen in manic episodes only exists as long as the mood state is present. Additional features of borderline personality disorder, including non-suicidal self-harm, dissociative experiences, and chronic feelings of emptiness, may help to further the distinction. Don't use treatment response to distinguish between bipolar disorder and borderline personality disorder, as antidepressants are ineffective in both conditions while mood stabilizers and antipsychotics can each provide some benefit in either disorder.

OTHER PERSONALITY DISORDERS
Certain symptoms of mania can easily be mistaken for evidence of specific personality disorders. In particular, grandiosity can be confused for **narcissistic** personality disorder, excessive emotionality can be confused for **histrionic** personality disorder, and irritability can be confused for **antisocial** personality disorder. As with borderline personality disorder, be careful not to confuse these state-dependent characteristics (which will come and go with the mood episode) with the **chronic and enduring** traits found in personality disorders.

SUBSTANCE-INDUCED MANIA
The behavioral effects of specific drugs can often resemble mania either during intoxication or withdrawal. For example, someone taking a stimulant like cocaine or methamphetamine can develop high levels of energy, activity, and sleeplessness that can closely mimic a manic episode, while withdrawal from depressants like alcohol or benzodiazepines can induce a state of anxiety, restlessness, and insomnia that can similarly be mistaken for a manic or mixed episode. Pay attention to the **timing** and **attributability** of symptom onset to differentiate bipolar mania from substance-induced mania. In addition, be mindful that even some prescription drugs (such as steroids) can induce a prolonged state of mania.

ANTIDEPRESSANT-INDUCED MANIA
While it is technically a form of substance-induced mania, antidepressant-induced mania deserves special mention. For a long time, it was believed that antidepressants, when given to someone with bipolar disorder, could "switch" them into mania. The evidence on this is **inconclusive**, with some studies showing a link between antidepressants and mania and others showing no relationship. The current standard is to avoid diagnosing bipolar disorder if the manic symptoms only developed in the context of antidepressant use and go away soon after the medication is stopped. Only in cases where mania persists for an extended period of time following antidepressant discontinuation should a primary diagnosis of bipolar disorder be considered.

ADDICTION
Bipolar disorder and addiction are frequently comorbid, with up to 70% of patients with bipolar disorder meeting criteria for a substance use disorder at some time in their lives. It is likely that the two disorders feed into each other, with the recklessness and impulsivity of mania predisposing towards use of addictive substances which can

later bloom into an addiction. Conversely, continued overuse of drugs can exacerbate the depression and irritability found in bipolar disorder, leading to a vicious cycle.

Because of this overlap, overdiagnosis and underdiagnosis of bipolar disorder in substance abusing populations are equally problematic. As many as two-thirds of people who have been diagnosed as having both bipolar disorder and a substance use disorder do not meet criteria for bipolar disorder when structured interviews are used, suggesting high rates of overdiagnosis in this population. Yet clinicians need to be mindful to screen for addiction in patients with bipolar disorder to avoid missing an important part of the picture. In nearly all cases, conducting a careful substance use history and requesting a urine toxicology screen can be helpful. Finally, be sure to carefully assess the **timing** and **attributability** of the relationship between mood symptoms and substance use (for example, if irritability and sleeplessness only appear when someone is withdrawing from alcohol).

MANIA DUE TO A MEDICAL CONDITION
A state resembling mania can be induced by a variety of medical conditions, including hyperthyroidism, Cushing's disease, and various intracranial conditions including tumors and infections. Consider the possibility of mania due to another medical condition in patients who do not have a personal or family history of bipolar disorder (especially if they are older and have not yet had a mania episode), where there is anything atypical about the clinical presentation, or when mania presents with unexplained neurologic or physical findings such as vital sign abnormalities.

ANXIETY DISORDERS
Anxiety is common in bipolar disorder but is generally more of a missed diagnosis than a misdiagnosis. However, in some cases the racing thoughts, irritability, and difficulty concentrating found in anxiety disorders can be mistaken for similar symptoms in bipolar disorder. The **episodicity** of bipolar disorder should help to distinguish these symptoms from the more chronic course associated with anxiety disorders.

ATTENTION DEFICIT HYPERACTIVITY DISORDER
Certain symptoms of ADHD, including racing thoughts and impulsivity, can resemble mania. However, in ADHD these symptoms will have been **continually present since childhood**, whereas in mania they will come and go in an episodic pattern.

SCHIZOPHRENIA AND SCHIZOAFFECTIVE DISORDER
The relationships between mood and psychotic disorders will be explored more fully in the next chapter. For now, just know that bipolar disorder can present with psychotic symptoms, so the presence of psychosis does not necessarily rule *in* schizophrenia, nor does it rule *out* bipolar disorder.

THE "MANIAS"
Several mental disorders in the DSM have the word "mania" in their name, including **kleptomania** (excessive stealing), **pyromania** (fire starting), and **trichotillomania** (compulsive hair pulling). Don't let the suffix confuse you: these conditions are not in any way related to bipolar disorder.

PUTTING IT ALL TOGETHER

In many ways, bipolar disorder is a paradox. It is characterized by opposite extremes of mood that can somehow happen at the same time. Its hallmark state is exceptionally easy to recognize clinically, yet diagnosing the disorder as a whole is incredibly challenging. It is somehow both overdiagnosed and underdiagnosed as well as both overtreated and undertreated, leading to pathologizing of normal emotions, perpetuation of stigma, and use of ineffective and harmful treatments.

Appropriate use of the bipolar diagnosis requires a firm understanding of the phenomenology of the disorder as well as its epidemiologic, prognostic, mechanistic, and treatment considerations. Use the **DIG FAST** and **SIGECAPS** mnemonics to recognize the specific signs and symptoms of bipolar mania and bipolar depression, respectively, while remembering that **MANIA** is associated with **M**ore **A**ctivity and is **N**ot **I**nherently **A**ffective. Consider that it is not always possible to differentiate bipolar depression from unipolar depression until someone has had their first manic or hypomanic episode. However, making this distinction is crucial as the prognosis differs significantly between the two conditions (with a much higher rate of recurrence after a first episode in bipolar disorder) and requires different treatment considerations. Both mania and depression are high-risk states and can often require immediate and intensive treatment. Treatment for bipolar disorder involves both **medications and therapy**, with mood stabilizers and antipsychotics being used for treatment and prevention of both mania and depression (although the specific medications used within these classes will differ depending on the mood state). Finally, use the **Reactive PLANETS** mnemonic to evaluate mood states in a structured way that allows for identification of potential misdiagnoses and missed diagnoses.

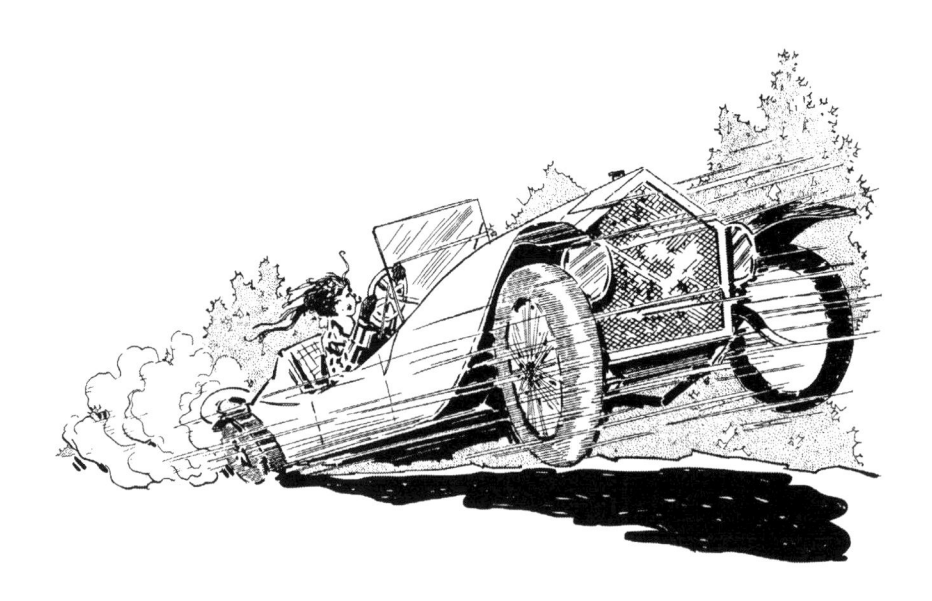

REVIEW QUESTIONS

1. A 22 y/o F is brought into the emergency department by police after she was involved in a physical altercation at a local supermarket. According to the police report, the patient hit another person in the head with a nutcracker while dancing in the aisles. Upon entering the room, the psychiatrist on-call sees that she is only wearing her underwear. She stands up and says, "You need to let me go! I have to get back to the store so that I can make my 'world's greatest pecan pie'!" She proceeds to detail her plans to bake the "the biggest, baddest pecan pie that man has ever seen" so she can qualify for a baking show competition on television. She speaks of these plans very rapidly but is easily distracted, saying, "Oh you're a doctor? Where did you go to school? Did you go to Harvard? I've been to Harvard, I taught there before. I taught them everything they know!" Her husband arrives who reports that the patient has no prior psychiatric history and takes no medications outside of oral contraceptives. While the psychiatrist is talking with her husband, she begins banging on the door and yelling, "That's the jerk who threw away my pie! I'm gonna kill him!" What is the most appropriate next step?
   - A. Start lithium
   - B. Start an anticonvulsant mood stabilizer
   - C. Start an antipsychotic
   - D. Start an antidepressant
   - E. Defer medications until the results of a urine drug screen are available

2. (Continued from previous question.) The patient is admitted to the hospital for further management. She consistently denies that there is any problem and declines any medication that is offered to her. The urine drug screen returns negative. For the first two days of hospitalization, the patient is seen walking around the unit shaking hands with other patients and inviting them on trips with her to Bermuda and Hawaii. While talking with one of the male nurses, she attempts to reach her hand down his pants and is escorted back to her room. During a family meeting that day, her husband breaks down in tears and says, "This isn't her. I don't know what happened to my wife. Is she going to be like this forever?" What is the most appropriate response?
   - A. "Yes, this is likely a permanent change in her personality."
   - B. "No, but it is very likely that she will have times like this in the future."
   - C. "No, but there is a 50-50 chance that she will have times like this in the future."
   - D. "No, and it is unlikely that she will have times like this in the future."
   - E. "No, this is likely the first and last time this will ever happen."

3. A 20 y/o M comes to a psychiatric clinic for an initial evaluation. He reports that over the past 5 weeks he has lost all interest in interacting with other people, saying that socializing "tires me out and I can't afford that right now." He has not been participating in soccer intramurals despite being team captain. His mood is "terrible," and he admits that he has been thinking of ways to kill himself over the past several days. When asked about his appetite, he responds by saying, "It is impossible for me to eat when I have spiders living in my throat." He denies that this is a metaphor and voices his belief that spiders have taken up residence in his vocal cords. He believes that the spiders sometimes "vibrate my vocal cords" to communicate with him while he is falling asleep at night. Further history taking reveals that his father and paternal grandmother have both been hospitalized for manic episodes. He has no personal psychiatric history and has never taken medications. Physical examination reveals no abnormalities other than slowed movements and speech. He lays motionless on the couch, avoids eye contact, and does not engage in spontaneous movement for most of the interview as seen in the image below:

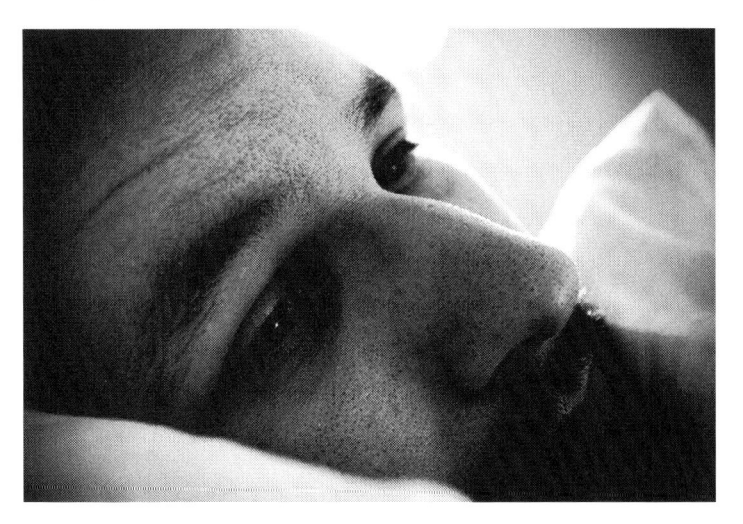

Which of the following features argues for a higher likelihood of bipolar rather than unipolar depression?
A. Onset during adolescence
B. Presence of psychomotor retardation
C. Presence of psychotic features
D. Family history of mania
E. All of the above predict a higher chance of bipolar depression
F. None of the above predict a higher chance of bipolar depression

4. (Continued from previous question.) Which of the following is the most appropriate statement to make at this time?
   A. "You have bipolar disorder. We should start a mood stabilizer."
   B. "You probably have bipolar disorder. We should avoid antidepressants."
   C. "It's possible you have bipolar disorder. Let's monitor closely and not prescribe any medications."
   D. "It's unlikely but not impossible that you have bipolar disorder. Let's start an antidepressant with an antipsychotic."
   E. None of the above

5. A 45 y/o F comes into the psychiatrist's office. She is being considered for promotion to an executive office at her company on Wall Street and has been asked to undergo a comprehensive mental health evaluation. On interview, she denies feeling depressed either now or in the past. She does endorse having times in her life when she is able to function at a higher level than usual, "writing reports and filling out spreadsheets like a madwoman." These episodes usually last for several weeks at a time. During these episodes, she often is able to function on "only a few hours, maybe 3 or 4 hours" of sleep per night but does not feel significantly fatigued during the day. She denies use of caffeine, nicotine, alcohol, or other substances. She denies auditory hallucinations, delusions, or paranoia other than saying "sometimes I think other people at work are jealous of me and would want nothing more than to see me dead, but that's Wall Street for you" with a laugh. She is married to her husband of 3 years and has a 5-year-old son at home. She has never taken psychiatric medications and is not aware of any medication allergies. What is the most likely diagnosis?
   A. Bipolar I disorder
   B. Bipolar II disorder
   C. Schizoaffective disorder, bipolar type
   D. Schizoaffective disorder, depressive type
   E. Major depressive disorder
   F. None of the above

1. **The best answer is C.** This patient is likely suffering from a manic episode, although due to a lack of history other causes like a substance-induced mood disorder cannot be ruled out. However, given the patient's high level of agitation and risk of violent behavior, it is appropriate to start treatment before diagnostic clarity is achieved (answer E). Out of the available options, antipsychotic medications are the most effective at rapidly reducing a state of mania and should be started first. Lithium or an anticonvulsant mood stabilizer can be started concurrently but should not be the only medication prescribed in an emergent situation like this (answers A and B). An antidepressant runs the risk of exacerbating manic symptoms or inducing rapid cycling and should be absolutely avoided in this situation (answer D).

2. **The best answer is B.** Mania is associated with a high chance (over 90%) of future mood episodes, even with treatment. For this reason, patients and their families should be counseled on the risk of recurrence and be advised on how to prepare for them, such as coming up with a safety plan and knowing who to contact in case of an emergency. Mania is an episodic condition, not a permanent change to someone's personality (answer A).

3. **The best answer is E.** All of these clinical features predict a higher chance of bipolar depression compared to unipolar depression.

4. **The best answer is D.** Despite a high number of risk factors that increase the likelihood of bipolar depression in this patient, first episodes of depression should be considered to be unipolar in origin until proven otherwise. Therefore, it is not appropriate to tell the patient that he has bipolar disorder with any degree of certainty (answers A and B). Considering that bipolar depression is significantly less common than unipolar depression, it is reasonable to say that it is unlikely that he has bipolar depression, in which case he would likely qualify for a diagnosis of major depressive disorder with psychotic features which is treated with a combination of an antidepressant and an antipsychotic (answer D). Given the severity of his current symptoms, it would not be appropriate to monitor without recommending treatment (answer C).

5. **The best answer is F.** This patient shows no evidence of distress or dysfunction in her life, precluding a diagnosis of a mental disorder. It is questionable whether she experiences hypomanic episodes, as her self-reported description of her behavior is at least consistent with hypomania. However, as there is no evidence of impairment from these episodes and no associated depressive episodes, they would not be diagnosed as being a disorder. It is possible that, in the future, she will develop depressive episodes, at which time a diagnosis of bipolar II disorder could be considered. Until that time, however, there is no justification for any psychiatric diagnosis for this patient (answers A through E).

7 SCHIZOPHRENIA

Psychosis is an abnormal mental state where someone is **unable to distinguish reality from falsehoods**. While the nature of reality can be debated, in a clinical sense it refers to a *shared* or *consensus* reality. For example, if 100 people are sitting silently in a room and only one of them says that they can hear people talking, then it is reasonable to suggest that that person does not share the same reality as the other 99 people in the room. The word "psychosis" is a broad term that can encompass many possible symptoms and causes. You could say that someone with delirium is psychotic, and under this broad definition you would be right. Within the field of psychiatry, however, the word often has a more specific meaning, referring to a state of **primary psychosis** that is not attributable to any other medical or psychiatric condition (compared to delirium, which would be a *secondary* psychosis).

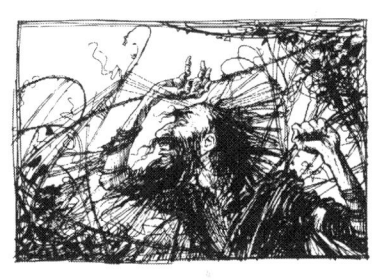

Primary psychosis is the hallmark state of **thoughts disorders** like **schizophrenia**. In this chapter, we'll review the phenomenology of schizophrenia including the specific forms of hallucinations, delusions, thought disorganization, and negative symptoms that are seen. From there, we will learn about the progression of schizophrenia across the lifespan as well as the possible mechanisms underlying the disorder. Finally, we will cast our eye on the misdiagnoses and missed diagnoses that must be considered when evaluating anyone with psychotic symptoms. Schizophrenia is among the most challenging mental disorders to diagnose, as many other conditions can mimic primary psychosis. Despite this challenge, understanding schizophrenia is crucial, as people with this disorder are often among the most vulnerable in all of medicine. By taking the time to understand the phenomenology of schizophrenia on a deeper level, you can make sure that the diagnostic "label" is only applied when it would be both accurate and beneficial to the patient.

SIGNS AND SYMPTOMS OF SCHIZOPHRENIA

Symptoms in schizophrenia are classically split into two groups: **positive symptoms** and **negative symptoms**. Positive symptoms are those that are **P**resent in schizophrenia but *absent* for most people, whereas **N**egative symptoms are those that are **N**ot present in schizophrenia but *are* for most people. When most people think of schizophrenia, it is the dramatic positive symptoms such as **hallucinations** and **delusions** that come most rapidly to mind. However, the dysfunction caused by schizophrenia owes as much to the *presence* of these positive symptoms as it does to the *absence* of normal abilities caused by negative symptoms.

You can use the phrase **HD BS Network** to remember the 5 core signs and symptoms of schizophrenia: **H**allucinations, **D**elusions, disorganized **B**ehavior, disorganized **S**peech, and **N**egative symptoms. (This phrase should be easy to link to schizophrenia, as auditory hallucinations are common in this disorder. These voices are incredibly clear and sound like real voices to the patient so they are very high definition or HD. However, they are also not real, so it's as if the patient is hearing radio waves spreading a network of fake BS.) Per DSM-5 criteria, **2 or more** of these symptoms must be present for a period of at least **6 months** to qualify for the diagnosis. You can remember this by thinking of it as **2-4-6-ophrenia**: you need **2** symptoms **for** at least **6** months.

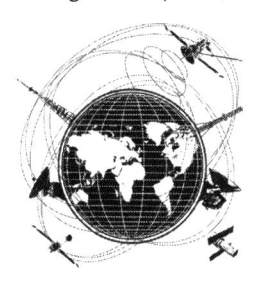

> The phenomenology of **schizophrenia** includes **hallucinations**, **delusions**, **disorganized behavior**, **disorganized speech**, and **negative symptoms**.
>
> **HD BS** *Network:*
> *H*allucinations
> *D*elusions
> *B*ehavior (disorganized)
> *S*peech (disorganized)
> *N*egative symptoms
>
> *2-4-6-ophrenia: you need* **2** *symptoms* **for** *at least* **6** *months.*

HALLUCINATIONS
In contrast to the **vis**ual hallucinations found in delirium (which are typically **vis**ceral in origin), the hallucinations associated with schizophrenia are primarily **auditory** (or **odd**-itory) in nature, reflecting the **odd**-ness of psychosis.

> **Hallucinations** related to **schizophrenia** are generally **auditory**, not visual.
>
> **Odd**-*itory hallucinations are linked to* **odd** *behavior, speech, and thoughts.*

People with schizophrenia "hear voices" in a **characteristic and recognizable way**. The voices typically take the form of a **running commentary** between several speakers (often a mix of **male and female voices**) who talk about the person in a **critical** or demeaning way. The voices are **intermittent** (rather than continuous) and are clearly perceived as coming from **outside their head** (as opposed to "voices *inside* my head"). These voices are not vague or nebulous; instead, people with schizophrenia hear what the voices say in a **clear** and vivid fashion. People with auditory hallucinations related to schizophrenia often experience them as **distressing** and will generally try to find specific **reducing behaviors** (such as listening to the radio, watching TV, or talking with others) that can decrease the intensity of the voices. People will also generally try to **hide** or minimize the fact that they experience auditory hallucinations and will generally not eagerly disclose the fact that they hear voices. People experiencing auditory hallucinations related to primary psychosis may be seen verbally or physically reacting to what the voices are telling them ("Shut up! You don't know what you're talking about!"), which is described on the mental status exam as **responding to internal stimuli**. Auditory hallucinations also almost never occur in the absence of other positive symptoms, with delusions being reported concurrently with auditory hallucinations nearly 90% of the time.

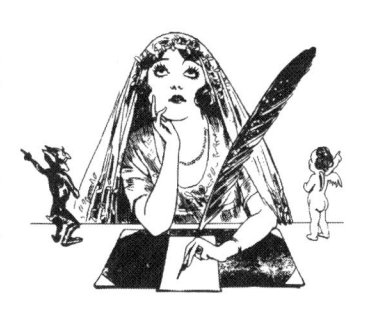

DELUSIONS

Delusions are the **most specific symptom** seen in schizophrenia. A delusion is defined as a **fixed false belief**: *fixed* because they are unchangeable even in the face of clear evidence to the contrary and *false* because the they are clearly incorrect or incompatible with reality. Delusions must also be clearly **outside the norms** of one's cultural or religious background. For example, followers of certain religions have beliefs that would be considered fixed and false by people who are not in that religion (such as a belief in reincarnation in Hinduism or the virgin birth in Christianity). However, these would not be considered delusions as they are shared by others in the same belief system.

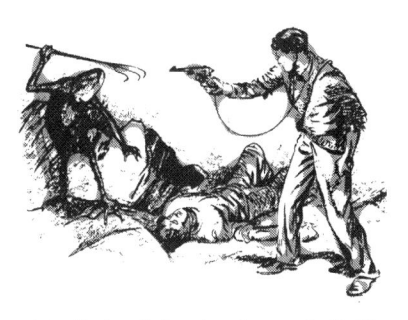

Delusions in schizophrenia often take specific and recognizable forms. In particular, schizophrenic delusions tend to be **paranoid** and **persecutory** in nature, such as someone believing that they are the target of a complex conspiracy ("Someone's watching me, I just know it. They mean to do me harm!"). Delusions can be classified as **bizarre** (beliefs that are so outlandish as to be strictly impossible, such as someone who believes that aliens from a nearby galaxy have sent detached eyeballs to watch their every move) or **non-bizarre** (beliefs that are highly unlikely to be true but are *technically* possible, such as someone who believes that the government has hacked their internet router and is broadcasting their internet history to their neighbors). These delusions often involve **ideas of reference** where random or everyday events are connected in a way that has some great or cosmic significance. For example, someone watching the news on television may believe that the anchors are blinking in Morse code in order to communicate a special coded message that only they can understand.

In addition to ideas of reference, delusions in schizophrenia also frequently involve beliefs that one's thoughts or actions are being manipulated by outside forces. These delusions include **thought broadcasting** (the idea that one's thoughts are being transmitted externally to be heard by others), **thought withdrawal** (the idea that one's thoughts are being taken out of their mind), **thought insertion** (the idea that thoughts are being inserted into one's head by others), and **delusions of control** (the idea that one's movements are not their own and that they are being controlled by someone else like a puppet). People with schizophrenia appear to have specific neural deficits that make it so that they have trouble recognizing that their own thoughts and actions are actually self-generated. As one notable example, many people with schizophrenia are able to tickle themselves. For most people, trying to tickle yourself is futile because your brain generates a signal that the sensory input it is receiving has originated from your own body. However, in schizophrenia this "self signal" is gone, leading to difficulties in recognizing when thoughts and behaviors are internally generated. This likely accounts for the variety of delusions people with schizophrenia experience that all involve a sensation of outside forces being in control. The ability to self-tickle also correlates with unusual perceptual experiences like hallucinations, suggesting a shared mechanism.

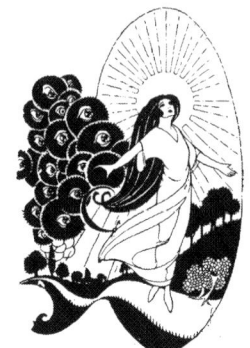

DISORGANIZATION
The final category of positive symptoms is **thought disorganization**. People with schizophrenia often have profound difficulty with maintaining a clear and coherent train of thought. While thought disorganization can be trickier to evaluate than either hallucinations or delusions (as it relies on thought *process* more than thought *content*), it is even more important for diagnosing schizophrenia as it is quite **specific** for primary psychosis (compared to auditory hallucinations and delusions which can also be found in other conditions such as delirium, depression, or mania).

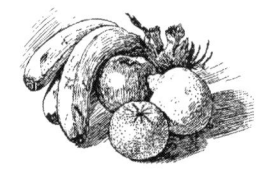

Because psychiatrists cannot read minds, thought disorganization must be inferred from disorganization in more objectively observed domains such as **speech** and **behavior**. Speech and behavior both follow rules that are so ingrained that most people don't even realize them until they are broken. For example, during a conversation most people go from one concept to another based on a **linear** train of thought involving logical associations between words and ideas. If you were to ask someone in a non-psychotic state what the relationship is between an orange and a banana, the answer will likely be, "They're both fruit." However, if you were to ask the same question to someone in a state of primary psychosis, the answer is almost *never* going to be, "They're both fruit." (They may instead say something like, "A banana is a cog and an orange is its place in the machine just like you and me!") In schizophrenia, the normal connections from one thought to the next are replaced by a **loosening of associations** in which thoughts are connected by less meaningful connections.

Disorganized speech is often quite noticeable when it is present. For example, someone in a psychotic state who is asked a question may answer based on the *sounds* of words rather than their actual meanings, known as a **clang association** ("What do you do at the beach?" "Beach? That's no leech, preach, let me teach."). In this case, the important part of the word (its meaning) is replaced by an irrelevant characteristic (its phonetic sound). Other ways in which thought disorganization can become apparent is when people simply make up words (*neologisms*), repeat what the other person said without any understanding of its meaning (*echolalia*), or say the same word repeatedly without any purpose (*perseveration*). In severe cases, thought disorganization can go so far that the words coming out of their mouth are complete non-sense (often called a *word salad*). In all of these cases, it is as if the train of thought has been hijacked and forced to make irrelevant connections.

In addition to speech, thought disorganization can manifest in **disorganized behavior**. Whereas most people behave in a way that is dictated by clear motivations, disorganized behavior in schizophrenia is notable for its **purposelessness**. People with schizophrenia may act bizarrely or unpredictably such as walking around endlessly from one corner of the room to the next, repeating the same motions over and over (*motor perseveration*), or copying a movement that someone else just did (*echopraxia*). The behavioral symptoms of **catatonia**, including negativism, catalepsy, and waxy flexibility, can also be seen in severe cases of schizophrenia.

NEGATIVE SYMPTOMS
In contrast to **P**ositive symptoms (things that are **P**resent but shouldn't be), **N**egative symptoms are things that *should* be present but are **N**ot, including deficits in the emotional, social, and cognitive skills that most people have. You can remember the main negative symptoms in schizophrenia by thinking of them as the **5 A's**:

A is for Affect. People in a state of primary psychosis often have a **blunted affect** as if their facial expressions are being constrained by an unseen force. Because of this, their affect is often completely incongruent to what they say they are saying. For example, you might think that someone who believed that their every thought was being transmitted to a secret society intent on destroying the world would appear quite distraught when talking about this. However, due to the blunting of affect seen in schizophrenia, they may instead talk about it passively without any change in their facial expressions. Affective deficits often begin prior to the onset of any positive symptoms of psychosis, and family members will often describe that a person looks "off" even months before an official diagnosis. Affective deficits also tend to be progressive, and older people with long-standing psychotic conditions may develop a completely flat affect with zero trace of emotional expression.

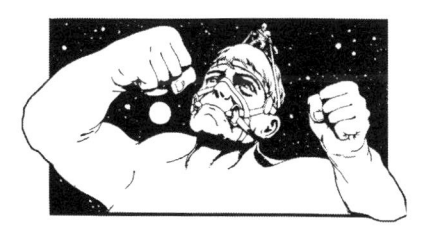

A is for Ambivalence. Another negative symptom in schizophrenia is **ambivalence** or extreme difficulty in making decisions. A certain amount of uncertainty in decision making is completely normal. However, in schizophrenia this ambivalence is severe and extends into many areas of life, preventing most meaningful or goal-directed behavior. Even when asked about things that should be relatively uncontroversial ("It's particularly cold tonight. Do you want a blanket?"), someone with schizophrenia-related ambivalence may still have trouble deciding ("Hmm... I'm not sure.").

A is for Alogia. While speech in schizophrenia can often be disorganized (which is a positive symptom), in many cases speech can be impaired, reduced, or even entirely absent as well, which is known as **alogia**. Alogia can range from small reductions in the amount of speech to being completely mute for months or years on end.

A is for Anhedonia. People with schizophrenia often experience **anhedonia** which is the inability to feel pleasure or engage in activities that they previously found enjoyable. Anhedonia can lead to a state of **amotivation** where people stop trying to pursue any form of goal-directed behavior and instead simply sit, stare, or lie down for hours on end. Despite sharing their name, anhedonia in schizophrenia likely differs from anhedonia on a mechanistic level. (Recall that while anhedonia is quite *sensitive* for depression, it is not necessarily *specific* and can be seen in other disorders as well.)

A is for Asociality. People with schizophrenia often develop severe difficulties relating to other people and instead are preoccupied with their own internal experiences, resulting in **asociality**. (While this phenomenon was classically known as "autism," in modern psychiatry the term autism generally refers to autism spectrum disorder, so for the sake of clarity we will not use the term in this way.) People with schizophrenia often appear completely disinterested in what is going on around them, even during major life events that would normally provoke strong emotions such as death, birth, and marriage. Many end up withdrawing socially and "live in their own world," leading to isolation and loneliness. These social difficulties may be due, at least in part, to the presence of positive symptoms, which can be disturbing or off-putting to others. However, the social deficits in schizophrenia often extend far beyond what would be expected from the effects of positive symptoms alone.

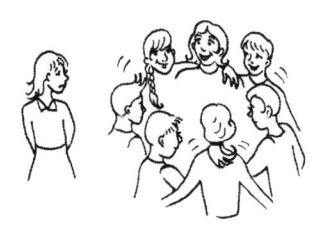

Negative symptoms in schizophrenia include **deficits** in emotional range, decision-making ability, speech, pleasure, and socialization.

The 5 A's:
Affect
Ambivalence
Alogia
Anhedonia
Asociality

SCHIZOPHRENIA ACROSS THE LIFESPAN

Learning about schizophrenia is more challenging than mood disorders like bipolar disorder or depression. Because mood disorders occur in discrete episodes, you only have to learn what the clinical picture looks like *during* an episode. In contrast, schizophrenia is *not* an episodic disorder, so you will need to pay particular attention to how the disorder appears across the entire lifespan and not just at a single moment in time.

EPIDEMIOLOGY

Schizophrenia is found in 0.5 to 1% of the population, giving it a **low base rate** and increasing the risk of overdiagnosis. **Men** are affected more frequently than women, with 3 men diagnosed for every 2 women. Interestingly, people born in cities and those with immigrant status in their current country of residency appear to be at higher risk.

Like bipolar disorder, schizophrenia is typically diagnosed in **early adulthood**. The age of onset is **earlier in men** (between 18 and 25) than it is for women (between 25 and 35). However, as many as 15% of people with schizophrenia do not develop symptoms until after the age of 40, with 5% doing so after the age of 60. For this reason, late-life onset generally argues *against* a diagnosis of schizophrenia but does not rule it out entirely.

While the characteristic symptoms of schizophrenia generally do not begin until early adulthood, many people who are diagnosed with schizophrenia showed signs even in childhood, including odd beliefs, social withdrawal, physical clumsiness, and poor performance in school. This pre-syndromal state is known as a **prodrome**. Although these symptoms are common in people who go on to develop schizophrenia, they are unfortunately not specific enough to allow for early diagnosis as only around one-third of patients diagnosed as having a prodrome actually go on to have a **first break** where active symptoms of psychosis emerge. As the other two-thirds do not develop schizophrenia, the risk of false positives from diagnosing and treating based only on prodromal symptoms is too high.

PROGNOSIS

Schizophrenia involves a lifelong pattern of **acute symptomatic exacerbations** on top of **progressive functional deterioration**. (The progressive nature of schizophrenia is underscored by the fact that it was originally called *dementia praecox* or "early dementia.") As a progressive illness, social and occupational functioning are often **significantly impaired** even when there are no active symptoms of psychosis. (This is in contrast to mood disorders, where functioning is generally *preserved* between episodes.)

Once a first break has occurred, the **chance of future symptom recurrence is high**, with 80 to 90% of people having another exacerbation in their lifetime (a recurrence rate as high as bipolar disorder). This has important implications both for educating patients and families about the nature of the illness as well as deciding on how long to continue with treatments. An earlier age of onset tends to predict a more severe course of illness.

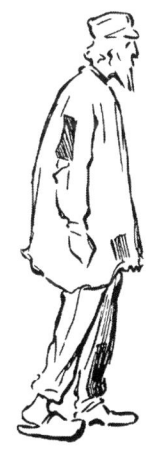

Psychotic symptoms do not have a built-in "expiration date" in the same way that manic or depressive episodes do. Studies have found that, without treatment, symptoms of psychosis can continue unabated for **years at a time**, although for some people symptoms naturally take on a more waxing and waning course.

People with schizophrenia often lead difficult lives. Less than 20% of people with schizophrenia are able to find employment, leaving them dependent upon others for support. Without this support, outcomes can be tragic, and people with schizophrenia are over 10 times more likely to be **incarcerated** or chronically **homeless**. On average, people with schizophrenia live 10 to 20 years less than their peers. A variety of explanations exist for this discrepancy, including the effects of chronic homelessness, a lack of interest in medical care, and a higher propensity for developing medical illness (either due to the disorder itself or from common side effects of medications). Some of this gap in life expectancy may be attributed to **suicide** as well. While not as common as in mood disorders, suicide still occurs in schizophrenia, with the diagnosis being found in around 15% of all fatal suicides. When suicide does occur, it tends to happen in an early stage of the illness when someone's insight is sufficiently preserved that they know that they are unwell and that they will likely not be able to live the life that they would have wanted to.

TREATMENT
Treatment of schizophrenia consists of **medications** and **psychotherapy**. Like bipolar disorder, the standard of care almost always involves medications, as psychotherapy alone is not considered sufficient for treating schizophrenia in most cases. With treatment, psychotic symptoms can be reduced in a matter of days or weeks.

Medications used to treat schizophrenia are known as **antipsychotics**. The majority of antipsychotics act as **dopamine receptor blockers** and lead to rapid reductions in positive symptoms with a **medium effect size** (around 0.5). While antipsychotics are effective at treating the *positive* symptoms of schizophrenia, they are much less effective at treating *negative* symptoms and may even worsen them by blocking the sense of motivation and drive that dopamine normally provides. Because of this, antipsychotics are much more effective at improving *symptomatic* outcomes than *functional* ones.

Antipsychotics are associated with some significant side effects that must be taken into account. Older (or "typical") antipsychotics are known for causing specific motor side effects known as **extrapyramidal symptoms**, including sudden uncontrollable muscle contractions (*acute dystonia*), motor restlessness (*akathisia*), slowed movement (*bradykinesia*), and uncontrollable movements (*tardive dyskinesia*). Newer (or "atypical") antipsychotics tend to have fewer extrapyramidal symptoms but can cause severe **metabolic** effects including obesity, diabetes, and hyperlipidemia. Typical and atypical antipsychotics are equally effective, so the decision to use one antipsychotic over another is generally based on the side effect profile.

In cases of **treatment-refractory schizophrenia**, a particular antipsychotic known as **clozapine** is significantly more effective, with a **large effect size** around 0.9. However, clozapine is associated with a small but significant risk of agranulocytosis, a rare but potentially deadly side effect that depletes the immune system and makes someone unable to fight off even small infections. Because of this, regular laboratory monitoring of blood cells is required for anyone on clozapine. While the risk of agranulocytosis makes clozapine impractical as a first-line treatment, in particularly severe or refractory cases it can be a life-saving treatment (as can ECT, which has a large effect size even for those already taking medications).

Hospitalization may be required for severe symptoms in schizophrenia. Even in cases where someone with psychosis is not actively dangerous to themselves or others, many states allow for involuntarily detainment of individuals who are **gravely disabled** to the extent that they are unable to secure basic provisions such as food, clothing, and shelter due to their condition. In cases where insight is severely impaired, a court order for involuntary treatment may need to be sought.

In addition to medications, psychotherapy can be an incredibly helpful adjunctive treatment. The best studied form of therapy in schizophrenia is **CBT for psychosis** which has been shown to reduce both positive and negative symptoms while improving the overall level of functioning with a **small effect size** (around 0.4).

The outcomes of schizophrenia treatment vary across the world. Paradoxically, countries with less access to mental health care have been found to have *better* functional outcomes for schizophrenia than those with more well-developed healthcare systems. The reasons for this are unclear, but it may have to do with the superior ability of communities to care for patients with psychotic illnesses in more family-oriented cultures compared to industrialized societies that tend to place a strong emphasis on independence and individuality. In addition, more frequent use of antipsychotics in developed nations may be partially to blame, as they may actually worsen functional outcomes (despite being effective for positive symptoms). However, this must be weighed against other evidence showing that the duration of untreated psychosis is itself predictive of poor long-term functioning, so it remains unclear what the optimal treatment strategy for maximizing long-term functional outcomes should be.

MECHANISMS OF SCHIZOPHRENIA

The experience of psychosis is not one that most people will easily understand. Unlike other psychiatric syndromes like depression where most of the symptoms (like fatigue or sadness) will be familiar to most people, in schizophrenia the most prominent symptoms of the disorder (like delusions or hallucinations) don't have any direct parallels in most people's lives. Because of this, schizophrenia can be an incredibly difficult disorder to comprehend, leading to misinformation, misconceptions, and misdiagnoses. However, by focusing on the underlying mechanisms of the disorder, we can avoid these pitfalls and improve our diagnostic skills.

At its core, a state of primary psychosis appears to involve abnormalities in the process of assigning **salience**. Salience is the "interestingness" of information and reflects how relevant we perceive that information to be. While reading a textbook, for example, you might highlight passages that you perceive to be particularly salient (maybe you're even doing it in this textbook). By highlighting certain words and not others, you are saying in effect that some words are more important or *salient* than the words around them. We use salience to filter information, giving salient items more attention and being more likely to act upon them. For example, if you were given ten random numbers (say, 1558378290) but not told anything about them, you probably wouldn't find them to be particularly salient and, without that salience, they would drop from your attention and quickly be forgotten. However, if you were told that these same ten numbers are from tomorrow's winning million dollar lottery ticket and that there's still time to enter, then suddenly the numbers become *very* interesting indeed. By being given this context, the *salience* of the information has increased even though the numbers themselves have not changed at all. This illustrates that salience is not an inherent property of the information itself; rather, it is assigned based on the context of the situation.

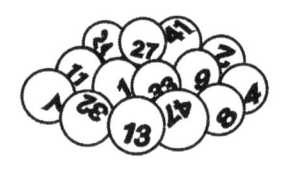

On a biological level, the neurotransmitter **dopamine** appears to be involved in assigning salience. When information is found to be salient, your brain releases dopamine which makes you more likely to pay attention to the information and act upon it.

Going back to schizophrenia, people with this condition are believed to be in a **pro-salient state** characterized by a tendency to assign salience indiscriminately without regard to context, leading to **connections and patterns being perceived in things that are not actually connected**. To help you understand what it is like to be in a pro-salient state, imagine that one morning as you're leaving your house you notice a black car parked across the street. As soon as you see it, the car starts and drives off quickly. You find this a little odd but ultimately don't think too much of it. However, the next day the exact same thing happens. It's enough to bother you slightly, but you are still able to put it out of your mind. When it happens for a third day in a row (and then a fourth and a fifth), however, it begins to get under your skin. After a week of seeing this black car drive off every day as soon as you walk out of your house, you are absolutely convinced that this is **no mere coincidence**—there *must* be some significance to what you are noticing. Maybe someone is spying on you. But why? You're just a regular person. Why would someone go through all this trouble?

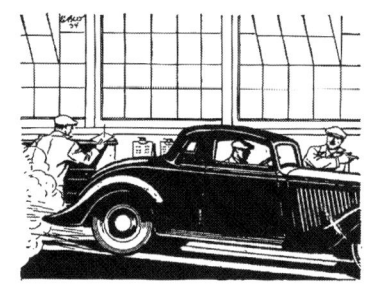

Unless… maybe you know more than you think you do? As you go throughout your day, you begin to notice things that you never noticed before. Your boss seems a little bit colder towards you than normal. *Is she in on this too?* While going home at night, you see four different police cars. *Are there normally that many? Am I a part of some vast international conspiracy? Do I have some kind of superpower that I am unaware of? What is going on?!?*

Take the way you are feeling right now and save it in a bottle labeled "pro-salient state." This feeling is exactly what people in initial stages of schizophrenia experience. When we perceive patterns in things, it causes us to assign salience to information more easily. In this way, pro-salient states can be adaptive by enabling us to make mental connections we otherwise would not have (like a detective putting together seemingly disparate clues to solve a murder case). However, when this process goes too far, confusion and dysfunction can result.

People with schizophrenia are believed to be in a state of **aberrant salience** where importance is assigned to every bit of new information without any clear connection to whether it is actually relevant or not. Returning to the lottery numbers from earlier, the sudden increase in the salience of those ten numbers upon revealing their significance was noticeable, but at least we knew *why* the salience had increased. However, having schizophrenia is like suddenly entering a world in which *every bit of information* had the potential to make you a million dollars in the same way as tomorrow's winning lottery ticket. This makes life initially quite vivid and dramatic for someone in a state of aberrant salience, and people in early stages of schizophrenia often report a distinct sense that everything, everywhere feels like a potential clue to solving some vast puzzle, saying things like:

"My senses were sharpened. I developed a greater awareness of the world and became fascinated by the little insignificant things around me."

"My senses seemed alive... Things seemed clear-cut, I noticed things I had never noticed before."

"I felt that there was some overwhelming significance in this."

"I felt like I was putting a piece of the puzzle together."

While this can initially be thrilling, a state of aberrant salience quickly becomes a confusing and unbearable way to live. In a pro-salient state, your mind is particularly likely to make connections even between unrelated or disparate events, setting the stage for the development of new (and often delusional) beliefs. If someone watches the news in a state of aberrant salience, they might come to believe that the president is using their State of the Union address to communicate a special coded message meant only for them. When listening to music, they may get the feeling that there must be a reason why that particular song came on the radio at that exact moment. On the internet, any random stimulus—like a pop-up ad about a new brand of lotion—may seem so special and compelling that it *must* somehow be the key to saving the world. To everyone else, these ideas sound, frankly, psychotic. For someone in a state of aberrant salience, however, these **delusions** help them to make sense out of a senseless mental environment where everything is suddenly imbued with a sense of world-changing importance.

Aberrant salience also explains the profound **thought disorganization** that occurs in schizophrenia. Our brains use salience to **filter incoming information** by focusing on what seems most important and giving less attention to the rest (like highlighting words in a book). A state of aberrant salience, however, is like reading a book where *every single word* is highlighted. Normally highlighting helps to organize information and allows you to focus on what is most important. When every word is highlighted, however, this system of organization breaks down, and you can no longer rely on a sense of salience to guide your attention. This is exactly what is seen in schizophrenia, with aberrant salience appearing to leave people in a state of perpetual **information overload**. When the filter of salience breaks, people become constantly bombarded by new information every second of the day with no way of making sense of it all. It would be like trying to watch dozens of TV screens all at the same time or listening to ten different conversations at once. In this state of confusion, it is no wonder that people with schizophrenia appear to have such profound difficulty following even a simple train of thought.

The concept of aberrant salience can inform not only our understanding of schizophrenia but also how we treat it. If aberrant salience is associated with excess dopamine, then using medications to block dopamine should reduce the symptoms of schizophrenia. This appears to be true, as all of the drugs prescribed for schizophrenia block dopamine receptors to some degree. This creates a state of **dampened salience** where information lacks the power to capture attention that it once had, leading to reductions in positive symptoms. However, this comes at a cost, as antipsychotics cause a *global* dampening of salience for all information that the brain processes (not just aberrantly salient information). This shows both the power and the limitations of using antipsychotics to treat schizophrenia: these drugs reverse the excess of dopamine driving a state of aberrant salience, but in doing so they can interfere with the normal ability of salience to guide attention, motivation, and goal-directed behavior as well. In contrast, therapies to treat schizophrenia like CBT for psychosis are more able to teach the patient how to recognize aberrant thought patterns, allowing for a more targeted and nuanced approach for patients.

Ultimately, no single theory is going to be able to explain a disease as complex as schizophrenia. While aberrant salience explains the delusions of reference and thought disorganization that are found in schizophrenia, other symptoms (such as auditory hallucinations or delusions of control) appear to be related to a profound inability to differentiate between self-generated stimuli and those coming from the external environment (the "self-tickling" hypothesis mentioned earlier). In addition, neither of these hypotheses account for the profound negative symptoms that are often found in advanced stages of the illness. Researchers currently point to the idea of a "two-deficit" model of schizophrenia in which multiple abnormalities are needed to explain the entirety of what we see. Nevertheless, the concept of aberrant salience is a good place to start, as it can provide a helpful framework for understanding the phenomenology of schizophrenia as well as the benefits and drawbacks to using dopamine-blocking medications to treat it.

HOW TO DIAGNOSE PSYCHOTIC DISORDERS

While a state of primary psychosis often implies a diagnosis of schizophrenia, there are a variety of related disorders that should be considered as well, including delusional disorder, schizoaffective disorder, and psychotic disorders related to mood, substance use, or medical conditions. We'll cover the most common types of psychosis-related disorders in this section.

SCHIZOPHRENIA

Diagnosing schizophrenia is based on the presence of certain signs and symptoms (as captured in the **HD BS Network** mnemonic) in combination with a characteristic course of illness across the lifespan, including an early prodrome, a slow functional decline, and active symptoms lasting at least 6 months. Specific findings on the mental status exam that argue for a diagnosis of schizophrenia include disorganized speech, disorganized behavior, blunted affect, delusions, paranoia, and/or auditory hallucinations. Insight and judgment are often impaired due to the inability to tell reality from fantasy (as people with schizophrenia genuinely believe in their delusions and are convinced that the voices they hear are real).

Research has shown that the **P**ositive symptoms of psychosis are highly s**P**ecific for schizophrenia. These **first-rank symptoms** include auditory hallucinations in the characteristic "critical running commentary," delusions of thought manipulation (including thought withdrawal, insertion, interruption, and broadcasting), and delusions of control (including a sense that one's actions are being manipulated by outside forces). While first-rank symptoms are **highly specific** for schizophrenia, they are not particularly sensitive. In contrast, the **N**egative symptoms of schizophrenia *are* quite se**N**sitive, and a lack of negative symptoms can help to rule out the diagnosis (particularly for someone who has had the diagnosis for several years, as the ratio of negative symptoms to positive symptoms tends to increase over time). However, negative symptoms are not very specific, as anhedonia, ambivalence, and lack of motivation can be found in non-psychotic illnesses like severe depression as well.

> **Positive symptoms** are those that are **present in schizophrenia**, while **negative symptoms** are functions that are **absent in schizophrenia**.
>
> *Positive symptoms = Things that are Present but shouldn't be = Specific!*
> *Negative symptoms = Things that are Not present but should be = SeNsitive!*

Historically, the DSM differentiated between several subtypes of schizophrenia, including paranoid, disorganized, catatonic, undifferentiated, and residual forms. However, in the DSM-5 these subtypes were removed as there did not appear to be any diagnostic or prognostic benefits to differentiating between the subtypes, and schizophrenia is now considered a **single diagnosis**.

BRIEF PSYCHOTIC DISORDER AND SCHIZOPHRENIFORM DISORDER

The primary distinction when making a diagnosis of a primary psychotic disorder is in regards to **timeframe**. Because a diagnosis of schizophrenia prognostically "commits" someone to a lifetime of symptoms, one should be cautious when assigning the diagnosis. For this reason, schizophrenia should only be diagnosed when psychotic symptoms are sustained for at least **6 months** (remember **2-4-6-ophrenia!**). Psychotic symptoms lasting less than one month should be diagnosed as **brief psychotic disorder**, while those lasting between 1 and 6 months should be diagnosed as **schizophreniform disorder**. The distinction between brief psychotic disorder, schizophreniform disorder, and schizophrenia appears to have prognostic value, as only a third of patients with brief psychotic disorder and two-thirds of patients with schizophreniform disorder progress to having "full-blown" schizophrenia. While the 6 month cut off is ultimately arbitrary, it underscores the point that the **duration of psychotic symptoms** matters for the prognosis of primary psychosis.

DELUSIONAL DISORDER

Delusional disorder is a condition in which people develop delusions that are similar to those found in schizophrenia. However, in delusional disorder the other signs and symptoms of schizophrenia (including disorganized thoughts, auditory hallucinations, and negative symptoms) are notably *absent*. In addition, the life course of individuals with delusional disorder does not mirror that of schizophrenia, as these people are often employed, married, and lacking in other features suggestive of a mental disorder. On interview, they are often coherent, sensible, and reasonable—until they begin talking about their particular delusions.

If all the other parts of schizophrenia are missing, then why is delusional disorder a disorder at all? After all, delusions may be entirely normal. However, for some people, their belief in these delusions is firm enough that it can cause significant problems in their lives *even in the absence of any other symptoms*. For example, if your spouse of 30 years suddenly started believing that they had been abducted by aliens working for the CIA and refused to stop talking about it, it may begin to strain the marriage (not to mention their ability to hold a job or maintain other friendships).

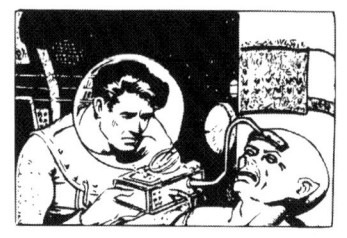

Pharmacologic treatments for delusional disorder are not very effective, with very limited benefit from antipsychotics (although they could be tried in severe cases). Cognitive behavioral therapy or other psychotherapies do not appear to reduce the intensity of the delusion itself, but they can nevertheless be helpful for mitigating the social or occupational dysfunction resulting from the delusions (such as teaching people the situations in which it is or is not appropriate to talk about the delusions).

SCHIZOAFFECTIVE DISORDER

Traditionally, the field of psychiatry made a distinction between psychotic disorders like schizophrenia and mood disorders like depression or mania, as these were thought to be entirely separate and distinct processes with different prognostic and treatment considerations. As time went on, however, this split between psychotic and affective disorders became harder to justify, as people with depression and mania often developed psychotic symptoms while those with schizophrenia sometimes had mood changes. In addition, there seemed to be people who clearly had mood episodes while also having discrete periods of psychotic symptoms.

To address this, the diagnosis of schizoaffective disorder was created to describe people who, by all appearances, genuinely experienced both psychotic and affective symptoms. The key with schizoaffective disorder is that **both processes need to have been present in the absence of the other** for at least some period of time. Someone who has only ever had psychotic symptoms *during* a mood episode would be diagnosed with a mood disorder with psychotic features. Only when there is a clear history of psychosis *in the absence of* an abnormal mood state and an *additional* history of mood episodes should the diagnosis of schizoaffective disorder be applied. Mood symptoms must be in excess of what would be expected from the psychotic disorder alone (such as the anhedonia or amotivation seen in schizophrenia).

Schizoaffective disorder is intended to be a **rare diagnosis**, and people who truly qualify for the diagnosis are few and far between. Because of its rarity, schizoaffective disorder is liable to rampant **overdiagnosis**, and studies have found that most people diagnosed with schizoaffective disorder have never actually met criteria for the disorder at any point in their lives. It is also a very **unstable diagnosis**, with only one-third of people diagnosed with schizoaffective disorder during a first hospitalization still having that diagnosis 6 months later (compared to over 90% for schizophrenia, over 80% for bipolar disorder, and over 70% for depression). These incorrect diagnoses often stem from **improper history taking** and a knee-jerk tendency to assume that any patient with both psychotic and mood symptoms has schizoaffective disorder (rather than more common disorders like a mood disorder with psychotic features). This is important enough that it bears repeating:

Mood + Psychosis ≠ Schizoaffective Disorder

In cases of "genuine" schizoaffective disorder, the prognosis lies at a sort of "halfway point" between schizophrenia and the mood disorders, as people with schizoaffective disorder often have *better* functioning between episodes compared to people with "pure" psychotic disorders but *worse* inter-episode functioning compared to people with "pure" mood disorders. Treatment almost always involves medications, including both antipsychotics and mood stabilizers. As with bipolar disorder, antidepressants should generally be avoided due to a risk of inducing rapid cycling. Recent revisions to the diagnostic criteria for schizoaffective disorder bring it closer to the mood disorders than the psychotic disorders, as it now requires that mood episodes be present for "the majority of the total active and residual course of illness from the onset of psychotic symptoms up until the current diagnosis." However, only time will tell what effect this has on the reliability and validity of schizoaffective disorder.

MOOD DISORDERS WITH PSYCHOTIC FEATURES
People in depressive or manic episodes can develop psychotic symptoms, especially when mood symptoms are severe. However, the presence of psychotic symptoms does not automatically imply a diagnosis of schizophrenia or schizoaffective disorder. Rather, a diagnosis of depression or bipolar disorder with psychotic features should be considered. This is more than just semantics: the prognosis and treatment considerations between mood disorders with psychotic symptoms and primary psychotic disorders differ so drastically that getting the diagnosis wrong could enter the patient into a long cycle of misinformation and incorrect treatments. As with schizoaffective disorder, the key is to look at the **relationship of psychotic symptoms to mood episodes**. Provided that psychotic symptoms have only occurred *during* mood episodes, a diagnosis of a mood disorder with psychotic features is appropriate.

Spend some time studying the schematics on the next page, as they will help to clarify the relationships between mood and psychotic disorders!

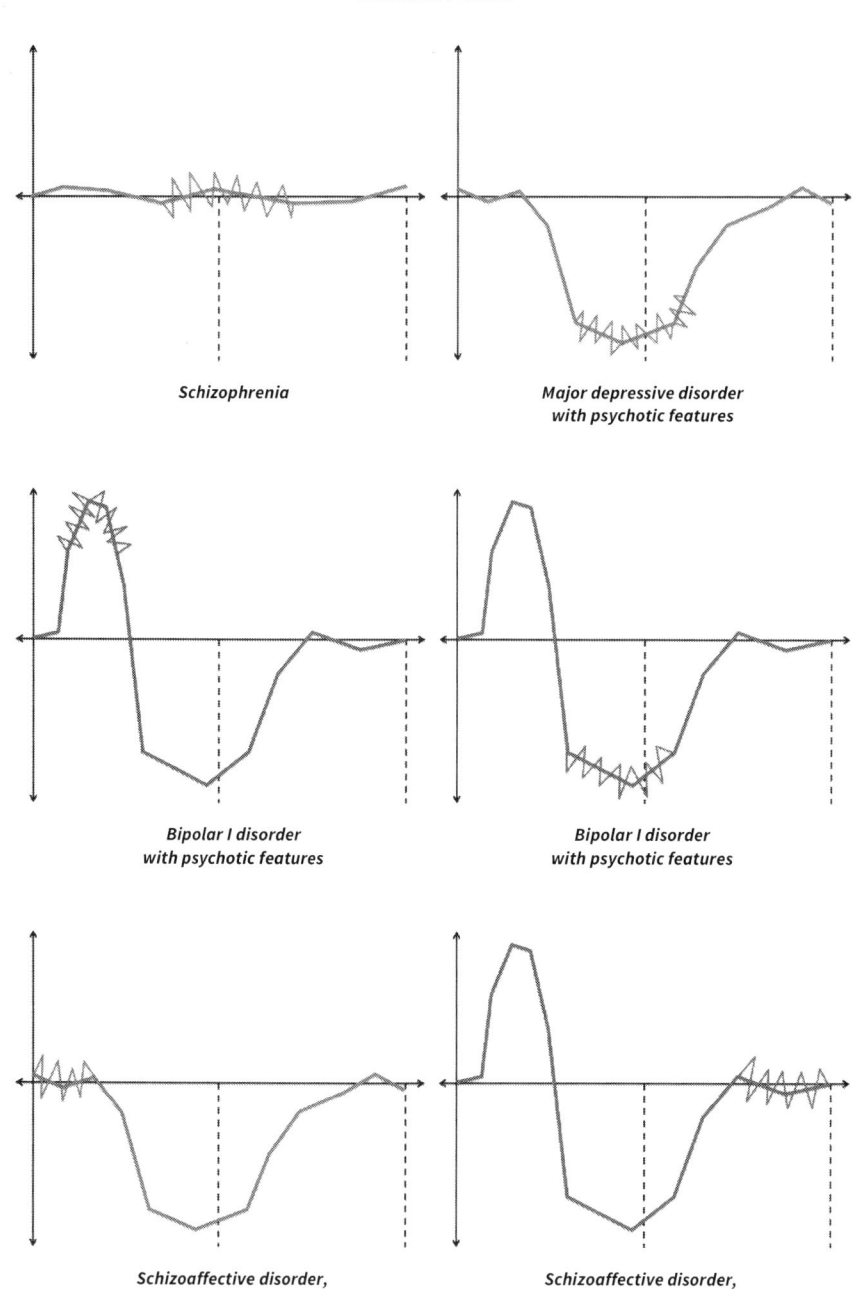

Schizophrenia

Major depressive disorder with psychotic features

Bipolar I disorder with psychotic features

Bipolar I disorder with psychotic features

Schizoaffective disorder, depressive type

Schizoaffective disorder, bipolar type

Schematic diagrams of various disorders featuring both mood and psychotic symptoms. The x-axis shows time in years (with individual years marked by a dotted line), the y-axis shows the patient's mood state (with euthymia set at the x-axis, manic symptoms above the x-axis, and depressive symptoms below the x-axis), and a jagged line indicates the presence of psychotic symptoms.

If there is a history of psychosis but no mood episodes, a diagnosis of schizophrenia should be given (top-left). If psychotic symptoms occur only during depressive episodes and there is no history of mania, a diagnosis of major depressive disorder with psychotic features is appropriate (top-right). If there is a history of manic episodes as well as psychosis but the psychotic symptoms have only occurred *during* a mood episode (either depression, mania, or both), the diagnosis would be bipolar disorder with psychotic symptoms (middle row). Only if psychotic symptoms have occurred even in the *absence* of a mood episode should a diagnosis of schizoaffective disorder be considered (bottom row). Schizoaffective disorder can be **depressive type** or **bipolar type** depending on the type of mood episodes present. (As a final note, there is no such thing as dysthymia or cyclothymia with psychotic features as, by definition, the presence of psychotic features implies a severe mood episode.)

DIFFERENTIAL DIAGNOSIS OF PSYCHOTIC DISORDERS

As a rare condition, schizophrenia is subject to **overdiagnosis** more often than underdiagnosis (especially considering that the positive symptoms of schizophrenia are often quite dramatic and bizarre, making them hard to miss). Overdiagnosis of schizophrenia can almost always be attributed to a focus on *content* over *context*. A diagnosis of schizophrenia should never be given on the basis of a single symptom (even "classic" symptoms like auditory hallucinations and bizarre delusions). Instead, the *context* in which those symptoms have come about, including the patient's level of functioning across the lifespan and the presence of aberrantly salient thought processes, are much more helpful in confirming a diagnosis. With this in mind, we will explore the most common misdiagnoses and missed diagnoses involving psychosis.

NORMALCY

Most of the symptoms of schizophrenia are not inherently pathological. For example, up to 10% of the population hears voices under normal circumstances but are not significantly impaired by this experience. In addition, many cultures and subcultures have specific beliefs that would likely be considered delusional by people coming from another worldview, which is why it's so important to consider the cultural context of a belief before calling it a delusion. Even people who have beliefs that are genuinely outside the norms of their society are not necessarily ill. For example, as many as 5% of Americans believe that they have been abducted by aliens, yet studies on these individuals have shown that the vast majority show no signs of psychiatric pathology. Therefore, it is imperative to avoid diagnosing schizophrenia in someone who reports auditory hallucinations or delusions *unless* there are additional features (such as thought disorganization or negative symptoms) to indicate a certain level of actual dysfunction.

In some cases, psychotic symptoms can represent a culturally accepted **idiom of distress**. For example, someone might tell their doctor that they are hearing voices as a way of bringing attention to an unpleasant life circumstance such as bereavement or abuse. As before, look for evidence of actual dysfunction across the lifespan to avoid overliteralizing and overmedicalizing these concerns.

DEPRESSION
Schizophrenia can often be misdiagnosed as depression, as a number of symptoms overlap between the two conditions (especially negative symptoms like apathy, anhedonia, and lack of motivation). This is especially true during the **prodromal state** before the characteristic first-rank symptoms of schizophrenia have emerged. Look for a pattern of episodicity and specific thought patterns such as guilt, hopelessness, or rumination, all of which would increase the likelihood of depression. In some cases, however, it is not always possible to "call" the diagnosis correctly from the get-go. Similar to cases of bipolar depression that present initially as depression, there may be times when you have to wait for schizophrenic symptoms to "declare themselves" before being certain about your diagnosis (although certain symptoms, such as odd or eccentric beliefs, may keep schizophrenia higher on your differential).

MANIA
Even in the absence of psychotic symptoms, mania can sometimes be misdiagnosed as schizophrenia. The source of confusion is often related to the presence of delusions in both disorders. People in a manic state may have delusions, but this does not automatically mean that they have schizophrenia or delusional disorder. Instead, the *nature* of delusions matters. In mania, delusions tend to be grandiose and reward-oriented while in primary psychosis they are more likely to involve classic first-rank delusions including conspiratorial thinking, paranoia, thought manipulation, or delusions of control by outside forces. The line between manic and psychotic delusions is not always clear, but the presence of other **distinguishing symptoms** (such as distractibility and flight of ideas in mania or thought disorganization and negative symptoms in schizophrenia) as well as careful consideration of the pattern of illness across the lifespan (whether it is episodic or progressive) can help as well.

FACTITIOUS DISORDER AND MALINGERING
Factitious disorder and malingering (discussed further in Chapter 13) both involve the intentional production of symptoms for specific gains such as wanting to be in the sick role or to obtain disability benefits. It is not uncommon for psychosis to be the condition feigned by people with factitious disorder or malingering, as schizophrenia only requires the production of subjective psychiatric symptoms (rather than physical signs, which are harder to fake). A key diagnostic feature of people who are producing or exaggerating psychotic symptoms is that they will often be **willing to volunteer these symptoms** during an interview whereas most people with schizophrenia will attempt to hide their symptoms and only talk about them when asked. In addition, people who are producing symptoms tend to focus on the symptoms of schizophrenia that are more easily fabricated (such as auditory hallucinations) while avoiding symptoms like thought disorganization that are more difficult to fake. (To get a sense of this, put down the book and record yourself trying to make neologisms, clang associations, or a world salad—it's not easy to do.)

Having a structured method of assessing auditory hallucinations can help to distinguish between genuine and feigned symptoms. Use the mnemonic **Vague AWD** (odd) **LIARS** when asking patients about their auditory hallucinations to get a better sense of their likely origin (this will also help you to review what we learned earlier about the phenomenology of schizophrenia!):

Vague is for Vague. Patients who are feigning auditory hallucinations will often say that the voices are vague or fuzzy, in contrast to schizophrenia where the content of the voices are quite clear.

AWD is for Associated With Delusions. Hallucinations in schizophrenia are almost always associated with delusions. In contrast, people who are feigning psychosis will tend to report auditory hallucinations as their sole symptom.

L is for Laterality. Voices in schizophrenia sound like they are coming from all around, whereas people feigning psychosis may say the voices are coming from one side of their head or the other.

I is for Inside. Patients with schizophrenia genuinely perceive their voices as coming from the outside world. In contrast, people who are feigning psychosis are more likely to talk about "voices inside my head."

A is for Able to resist. Command auditory hallucinations can occur in schizophrenia. However, the patient is generally able to resist what they tell them to do, especially if doing so would be dangerous. In contrast, people who are feigning psychosis are more likely to say that they are forced to do what the voices tell them to do.

R is for Reducing strategies. Most patients with schizophrenia find their voices to be distressing and will have found specific strategies to help reduce the intensity of the voices. In contrast, people who are feigning psychosis will often not be able to describe any strategies to reduce hallucinations.

S is for Secondary gain. Finally, feigned psychosis should be high on your differential when there is a clear reward to be gained by reporting auditory hallucinations.

> Feigned psychosis differs significantly from the **typical phenomenology** of auditory hallucinations in schizophrenia.
>
> ***Vague AWD LIARS:***
> *Vague*
> *Associated With Delusions*
> *Laterality*
> *Inside*
> *Able to resist*
> *Reducing strategies*
> *Secondary gain*

CLUSTER A PERSONALITY DISORDERS

Schizophrenia and personality disorders can be difficult to disentangle, as both are chronic and life-long conditions (as opposed to episodic disorders like depression and bipolar disorder). In particular, the cluster A personality disorders have symptoms that overlap significantly with schizophrenia, including paranoia (**paranoid** personality disorder), social isolation (**schizoid** personality disorder), and strange beliefs (**schizotypal** personality disorder). Of these, only schizotypal personality disorder appears to be actually related to schizophrenia, with genetic links between the two disorders. In addition, about a third of people with schizotypal personality disorder will go on to develop "full-blown" schizophrenia. In contrast, the other cluster A personality disorders (paranoid and schizoid) may superficially resemble schizophrenia but ultimately should be seen as unrelated conditions.

CLUSTER B PERSONALITY DISORDERS

Cluster B personality disorders and in particular **borderline personality disorder** are frequently missed on the differential for psychosis. However, it is not at all uncommon for people with borderline personality disorder to report psychotic symptoms (including auditory hallucinations and paranoia) that can resemble schizophrenia. In fact, up to 20% of patients in primary care settings who report psychotic symptoms meet criteria for borderline personality disorder rather than schizophrenia.

We'll go over borderline personality disorder in more detail in Chapter 15, but for now just know that it differs from schizophrenia in a few key ways. First, people with schizophrenia tend to experience a **progressive decline** over time whereas those with borderline personality disorder tend to have a stable (or even improving) level of dysfunction after early adulthood. Borderline personality disorder also tends to lack the thought disorganization or negative symptoms that characterize schizophrenia. Self-reported psychotic symptoms in borderline personality disorder are often more in line with **idioms of distress** than they are with the classic phenomenology of auditory hallucinations and paranoid delusions related to schizophrenia. These so-called "micropsychotic" symptoms are often experienced during times of extreme stress and are sometimes accompanied by dissociative symptoms, discussed next.

DISSOCIATIVE DISORDERS

We'll discuss dissociation more in Chapter 12, but briefly this term refers to a transient state of feeling detached from reality. Any condition involving the words "feeling detached from reality" is naturally going to invite comparisons to (and confusion with) schizophrenia and other psychotic disorders. However, dissociation and psychosis are ultimately very different states. The key is that someone in a state of dissociation will say that their experience *feels* unreal but will still be able to distinguish between their own internal experiences and the objective reality of the outside world. In contrast, someone in a state of psychosis is *genuinely unable* to tell that their subjective experiences do not represent a shared reality. The concept of "**reality testing**" (or the ability to tell what is real from what is fake) is used to distinguish between these two experiences, as this ability is impaired in psychosis but intact in dissociation.

DEMENTIA

On the surface, one may think that dementia and schizophrenia would rarely be confused, especially since dementia tends to begin much later in life compared to schizophrenia. However, there are overlapping features of the disorders that can cause confusion. For one, dementia can often present with psychotic symptoms (including hallucinations and delusions), especially in advanced stages. In addition, schizophrenia itself is associated with cognitive deficits that may resemble dementia (keep in mind that the original name for schizophrenia was "premature dementia").

If you focused only on content, it may be tempting to diagnose new-onset psychotic symptoms as signs of a late-onset schizophrenia (which, while rare, does occur). However, looking at the *context*, a late-life onset and a lack of prior psychiatric history both point towards dementia. People with late-life schizophrenia also tend to be socially isolated and unmarried, whereas those with dementia would match the average population in this regard. Further, hallucinations in dementia are primarily visual rather than the classic "running commentary" auditory hallucinations reported in schizophrenia, while delusions tend to take specific forms in dementia (including **delusional misidentifications** such as someone believing that their son is trying to kill them even though he is only coming over to help with gardening).

For particularly unclear cases, cognitive testing such as the MoCA or MMSE (discussed more in Chapter 22) can be performed. While patients with schizophrenia do have some cognitive deficits, they have relatively intact recall of learned information and visuospatial ability (two things that patients with dementia frequently struggle with). Assessing one's level of orientation can be helpful as well, as patients with schizophrenia often still know their name, location, and time (although their understanding of the situation may be impaired due to poor insight).

DELIRIUM AND PSYCHOSIS DUE TO A GENERAL MEDICAL CONDITION

Broadly speaking, schizophrenia and delirium are both "psychosis" in that they share an inability to distinguish fantasy from reality. However, delirium would be considered a case of **secondary psychosis** as opposed to primary psychosis. It is generally not too difficult to distinguish delirium from schizophrenia, as the mental changes in delirium are often of an **acute onset** (as opposed to a slow onset in schizophrenia), represent a dramatic **change from baseline**, and are accompanied by **other signs and symptoms** of a medical illness such as fever, vital sign abnormalities, and/or focal neurologic deficits. In addition, the mental state in delirium tends to fluctuate (waxing and waning from one hour to the next), while it is more stable across days or weeks in schizophrenia. The hallucinations in delirium also tend to be **visual** rather than auditory (recall that **vis**ual hallucinations are typically **vis**ceral in origin). Finally, keep in mind that a history of schizophrenia does not preclude someone from developing delirium: it is absolutely possible for someone with schizophrenia to develop delirium as the result of a medical illness!

A variety of medical conditions can also cause a state of secondary psychosis, including malignancies (such as brain tumors), infections (syphilis), genetic disorders (Wilson's disease), neurologic conditions (multiple sclerosis), endocrine diseases (hyperthyroidism), and many others. As with delirium, it is exceedingly rare for a medical condition to cause psychosis as defined in terms of schizophrenia (including the classic "running commentary" auditory hallucinations, paranoid delusions, and thought disorganization), and the same features of the history (including sudden onset, decreased levels of orientation, and lack of prior psychiatric history) can help as well. In cases where a medical etiology is suspected, a complete work-up should be considered. Brain imaging may be helpful in cases where there is reason to suspect central nervous system involvement such as patients who report a headache, have a history of recent head trauma, or exhibit focal neurologic deficits on exam.

ANTI-NMDA RECEPTOR ENCEPHALITIS

Anti-NMDA receptor encephalitis is technically a form of secondary psychosis due to a general medical condition, but it deserves special mention because (unlike most other medical conditions) it can and does present with psychotic symptoms that *are* highly reminiscent of "textbook" psychosis as seen in schizophrenia, including delusions, auditory hallucinations, and even catatonia. In addition, psychiatric symptoms may be present for several weeks before any focal neurologic signs like memory loss or seizures occur, making it possible that a psychiatrist may evaluate someone with this condition before any other medical specialty.

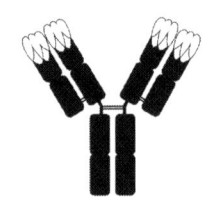

Anti-NMDA receptor encephalitis can occur when someone's immune system generates autoantibodies that target a specific type of glutamate receptor in the brain. Often, this is caused by microstructural similarities between NMDA receptors and **teratomas**, or tumors made up of multiple types of tissues. Anti-NMDA receptor encephalitis is most often associated with **ovarian** teratomas, making it much more common in women compared to men. While anti-NMDA receptor encephalitis is rare, consider the diagnosis in cases of new-onset psychosis with any focal neurologic deficits, alterations in sensorium, or vital sign instability, especially if there is no prior psychiatric history. Treatment involves immunotherapy and surgical removal of the tumor, if present.

ADDICTION AND SUBSTANCE-INDUCED PSYCHOTIC DISORDER

People with schizophrenia use substances at a rate that far exceeds that of the general population. Because of this, an assessment of current and past substance use should be done for every patient diagnosed with schizophrenia. Similar to mood disorders, the relationship between substance use and schizophrenia is a **two-way street**. The stress of having schizophrenia likely increases the chances of using drugs, but use of drugs can also increase the chance of developing psychosis. Three classes of drugs in particular deserve special mention: **stimulants**, **hallucinogens**, and **cannabis**. Stimulants like methamphetamine can create a mental state that strongly resembles psychosis, including paranoia and hallucinations (likely due to the increased release of dopamine). A state resembling psychosis can also occur with certain types of hallucinogens, particularly dissociative hallucinogens such as phencyclidine. In the majority of cases, this substance-induced psychosis tends to be self-limiting and lasts only as long as the drug is in one's system. However, in cases of prolonged use (especially of methamphetamine), there may be permanent symptoms and functional impairment even during periods of sustained sobriety.

In contrast, the acute mental state changes produced by cannabis are rarely confused for psychosis even though some degree of paranoia can occur. (This does not hold true for high potency forms of cannabis, including synthetic cannabinoids, which may be associated with an acute psychotic state.) However, prolonged use of cannabis has been found to be a risk factor for developing a state of chronic psychosis that can be nearly indistinguishable from "ordinary" cases of schizophrenia. It appears that in some individuals who are biologically vulnerable to developing schizophrenia, exposure to cannabis can "unmask" the disorder and cause it to develop earlier than it might have otherwise. While this does not apply across the board, individuals with a strong genetic predisposition towards schizophrenia should be counseled about the risk of developing psychosis with cannabis use, especially during adolescence.

Finally, a variety of prescription medications, including steroids, prescription stimulants, immunomodulators, anticholinergics, and drugs that increase dopamine transmission in the brain (such as L-dopa and amantadine) can cause psychotic symptoms in some individuals.

OBSESSIVE-COMPULSIVE DISORDER

Obsessive-compulsive disorder (OCD) is a condition characterized by obsessive thoughts and beliefs that are often not consistent with reality. The beliefs seen in obsessive-compulsive disorder may be occasionally confused for the delusions seen in schizophrenia as both involve thoughts that persist even when presented with clear and convincing evidence to the contrary. However, the key differentiating factor is that the obsessions in obsessive-compulsive disorder are **ego-dystonic** (meaning that the person recognizes that they are excessive or unreasonable) whereas the delusions in schizophrenia are **ego-syntonic** (as the person truly believes them). We will discuss this distinction further in Chapter 10.

POST-TRAUMATIC STRESS DISORDER

Post-traumatic stress disorder (PTSD) can be confused with schizophrenia for a number of reasons. Combat veterans returning from active duty are often in the same age range as the average onset of schizophrenia in men. In addition, some symptoms including paranoia and affective blunting (the characteristic "thousand yard stare" in returning combat veterans) are seen in both schizophrenia and PTSD. Flashbacks and re-experiencing episodes related to PTSD can sometimes take on an intensity that resembles a psychotic state, although one's reality testing ability remains intact during these periods. As with nearly all of the disorders that are confused for schizophrenia, the key to differentiating between the two lies in the *context* of the disorder rather than its content. A traumatic event is required for a diagnosis of PTSD (although this does not necessarily rule out schizophrenia, as trauma appears to increase one's risk for developing schizophrenia). When paranoia occurs in PTSD, it is often **related to the traumatic event** rather than being bizarre or hypersalient in nature. In addition, disorganization and negative symptoms are often lacking in PTSD but present in schizophrenia.

AUTISM

Autism is a condition characterized by difficulties in social communication combined with restricted interests and behaviors. Individuals with autism begin exhibiting signs in early childhood, including poor eye contact, social withdrawal, and flat or inappropriate affect. Given that these exact same symptoms are found during the prodrome of schizophrenia (and at the same time of life), it is perhaps not surprising that there is some diagnostic confusion between autism and schizophrenia. However, some factors can point more towards one or the other. It is rare for schizophrenia to have "full blown" psychotic symptoms beginning before the age of 13, so onset of clinically significant symptoms during early childhood suggests autism (though does not rule out schizophrenia entirely). In addition, there is nothing that suggests that someone cannot have both autism and schizophrenia, and indeed some studies have found that autism may be an independent predictor of later development of a psychotic disorder, suggesting shared genetic and environmental contributors to both. In general, though, be cautious about diagnosing schizophrenia in someone with autism unless it is clear that the signs and symptoms observed exceed what would be expected from autism alone and are directly in line with what is known about the phenomenology of a primary psychotic disorder.

PUTTING IT ALL TOGETHER

Schizophrenia is an incredibly disabling, stigmatizing, and tragic condition. Despite new cases being relatively rare compared to other disorders like depression and anxiety, schizophrenia still takes a large toll on society due to its early age of onset and its progressive, unremitting course. Because of this, a diagnosis of schizophrenia should be considered only when there is a high degree of diagnostic certainty. The DSM has built in at least one safeguard (the 6 month requirement – remember **2-4-6-ophrenia**!) to prevent against overdiagnosis. However, the best defense against misdiagnosis is to develop a firm knowledge of the clinical features that suggest schizophrenia rather than other forms of psychosis, including an understanding of the key role that salience plays in schizophrenia. Diagnostic criteria (as captured in the **HD BS Network** mnemonic) are tools to help remember major symptom domains, but they should be used with caution. Indeed, the presence of any of these symptoms should be the *starting point* for further investigation rather than the end process. For example, if someone says that they hear voices, you should not place a checkmark next to "Auditory Hallucinations" and move on. Instead, the presence of this symptom requires further characterization. Are the voices inside or outside the head? Are they associated with delusions? Are they hidden or eagerly volunteered during the interview? What evidence is there that these voices are causing any sort of distress or impairment? More than most psychiatric disorders, schizophrenia requires a deep understanding of what exactly is meant by each of these symptoms.

When psychotic symptoms overlap with mood disturbances, a high degree of care should be taken to characterize the exact relationship of these symptoms to each other to avoid overdiagnosing schizophrenia or schizoaffective disorder. Review the diagrams on page 116 to solidify your understanding of these relationships.

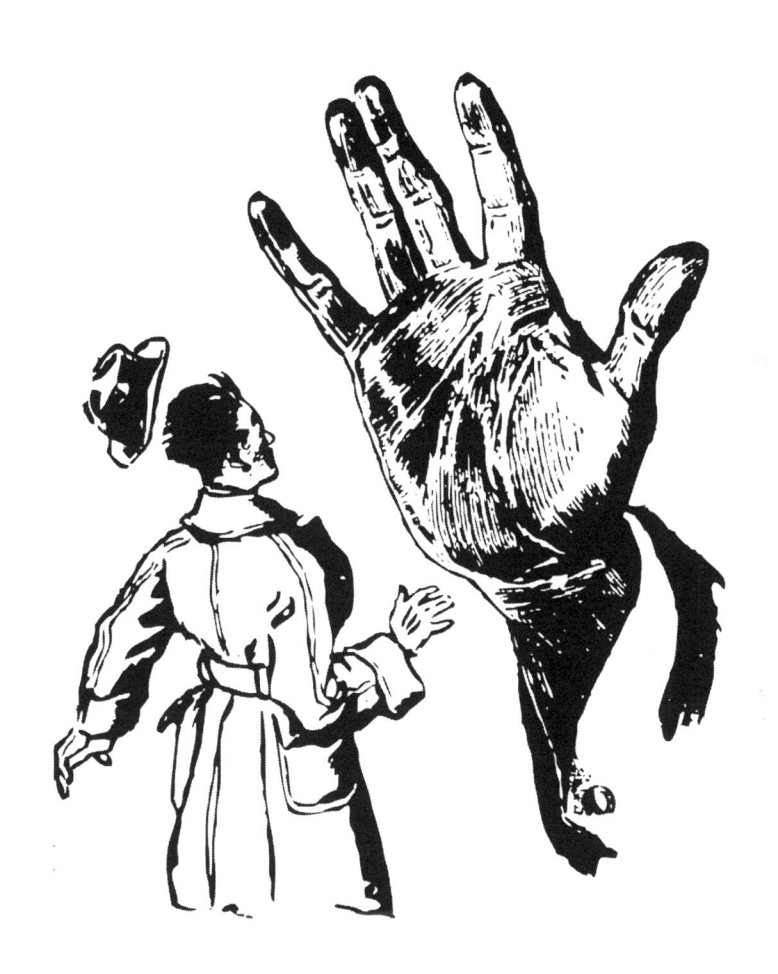

REVIEW QUESTIONS

1. A 21 y/o M is brought into the hospital by his roommates who are concerned that he has been "acting crazy" since last night. They say that he has been "talking endlessly" about how the government has sent spies to poison him because he is "an agent of impending destruction." On exam, the patient appears highly suspicious and gives very short answers to any questions asked. He is noted to be perseverative on thoughts related to the government and often returns to this topic no matter what kinds of questions he is asked. He denies visual or auditory hallucinations. His roommates, one of whom has known the patient since he was a child, said that he has never acted like this before. He works as a salesman at a local shoe store and has a girlfriend. Which of the following aspects of the history argues most strongly *against* a diagnosis of a primary psychosis for this patient?
    A. Non-bizarre nature of delusions
    B. Presence of paranoia
    C. Sudden onset of symptoms
    D. Age of the patient
    E. Absence of auditory hallucinations

2. A 37 y/o F is brought into the emergency department after she was detained for walking into oncoming traffic. On interview, the patient asks the psychiatrist if he is a surgeon. When the psychiatrist responds no, the patient asks for someone who can remove the "reverse hearing aids" in her ears. When asked about this further, the patient says that she has been fitted with "reverse hearing aids" by a television news anchor who is attempting to extract her innermost thoughts on how to create a vaccine for HIV. Otological exam is unremarkable. What term best describes this patient's belief?
    A. Thought broadcasting
    B. Thought withdrawal
    C. Thought insertion
    D. Delusions of control
    E. Not a delusion

3. (Continued from previous question.) The patient's sister arrives at the hospital. She says that the patient has never had symptoms like this before and was "completely normal" 3 months ago. However, she started to behave oddly after losing her job as a clerk at a local grocery store 2 months ago. The sister then asks, "I work as a nurse at another hospital and have seen people come in with schizophrenia. Do you think that's what my sister has?" Assuming that the patient meets criteria for an episode of primary psychosis, what is the best response?
    A. "Your sister almost certainly will develop schizophrenia."
    B. "Your sister is more likely than not to develop schizophrenia."
    C. "Your sister has about a 50% chance of developing schizophrenia."
    D. "It is possible but unlikely that your sister will develop schizophrenia."
    E. "Your sister definitely will not develop schizophrenia."

4. (Continued from previous question.) The patient is admitted to the hospital and started on an antipsychotic. She improves to the point where the patient's family feels comfortable with her discharging from the hospital to live with them at home. Which of the following signs and symptoms that were present at the time the patient was admitted to the hospital is most likely to still be present at the time of discharge?
   A. Having a facial expression that does not change
   B. Appearing to engage in conversations when no one else is in the room
   C. Believing that she has "reverse hearing aids" in her ears
   D. Saying words like "flearing" or "teck neck"
   E. Feeling that there is some "overwhelming significance" to events

5. A 26 y/o M with a history of schizophrenia since age 19 is brought to a clinic for an intake evaluation after his family moved across the country. He has had a long and unremitting course of the disorder with over 10 hospitalizations related to aggressive behavior in the context of paranoid delusions. He is currently taking two different antipsychotics, including risperidone 6 mg/day and quetiapine 400 mg/day. Despite this, he continues to have severe psychotic symptoms, including bizarre delusions, auditory hallucinations, and thought disorganization. He lives at home, and his mother (who was previously employed as a lawyer) is unable to work due to his need for constant supervision. He has previously taken multiple other antipsychotic medications, including olanzapine, ziprasidone, and haloperidol, none of which resulted in sustained decreases in symptom severity or increases in functional status. What is the next best step?
   A. Increase the dose of risperidone
   B. Increase the dose of quetiapine
   C. Discontinue risperidone
   D. Discontinue quetiapine
   E. Replace the existing antipsychotics with a new medication

1. **The best answer is C.** Symptoms related to a primary psychotic disorder such as schizophrenia rarely have an acute onset. Instead, signs of symptom progression are often apparent for several weeks or months before they become clinically significant. In addition, there is often a prodromal state characterized by cognitive and social deficits that result in social and occupational dysfunction (neither of which appear to be present here). An acute onset of symptoms usually argues for a substance-induced psychotic disorder. While the patient's delusions are notably non-bizarre, this does not rule out a diagnosis of primary psychosis as many patients with schizophrenia have non-bizarre delusions (answer A). Paranoia is common in primary psychosis and would argue *for* the diagnosis, not against it (answer B). The patient's age is within the normal window of developing schizophrenia in men (answer D). Finally, the absence of auditory hallucinations does not effectively rule out a diagnosis of primary psychosis, as this is not a required symptom and is more specific for the diagnosis than it is sensitive (answer E).

2. **The best answer is A.** This describes a clear example of thought broadcasting where someone in a state of primary psychosis believes that their thoughts are being transmitted to others.

3. **The best answer is B.** Assuming that this patient meets criteria for primary psychosis, she would likely be diagnosed as having schizophreniform disorder given that her symptoms have been present for around 2 months. Around two-thirds of cases of schizophreniform disorder progress to having schizophrenia, making her chances "more likely than not."

4. **The best answer is A.** Out of the answer choices, only a flat affect is considered to be a negative symptom. Negative symptoms are the least likely to respond to treatment with antipsychotic medications. Auditory hallucinations (answer B), delusional beliefs (answer C), disorganized speech (answer D), and a pro-salient state (answer E) are all considered to be positive symptoms that would generally respond to medications.

5. **The best answer is E.** This patient appears to be suffering from treatment-refractory schizophrenia as evidenced by continued symptoms and dysfunction despite treatment with two different antipsychotics at effective doses. Given this, a trial of clozapine appears to be warranted, as this medication is the most effective option for treating treatment-refractory cases of schizophrenia. Simply increasing the dose of his existing medications (answers A and B) would be unlikely to result in improvement, while discontinuing either medication (answers C and D) can precipitate further psychotic symptoms.

8 ADDICTION

Use of **psychoactive substances** is common, with over 90% of people in the United States taking at least one on a regular basis. While many people are able to use psychoactive substances without major negative effects on their physical or mental health, a significant minority will develop problems as a direct result of substance use. People experience problems related to substances in three distinct ways: intoxication, withdrawal, and addiction. These three things are closely related, but they are ultimately separate conditions so it's important to get them straight right from the get-go!

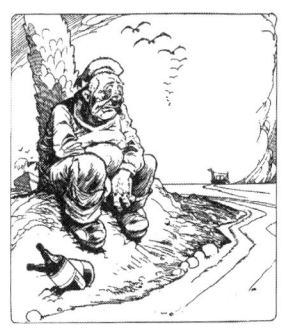

Intoxication is an *acute* state of being under the influence of a psychoactive substance, with the specific constellation of signs and symptoms associated with each substance being known as its toxidrome. **Withdrawal** is also an *acute* state, but this time it involves the physiological and psychological effects of suddenly discontinuing a substance, which are often the opposite of what you see in a state of intoxication with that same substance. In contrast to intoxication and withdrawal, addiction is a *chronic* condition characterized by repeatedly engaging in a specific activity despite suffering negative consequences as a result. When this involves drugs, it is known as a **substance use disorder**. However, addiction can also involve specific behaviors such as gambling that have similar effects in the brain as addictive substances. Because not all addictions involve drugs, the term **reinforcer** will instead be used to refer to the various substances and behaviors that can be the targets of addiction.

We will begin this chapter by exploring the specific states of intoxication and withdrawal associated with each of the most common types of psychoactive substances. From there, we will turn our attention to understanding the phenomenon of addiction, including how it presents on a clinical level, its trajectory across the lifespan, and how to approach treatment.

PSYCHOACTIVE SUBSTANCES

Psychoactive substances can be divided into a few broad categories, including **stimulants** (those with a net *activating* effect on the central nervous system), **depressants** (which have a net *inhibiting* effect), **opioids** (pain-relieving compounds), **cannabinoids** (which are found in marijuana and have a distinct set of effects), **hallucinogens** (which cause perceptual disturbances), and **inhalants** (which cause a characteristic "head rush"). It's important to be able to recognize states of intoxication and withdrawal related to each of these substances, especially considering that some (especially alcohol and opioids) can be incredibly dangerous and may require emergency treatment.

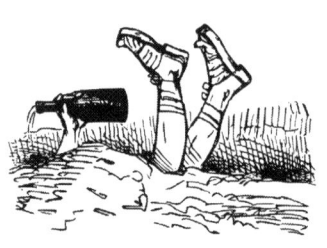

A diagnosis of intoxication is based on the presence of particular signs and symptoms as well as someone's reported history of substance use (although this cannot always be assumed to be accurate). Urine toxicology tests, which screen for common substances of abuse, can provide objective evidence to aid the diagnosis. Intoxication exists on a continuum with **overdose** in which so much of a particular substance is taken that it results in disease, disability, or death. Overdoses can be intentional (as in a suicide attempt) or accidental (as in someone who underestimated how much of the drug they were taking). The problems caused by overdosing vary drastically from substance to substance, with some (like opioids) being highly toxic in overdose while others (like cannabinoids) being relatively safe.

Following intoxication, drugs are metabolized out of the body according to their half-life. Abrupt discontinuation of a drug can lead to a state of withdrawal which, for many substances, often produces the **opposite** effects of what is seen during intoxication. For example, withdrawal from stimulants produces a state of fatigue and lethargy while withdrawal from depressants leads to restlessness and anxiety. You can remember this by thinking that *what goes up must come down and what goes down must come back up*. Not all substances have clinically significant withdrawal states, and for those that do, the dangerousness of withdrawal varies widely from being potentially lethal (like alcohol) to being merely uncomfortable (like cocaine).

Because the intoxication and withdrawal states of certain substances can mimic mental disorders so closely, differentiating between a primary psychiatric disorder and a substance-induced condition can be a challenge. The key is to focus on the **timing** of symptom onset. For example, someone with a methamphetamine-induced psychotic disorder may look and sound *exactly* like someone in an agitated psychotic or manic state, yet within 24 hours their thought process and level of psychomotor activity are largely back to normal. In contrast, symptoms of a primary psychiatric disorder will rarely resolve this quickly. Because of this, **rapid onset or resolution of symptoms** is highly suspicious for a substance-induced syndrome.

STIMULANTS

Stimulants, also known as "uppers," include a wide range of substances ranging from mild stimulants such as **caffeine** and **nicotine** to moderate stimulants including prescription drugs such as **methylphenidate** (Ritalin) and **amphetamine** salts (Adderall) and finally up to incredibly powerful stimulants like the illegal drugs

cocaine (coke or crack), **methamphetamine** (speed or crystal), and **MDMA** (ecstasy or molly). What these stimulants all share in common is that they increase the amounts of the neurotransmitters **dopamine** and **norepinephrine** in the central nervous system, leading to an overall activating effect.

People taking stimulants generally feel *fantastic*: they have increased energy, are better able to focus, feel less inhibited around other people, and are able to perform tasks better (a state that bears a striking resemblance to mania). Physiologically, the effects of stimulants are largely mediated by the **sympathetic nervous system** and include increases in vital signs (such as heart rate, blood pressure, breathing rate, and temperature) as well as mydriasis (or dilation of the pupils). At high doses, increased psychomotor energy can turn into restlessness, anxiety, paranoia, and aggression while overactivation of the sympathetic nervous system can lead to hypertension, hyperthermia, cardiac arrhythmias, or seizures. A state of **substance-induced psychosis** is commonly associated with high doses of stimulants like methamphetamine and can be clinically indistinguishable from either mania or primary psychosis.

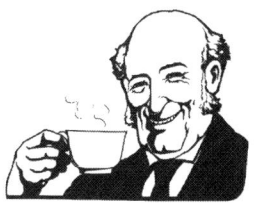

In contrast to the activating effects seen during intoxication with stimulants, stimulant withdrawal generally involves feelings of low energy, poor mood, and apathy (remember that *what goes up must come down*). Despite being uncomfortable, stimulant withdrawal is rarely life-threatening.

DEPRESSANTS

Depressants, also known as sedatives or "downers," include **alcohol** and the prescription drug classes **benzodiazepines** and **barbiturates**. These drugs work by binding to the **GABA** receptor which *inhibits* neuronal firing in the brain and causes a global *decrease* in central nervous system activity.

Depressant intoxication is associated with sleepiness, low energy, difficulty focusing, cognitive impairment, muscle relaxation, slowed motor activity, and poor muscle coordination (all of which together can strongly resemble a state of depression—hence the name "depressant"). Depressant overdoses present with severe sedation and slowed vital signs. In contrast to stimulants, depressants are significantly more **dangerous in overdose**. In the case of alcohol and barbiturates, overdose can even lead to coma or death. In fact, alcohol remains one of the leading causes of substance-related death in the United States, and barbiturates have even been used in lethal injections for many years. (Benzodiazepines are the exception here and are generally much safer in overdose.)

Withdrawal from depressants often involves feelings of restlessness, anxiety, and insomnia accompanied by increases in vital signs (*what goes down must come back up*). In severe cases of withdrawal, hallucinations, seizures, vital sign instability, or even death can occur. Alcohol withdrawal in particular deserves special mention, as it can be a potentially deadly state especially for people who have used alcohol regularly for long periods of time. Complicated alcohol withdrawal often requires admission to the hospital for close monitoring of vital signs and treatment with benzodiazepines to allow for a slow, steady return to baseline. The window for complicated withdrawal is usually **one week** following the last drink.

There are two clinical conditions related to alcohol withdrawal that you must be able to recognize and differentiate between. The first, **alcoholic hallucinosis**, is a generally *benign* state in which people experience transient visual, auditory, or tactile hallucinations within the first 24 hours of their last drink. Aside from monitoring for signs of complicated withdrawal, no specific treatment is needed. In contrast, the second condition, known as **delirium tremens** or DTs, is a *potentially deadly* state associated with severe vital sign instability, confusion, and both visual and auditory hallucinations (the classic "seeing pink elephants") that occurs around 24 to 72 hours after the last drink. In severe cases, seizures or death can occur. There are often objective signs of stress and organ damage as well, including markers of inflammation (such as elevated ESR and white blood cell count) and liver damage. You can remember the syndrome using the mnemonic **DTS are HELL**, which stands for **D**elirium, **T**remor, **S**eizures, **H**allucinations, **E**SR, **L**eukocytosis, and **L**iver function tests.

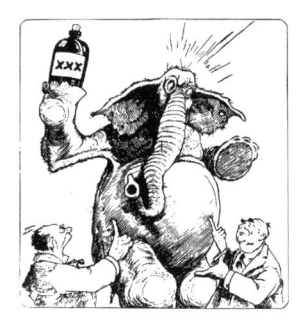

> **Delirium tremens** is a **potentially fatal** outcome of **alcohol withdrawal** that must be differentiated from **alcoholic hallucinosis**, which is more benign.
>
> *DTS are **HELL**:*
> **D**elirium
> **T**remor
> **S**eizures
> **H**allucinations
> **E**SR
> **L**eukocytosis
> **L**iver function abnormalities

OPIOIDS

Opioids include both **prescription painkillers** like morphine and oxycodone (OxyContin) as well as "street" drugs like **heroin**. (Despite differences in how they are handled legally, on a biological level there is no difference between prescription and recreational opioids.) Opioids are often lumped together with "downers" because they can cause sedation, but their pharmacologic effects differ enough from depressants to warrant separate consideration. Opioids bind to **opioid receptors** (rather than GABA receptors), leading to a state of reduced pain perception, drowsiness, and euphoria. Physiologically, use of opioids constricts the pupils (known as miosis), slows down the gastrointestinal tract (leading to constipation), and depresses the respiratory drive. It is this latter effect that makes opioids **extremely dangerous in overdose**, as the decrease in respiratory rate combined with a general stupor can lead to hypoxemia and death. To remember the functions of opioids, think of the 19th century disputes over British trade in China known as the Opium Wars. This will help you connect opioids to the mental image of an **ARMED C**olonialist, which stands for **A**nalgesia, **R**espiratory depression, **M**iosis, **E**uphoria, **D**rowsiness, and **C**onstipation.

Drugs that bind to **opioid receptors** are clinically useful as painkillers but can cause **respiratory depression, miosis, euphoria, drowsiness,** and **constipation** as well.

> *ARMED Colonialist:*
> *Analgesia*
> *Respiratory depression*
> *Miosis*
> *Euphoria*
> *Drowsiness*
> *Constipation*

As expected, opioid withdrawal produces the opposite signs and symptoms seen during intoxication, with *increased* pain perception, hyperventilation, mydriasis, dysphoria, restlessness, and diarrhea. In contrast to opioid intoxication and overdose, withdrawal from opioids is rarely dangerous (although it can be very uncomfortable).

CANNABINOIDS

Cannabinoids are the major psychoactive ingredients in **cannabis** or **marijuana**. In particular, **tetrahydrocannabinol** (THC) is the molecule responsible for producing the "high" that is commonly associated with use of cannabis. However, a variety of other effects are noticeable as well, including short-term memory loss, increased hunger, paranoia, decreased energy and motivation, and redness of the eyes.

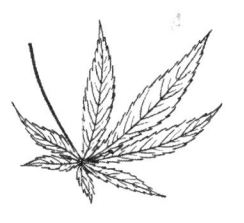

Notably, THC is not the only active cannabinoid found in cannabis. One of the most important to know about is **cannabidiol** (CBD) which actually *opposes* some of THC's effects. The particular balance between THC and CBD accounts for the different effects found in various strains of cannabis. Strains that have more THC tend to produce a greater "high," while those with more CBD tend to have greater analgesic, anti-inflammatory, and anti-anxiety effects. Because it opposes many of the effects that cannabis is known for, you can think of **CBD** as a **C**annabis **B**ringer **D**owner."

> **Tetrahydrocannabinol** is the active ingredient in **cannabis** while **cannabidiol** acts as a cannabinoid receptor **antagonist**.
>
> *THC is The High Chemical, CBD is the Cannabis Bringer Downer.*

Cannabinoids are relatively safe in overdose and have few, if any, negative effects in withdrawal. However, cannabinoids should also not be seen as entirely benign drugs, as long-term use (especially beginning in adolescence) has been linked not only to decreases in intelligence but also to an increased risk of developing a psychotic illness that can sometimes continue even after the drug has been stopped. Increasing clinical attention to negative psychiatric effects of cannabinoids may be due in part to increasing concentrations of THC in plants grown over the past few decades, which may warrant reconsideration of cannabis's status as a "benign" drug.

HALLUCINOGENS

Hallucinogens consist of two distinct classes of drugs: **serotonergic hallucinogens**, which include LSD (acid), psilocybin (mushrooms or shrooms), and mescaline (peyote), as well as **dissociative hallucinogens**, which include dextromethorphan, ketamine, and phencyclidine (PCP). Both classes of hallucinogens share the ability to profoundly affect one's senses, but they are ultimately quite different in their effects and clinical significance.

Serotonergic hallucinogens tend to cause **perceptual abnormalities** such as visual hallucinations, movement of inanimate objects, and a feeling that different senses are merging together. Serotonergic hallucinogens are not particularly dangerous in either intoxication or withdrawal and are not considered to be addictive.

In contrast, dissociative hallucinogens distort perceptions of sight and sound and produce feelings of detachment from one's **sense of reality** and **sense of self**. (The state of dissociation will be discussed more fully in Chapter 12.) Often, people taking dissociative hallucinogens report feeling that they are in a trance or **dream-like state**. Suppression of pain signals is often noted as well (with ketamine in particular finding use in clinical settings as an emergency anesthetic). Depending on the dose and the specific drug involved, other symptoms such as sedation, amnesia, and loss of coordination may be reported as well. The safety of dissociative hallucinogens varies from one substance to the next, with some (like dextromethorphan) being relatively benign and others (like ketamine and phencyclidine) being associated with a state of excited delirium that can resemble stimulant intoxication.

INHALANTS

Inhalants are a diverse class of substances that comprise everything from common household products like paint and glue to anesthetics like nitrous oxide or diethyl ether. Inhalants generally produce a transient "**head rush**" or "numbing" effect which lasts for only a few seconds or minutes. Given the short duration of action, it is unlikely that you will ever diagnose *acute* inhalant intoxication. In contrast, you may see people suffering the medical consequences of *chronic* inhalant use. While the negative effects vary depending on the specific compounds used, they can be quite severe, including permanent damage to the nose and lungs, increased risk of infection, and hypoxic brain damage. Due to their readily available and generally inexpensive nature, inhalants are often used by children, teenagers, and institutionalized or impoverished people who lack access to other psychoactive substances.

SIGNS AND SYMPTOMS OF ADDICTION

Now that we have an understanding of the states of intoxication and withdrawal associated with each type of substance, we can begin learning about the signs and symptoms of addiction. Intoxication and addiction are closely related concepts, as addiction typically involves repeated episodes of intoxication. However, from a diagnostic perspective they should be considered **separate diagnoses**, as not everyone who is intoxicated with a particular substance is necessarily addicted to it and not everyone who has an addiction is currently intoxicated.

The DSM-5 lists 11 distinct criteria for substance use disorders and other forms of addiction which you can remember using the phrase **Time 2 CUT DOWN PAL**. The 2 will remind you that **2 or more** of these criteria are required for diagnosis. The rest of the phrase will remind you that patients spend a lot of **T**ime using or obtaining the substance, experience **C**ravings or urges to continue using, are **U**nable to cut down on using the substance even after repeated attempts, experience **T**olerance to the effects of the substance so they need more and more to get the same effect, can have **D**angerous results of use, affect **O**ther people through their use resulting in interpersonal or social problems, experience **W**ithdrawal when they stop using the substance, end up **N**eglecting major roles and responsibilities such as work or family, have physical or psychological **P**roblems that have been created and/or made worse by substance use, have given up **A**ctivities like socializing or hobbies due to excessive use, and finally have used **L**arger amounts of the substance or for longer than wanted.

Addiction presents with a variety of signs and symptoms resulting in **distress** and **functional impairment.**

Time 2 CUT DOWN PAL:
Time spent
2 or more of these symptoms
Cravings
Unable to cut down
Tolerance
Dangerous use
Others affected
Withdrawal
Neglect of roles/responsibilities
Problems created or made worse
Activities given up
Larger amounts or for longer

However, these 11 criteria are a lot to remember, and you can recognize the overall pattern of addiction using just 3 things which we will refer to as the **3 Reapers: rep**eated use of **re**inforcers (**p**ositive) despite negative **rep**ercussions. If those eight words describe the pattern of someone's behavior, then in most cases you can diagnose addiction. Let's go ahead and break the 3 Reapers down into their three components:

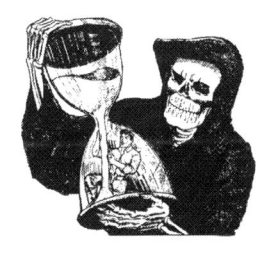

Repeated use. Addiction involves doing something repeatedly. This can involve use of substances, such as alcohol, or specific items or behaviors, such as gambling at slot machines.

Positive reinforcers. The specific substances and behaviors in addiction must be positively reinforcing. To understand what is meant by this, we will need to discuss the concept of **operant conditioning**. Operant conditioning describes how a behavior can be modified by the response it gets. **Reinforcement** is any response that *increases* the frequency of the behavior, while **punishment** is any response that *decreases* its frequency. As one example, picture a boy trying to sneak a cookie from the cookie jar before dinner. If he is caught, he will get a swat on the hand (a punishment meant to decrease that particular behavior). On the other hand, if he gets away with it, the deliciousness of the cookie may act as a reinforcer of that behavior, and he is likely to try and sneak more cookies in the future.

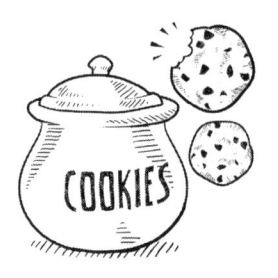

Reinforcements and punishments can be described as either **positive** or **negative**. Positive and negative refer to whether something is *introduced* or *taken away*. In the cookie example, both the reinforcer (the cookie) and the punishment (a slap on the hand) would be considered *positive* because they both introduce something into the situation. However, if the mother had taken away something that the boy desired (such as access to the TV), this would be considered a *negative* punishment as the behavior was made less frequent by taking something away. In contrast, if the boy was incredibly hungry and the cookie's primary effect was to remove hunger, this would also be a *negative* reinforcement. A negative reinforcer can also act by *preventing* an aversive experience. For example, someone who studies hard for a test may be negatively reinforced by avoiding the upsetting experience of getting a bad grade, and they will likely continue to study hard in the future.

Negative repercussions. Finally, negative repercussions of use, such as losing a job, alienating family and friends, getting into legal trouble, or jeopardizing one's health, are a key part of the equation for addiction, and addiction cannot be diagnosed in their absence.

Addiction involves **repeated use** of **positive reinforcers** despite **negative repercussions**.

The 3 Reapers: Repeated use of Reinforcers (positive) despite negative Repercussions.

None of these components on their own are sufficient to diagnose addiction. Even *any two* of them combined is not enough. It is only when *all three* components combine that the specific state of addiction emerges. To demonstrate this, let's see what happens when we remove any one of these components from the definition:

Repeated use of positive reinforcers (but no negative repercussions). Repeated use of positive reinforcers is not a problem as long as there are no repercussions. Technically speaking, things like eating an apple a day could fall under the banner of "repeated use of positive reinforcers," but because they cause no negative repercussions, they would not satisfy any reasonable definition of addiction.

Use of positive reinforcers with negative repercussions (but not repeated). This is slightly more problematic, as even a one-time exposure to specific substances can cause damage. However, if it is not repeated—if the person is able to avoid the problematic reinforcer in the future—then by definition it cannot be an addiction. For example, someone with a severe nut allergy who ate trail mix (a positive reinforcer) could potentially end up in the hospital (a negative repercussion). However, this person would likely try to avoid trail mix in the future and make sure this experience is not repeated, so it would not make sense to call this an addiction.

Repeated use of things (that are not positively reinforcing) despite negative consequences. This is the behavior that is *most* tempting to call an addiction, but it is more accurately characterized as a **compulsion** (which we will talk about more in Chapter 10). To understand what a compulsion is, picture someone who is perpetually worried about exposure to germs and frequently uses hand sanitizer throughout the day (repeated use). Perhaps they use it so much that they begin to erode the skin on their hands, making them more susceptible to infections (negative repercussions). However, this person is not using hand sanitizer because it is inherently pleasurable in the same way that someone using cocaine and heroin would be. Instead, they are using it as a *negative* reinforcer to calm an internal sense of anxiety, making it a compulsive (rather than addictive) behavior. While differentiating between compulsive and addictive behavior may seem like a minor technicality, from a clinical standpoint these two entities are associated with completely different prognoses and treatment requirements, making such a distinction crucial.

Having this behavioral framework can help us understand two of the patterns brought up in the **Time 2 CUT DOWN PAL** mnemonic: tolerance and withdrawal. **Tolerance** occurs when the same reinforcer feels less and less pleasurable each time it is used. Someone who tries heroin for the first time may experience "the most perfect feeling of bliss" that they have ever experienced in their life—everything is wonderful, peaceful, perfect, and pleasantly numb. However, several hours later this state begins to wear off. Wanting to return to this wonderland, they take another hit. While some of the effect comes back, it's not as good as the first time. Frustrated, they try taking a larger hit but still can't quite get back to where they were before. After a while, they are using heroin more often and via more direct methods (such as injecting directly into their veins). They have sold their possessions, estranged all family and friends, and are living on the street. Still, that perfect dream world that they experienced the first time remains as elusive as ever. (This is sometimes called "chasing the dragon.")

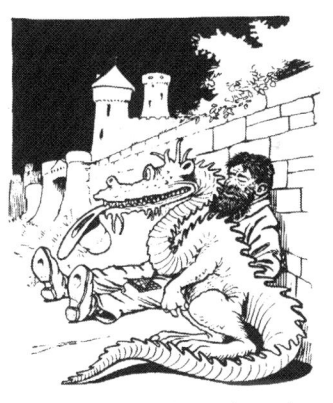

We learned earlier that **withdrawal** is a state of distress and discomfort when one attempts to quit using. For example, someone who is addicted to heroin may experience a withdrawal state involving high levels of anxiety, restlessness, insomnia, muscle aches, cramping, diarrhea, nausea, and vomiting. In someone who is highly tolerant to the drug, they may continue using it largely to avoid a withdrawal state rather than for any euphoric rush (which may have long since disappeared). This illustrates an important point regarding addiction: while the object of an addiction is often positively reinforcing at the beginning, in most cases the *positive* reinforcement wanes over time and is replaced by primarily *negative* reinforcement.

Tolerance and withdrawal together help to explain why addictions are so powerful, as they involve *both* positive and negative punishments for stopping as well as *both* positive and negative reinforcements for using it again. Someone who attempts to quit heroin not only loses the intensely pleasurable state of euphoria from the drug (a negative punishment) but also experiences an incredibly uncomfortable withdrawal state (a positive punishment). Using heroin again removes this withdrawal state (a negative reinforcement) and provides that sense of euphoria which, while lesser than the first time they used, remains intrinsically rewarding (a positive reinforcement). This combination of **all four kinds of reinforcement** is so potent that it can overwhelm the ability of other interventions to decrease the behavior. This explains why many people who are addicted to specific reinforcers often continue to use them despite repeatedly being severely punished for their use and are resistant to interventions (such as going to jail or being paid cash to not use drugs) that involve only a single kind of reinforcement.

ADDICTION ACROSS THE LIFESPAN

More than any of the conditions we have talked about so far, addiction is a **highly variable disorder** that is dependent upon multiple factors. Most important among these is the **specific reinforcer** involved, as tobacco use disorder differs from alcohol use disorder which differs from opioid use disorder which differs from gambling disorder and so on. Nevertheless, despite this wide variation, a few consistent themes emerge when looking at addiction across the lifespan.

EPIDEMIOLOGY

Taken as a whole, addiction is one of the most common psychiatric conditions with a lifetime prevalence of around 10% of people in the United States. This gives it a relatively **high base rate** in the population, making it liable to **underdiagnosis** rather than overdiagnosis. The risk of underdiagnosis is compounded further by the fact that many people will attempt to minimize or hide addictive behaviors from their providers due to the stigma and prejudice that often occur.

Most addictions begin during **adolescence** or early adulthood, with some arguing that substance abuse is in many cases a pediatric disease. However, in many cases, addictive behavior can continue on into adulthood or older age as well. In systematic studies, **men and women** appear to be equally vulnerable to addiction. However, in clinical settings, men are treated for addictive disorders more than twice as often as women. This difference in gender ratio is likely due to the fact that men tend to use illegal substances more often than women (who may be more prone to addictions involving legal substances such as alcohol or benzodiazepines that are less likely to come to clinical attention even if they can be equally harmful).

Addiction is **frequently comorbid** with other mental disorders. In fact, up to half of all people with a mental disorder will meet lifetime criteria for a substance use disorder and vice versa. The presence of both an addiction and a separate mental disorder (known as **dual diagnosis**) worsens the prognosis for both types of disorders considerably. This makes screening for addictive behaviors important for every patient presenting with mental health concerns. While the specific reinforcer that is the target of the addiction carries important implications for both prognosis and treatment, ultimately the diagnosis of addiction is independent of the particular reinforcer involved, as the core features of the disorder (including frequent use, cravings, tolerance, and severe consequences of use due to the increasing time and effort spent on obtaining the reinforcer) are found across all addictions.

PROGNOSIS

Like other aspects of addiction, the prognosis for addictive disorders is **highly variable**, with the strongest predictor of prognosis being the specific reinforcer involved. Reinforcers differ significantly in regards to how addictive they are, with some being incredibly addictive and others having only minimal addictive properties. For example, less than 10% of people who try cannabis become dependent upon it, but this increases to 15% for cocaine, 25% for heroin, and more than 67% for nicotine. A couple of factors, including the speed at which the drug reaches the brain and how strongly it interacts with the dopamine receptor, are strongly correlated to how addictive a substance is. These variations lead to clinically significant differences in prognosis, with certain drugs becoming more addictive when they are inhaled (consider that injected heroin is significantly more addictive than orally ingested heroin). The inherent addictiveness of the reinforcer also plays a large role in how easy it is to quit, with cannabis use disorder taking on average 5 years to enter remission while tobacco use disorder takes 25 years.

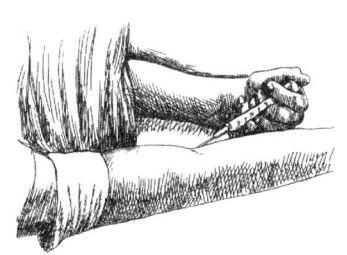

Despite common stereotypes of "lifelong junkies," the prognosis for addiction is actually not as bad as widely believed. This is due to the fact that most studies on patients with addiction were conducted on people who were receiving treatment for addiction within the health care system, where severe and treatment-resistant addictions tend to be overrepresented. In reality, the majority of people who struggle with addiction are able to enter remission without ever coming to medical attention. That is not to say that there are not cases where the outcomes of addiction are very dire! In fact, the personal, social, and societal harm caused by addiction places it up there with some of the biggest killers in medicine, including diabetes and cancer. However, it's important to remember that a diagnosis of addiction does not make someone "an addict" or doom them to a life of misery. For many people, it is entirely possible to overcome addiction with or without treatment.

TREATMENT

Like prognosis, treatment for addiction is also **highly variable**. For some people, quitting an addiction is as simple as deciding to stop. For others, the initial desire to quit is followed by decades of bouncing between abstinence and relapses. For still others, the desire to quit is never there at all. Because of this variability, statistics on the efficacy of addiction treatment are not very informative until they are broken down by the specific reinforcers involved.

As a general process, treatment of addiction involves facilitating the initial transition to *achieving* sobriety (known as **detoxification** or "detox"). This is followed by treatment focused on *maintaining* sobriety (known as **rehabilitation** or "rehab"). For some reinforcers, detoxification is as easy as just stopping. For others (like alcohol), detoxification may require admission to a medical facility for intensive monitoring. Following detoxification, rehabilitation can be accomplished using a variety of treatment modalities. **Individual and group therapy** can teach skills to decrease cravings and impulsivity. For certain reinforcers such as opioids and alcohol, **medications** can play a role by preventing withdrawal, reducing cravings, and blocking the positive effects of the reinforcer. However, for other reinforcers like methamphetamine or cocaine, no medications have yet proven to be helpful.

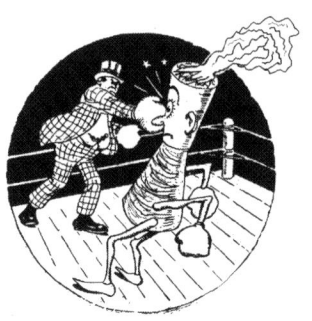

Of course, even beginning the process of detoxification and rehabilitation requires that the patient is motivated for treatment. However, in many cases, addiction can significantly impair one's insight that their use is problematic, even in the face of significant evidence to the contrary (someone can go from being a good father with a stable career to a homeless person living on the street in the span of a year and *still* deny that there is any kind of problem). In fact, it is estimated that less than 20% of people struggling with addiction will seek treatment on their own. To address this, a specific counseling technique known as **motivational interviewing** can be used to increase a patient's motivation to treat their addiction. Rather than approaching all patients with addiction in the same way, motivational interviewing encourages providers to identify the **stage of change** that the patient is in and use specific techniques that are appropriate for that stage. For example, when working with someone who doesn't think that their alcohol use is a problem, asking them to set a quit date is unlikely to be effective. Instead, asking the patient to think of ways in which their drinking may be harmful is more likely to be effective. By matching interventions to the stage of change, patients are more likely to quit. Motivational interviewing has a **large effect size** of 0.8 compared to treatment as usual.

Relapses are common in addiction treatment, and **relapses should not be viewed as failure** either on the part of the patient, the provider, or the treatment itself. In fact, placing too strong of an emphasis on sobriety as the only end-point of treatment can be counterproductive. Instead of merely *eliminating* the addiction, it is more helpful to *replace* it with other activities that the patient finds satisfying. For many people, engaging in meaningful work, hobbies, or social activities can help to prevent the sense of boredom or emptiness that often leads to relapses. Some evidence suggests that social support is one of the most important, if not *the* most important, predictor of successful treatment. Because of this, it is helpful to think that **the opposite of addiction is not sobriety but connection and community**.

MECHANISMS OF ADDICTION

While the concepts of operant conditioning can help us to understand the behavioral processes at work in addiction, they don't explain why some individuals develop an addiction after even a single exposure to a reinforcer while others remain functional despite decades of use. As with many parts of psychiatry, *it's never just one thing*. While we have already explored how different drugs vary in their addictiveness, different people also appear to vary in their inherent **vulnerability to addiction**.

The precise reasons why some people are more prone to addiction than others are unclear. Some evidence has suggested that people who are prone to addiction are more likely to experience **negative emotions at baseline**. This makes use of substances *both positively and negatively reinforcing* from the very first use by not only inducing a pleasurable feeling but also relieving the state of chronic dysphoria in which the person lives. (Compare this to someone who is generally happy with their life and would therefore only receive positive reinforcement from use of substances.)

However, some additional factors have also been found to stratify the risk of developing an addiction. In particular, **impulsivity** also appears to be a significant risk factor for addictive disorders. In a classic experiment, children were given access to a sweet treat (a marshmallow) and told that they could either eat it immediately or wait 15 minutes to be given a second marshmallow. Children who were able to delay gratification for longer (an indicator of low impulsivity) were found to have lower rates of addiction as adults, suggesting that impulse control and the ability to delay gratification are protective against developing addictive disorders. In contrast, the children who ate the marshmallow right away were noted to be at much higher risk of addiction later in life, suggesting that their inability to refrain from activities which provided **im**mediate **pos**itive reinforcement is related to problems with impulse control (which you can write as "**impos** control" to connect the two concepts).

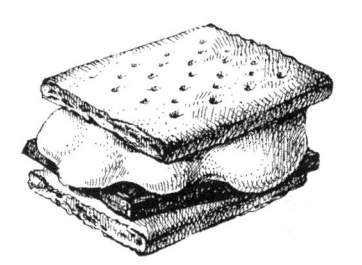

> **Addiction** often involves **poor impulse control** or a tendency to seek **immediate positive reinforcers** without consideration of consequences.
>
> *Impos control problems are related to immediate positive reinforcement (even if there are long-term negative consequences later).*

However, a later variant of this experiment found that intrinsic personality factors do not tell the whole story, as people's perceptions of how reliable their environment is also plays a strong role. For example, if prior to the experiment a child is made a similar promise by an adult ("If you wait, then you will be rewarded") but then fails to receive it ("I'm sorry, we are out of any additional marshmallows today"), they are more likely to decide against delaying gratification again and would instead eat the marshmallow right away, as they now believe that promises of future gains cannot be reliably counted on. This suggests that growing up in chaotic or unstable environments can also play a large role in impulsivity and the later development of addictive disorders. Under these kinds of conditions, a greater focus on immediate gains may actually be an adaptive response to an unreliable environment.

The combination of a tendency towards negative emotions (which makes use of drugs both positively *and* negatively reinforcing from the get-go) along with a greater focus on immediate rewards over long-term gains appears to predispose certain individuals over others to developing addictive behaviors. Once exposure to these reinforcers has occurred, however, a different set of processes involving the protein **Delta FosB** (or ΔFosB) take over. ΔFosB appears to play a critical role in all forms of addiction by acting as a "**molecular switch**" that is turned on following exposure to a reinforcer. Interestingly, ΔFosB appears to be involved in *all* addictions regardless of the specific reinforcers involved, including drugs like heroin and cocaine or behaviors like gambling and shopping. You can remember the association of ΔFosB with addiction by thinking of the Δ as a triangle with the **3 Reapers** in each corner:

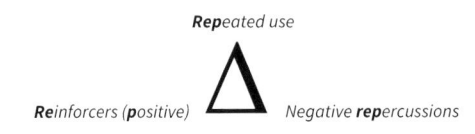

Repeated use

Δ

Reinforcers (positive)   *Negative repercussions*

ΔFosB is involved in both substance-related and behavioral addictions.

*Think of the Δ in ΔFosB as a **triangle** with the **3 Reapers** at each corner.*

ΔFosB acts to stimulate neuronal growth in dopamine-producing neurons in the **ventral tegmental area** which itself projects to the **nucleus accumbens**, the primary region of the brain where many addictive substances act. These brain areas, known collectively as the **reward circuitry**, have played a key role in the evolutionary success of our species as they are involved in promoting many of the behaviors (such as eating nutrient-rich food, seeking sexual partners, and gaining possessions) that are not only pleasurable but also necessary for survival. When these brain regions are hijacked by specific substances, however, the normally adaptive seeking behaviors can become pathological and lead to distress and dysfunction. With enough exposure, the reward circuitry soon becomes non-responsive to anything *but* that particular reinforcer, leading to a state of anhedonia ("Nothing else in my life feels good—only heroin."). This anhedonia can be a major obstacle to abstinence, as the things that normally bring pleasure have been rendered ineffective. This has important implications for treatment, and healthcare providers must be mindful to help their find specific things (like socializing or exercise) that still feel good.

Overall, the mechanisms of addiction are varied and complex, involving psychological concepts (operant conditioning), personality factors (impulsivity and the tendency to experience negative emotions at baseline), environmental influences (the predictability and stability of one's circumstances), molecular biology (ΔFosB), and brain circuity (the ventral tegmental area and nucleus accumbens). By taking the time to understand the role that each of these mechanisms plays, we can better understand our patients and get them the help that they need.

HOW TO DIAGNOSE ADDICTIVE DISORDERS

Addiction is not hard to diagnose. As long as all 3 Reapers are there (**rep**eated use, **p**ositive **re**inforcers, and negative **rep**ercussions), you can diagnose addiction. In clinical practice, a diagnosis of addiction is often made on the basis of supporting history, including psychological symptoms (like cravings), specific behaviors (such as spending a lot of time attempting to obtain the reinforcer), and consequences of that behavior (including lost jobs, legal penalties, and medical problems). You can systematically gather a complete substance history using the mnemonic **TRAPPED** which stands for **T**reatment history, **R**oute of administration, **A**mount used, **P**attern of use, **P**rior abstinence, **E**ffects of use (both positive and negative), and **D**uration of use.

> A **complete substance history** should systematically evaluate the **pattern of the patient's substance use** and their **attempts at sobriety**, if any.
>
> *TRAPPED:*
> *Treatment history*
> *Route of administration*
> *Amount used*
> *Pattern of use*
> *Prior abstinence*
> *Effects of use*
> *Duration of use*

Historically, the DSM made a distinction between substance **abuse** (repeated use of a substance despite adverse consequences) and **dependence** (needing to use a substance to avoid a withdrawal state). However, in the DSM-5 this distinction was dropped in favor of a single diagnosis: **substance use disorder**. A diagnosis of a substance use disorder should specify the specific substance involved (such as alcohol use disorder or opioid use disorder). People with multiple substance use disorders should have them listed separately, as each can be at a different level of severity. For example, someone could have "alcohol use disorder, severe, active," "opioid use disorder, in partial remission on maintenance therapy," and "methamphetamine use disorder, in long-term remission" all at the same time. Because of this, for a patient with multiple substance use disorders, you should list each of them separately rather than using a broad and unhelpful term like "polysubstance use disorder."

In this section, we will revisit each of the major classes of psychoactive drugs through the lens of how they appear in cases of addiction, including their diagnosis, prognosis, and treatment. We will also touch briefly on behavioral addictions.

STIMULANT USE DISORDER

Stimulant use disorder generally refers to addiction to either **methamphetamine** or **cocaine**, as caffeine use generally does not result in significant pathology and nicotine addiction differs enough in its prognosis and treatment that it is considered separately as tobacco use disorder. Because stimulants provide a subjective sense of energy and euphoria, they can be very positively reinforcing, making stimulants among the most addictive substances. Despite several studies, **no medications** have been shown to be helpful with treating stimulant use disorder. Instead, a variety of interventions (such as cognitive behavioral therapy, motivational interviewing, or even just paying people for negative drug tests) have shown some efficacy. Overall, stimulant use disorder tends to have a **good prognosis**, with around 80% of methamphetamine-dependent patients achieving remission within 5 years of diagnosis.

TOBACCO USE DISORDER

Nicotine (the active ingredient in tobacco products like cigarettes) is the single **most addictive substance** in the world. Not only is nicotine incredibly addictive through its rapid absorption into the brain, it is also widely available, making maintaining abstinence even more challenging. Nicotine withdrawal is also associated with particularly **severe cravings**. All of this makes smoking cessation incredibly difficult. However, it is important to encourage your patients to quit smoking, as tobacco use is associated with a host of health problems, including an increased risk of cardiovascular disease and various types of cancer. In fact, smoking cessation is the single **most effective lifestyle modification** you can encourage for your patients in nearly all cases!

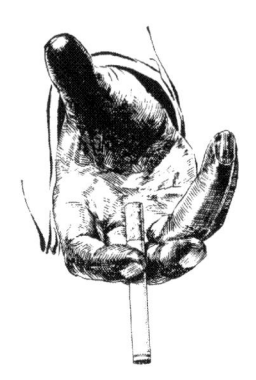

Effective treatment strategies for tobacco use disorder exist and include **medications**, **therapy**, or both. **Nicotine replacement therapy** (including nicotine gums or patches), the nicotinic receptor partial agonist **varenicline**, and the antidepressant **bupropion** have all shown efficacy at improving quit rates, with varenicline being the most effective. **Psychosocial treatments** are also helpful by providing personal support and teaching patients how to cope effectively with cravings. However, even with treatment, smoking cessation is a long process. For many people, it can take several years and multiple attempts to quit before sustained abstinence is achieved.

ALCOHOL USE DISORDER

Alcohol causes the most harm of any single psychoactive substance due to its legal status, wide availability, and severe medical, social, and societal consequences of misuse. Because of this, identifying and treating alcohol use disorder is of primary importance. A specialized screening tool has been developed to help identify patients with an active alcohol use disorder. Anyone who answers "Yes" to 2 or more of the following **CAGE** questions has a high likelihood of having an alcohol use disorder: "Have you ever felt you ought to **C**ut down on your drinking?" "Have people **A**nnoyed you by criticizing your drinking?" "Have you ever felt **G**uilty about your drinking?" and "Have you ever had an **E**ye-opener (a drink first thing in the morning)?"

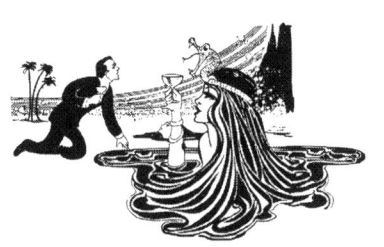

> Screen for **alcohol use disorder** using the four **CAGE questions**.
>
> *CAGE ("yes" to 2 or more is a positive screen):*
> **C**ut down
> **A**nnoyed
> **G**uilty
> **E**ye-opener

Alcohol is a highly toxic substance that has been linked to increased rates of metabolic diseases, brain damage, and various kinds of cancer. However, the most commonly affected organ is the **liver**, which metabolizes alcohol. People with extensive histories of alcohol use often have signs of liver damage including elevated hepatic enzymes. While there are increases in both aspartate transaminase (AST) and alanine transaminase (ALT), a greater increase in AST compared to ALT (known as the **AST/ALT ratio**) is characteristic of chronic alcohol abuse. You can remember the greater increase in **AST** by thinking that getting w**AST**ed raises your **AST**.

> A **high AST-to-ALT ratio** is characteristic of **alcohol use disorder**.
>
> *Getting w**AST**ed raises your **AST**.*

Another liver enzyme known as gamma-glutamyl transferase (GGT) is a highly *sensitive* marker of chronic alcohol use. Combined with a high AST/ALT ratio, it is highly suggestive of excessive alcohol intake. You can remember the association of **GGT** with alcohol by thinking that it is elevated in people who are **G**onna **G**et **T**rashed.

> Elevated **gamma-glutamyl transferase** is a sensitive index of **alcohol use disorder**.
>
> ***G**onna **G**et **T**rashed and raise my **GGT**!*

Effective treatments are available for alcohol use disorder. As mentioned previously, alcohol withdrawal is potentially deadly, so detoxification programs with close monitoring of vital signs is often necessarily (particularly in cases where there is a history of complicated withdrawal). **Benzodiazepines** can be used to treat vital sign abnormalities or seizures if they occur. Once the patient is successfully detoxified off of alcohol, a variety of **rehabilitation** strategies are available, including both individual and group therapy. A variety of medications are also available for chronic treatment of alcohol use disorder, although these must generally be paired with other forms of support to be effective. These medications work by a variety of mechanisms. Some, like **disulfiram**, introduce an element of positive punishment to drinking by causing a build-up of toxic metabolites whenever someone drinks, making them feel incredibly sick. Another drug known as **naltrexone** blocks the ability of alcohol to activate opioid receptors and thereby reduces the pleasurable sensation that one gets from drinking. Finally, **acamprosate** acts by opposing glutamate, a neurotransmitter that is hyperactive in people who have previously been alcohol dependent, and helping to make a state of chronic alcohol withdrawal more bearable. These three medications each can play a role in treatment of alcohol use disorder, though generally they have **low effect sizes** in the range of 0.1 to 0.4.

BENZODIAZEPINE USE DISORDER
Use of benzodiazepines is common, with up to 15% of adults having taken at least one dose in the past year. When used on a short-term basis for treatment of anxiety, these medications can be very effective. However, with long-term use a number of worrying patterns emerge, including memory impairment, disinhibition, depression, emotional blunting, and psychological and physiologic dependence resulting in a tendency to make anxiety *worse* rather than better. The majority of benzodiazepine misuse also occurs in the context of use of other substances (often alcohol and opioids) that can increase the toxicity of these drugs in overdose significantly. While *dependence* upon benzodiazepines is common, *addiction* is rare because the desired effect of these medications is to *remove* a state of anxiety, making them *negatively* (rather than positively) reinforcing. For this reason, chronic misuse of benzodiazepines represents a *compulsive* behavior rather than an addictive behavior in most cases (people take them to *not feel bad* rather than to *start feeling good*).

The best way of preventing benzodiazepine misuse is to avoid prescribing them in anything but short courses with the smallest amount possible and only when there are no better alternatives. For someone who is already misusing benzodiazepines, a taper should be scheduled. While this can result in an uncomfortable and protracted withdrawal state, many people notice that their depression and anxiety both improve considerably once the taper is completed, making it a worthwhile effort.

OPIOID USE DISORDER
Misuse of opioids is increasingly common in the United States, with up to 2% of adults having used heroin at some point in their lives. On a clinical level, there is no difference between prescription painkillers and illicit narcotics, and many people will transition from one to the other. Opioids can be **extremely dangerous in overdose** due to their tendency to cause respiratory depression, and deaths related to opioid overdoses have reached crisis levels in many parts of the country.

Treatment for opioid use disorder involves an initial phase of detoxification. Opioid withdrawal can be incredibly uncomfortable, including emotional dysphoria, restlessness, muscle aches, nausea, vomiting, abdominal cramping, and diarrhea. While this is not dangerous, treating withdrawal symptoms with medications can facilitate abstinence by removing the positive punishment for abstinence. Following detoxification, patients with opioid use disorder often need long-term efforts to prevent relapse. The evidence suggests that the best treatments involve a combination of **medications** and **psychosocial treatment** rather than either alone. Medications can either block the opioid receptor directly, as in **naltrexone**, or bind to the opioid receptor in a way that doesn't induce euphoria or interfere with functioning in the way that addictive opioids do, as in **methadone** or **buprenorphine**.

CANNABIS USE DISORDER
Cannabis is significantly less addictive compared to other substances like opioids or nicotine. However, because cannabis is widely used (with over half of American adults having tried it at some point), cannabis dependence has a relatively high base rate in the population at around 4%. The majority of people who are dependent upon cannabis begin before the age of 25, and most use it in addition to other substances. While cannabis is not particularly dangerous in either overdose or withdrawal, it can lead to dysfunction in life due to persistent apathy and low motivation. Treatment strategies for cannabis use disorder have been poorly studied, although motivational interviewing and CBT appear most effective so far.

BEHAVIORAL ADDICTIONS
Behavioral addictions involve specific reinforcers that are not *biologically* active in the same way that drugs are but can still be powerfully rewarding. While the DSM-5 makes a distinction between substance use disorders and behavioral addictions, research on the underlying neural mechanisms has shown that substance use disorders and behavioral addictions are much more alike than they are different, as both activate ΔFosB and stimulate neuronal changes in the reward circuitry.

Gambling is the best studied of the behavioral addictions and is the only one listed as a discrete diagnosis in the DSM-5. Gambling is particularly addictive because it operates on a **variable reinforcement schedule**. To better understand what is meant by this term, compare a slot machine to a vending machine. A vending machine acts in the same way every time: if you put in $1, you will get a can of soda. Therefore, you go to a vending machine when you want a drink but not at any other times. In contrast, a slot machine is inherently *unpredictable*: if you put in $1, you don't know if you will get $0, $1, or $100 back. Variable reinforcement schedules seem to intrinsically be much more addictive than predictable reinforcement schedules and make the rewards seem much more enticing and valuable. This unpredictability is incredibly **salient** to our brains and motivates us to act, and for this reason variable reinforcement schedules are often highly addictive. Because of this, addiction to slot machines and other forms of gambling are much slower to go away than addiction to vending machines. While a slot machine is a classic example, variable reinforcement schedules are increasingly found in other media, including video games.

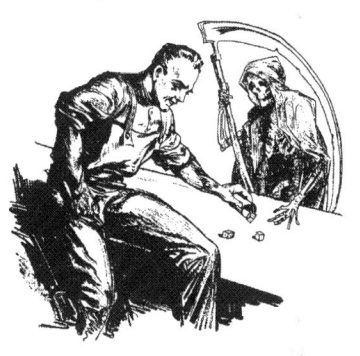

Variable reinforcement schedules can lead to **behavioral addictions**.

Veri-able reinforcement schedules are ***very able*** to addict people!

While gambling is the only behavioral addiction officially recognized in the DSM, a variety of other behavioral addictions have been studied including addiction to food, **pornography**, **shopping**, and the **internet**, among other things. What each of these things has in common is that they represent a **supernormal stimulus**, or something that has long been adaptive for humans to desire but is now available in such concentrated form that our attraction to it leads to unhealthy patterns.

Let's use food as an example. Throughout our species' history, we had access to naturally occurring foods like meat, nuts, fruits, and vegetables. Our brains are finely tuned so that these "normal" reinforcers are *just* rewarding enough that we will spend *some* of our time seeking it (but not *so* rewarding that we spend *all* of our time seeking it). However, in the modern day there are cookies, chips, and ice cream, each of which combines fat, sugar, and salt into a hyper-appetizing delicacy that evolution has not prepared us for. Exposure to these supernormal foods hijacks this our otherwise helpful reward circuitry and, for some people, turns food an all-consuming obsession.

Pornography is another example. It is evolutionarily advantageous for humans to place a high priority on seeking out sexual partners and to devote time and resources to attracting a mate. However, in an age where the internet provides easy access to millions of perceived potential sexual partners at all times of the day, our adaptive desire to bond and procreate has been co-opted by concentrated stimuli that, for some, becomes excessive and unhealthy, leading to addictive patterns.

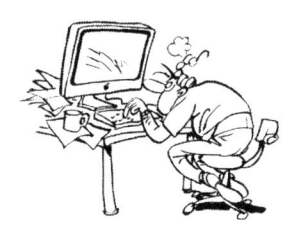

While there is controversy in the field of psychiatry about whether behavioral addictions are "true" addictions in the same way as substance use disorders, the fact that they fit the same pattern (repeated use of positive reinforcers despite negative repercussions) and involve the same biological mechanisms (ΔFosB and the reward circuitry) argues for a shared diagnostic approach. Treatment for behavioral addictions also resembles substance use disorders to a large degree, with motivational interviewing, CBT, and psychosocial therapies being helpful. While no medications have been approved specifically for treating behavioral addictions, some (including naltrexone) have been shown in a few studies to reduce pathological gambling, shopping, sexual behavior, and internet use.

DIFFERENTIAL DIAGNOSIS OF ADDICTIVE DISORDERS

Unlike depression, bipolar disorder, and schizophrenia where a precise understanding of the phenomenology of these conditions is necessary ("Is it decreased sleep or decreased *need* for sleep?" "Are the voices coming from *inside* or *outside* their head?"), cases of addiction can largely be diagnosed using easily understandable signs and symptoms (such as those in the **Time 2 CUT DOWN PAL** mnemonic) or, even more simply, by using the **3 Reapers**. Because of this, the primary pitfalls to avoid when diagnosing addiction are *missed* diagnoses rather than *mis*diagnoses. Due to the high comorbidity between addiction and other mental disorders, anyone presenting with an addiction should be carefully screened for the presence of other psychiatric syndromes (such as mood disorders, anxiety, schizophrenia, personality disorders, PTSD, and OCD) and vice versa.

While misdiagnosing an addiction as a different disorder is rare, misdiagnosing the effects of substance use as a primary psychiatric disorder is more common. This is because the effects of specific substances can not only mimic nearly every psychiatric syndrome but also can increase the risk of developing various mental disorders (such as alcohol-induced depressive disorder or cannabis-induced psychotic disorder). There is often a "chicken or egg?" question intrinsic to the discussion of any substance-induced disorder ("Did this person become depressed because of their addiction, or did they get addicted because they were depressed?"). While the answer to this question can be helpful to guiding treatment ("Do we treat the depression or alcoholism first?"), a clear and unambiguous answer is not always found. In these cases, it is generally best to **treat the addiction first** and see whether the psychiatric symptoms resolve accordingly. In cases where they do not, separate treatment of a mental disorder may be necessary.

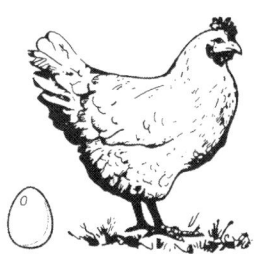

NORMALCY

Engaging in "vices" like drug use or gambling is not inherently pathological. Recall from the 3 Reapers that negative repercussions are a necessary component for diagnosing addiction, so in the absence of any significant consequences, you should not diagnose addiction even if someone is engaging in repeated use of positive reinforcers. It's also worthwhile to keep in mind that negative repercussions from substance use do not exist in a vacuum. For example, someone who has a medical condition like multiple sclerosis may use cannabis as an evidence-based way of relieving spasticity. However, in many places, use of cannabis for *any* reason remains illegal, making it possible that this person could get fired from their job or sent to prison. If this happens, can we now diagnose this person as having a *disorder*? This position seems difficult to hold, especially considering that this exact same person would not have had the same repercussions if they lived in a different place where cannabis use was legal. In these cases, the negative repercussions of addiction can be more accurately attributed to *societal* (rather than personal) dysfunction, yet our diagnostic system is designed in such a way that a diagnosis is always *personal* (rather than societal). These grey areas reveal the limits of an artificial diagnostic scheme that attempts to impose strict limits upon an inherently messy subject. For this reason, always use your judgment on where to draw the line between normalcy and addiction, and try your best to avoid knee-jerk diagnoses of addiction (such as diagnosing cannabis use disorder for someone who uses cannabis but has no problems from it).

MOOD DISORDERS

The specific behavioral effects of particular substances can often be mistaken for mood disorders. Stimulants like methamphetamine can resemble mania, while depressants can obviously resemble depression. Paying close attention to the **timing** of symptom onset in relation to substance use can help to resolve this ambiguity.

Mania deserves special mention, as the impulsivity and hyperhedonia seen in mania can manifest in excessive use of drugs and other reinforcers. For some people, this "pseudoaddictive" behavior will go away with resolution of mania, making it more likely that the addictive behaviors can be attributed entirely to the recklessness of mania. However, in other cases, substance use that began during mania can develop into a "full blown" addiction that persists even after the mood episode resolves. Be cautious when diagnosing addiction during a manic state, but don't rule out the possibility entirely.

PSYCHOSIS
A variety of drugs can induce a state that strongly resembles psychosis, including drugs like methamphetamine that result in excessive release of dopamine. Always have substance-induced psychotic disorder on the differential for anyone presenting with psychotic symptoms, especially if they **appear suddenly**, **resolve quickly**, or occur along with other features (such as increased vital signs) that suggest that something more may be going on. In addition, keep in mind that chronic use of methamphetamines and cannabis can lead to *persistent* psychotic syndromes, so in these cases the symptoms may remain even once the substance is stopped.

OBSESSIVE-COMPULSIVE DISORDER
The repetitive harmful behaviors seen in OCD can often be mistaken for the repetitive harmful behaviors seen in addiction. Pay close attention to whether the behavior is *positively* reinforcing (as in addiction) or *negatively* reinforcing (as in OCD or related disorders). While this point can seem technical, it matters a lot for prognosis and treatment, with medications that work on reward circuitry (like naltrexone) being more helpful for addictive behaviors while medications that modulate serotonin (like SRIs) being more helpful for compulsive behaviors.

ANXIETY
Use of stimulants and withdrawal from depressants can both induce very strong feelings of anxiety that may be mistaken for a primary disorder. In addition, people with an anxiety disorder are at higher risk of substance misuse, particularly with substances like alcohol or benzodiazepines that are intrinsically anxiety-relieving (making them both positively and negatively reinforcing at the same time).

PAIN
Reasonable use of opioids to relieve pain is medically and ethically justified. In these cases, opioids are being used for their *negatively* reinforcing qualities (removing pain) instead of their *positively* reinforcing traits (inducing a feeling of euphoria). Because of this, don't assume that everyone who seeks out opioids is suffering from an addiction. However, it's worth remembering as well that even someone who starts out using opioids for "legitimate" medical reasons can transition to problematic use.

TRAUMA
Trauma and addiction often go together, with current symptoms of PTSD being 3 times more common in people suffering from an addiction. In addition, it is more difficult to treat addiction in people who have untreated symptoms related to trauma. For this reason, it is helpful to keep PTSD (as well as closely related disorders that also are linked to trauma including cluster B personality disorders, somatoform disorders, and dissociative disorders) on the differential for anyone with an addiction.

PUTTING IT ALL TOGETHER

Addiction is one of the largest problems facing society today, and it is estimated that 20% of all deaths in the United States are related to this disorder. Addiction exacts further costs on society in terms of high medical costs, broken families, and increased rates of accidents, overdoses, suicide, and violence. Despite these costs, barely over 10% of people struggling with addiction receive high-quality treatment. Because of this, it is essential to evaluate for addiction in every patient presenting with a psychiatric issue (remember the **S** in **CHAMPION'S PSYCH EVAL**!).

When assessing for substance use, it is helpful to have a systematic framework to screen for each of the major reinforcers. To give you a mnemonic for this framework, picture someone who is currently destroying their life due to an uncontrolled addiction. His friends stage an intervention and successfully get him into rehab. However, they realize that now there is no one to take care of his dog. The friends look at each other, with nobody quite yet willing to step up and volunteer to care for the dog. The question on everyone's mind, naturally, is, "This guy's out of control, but **CAN HIS DOG Behave**?" This phrase can remind you of the major classes of addictions to remember: **C**annabis, **A**lcohol, **N**icotine, **H**allucinogens, **I**nhalants, **S**timulants, **D**epressants, **O**pioids, **G**ambling, and other **B**ehavioral addictions.

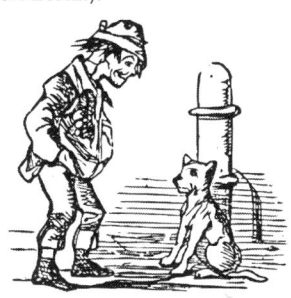

> Having a framework for the various **types of addictions** can be helpful when taking a **complete substance history**.
>
> *CAN HIS DOG Behave?*:
> *C*annabis
> *A*lcohol
> *N*icotine
> *H*allucinogens
> *I*nhalants
> *S*timulants
> *D*epressants
> *O*pioids
> *G*ambling
> *B*ehavioral

REVIEW QUESTIONS

1. A 44 y/o M comes into an addiction medicine clinic for an initial evaluation. He recently went through a divorce and lost custody over his two twin daughters in the process ("The judge says it was mostly due to my drinking"). He reports alcohol intake on most days. He is asked several times to quantify exactly how much he drinks per day but consistently avoids the question by giving tangential responses; the clearest answer he gives is "a lot." When asked about his reason for drinking, he says that he finds that drinking "has always been there at the happiest moments of my life" and that he finds himself going to bars primarily out of boredom and a desire to socialize. He is motivated to stop drinking ("I don't give a shit about my ex but I have to get my daughters back") and has been attending Alcoholics Anonymous meetings every day for the past week. His last drink was 10 days ago. He has never seen a psychiatrist before or taken psychotropic medications. Vital signs are all within normal limits. Which of the following is the best single treatment recommendation at this time?
    A. Refer for inpatient detoxification
    B. Prescribe a benzodiazepine
    C. Prescribe naltrexone
    D. Prescribe acamprosate
    E. Prescribe disulfiram
    F. Psychosocial support and therapy

2. (Continued from previous question.) To rule out medical complications of alcohol use, a variety of blood tests are ordered. Which of the following laboratory values is *least* likely to be elevated in this patient?
    A. Gamma-glutamyl transferase (GGT)
    B. Aspartate transaminase (AST)
    C. Alanine transaminase (ALT)
    D. ALT-to-AST ratio
    E. All of these are likely to be elevated

3. (Continued from previous question.) The patient reports increasing feelings of depression over the past 2 weeks since being told that he was losing custody of his daughters. His specific symptoms include poor appetite, difficulty falling and staying asleep, feeling guilty, having poor energy, and finding it difficult to concentrate on other things. He denies suicidal ideation, and there is no evidence of psychomotor slowing on exam. In addition to alcohol use disorder, which of the following diagnoses is most appropriate at this time?
    A. Major depressive disorder
    B. Bipolar depression
    C. Substance-induced mood disorder
    D. Adjustment disorder
    E. No additional diagnoses should be assigned

4. A 35 y/o M begins seeing a therapist for "sex addiction." He reports spending up to 5 hours each day on the internet looking for potential sexual partners. He typically contacts several hundred women per day and meets with new partners two or three times each week, although he says "sometimes it's like a buffet and other times it's a drought." He has contracted several sexually transmitted infections as he prefers not to use condoms because "it dulls the fireworks." He has occasionally attempted to "play it straight" and see the same partner multiple times but finds that he often suffers from erectile dysfunction when he does so. He feels guilty about his behavior but finds himself unable to stop. Which of the following features of his behavior makes it most difficult for him to stop?
   A. Ease of looking for partners online
   B. Unpredictable nature of seeking new partners
   C. Pleasurable sensation of orgasm
   D. Sense of danger from contracting sexually transmitted infections
   E. Presence of erectile dysfunction when seeing the same partner

1. **The best answer is F.** This patient is likely suffering from an alcohol use disorder. While he does not quantify the amount he is drinking, it is clear that there is repeated use of alcohol despite negative repercussions (such as losing custody of his daughters). Treatment for alcohol use disorder involves an initial period of detoxification. However, the window for acute withdrawal symptoms is generally one week after the last drink. Given that his last drink was over on week ago, it is likely unnecessary in this case (answer A). Benzodiazepines would also be unnecessary given his lack of vital sign instability or other symptoms suggestive of withdrawal (answer B). Each of the other listed medications can play a role in treatment of alcohol use disorder; however, they must generally be paired with psychosocial rehabilitation to be effective (answers C, D, and E). Therefore, the best *single* treatment option for this patient is psychosocial rehabilitation.

2. **The best answer is D.** Chronic use of alcohol is associated with increases in multiple laboratory values, including gamma-glutamyl transferase (answer A), aspartate transaminase (answer B), and alanine transaminase (answer C). However, it is the ratio of AST to ALT that is reliably elevated in alcohol use disorder, not the ratio of ALT to AST.

3. **The best answer is C.** While the patient technically meets criteria for a major depressive episode (including 5 out of 9 symptoms for at least 2 weeks), the presence of excessive alcohol intake around the same time period precludes a diagnosis of a primary mood disorder, including both major depressive disorder (answer A) and bipolar depression (answer B). Instead, a diagnosis of a substance-induced mood disorder should be given. It is possible that these symptoms will persist even once sustained abstinence from alcohol has been achieved, at which time a diagnosis of a primary mood disorder could be considered; for the time being, however, the most likely explanation for his mood symptoms is his recent substance use, especially considering his lack of prior psychiatric history. While there is a recent major life stressor, the patient's current symptoms are too severe to qualify for a diagnosis of adjustment disorder which by definition is subsyndromal (answer D) or for no additional diagnosis to be given (answer E).

4. **The best answer is B.** With the exception of a sense of danger from contracting new infections (answer D), all of these factors likely play a role in maintaining this patient's behavior. However, it is the unpredictability of a variable reinforcement schedule that has been found to correlate most strongly with which behaviors develop into an addiction. The pleasure of an orgasm (answer C) acts as a positive reinforcer for sex while the presence of erectile dysfunction (answer E) acts as a negative punishment for seeing the same partner, which can support the current pattern of the patient's behavior but likely does not contribute to his high degree of use to the same extent as the variable reinforcement schedule. The ease of looking for new partners online (answer A) may have played a role in initiating this behavior but likely does not account for why it has developed into an addiction.

9 ANXIETY

Anxiety is an unpleasant mental state involving persistent **worrying** about the possibility of future dangers, threats to safety, or upsetting events. Anxiety manifests **physiologically**, **psychologically**, and **behaviorally** with specific signs and symptoms, including an increased heart rate, pessimistic thought patterns, and avoidance of particular places or situations. Despite being unpleasant, anxiety is not intrinsically harmful or pathological. In fact, anxiety is often adaptive by allowing us to foresee possible negative outcomes and take steps to avoid them. For example, someone who begins going to the gym and eating a better diet is likely motivated at least in part by anxiety about becoming unhealthy. In this way, anxiety is similar to pain: both are experienced as distressing and unpleasant, but both serve a practical purpose by motivating us to avoid harmful things or situations.

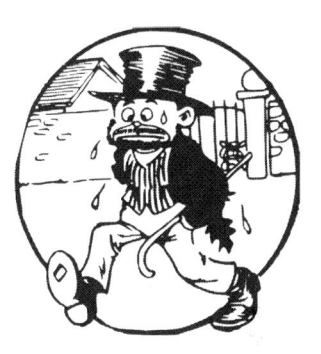

However, for some people anxiety becomes extreme and excessive to the point that it is no longer helpful but instead causes the person to act in a maladaptive way. These people are said to be suffering from **anxiety disorders**. Anxiety disorders involve exaggerations or abnormalities in the way that humans process **alarm signals**, leading to the development of **irrational beliefs** as well as maladaptive **coping behaviors** that, while intended to avert bad outcomes, instead end up *causing* more dysfunction than they prevent. The goal in diagnosing and treating anxiety disorders is not to eliminate anxiety altogether, as a life that is completely free of anxiety would likely be equally problematic (not to mention unattainable). Instead, the goal should be to restore a pattern in which anxiety is a *helpful* signal rather than a harmful one.

SIGNS AND SYMPTOMS OF ANXIETY

The signs and symptoms of anxiety are not hard to recognize, as nearly everyone has experienced them at some point in their lives. The core symptom here is a feeling of **worry**, meaning that the patient is concerned that something bad will happen in the future. However, this thought pattern is accompanied by bodily sensations as well.

Anxiety is **both a state and a trait** in that it can be both an immediate mental state in response to current circumstances ("I'm feeling very anxious right now") as well as a chronic and enduring disposition towards anxiety ("I'm kind of an anxious person"). Anxiety can also manifest differently depending on whether it is experienced as an acute episode (as in a panic attack) or as a chronic state (as in generalized anxiety). We'll look at each of these in turn.

Acute anxiety presents with both physiological signs, including a racing heartbeat, shortness of breath, tingling sensations, and nausea, as well as psychological symptoms, including racing thoughts, fear of dying, and feelings of impending doom. The complete list of core signs and symptoms for acute anxiety are encompassed in the mnemonic **STUDENTS Fear C's** which stands for **S**weating, **T**rembling, **U**nsteadiness or dizziness, **D**issociation, **E**levated heart rate, **N**ausea, **T**ingling, **S**hortness of breath, **Fear** of dying, losing control, or going crazy, **C**hest pain, **C**hills, and **C**hoking sensations. You can easily link this mnemonic to anxiety by thinking of a pre-medical student having a panic attack because they think that they have gotten a C on their biology test. All of these symptoms are seen during a panic attack (which we will discuss further later in this chapter).

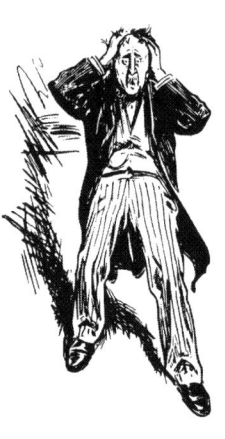

Acute anxiety manifests in both **physical signs** and **physiologic symptoms**, including vital sign changes, feelings of fear, and racing thoughts.

STUDENTS Fear C's:
Sweating
Trembling
Unsteadiness
Dissociation
Elevated heart rate
Nausea
Tingling
Shortness of breath
Fear of dying, losing control, or going crazy
Chest pain, Chills, and Choking sensations

In contrast, the core signs and symptoms of **chronic anxiety** are less immediate but are still highly distressing. You can remember these using the mnemonic **MISERA**-ble, which stands for **M**uscle tension, **I**rritability, difficulty with **S**leep, low **E**nergy, **R**estlessness, and poor **A**ttention. Other psychological symptoms, including ruminative thoughts and somatic complaints, are very common as well. (If these symptoms sound familiar, that is because we have discussed many of them previously in the context of depression! Indeed, depression and chronic anxiety appear to share many mechanistic features which likely accounts for the similar symptoms, overlap in treatments, and links to adverse childhood events that are shared between the two disorders.)

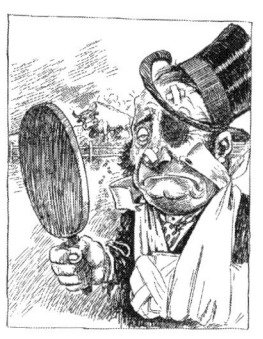

Chronic anxiety is associated with both **physical** and **physiologic** symptoms, including muscle tension, restlessness, and irritability.

MISERA-ble:
Muscle tension
Irritability
Sleep (decreased)
Energy (decreased)
Restlessness
Attention (decreased)

ANXIETY ACROSS THE LIFESPAN

EPIDEMIOLOGY
Anxiety is **common**, with over 10% of people having had an anxiety disorder within the past year and up to 30% meeting criteria for one during their lifetime. This makes anxiety disorders the most common *group* of mental disorders (although depression is still the most common *individual* mental disorder). This gives anxiety a **high base rate** in the population, making it liable to **underdiagnosis** (especially considering that the symptoms of anxiety are often less noticeable or overtly impairing than those seen in mania or psychosis). Like depression, **women** are diagnosed with anxiety disorders more than twice as often as men. Anxiety disorders often begin during **childhood and adolescence**, with almost all cases beginning by the age of 25.

PROGNOSIS
Without treatment, anxiety disorders tend to become **chronic** and persist throughout life (rather than being episodic in the same way that mood disorders are). While some degree of anxiety is almost always present for someone with an active disorder, there is often a natural waxing-and-waning of severity from day to day or even year to year.

The severity of symptoms often levels off with aging, as the prevalence of clinically significant anxiety disorders begins to decrease after the age of 55. However, some degree of impairment often remains even into old age.

While anxiety disorders are associated with a lower risk of suicide compared to mood disorders, the risk is still present. In addition, untreated anxiety disorders often lead to more social and occupational **disability** than mood disorders by virtue of their being a chronic (rather than episodic) disorder. The disability associated with depression, for example, often resolves once the depressive episode ends whereas for an anxiety disorder the dysfunction can continue unabated for years on end.

TREATMENT

As with most mental disorders, treatment involves **psychotherapy** and **medications**. However, in contrast to both depression (where either medications, therapy, or both are appropriate) as well as bipolar disorder and schizophrenia (where medications are almost always used with therapy being an adjunct), for anxiety disorders **therapy should almost always be the first-line treatment**. CBT in particular shows a **large effect size** (above 0.8) for the majority of anxiety disorders and is associated with enduring improvements that last long after the treatment has stopped.

Medications should be used more sparingly, as they tend to have smaller and more transient effects on anxiety. Antidepressants like **SRIs** are most commonly used and have a **small effect size** (around 0.3 or 0.4). They appear to be effective regardless of the specific anxiety disorder that is diagnosed (you might say they are "broad-spectrum antineurotics"). **Benzodiazepines** are often used for acute treatment of panic attacks, but they should *not* be used for chronic treatment of any anxiety disorder as they tend to actually **worsen long-term outcomes**. Benzodiazepines not only induce a state of psychological and physiologic tolerance that makes someone more susceptible to anxiety but they can also interfere with their ability to engage in the psychotherapy that is required for definitive treatment of an anxiety disorder. Because of this, benzodiazepines should be avoided for chronic treatment of anxiety in most cases.

MECHANISMS OF ANXIETY

In understanding the mechanisms of anxiety, it is important to distinguish between the states of **anxiety** and **fear**. Anxiety and fear are both part of our body's **stress response**, or the physical and mental changes that occur when encountering a challenge in our environment. However, in anxiety the focus is a perceived *future* threat whereas in fear the focus is on a *current* threat. For example, a deer who is suddenly attacked by a cougar jumping at them from behind the bushes will enter a state of *fear*, while a deer who walks around worrying about a cougar jumping out at any time is experiencing *anxiety*. While both are uncomfortable, fear and anxiety can each serve a purpose by motivating the organism to behave in an adaptive way (such as encouraging the deer to run away from the cougar or to avoid places where cougars are more likely to be found).

Fear   *Anxiety*

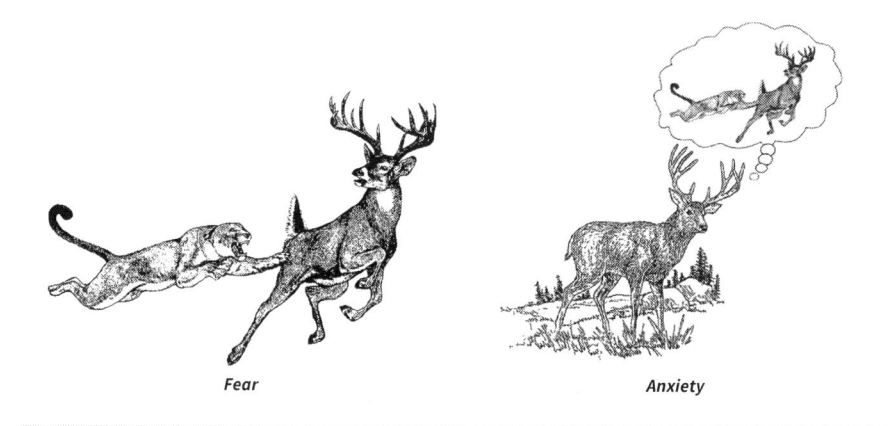

> **Fear** is related to **current threats**, while **anxiety** focuses on **future threats**.
>
> *Fear is about what's **here**, while anxiety is about the future.*

    Biologically, both anxiety and fear activate the fast-acting **sympathetic nervous system** which immediately puts the body into "fight or flight" mode. In response to the release of **epinephrine** and **norepinephrine**, the patient experiences all of the **STUDENTS Fear C's** signs and symptoms which is their body's attempt to prepare to either face down its threat or get away from it as quickly as possible. On a cognitive level, fear and anxiety are often experienced as "racing" or "loud" thoughts as well as a feeling of extreme unease. Compared to fear, anxiety tends to activate the sympathetic nervous system to a lesser extent (which makes sense, as the body's response to the *thought* of a cougar jumping out at you should naturally be less than a cougar *actually* jumping out at a you).

    While activation of the sympathetic nervous system explains the signs and symptoms of anxiety in the *acute* sense, it does little to account for *chronic* anxiety lasting months or years. For this, we need to turn to the slower-acting **hypothalamic-pituitary-adrenal axis** (or HPA axis). Activation of the HPA axis induces long-term changes in physiology, cognition, and behavior via the release of the hormone **cortisol**. Cortisol has many functions, including reducing inflammation, breaking down connective tissues, regulating blood pressure, and altering the metabolism of carbohydrates, protein, and fat. Chronic activation of the HPA axis has been linked to the specific signs and symptoms captured in the **MISERA**-ble mnemonic as well as an increased risk of depression which involves overactivation of the HPA axis as well.

> The **sympathetic nervous system** is involved in **acute fear and anxiety**, while the **hypothalamic-pituitary-adrenal axis** is activated in **chronic anxiety**.
>
> *The SN**S** is activated by both types of **S**tress, while the HP**A** is activated only by **A**nxiety.*

Now that we understanding the underlying pathophysiology for both acute and chronic anxiety, we can present a mechanistic framework that encompasses each of the specific anxiety disorders we will talk about in this chapter. The **alarm—beliefs—coping (ABC) model** of anxiety disorders provides a helpful framework for understanding the specific symptoms and behaviors seen in each individual type of anxiety disorders. In this model, the starting point for any and all anxiety disorders is an internal **alarm** signal. Something (either in the environment or an internal sensation) is telling us that there is cause for concern. Perhaps it is an oddly colored mole on our skin that we never noticed before or the sound of a window breaking at night. Regardless of the specific stimulus that triggers it, the alarm signal instantly activates the sympathetic nervous system, leading to the immediate symptoms of anxiety. Psychologically, thoughts tend to become focused on interpreting the alarm signal and developing a set of specific explanatory **beliefs** about the alarm ("Does this mole mean I have cancer?" or "Is someone breaking in?"). These beliefs form the basis upon which we consciously act in response to the alarm signal ("I need to go see a doctor," or "I have to get out of here!"). This experience then forms the basis of our **coping** strategies, including taking steps to either avoid this situation in the future or plan for what we should do if we ever find ourselves in a similar situation again ("I should wear sunscreen," or "I'm buying a security system!").

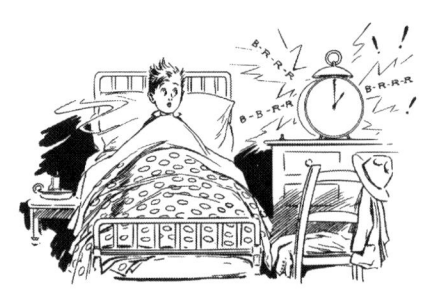

Viewed from this perspective, all anxiety disorders are characterized by a **defective alarm signal**, including "false alarms" that go off for unknown reasons and overactive alarms that won't turn off. All of the variations in thought and behavior that define the traditional separations between different types of anxiety disorders are ultimately just downstream consequences of this core abnormality. On a biological level, hyperactivity of the HPA axis appears to be the mechanism by which a defective alarm signal arises, and individuals with a wide variety of anxiety disorders all appear to share some degree of overactivity in one or more components of the HPA axis. A hypersensitive HPA axis has been linked to adverse events during childhood, including abuse, neglect, parental death, or a caregiver with a severe mental illness. Exposure to adverse events appears to induce long-lasting changes during the development of the HPA axis, leading to the hypersensitivity seen in anxiety disorders.

As we explore each of the specific patterns of anxiety disorders (including generalized anxiety disorder, panic disorder, specific phobias, and social anxiety disorder), try to view each of them through the lens of the **ABC model** and look closely at how the alarm system has become dysfunctional in each.

Anxiety disorders involve a consistent pattern of a defective **alarm signal** followed by **explanatory beliefs** and compensatory **coping strategies**.

*Anxiety is as easy as **ABC**: Alarm—Beliefs—Coping.*

HOW TO DIAGNOSE ANXIETY DISORDERS

Like most mental disorders, anxiety disorders are diagnosed using the psychiatric interview and mental status exam. While the current signs and symptoms of anxiety that are elicited during the evaluation process (the "state") are important in pointing towards a diagnosis, you must take into account the longitudinal pattern of anxiety across the lifespan as well (the "trait").

Unlike depression, mania, and psychosis, there is **no single disease prototype** to which all other related disorders can be compared. Instead, the major types of anxiety disorders (including generalized anxiety disorder, panic disorder, specific phobias, and social anxiety disorder) are a **heterogeneous** group of conditions, each with their own diagnostic, prognostic, and treatment considerations. However, they all share a similar fundamental pattern: an overactive alarm signal with explanatory beliefs and maladaptive coping strategies that lead to dysfunction.

Because of this shared pattern, it is perhaps no surprise that the majority (over two-thirds) of people who are diagnosed with one anxiety disorder also meet criteria for another. This makes being diagnosed with a single anxiety disorder the exception rather than the rule. In addition, people with one anxiety disorder will often "convert" to another during their lifetime, reinforcing further the notion that someone's anxiety *trait* (an overactive alarm signal) can produce various *state* abnormalities (the specific beliefs and coping behaviors that characterize each individual anxiety disorder).

In clinical practice, you will run into patients who seem to have "read the textbook" on each of these disorders and fit their patterns to a tee. However, you will also encounter many people who clearly suffer from excessive and debilitating anxiety but do not quite fit a particular diagnosis. Don't let this bother you too much. It's ultimately more important to identify the overall process of pathologically extreme or dysfunctional levels of anxiety than it is to "nail the diagnosis" based on the criteria found in the DSM.

GENERALIZED ANXIETY DISORDER

Generalized anxiety disorder (GAD) is characterized by **excessive and generalized anxiety in multiple areas of life**, including—but not limited to—work, home, family, friends, finances, health, politics, and transportation. (This places generalized anxiety disorder in contrast to other anxiety disorders that we will talk about later, such as specific phobias or social anxiety disorder, where severe anxiety is limited only to a single domain.) It is the persistence and pervasiveness of the anxiety that truly defines generalized anxiety disorder, which in the ABC model of anxiety is akin to an **alarm that rings all the time for no clear reason**.

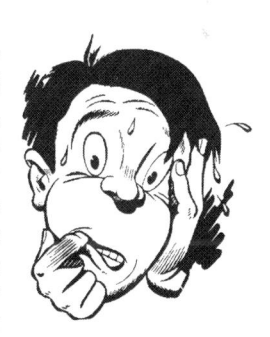

These worries are not only distressing to the patient but can also result in significant impairment. For example, someone with generalized anxiety disorder may end up having problems with social relationships ("I can't get married, she will cheat on me!"), difficulty at work ("I can't do this project, I'll screw everything up!"), trouble getting around ("I can't drive, the bridge will collapse!"), and complications even with things that most people would find exciting ("I can't buy a house, a hurricane is bound to hit soon!"). Left unchecked, these worries can prevent someone from engaging in the very parts of life that people find meaningful.

Patients with generalized anxiety disorder also suffer from the symptoms related to chronic overactivation of the HPA axis, including the **M**uscle tension, **I**rritability, impaired **S**leep, low **E**nergy, **R**estlessness, and poor **A**ttention captured in the **MISERA**-ble mnemonic.

In the DSM, you need both the anxious thought patterns and the specific symptoms to diagnose generalized anxiety disorder. You can remember the diagnostic criteria for this disorder using the mnemonic "**EGADS!** I'm **MISERA**-ble!" The first part will remind you that the disorder involves **E**xcessive and **G**eneralized **A**nxiety that is chronic, occurring on most **D**ays for at least **S**ix months. The second part will remind you that the DSM requires **3 or more symptoms** from the **MISERA**-ble mnemonic to be present.

> **Generalized anxiety disorder** is diagnosed when someone has **anxiety about most things** as well as specific **symptoms of chronic anxiety**.
>
> *"EGADS! I'm MISERA-ble!":*
> *Excessive and Generalized Anxiety occurring on most Days for at least Six months plus 3 or more of the MISERA-ble symptoms.*

For busy clinicians, asking a single question ("Do you worry excessively about minor matters?") has been found to be a **highly sensitive** screening instrument for generalized anxiety disorder, making it a quick and easy way to rule out the disorder. For people who answer yes, the presence of chronic anxiety symptoms can help to rule in the diagnosis provided that they have been present for at least 6 months.

Generalized anxiety disorder affects around 1-3% of the population at any given time, making it **relatively uncommon** (though by no means rare). As with most anxiety disorders, women are diagnosed twice as often as men. The diagnosis is highly comorbid with depression and dysthymia which suggests shared genetic, mechanistic, and environmental vulnerabilities. It is also often found in combination with addiction to specific substances, especially those that are inherently anxiety-relieving such as alcohol and benzodiazepines. Without treatment, the symptoms of generalized anxiety disorder tend to persist for years, if not decades.

Treatment for generalized anxiety disorder consists of **psychotherapy**. CBT is a particularly effective modality with a **large effect size** around 0.7 or 0.8. Medication treatment for generalized anxiety disorder generally involves either an **SRI** or **buspirone**, a medication that also interacts with serotonin receptors. While both have been shown to be helpful (with a **small effect size** around 0.2 or 0.3), like most medications for anxiety they should primarily be used in combination with therapy to ensure that the effects of treatment are sustained.

PANIC ATTACK

A panic attack is a brief period of intense **mental and physical discomfort** that results from sudden activation of the **fear response**. Symptoms during a panic attack are consistent with overactivation of the sympathetic nervous system and include all of the symptoms from the **STUDENTS Fear C's** mnemonic including **S**weating, **T**rembling, **U**nsteadiness or dizziness, **D**issociation, **E**levated heart rate, **N**ausea, **T**ingling, **S**hortness of breath, **Fear** of dying, losing control, or going crazy, **C**hest pain, **C**hills, and **C**hoking sensations. In fact, these symptoms are so linked to panic attacks that the DSM lists these as the core diagnostic criteria! These symptoms tend to follow a **crescendo-decrescendo pattern** where symptoms peak within a few minutes and then slowly subside after that. Panic attacks typically last for 5 to 10 minutes, although they can be as short as 1 minute or as long as an hour.

Panic attacks differ from normal fear reactions in terms of their **severity**. It is natural that the fear response should be greater or lesser depending on the circumstances. For example, seeing a spider across the room should naturally provoke a lesser fear response than pulling back the shower curtain to reveal a killer clown holding a knife. During a panic attack, however, the fear response loses its connection to the external circumstances and hits its maximum severity *every time*. (With apologies to Spinal Tap, during a panic attack the fear response goes to 11!) To use a real-world example, people with panic attacks who have lived through natural disasters like earthquakes have reported that what they felt during the disaster was nothing compared to what they experience during a panic attack.

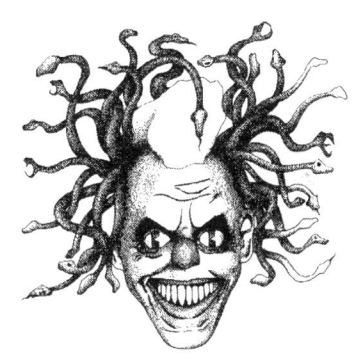

Panic attacks also differ from natural fear in their **timing**. A normal fear response occurs in direct response to an external stressor. However, while some panic attacks can be provoked by stress, the majority come "out of the blue." This is especially true for people who have had multiple previous panic attacks: the more panic attacks that someone has had, the more likely they are to be uncued. Being in this state of panic often leads people to believe that there must be something wrong, and many will call 911 or go to the hospital. However, even with extensive history taking, no trigger for the fear response is found in most cases. (With further apologies to Franklin D. Roosevelt, in the case of panic attacks the only thing to fear is the fear response itself!)

Panic attacks are **quite common**, with over 25% of all people having had a panic attack in their lifetime. Despite being incredibly aversive, panic attacks are not in and of themselves an anxiety disorder, as they do not involve anxiety (they involve *fear*), and there is often no evidence of dysfunction (many people who have had panic attacks continue to lead normal lives). However, for some people this dysfunctional alarm signal goes on to produce disabling beliefs and coping strategies that *do* represent a disorder, as we will explore next.

PANIC DISORDER

While not everyone who has panic attacks is disabled by them, for some people a consistent pattern of sudden, unexpected, and recurrent panic attacks gives rise to specific beliefs and coping strategies, including constant worrying about when they will have their next attack and avoiding places where they have previously had attacks. This is when panic *disorder* emerges. In this way, the distinction between fear and anxiety becomes important: while a panic attack is a state of extreme *fear*, panic disorder results from *anxiety* about having future panic attacks. Following the ABC model of anxiety disorders, panic disorder is akin to an **overactive alarm system that goes off randomly**, leading to a state of perpetual anxiety about when the alarm will ring next. While these beliefs and coping strategies are in many ways a logical response to the experience of having panic attacks, the constant anxiety and avoidance of going to specific places (including work, school, or even the grocery store) can become incredibly impairing and directly impact one's ability to lead a normal life. You can remember the overall pattern of panic disorder by thinking of the word **SURPrise**: **S**udden **U**nexpected **R**ecurrent **P**anic attacks that give **rise** to excessive and dysfunctional anxiety even between attacks. Just having panic attacks is not enough for the diagnosis; you need both the **SURP** and the **rise**.

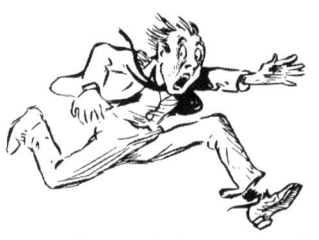

Panic disorder is when **sudden unexpected recurrent panic attacks** give rise to long-lasting **negative consequences**.

SURPrise! **S**udden **U**nexpected **R**ecurrent **P**anic *attacks that give* **rise** *to anxiety.*

While over a quarter of the population has had a panic *attack*, only one in six go on to develop panic *disorder*, giving it a **moderate base rate** of around 5% of the population. Like most anxiety disorders, panic disorder is diagnosed in women twice as often as in men. It generally begins in the late teenage years or young adulthood.

While panic *attacks* do not necessarily become more severe or frequent with each additional occurrence, the *anxiety* surrounding the panic attacks and the resultant dysfunction can worsen over time and become increasingly impairing. However, panic disorder also has a high rate of spontaneous remission, with over 75% of people diagnosed with panic disorder becoming free of symptoms within 3 years.

On an acute basis, **benzodiazepines** are very effective at rapidly terminating panic attacks. However, while helpful for short-term treatment, over the long-term chronic use of benzodiazepines often makes panic attacks more frequent and severe. Preventive treatment involves looking for any contributing lifestyle changes (such as caffeine intake) and modifying them. **SRIs** are helpful for reducing the frequency and severity of panic attacks when taken daily, with a **moderate effect size** of around 0.5. However, like most anxiety disorders, the best treatment for panic disorder is **CBT**, with the vast majority of patients achieving full remission from panic attacks within several months of initiating treatment (with a **large effect size** around 0.7) and maintaining these benefits even years after finishing therapy.

AGORAPHOBIA

Agoraphobia (literally "fear of the marketplace") is a disorder where people feel extreme anxiety in public places, causing them to remain in the safety of their own home. In severe cases, people with agoraphobia have not left their home for several years. Agoraphobia is almost always preceded by a history of panic attacks and can best be understood as a *specific coping strategy* that a**rise**s in response to **S**udden **U**nexpected **R**ecurrent **P**anic attacks. Staying home is a viable coping strategy because panic attacks tend to happen less frequently at home and, if they do happen, are often less severe because the person feels that they are in a safe place. In contrast, when a panic attack happens in a public place where the patient does not feel that they can escape from easily (like in a shopping mall), it can lead to feelings of being trapped or vulnerable, increasing the level of anxiety and making the panic attack even more aversive. This creates a pattern of **avoidance** of places that people have had a panic attack in the past, and for some this pattern becomes overgeneralized to the point where it includes avoiding any and all places that are not their own home.

Agoraphobia develops in around a quarter of all people with panic disorder, giving it a base rate of around 1%. It is generally considered to be a marker of severe panic disorder as evidenced by a spontaneous remission rate of only 25% (compared to 75% for panic disorder *without* agoraphobia). Treatment is the same as for panic disorder, although CBT is generally less effective, with an effect size under 0.3.

SPECIFIC PHOBIA

Specific phobias are characterized by an **intense fear response to a specific object or situation** that approaches the level of (or can even turn into) a "full blown" panic attack. In the ABC model of anxiety disorders, it is akin to an **alarm that goes off too strongly in response to a specific stimulus**. Specific phobias involve a variety of feared objects, each with its own fun-to-memorize name such as *ophidiophobia* (fear of snakes), *thalassophobia* (fear of the ocean), *nyctophobia* (fear of the dark), or *trypanophobia* (fear of needles). This dysfunctional alarm signal gives rise to particular beliefs and coping strategies aimed at avoiding the stimulus, and many people with a specific phobia will put forth significant effort to avoid any situation that could possibly result in exposure to it, such as a woman with *gephyrophobia* (fear of bridges) driving two extra hours per day to avoid going over the bridge that is the shortest route between her home and her work.

Specific phobias are likely adaptive to some degree. For example, someone with *arachnophobia* (fear of spiders) is more likely to survive than someone who has no fear of spiders. However, where specific phobias diverge from adaptive fear is in terms of **severity**, as the fear response experienced by those with a specific phobia is greatly out of proportion to what is helpful for survival. Many people with a specific phobia report an inciting incident that likely led to the development of that phobia, such as a child who is attacked by a duck who later develops *anatidaephobia* (fear of ducks). However, this isn't found in every case, and some specific phobias appear to develop completely "out of the blue."

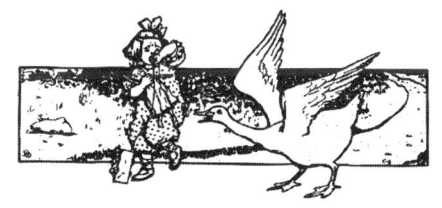

Specific phobias are **common**, with around 10% of people having a specific phobia at some time during their life. They usually begin in childhood or adolescence and affect women twice as often as men. Treatment consists of a specific type of CBT known as **exposure therapy** in which the patient is intentionally exposed to the object of their fear with gradually increasing intensity. For example, someone with a fear of snakes may play with a toy snake until they no longer feel afraid around it, at which point they would progress to looking at pictures of real snakes. The goal of exposure therapy is to make the patient feel *uncomfortable but not overwhelmed* with each exposure so they can gradually be able to tolerate being in the presence of the object of their fear. Exposure therapy is extremely effective at treating specific phobias, with a **large effect size** over 1.0 and benefits that last even after the therapy is completed. Medications do not play a significant role in treating specific phobias.

SOCIAL ANXIETY DISORDER

People with social anxiety disorder have chronic and persistent anxiety. However, unlike generalized anxiety disorder, this anxiety is focused entirely around one specific area: the possibility of **interpersonal rejection**. People with social anxiety disorder constantly worry that they will say or do something embarrassing or humiliating, leading to severe discomfort during even routine social situations. This hyperactive alarm system leads to specific beliefs ("I am unlikable, boring, and stupid") and coping strategies, including avoiding most or even all social situations. People with social anxiety disorder often have particularly pronounced anxiety about specific situations (such as public speaking or musical performances) that could potentially invite criticism from many people at once.

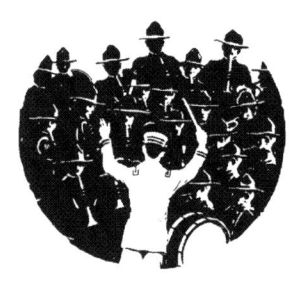

Social anxiety disorder is **common**, affecting around 10% of the population. It must be carefully differentiated from introversion or shyness which are normal personality traits. Separating social anxiety disorder from shyness requires clear evidence that the trait is impairing one's ability to function. While it is important to be mindful of the potentially stigmatizing nature of diagnosis, diagnosing social anxiety disorder can also have positive effects by providing a pathway for treatment, as **CBT** for social anxiety disorder is very effective (with a **large effect size** over 0.9) and produce long-lasting results. **SRIs** can also help (with a smaller effect size in the range of 0.3 or 0.4) but should generally be seen as a second-line intervention.

SELECTIVE MUTISM

Selective mutism is a condition in which people who are physically capable of speech have difficulty speaking in specific situations, often out of fear of being seen as stupid or silly. Paradoxically, being silent can itself lead to social judgment, creating a vicious cycle. It is most often diagnosed in children. Despite being listed by the DSM as a separate disorder, selective mutism is more likely a specific behavioral manifestation of **severe social anxiety disorder**, as nearly 100% of people who are diagnosed with selective mutism also meet criteria for social anxiety disorder. In addition, treatment strategies and response rates are largely the same between the two. You can think of selective mutism as a particular manifestation of severe social anxiety disorder.

DIFFERENTIAL DIAGNOSIS OF ANXIETY DISORDERS

There are a variety of psychiatric conditions that closely resemble anxiety or have anxiety as a prominent symptom, including depression, OCD, PTSD, somatoform disorders, and certain personality disorders (particularly those in cluster C). In the case of OCD and PTSD, both were actually considered to *be* anxiety disorders for a long time even though they are now conceptualized as being on their own spectrum. To help make sense of this, we will first develop a framework for assessing someone who comes to us with severe or persistent anxiety and then explore the specific misdiagnoses and missed diagnoses that are often associated with anxiety.

It is incredibly common for anxiety to be the primary presenting complaint of a patient seeking psychiatric treatment. However, just like depression (where someone saying that they are "depressed" is no guarantee that they will ultimately be diagnosed with depression), a chief complaint of "anxiety" does not guarantee that the person in front of you actually has a diagnosable anxiety disorder. Even once normalcy has been ruled out, there are a variety of mental disorders that can present with anxiety as a chief complaint. Having a structured framework for approaching these patients can be essential. To systematically evaluate any patients presenting with anxiety, use the mnemonic **ONSTAGE** to remind yourself to check whether their symptoms stem from **O**CD (or related disorders), are consistent with **N**ormalcy, are related to **S**omatization, can be ascribed to **T**rauma, are **A**ttributable to some external factor (such as a medical problem, substance use, or life events), are **G**eneralized (versus specific to certain situations or stimuli like in specific phobia and social anxiety disorder), or are **E**pisodic (as in panic attacks). We will use each of these as we review the various misdiagnoses and missed diagnoses associated with anxiety disorders.

Disorders that commonly present with **anxiety as the chief complaint** include **obsessive-compulsive**, **traumatic**, and **somatoform** disorders.

Use **ONSTAGE** to characterize the nature of anxiety:
OCD
Normalcy
Somatization
Trauma
Attributable
Generalized
Episodic

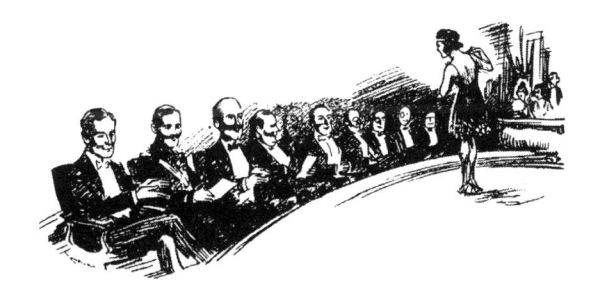

NORMALCY
Fear and anxiety are both normal and adaptive states that everyone experiences throughout their lives. Therefore, the mere presence of either fear or anxiety is not enough to diagnose an anxiety disorder. In fact, the majority of people experience anxious thoughts throughout the day, and this is not inherently impairing or pathological. However, when anxiety becomes extreme, the *quantitative becomes qualitative* (remember the principles of psychodiagnostic introduced in Chapter 2!), and certain people absolutely qualify for a diagnosis of an anxiety disorder.

The line between adaptive and maladaptive anxiety is not always clear, and careful consideration of both the advantages and disadvantages of diagnosis should be given at all times. For example, diagnosing an extremely shy person who doesn't think that their behavior is a problem with social anxiety disorder may instead stigmatize and alienate the patient. In contrast, if that same person had come to you specifically for help with this problem, then the diagnosis may be more appropriate as it allows them to access helpful treatments.

Anxiety can also intersect with normalcy in that the language of anxiety can be an **idiom of distress** as often as it is a disorder in and of itself. The language of anxiety is frequently used to communicate distress, such as someone saying that they are having a panic attack due to a bad day (even though, objectively speaking, there are no objective signs that what they are experiencing is in any way a panic attack). Keep in mind that *taking someone seriously does not always mean taking them literally*. You should always take the distress of someone you are treating seriously, but that does not mean abandoning the knowledge of these disorders that is necessary for clarity in diagnosis, treatment, and research.

ADJUSTMENT DISORDER
Anxiety is frequently reported as a primary symptom in adjustment disorder. The same rules apply here as for depression: the patient must not meet criteria for a "full blown" anxiety disorder, and the anxiety must have started after (and be directly related to) a significant life change or stressor. Adjustment disorder is best thought of as a non-stigmatizing "**diagnosis of normalcy**" that allows the patient to access helpful treatment (in this case, a type of psychotherapy known as supportive therapy).

DEPRESSION
Depression is so **frequently comorbid** with anxiety disorders that the presence of one should always prompt an assessment for the presence of the other. There appears to be a shared pathophysiologic mechanism between depression and anxiety, as HPA axis abnormalities are seen in both and could account for many of the symptoms that they share in common (including irritability, fatigue, insomnia, and difficulty concentrating). In addition, many of the same treatments (including SRIs and CBT) are highly effective for both. However, we should not go so far as to assume that depression and anxiety are the same disorder. The **episodic** nature of depression is distinctly different from the enduring and persistent nature of symptoms seen in many anxiety disorders. In addition, while comorbidity is the rule rather than the exception, we cannot ignore the fact that many people have "just depression" or "just anxiety."

POST-TRAUMATIC STRESS DISORDER
The relationship between PTSD and anxiety is complex. Indeed, for many years PTSD was considered to be an anxiety disorder. However, recent research has suggested that, while fear and anxiety can be core symptoms of PTSD, they are not the *only* emotions experienced by survivors of trauma and, indeed, it is possible to have PTSD without experiencing either fear or anxiety (which makes it really hard to argue that PTSD is an *anxiety* disorder). Instead, the predominant symptom of PTSD is the **re-experiencing of trauma**. For some, this manifests as fear and anxiety, but not necessarily for everyone. Nevertheless, be on the lookout for a history of trauma if a patient presents with anxiety, as anxiety may be the presenting symptom of PTSD.

OBSESSIVE-COMPULSIVE DISORDER
OCD is another disorder that was long thought to be an anxiety disorder. After all, the obsessions found in OCD are often clearly definable as anxiety ("If I don't wash my hands, then I will get sick and die!"). However, obsessional thoughts do not *always* involve anxiety. For example, someone who needs to count up the number of letters in each sentence they speak is not necessarily *anxious* about something bad happening; it just bothers them severely if they don't. In this way, OCD is revealed as a disorder of **error signaling** rather than a dysfunctional alarm system. In some cases, error signaling and alarm signaling overlap, but not always. Making a distinction between the error signaling of OCD and the dysfunctional alarm system in anxiety disorders is supported by a growing body of evidence showing that OCD and related disorders comprise their own "OCD spectrum" of disorders with substantially different diagnostic, prognostic, and treatment-related considerations.

PERSONALITY DISORDERS
Cluster C personality disorders (including avoidant, obsessive-compulsive, and dependent personality disorders) all feature worrying and anxiety to some degree, but each of them has a different link to existing anxiety disorders. As we will discover in Chapter 14, avoidant personality disorder is best conceptualized as a particularly severe variant of social anxiety disorder (similar to selective mutism), while obsessive-compulsive personality disorder is more similar to conditions like anorexia nervosa than it is to anxiety disorders. Finally, dependent personality disorder is a manifestation of an extremely high level of trait agreeableness which can present with significant anxiety symptoms ("I worry all day that my partner is going to leave me"). However, these worries all fall within the domain of interpersonal dependency.

SOMATIZATION
People with somatoform disorders (discussed further in Chapter 13) experience frequent physical symptoms for which no underlying medical cause can be found. Because physical symptoms are often taken to be a sign of medical illness, people who somatize often come in with anxiety as a presenting symptom. In cases of somatization, however, the anxiety is limited to only physical symptoms. Somatization differs enough from primary anxiety disorders in its prognosis and treatment requirements that it warrants separate consideration.

SUBSTANCE-INDUCED ANXIETY DISORDER

Anxiety (including both formal diagnoses like panic disorder and generalized anxiety disorder as well as people with an overall trait of high anxiety) can often be related to substance intake. Anything with a stimulating effect on the central nervous system can create anxiety, including prescription medications like thyroid hormone, albuterol, steroids, and stimulants. However, any discussion of substance-related anxiety would be incomplete without mentioning **caffeine**. Caffeine is ubiquitous, with over 85% of the United States population consuming at least one caffeinated beverage per day. Given this, it is *by far* the most common reason for substance-induced anxiety disorders. Multiple studies have shown a clear link between caffeine use and anxiety. In many cases, anxiety disorders can be treated or even cured completely by stopping all caffeine intake, so it is worthwhile to ask any patients suffering from an anxiety disorder to consider keeping of log of caffeine intake to see if there is any correlation.

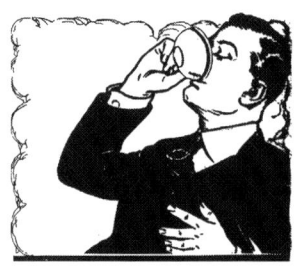

ANXIETY DISORDER DUE TO A GENERAL MEDICAL CONDITION

A host of physical diseases can produce symptoms that closely resemble primary anxiety disorders. At times, the conditions themselves (such as hyperthyroidism and pheochromocytoma) produce hormones that have a net stimulating effect on the central nervous system. In other cases, the pathophysiologic link between the physical disease and the patient's symptoms of anxiety are not as clear. In any case, you can remember some of the most common medical diseases that frequently present as anxiety using the mnemonic **Ph**ysical **Di**seases **T**hat **H**ave **C**ommonly **A**ppeared **A**nxious, which stands for **Ph**eochromocytoma, **Di**abetes mellitus (typically during hyper- or hypoglycemic episodes), **T**emporal lobe epilepsy, **H**yperthyroidism, **C**arcinoid, **A**lcohol withdrawal, and **A**rrhythmias. Clues that someone may be suffering from a medically-induced anxiety disorder include an atypical onset of symptoms (such as someone in their late sixties who never had problems with anxiety until a month ago), the presence of objective physical findings or vital sign abnormalities, or an episodic (rather than chronic) pattern of anxiety symptoms.

Several **medical conditions** can produce symptoms resembling **anxiety disorders.**

Physical Diseases That Have Commonly Appeared Anxious:
*Ph*eochromocytoma
*Di*abetes mellitus
*T*emporal lobe epilepsy
*H*yperthyroidism
*C*arcinoid
*A*lcohol withdrawal
*A*rrhythmias

PUTTING IT ALL TOGETHER

Anxiety disorders are best conceptualized as **various beliefs and coping strategies that arise in response to a dysfunctional alarm system**. The alarm either goes off all the time (generalized anxiety disorder), goes off randomly for unclear reasons (panic disorder), or rings at a volume that is vastly out of proportion to the trigger (specific phobia and social anxiety disorder). Given that a dysfunctional alarm signal is at the heart of each of these conditions, it is no surprise that someone with one anxiety disorder is likely to have another, and this is exactly what we see, with comorbidity being the rule rather than the exception.

Use the **STUDENTS Fear C's and MISERA**-ble mnemonics to remember the signs and symptoms of both acute and chronic anxiety. From there, use the **ONSTAGE** mnemonic to systematically approach the diagnosis for anyone coming in with anxiety as a major or presenting symptom, including assessing the **N**ormalcy, **A**ttributability, **E**pisodicity, and **G**eneralizability of the complaint (as well as whether a different type of condition that commonly presents with anxiety, such as **O**bsessive-compulsive, **T**raumatic, or **S**omatoform disorder, would be more diagnostically appropriate). For most forms of anxiety, **CBT** is going to be your first-line intervention, although in some cases SRIs or other medications can be used as well. Benzodiazepines are incredibly helpful for rapid treatment of anxiety (like during a panic attack) but tend to make anxiety worse in the long-term and should generally be avoided as a chronic treatment.

REVIEW QUESTIONS

1. A 10 y/o F is brought to see a psychologist for an initial evaluation by her mother. The girl has tears on her face and looks drowsy; she refuses to speak to the psychologist. The mother reports that the patient has stopped leaving the house for the past 2 weeks after a friend's pet parrot flew out of its cage and bit her several times on the arm. The mother says that even bringing her to the psychologist's office was a struggle ("I had to sneak Benadryl into her food or else there would be no way I could get her here!"). Prior to the incident 2 weeks ago, the patient was doing well in school and was well-liked by her peers. Because the patient is not talking to the psychologist, he brings in some stuffed animals for her to play with. She then begins screaming loudly and hyperventilating after picking up a stuffed bird as seen below:

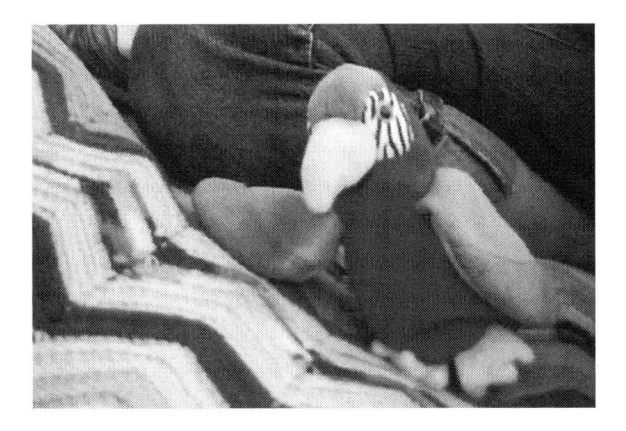

    What is the most likely diagnosis?
    A. Generalized anxiety disorder
    B. Panic disorder
    C. Specific phobia
    D. Social anxiety disorder
    E. Selective mutism
    F. None of the above

2. (Continued from previous question.) At the next appointment, the psychologist asks the girl to write down ten bird-related objects or situations that cause her to feel fear and then rank them in terms of how much fear they make her feel. She indicates that drawing a bird is associated with "a little fear," seeing a toy bird is associated with "some fear," and having a bird sit on her arm would make her feel "like I'm going to die." Which of the following would be the next best step?
    A. Ask her to draw a bird
    B. Bring in a toy bird
    C. Bring in a real bird
    D. Prescribe a benzodiazepine
    E. Discontinue treatment

3. A 25 y/o M presents to his primary care provider complaining of insomnia. He says that he first noticed difficulty sleeping one year ago but that it has steadily gotten worse since then. He primarily has difficulty falling asleep as he "cannot shut my brain off." He reports constant ruminative thoughts that his parents will die somehow ("like in a car crash, or they'll both get cancer, or someone will break in and murder them in their sleep"). He has not applied for a job since graduating from college last year as he is "sure that any employer is going to laugh at my paltry résumé." He describes feeling "stressed" most of the day and feels that he cannot relax. He has yelled at his parents several times over the past month when they ask him about his life, which he says he has never done before. He denies use of substances. He has never taken psychiatric medications before but saw a therapist for several years as a teenager after the death of his grandmother. Which of the following systems is most likely overactive in this patient?

    A. The hypothalamic–pituitary–adrenal axis
    B. The sympathetic nervous system
    C. The parasympathetic nervous system
    D. The orbitofrontal cortex
    E. The ventral tegmental area
    F. None of the above

4. A 19 y/o F is brought to the emergency department by her roommate after she started experiencing chest pain, difficulty breathing, dizziness, and "feeling like I was going to die." It took them 20 minutes to drive to the hospital, and by the time they arrived the patient reported that her symptoms had resolved. Vital signs at the time of initial examination are HR 118, BP 128/72, RR 20, and T 98.9°F. On interview, she describes having had similar episodes three times over the past month, including at work, at school, and while visiting friends. She denies having any major changes during that time period other than taking a new job; however, she says that overall she enjoys her job and doesn't feel that this is a major stress. Outside of needing to leave work early once, she has remained functional at her job and is performing well in her evening classes. She feels that overall her life is "good except for when stuff like this happens." Chest x-ray, EKG, and cardiac markers are all normal. She desires an explanation for her current symptoms. What is the most likely diagnosis?
    A. Panic disorder without agoraphobia
    B. Panic disorder with agoraphobia
    C. Generalized anxiety disorder
    D. Specific phobia
    E. None of the above

1. **The best answer is C.** This girl appears to have developed a specific phobia of birds (ornithophobia). People with specific phobias sometimes, but not always, develop this fear response following a specific incident. While the signs and symptoms seen in someone who is exposed to the object of their fear can be the same seen during a panic attack, the fact that these attacks only happen when exposed to the object rules out panic disorder (answer B). While the phobia has caused impairment even when the girl is not exposed to the object (she has stopped leaving the house or going to school), this is not consistent with generalized anxiety disorder as there is only a single object that is feared (answer A). The girl is not speaking which raises the possibility of selective mutism, but the fact that this has only occurred in the past 2 weeks and is not accompanied by any evidence that she suffers from a fear of interpersonal rejection or humiliation argues against either selective mutism or social anxiety disorder (answers D and E) as the explanation for her behavior.

2. **The best answer is A.** The psychologist is attempting to perform exposure therapy, which is an effective treatment for specific phobias. With each exposure, the goal is for the patient to feel "uncomfortable but not overwhelmed" to allow them to gradually reduce the fear response associated with the feared stimulus. In this case, starting with the stimulus that provokes the least fear (drawing a bird) would be the next best step. Medications do not play a significant role in treating specific phobias (answer D), while treatment should not be discontinued when there is an effective form of therapy available (answer E).

3. **The best answer is A.** This patient appears to be suffering from generalized anxiety disorder as evidenced by the presence of anxiety about multiple areas of his life that manifest in chronic symptoms of HPA axis activation including insomnia, restlessness, muscle tension, and irritability. The sympathetic nervous system is generally more involved in acute fear states like a panic attack (answer B), while the parasympathetic nervous system tends to *reduce* arousal rather than increase it (answer C). The orbitofrontal cortex is involved in prediction of rewards and is generally associated with mood episodes such as depression and mania (answer D), while the ventral tegmental area is implicated in addictive disorders (answer E).

4. **The best answer is E.** This patient has likely experienced a panic attack as evidenced by the presence of signs and symptoms of sympathetic nervous system activation, including tachycardia, chest pain, dizziness, and a feeling of impending doom. However, while she suffers from sudden, unexpected, and recurrent panic attacks, it is not clear that these have directly caused distress or dysfunction nor have they given rise to maladaptive behaviors (such as avoiding places like work or school where she has had a panic attack before). Therefore, it is not correct to say that she suffers from panic *disorder* (answers A and B). There is no evidence of chronic anxiety as would be seen in generalized anxiety disorder (answer C), nor do the panic attacks appear to be directly associated with specific objects or situations as would be seen in a specific phobia (answer D).

10 OCD

Obsessions are intrusive and unwanted thoughts that continue to recur despite attempts to resist them. Obsessive thoughts are disturbing and unpleasant, and someone who experiences obsessive thoughts often begins to feel distressed as result. This leads them to use **compulsions**, or specific behaviors that help to reduce the distress caused by obsessions. While compulsions are effective at reducing this distress, this relief is only temporary. In addition, because compulsions don't actually eliminate the obsessions driving the distress (if anything, obsessions are *reinforced* by compulsions), they create the potential for an **endless loop** between obsessions and compulsions that begins to take up more and more time, leading to dysfunction and disability.

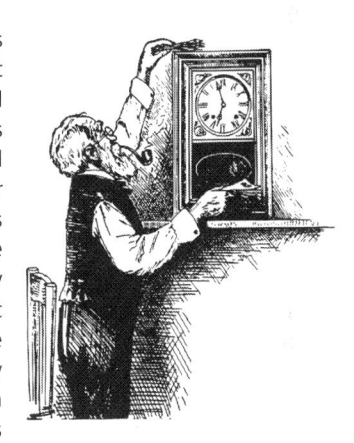

This is the basis of **obsessive-compulsive disorder** (commonly abbreviated as OCD), and we will start off our chapter by learning about this disorder in great detail. However, there are a number of other disorders that also involve obsessive thoughts, compulsive behaviors, or a combination of the two, including body dysmorphic disorder, hypochondriasis, trichotillomania, and tic disorder. These disorders are considered to be part of an **obsessive-compulsive spectrum** that bears a strong resemblance to "textbook" OCD in terms of phenomenology, prognosis, and treatment response. We will also look closely at the underlying mechanisms of obsessions and compulsions which will help us to understand how all of the disorders on the obsessive-compulsive spectrum fit together.

SIGNS AND SYMPTOMS OF OCD

Because obsessions and compulsions are central to understanding OCD, let's start off by making sure that we know exactly what we mean when we use these two terms.

OBSESSIONS

Obsessions are not normal thoughts. Instead, they have a number of characteristics which set them apart from the usual stream of consciousness that people have. To get a better feel for what an obsessive thought is like, imagine a young mother playing with her newborn baby outside. Suddenly, a random thought passes through her mind: *"You should kill your baby..."* She immediately reacts to this thought with a feeling of revulsion as well as some anxiety about what the thought might mean ("Why am I having this thought? Am I a baby murderer?"). She tries to reassure herself by saying, "That's ridiculous, that's not the kind of person I am" and reminding herself that she has never done something that like before. While this initially works to bring her anxiety down, soon the thought comes back (*"You should kill your baby..."*) which causes her to feel even more distress, as she now worries about what it means that the thought has come back *twice*. Her anxiety continues to rise, making the thought seem even scarier than it initially was. Over the next few days, she finds herself constantly haunted by this thought (*"You should kill your baby..."*), and she has even started avoiding going near her child out of fear that she might act on these thoughts (even though she has no desire to). These intrusive thoughts have now become an obsession.

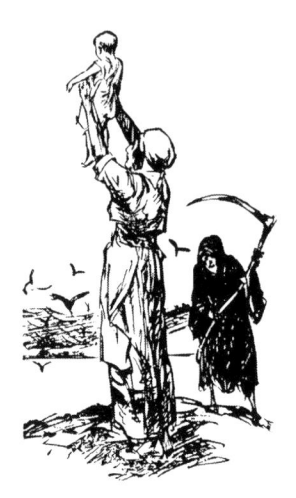

Let's go back through this story and use it to illustrate each of the characteristics of obsessive thoughts. Specifically, obsessive thoughts are **intrusive, mind-based, unwanted, resistant, distressing, ego-dystonic**, and **recurrent**. Handily, these attributes form the mnemonic "**I MURDER?**" (a question which you can imagine this poor woman asking herself over and over). Let's break these down one by one:

I is for Intrusive. Obsessive thoughts are experienced as intrusive, meaning that they enter the mind suddenly and without warning. This woman was minding her own business when suddenly this unpleasant thought entered into her mind.

M is for Mind-based. People with obsessional thoughts recognize that they originate from their own mind. This sets them apart from the auditory hallucinations found in schizophrenia which are experienced as originating outside of one's head and are genuinely believed to be an accurate perception of the real world.

U is for Unwanted. Obsessions are unwanted, and people who have these thoughts often try to ignore them or put them out of their mind. Paradoxically, any attempts to suppress obsessive thoughts often seem to make them even *stronger*, and in severe cases no amount of self-reassurance can make a dent in how frequent or intrusive the obsessions are.

R is for Resistant. Obsessive thoughts are remarkably resistant to efforts to ignore or suppress them. If the thought of killing your baby could be resisted easily through self-reassurance (as this woman initially tried to do), then it would likely be regarded as an unpleasant but ultimately meaningless occurrence (a bit of "flotsam in the stream of consciousness"). However, with obsessions, these thoughts aren't defeated so easily.

D is for Distressing. Obsessional thoughts are upsetting and cause distress to the person experiencing them. While most people have intrusive thoughts from time to time, it is the thoughts that are most distressing—those that are felt to be highly **inappropriate**, **disgusting**, or **immoral**—that are the most likely to develop into obsessions. (No one comes into clinic complaining of intrusive thoughts about cute kittens.) This explains why obsessional thoughts so often fit the worries and anxieties of the person who develops them, with someone growing up in a clean household being more likely to develop obsessions about orderliness and someone from a religious home being more likely to develop obsessions about blasphemous thoughts.

E is for Ego-dystonic. Someone having obsessional thoughts is generally able to recognize that, despite being based in their own mind, the intrusive thoughts are not reflective of their true desires. In this example, the mother is able to say very clearly that she has no desire to act upon these thoughts and that she finds them incredibly disturbing ("That's not the kind of person I am!"). The word **ego-dystonic** is used to describe these thoughts, as they are discordant with someone's self-concept (or their "ego" in psychiatric jargon).

R is for Recurrent. It is the recurrent nature of obsessive thoughts that truly defines them as a disorder. After all, even the most disturbing thoughts will be quickly forgotten unless they begin to happen repeatedly. The frequent recurrence of obsessive thoughts directly sets the stage for someone to seek out specific things they can do to help fight these thoughts when they recur, creating fertile ground for the development of compulsions (discussed next).

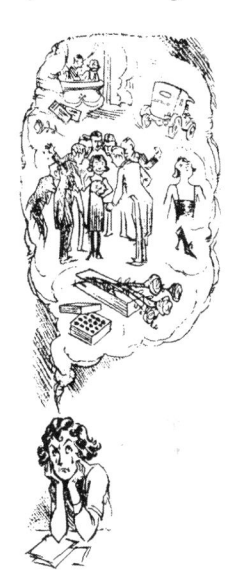

> Obsessions are **intrusive, mind-based, unwanted, resistant, distressing, ego-dystonic, recurrent** thoughts.
>
> *"I MURDER?":*
> **I**ntrusive
> **M**ind-based
> **U**nwanted
> **R**esistant
> **D**istressing
> **E**go-dystonic
> **R**ecurrent

In the real world, obsessions can take on a variety of specific forms. The most common forms include **checking** ("Did I forget to turn off the stove?"), **contamination** ("I will get sick if I don't clean my hands after touching a doorknob"), **symmetry** ("These books have to line up *exactly*"), and **taboo thoughts** involving topics such as sex and religion ("I can't stop thinking about having sex with the Virgin Mary"). The majority of people with OCD will have obsessions in more than one of these forms. However, despite these variations in content, all types of obsessive thought patterns will still fit the same underlying pattern as captured in the **I MURDER?** mnemonic.

COMPULSIONS

Because obsessions tend to provoke feelings of intense anxiety or distress, people with obsessions will try to find any thoughts or actions that they can do to relieve this distress. These **neutralizing behaviors** are known as **compulsions** (although you can think of them as **calm**-pulsions to help you remember that their intended purpose is to **calm** distress related to obsessions!).

> Compulsions are **neutralizing behaviors** that help to **reduce distress** related to obsessions.
>
> *Calm-pulsions help to calm obsessive thoughts.*

Let's illustrate this with an example. A young man is about to go to bed, as he has an important exam early the next morning. As his head hits the pillow, he has a sudden thought: "Did I forget to lock the front door?" He initially puts the thought out of his mind, but it won't go away and he begins to feel increasingly anxious about what might happen if the door is left unlocked the whole night. To counter this anxiety, he gets up to check the door (a compulsion), which immediately relieves his anxiety (making the compulsion a **negative reinforcer**). However, as soon as he climbs back into bed, the thought suddenly comes back: "Did I forget to lock the door?" Despite telling himself over and over that he *knows* that he checked the lock, he cannot put the thought out of his mind (the thought is *resistant*). His anxiety continues to rise until he cannot take it any longer, and he gets up to check the lock again. This again temporarily reduces his anxiety. However, just like before, this relief is not sustained, and the obsession recurs the moment he returns to his room. He becomes increasingly frustrated with himself for continuing to check the door over and over, but due to his ever-rising levels of anxiety, he cannot actually keep himself from doing so. (As with obsessions, compulsions are typically ego-dystonic: someone *knows* that their behaviors are excessive, but they are unable to stop themselves from engaging in them.) As a result, he spends the next five hours repeating this cycle, which keeps him up all night and prevents him from getting any rest. The next morning, he fails his test as he is too fatigued to concentrate on the questions. In this way, the loop between obsessions and compulsions has set the stage for a pattern of behavior that leads to distress, disability, and dysfunction.

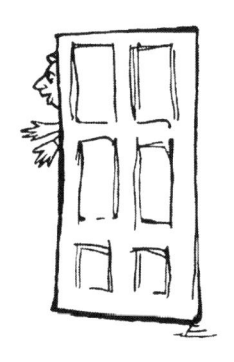

As this example illustrates, compulsions work, but they don't work for very long. (If they did, this poor student would have been able to get back to sleep after checking the lock just once!) Instead, people with OCD find that the same obsessive thoughts just come back again, often at a higher intensity than before. This leads to further use of compulsions to neutralize these thoughts, creating a vicious cycle between obsessions and compulsions. Research has shown that people with OCD have difficulty recognizing that tasks have been completed, and the "feeling of knowing" that something has been done (the door has been locked, your hands have been cleaned, the books are lined up perfectly, and so on) never comes. In anything, compulsions often reinforce the obsessive thoughts that necessitated them in the first place, effectively feeding the very beast that they were intended to defeat. This is what truly sets the stage for the **disordered loop** that is at the center of OCD.

THE IMPULSIVE COMPULSIVE-SPECTRUM

Before we move on, let's spend a few moments differentiating compulsivity from impulsivity, as both involve the **inability to inhibit an action** (as in someone can't *not* do something). However, compulsivity and impulsivity differ in regards to the reason *why* the person can't not do the behavior. As discussed in Chapter 8, impulsivity involves repeated use of *positive* reinforcers despite negative repercussions, resulting in the prioritizing of short-term benefits over long-term consequences. In contrast, compulsivity involves repeated use of *negative* reinforcers despite negative repercussions. Unlike the pleasurable activities that form the targets for addiction, compulsive behaviors are not inherently enjoyable (there is no "thrill" or "rush" to be found in checking a lock repeatedly). Instead, it is a compulsion's ability to *take away* distress (at least temporarily) that makes it so difficult to resist. It is this calming function that makes compulsions so difficult to resist. To remember this distinction, remember that **calm**pulsions work to **calm** an internal sense of anxiety. In contrast, **impos**'es provide **im**mediate **pos**itive reinforcement when they are indulged.

> **Impulses** and **compulsions** both involve an **inability to inhibit an action** but differ in whether the behaviors are **positively reinforcing** or **negatively reinforcing**.
>
> *Impos'es provide immediate positive reinforcement when they are indulged.*

To be clear, the line between impulsivity and compulsivity is not always neatly defined. Some behaviors are initially quite pleasurable but lose their pleasurable properties over time, turning them from an action done impulsively into one done compulsively. For example, someone who takes heroin for its euphoric rush may soon find that they are now using it primarily to avoid the uncomfortable state of withdrawal. In other cases, specific behaviors can be *both* positively and negatively reinforcing. For example, someone who is so angry after an argument with their spouse that they punch a wall may experience not only a lessening of their internal sense of agitation (a negative reinforcement) but also an emotional "thrill" that feels inherently pleasurable (a positive reinforcement). Despite the boundaries between these concepts not being completely clear cut, knowing these definitions can still help to guide diagnosis and treatment decisions in many cases.

OCD ACROSS THE LIFESPAN

EPIDEMIOLOGY
OCD is a relatively **rare** disorder with a **low base rate** in the population, with around 1% of people having clinically significant symptoms of OCD at any given moment and up to 3% being diagnosed at some point in their lifetime. This makes it more liable to **overdiagnosis** than underdiagnosis. **Men and women** have an equal chance of being affected. Onset of symptoms is often during **childhood or young adulthood**, with most people developing symptoms before the age of 20 and almost all before age 30.

PROGNOSIS
Symptoms generally come on gradually but soon become **chronic and enduring**. OCD is not considered an episodic disorder, although there may be times when symptoms can temporarily worsen or abate. The severity of OCD is on a spectrum, as some people are only mildly affected while others are completely disabled. The **amount of time** that someone spends thinking about obsessive thoughts and/or engaging in compulsive behaviors can be a helpful proxy for assessing how severe their disorder is. For example, if someone is spending 8 hours each day checking to see if the door is locked or washing their hands, it will be practically impossible for them engage in any kind of work, school, or social life. Beyond just time spent, OCD can severely disrupt one's quality of life in other ways. For example, a patient with OCD may not have touched another human being for years due to fear of contamination, leading to frayed relationships and unimaginable loneliness. Left untreated, OCD can reduce one's quality of life and ability to function for **years or even decades**. However, even without treatment, a small but noticeable lowering of symptoms may occur over time.

TREATMENT
The first-line treatment for OCD is psychotherapy, with **CBT** being the best-studied method. In particular, patients with OCD benefit from a form of CBT known as **exposure and response prevention** in which they are encouraged to expose themselves to the object of their obsessional thoughts without resorting to use of compulsions to reduce their anxiety. For example, someone who believes that all doorknobs are contaminated and feels the need to wash their hands after touching one would be encouraged to touch a doorknob and then delay hand washing for as long as possible. The length of time between the obsession and compulsion is made longer and longer until the link between them is eventually broken. By doing this, people with OCD begin to learn that the obsession does not actually lead to the feared outcome (they don't actually get sick if they don't wash their hands) and that the compulsions are unnecessary for preventing harm. Even in cases where exposure to the object of the obsession cannot be done directly (you can't ask someone to hold a knife to their baby in the same way that you could ask them to avoid washing their hands), just imagining the feared scenario via talking or writing about it can cause significant reductions in symptoms. Exposure and response prevention is incredibly effective at treating OCD, with a **very large effect size** over 1.0!

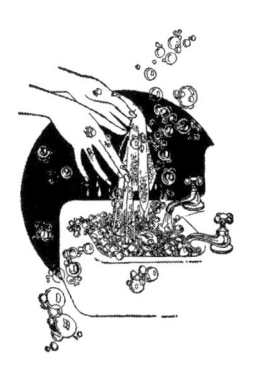

Medications can also be used to treat OCD. **Serotonergic medications** are most helpful, with SRIs being frequently used. These medications must often be used at **higher doses** than those used for depression. The use of SRIs for OCD has a **large effect size** (compared to the small to medium effect size seen when using SRIs for depression or anxiety). Compared to CBT, however, medication treatment of OCD has a few drawbacks. It produces only transient improvement in symptoms and is associated with a high recurrence rate when the medications are discontinued. In addition, it is unclear that combining medications with therapy leads to improved outcomes over therapy alone. Because of this, medications should mostly be used as a second-line option in cases where therapy has been ineffective, more rapid treatment is necessary, or the patient is unable to participate in therapy for whatever reason.

MECHANISMS OF OCD

The key to understanding OCD and other disorders on the obsessive-compulsive spectrum (which we will discuss in the next section) is to focus in on the **underlying pattern** of the disorder. This pattern has been known from the very first descriptions of OCD, including a line from the early 1900s that described people with the disorder as being "continually tormented by an **inner sense of imperfection** connected with the perception that actions or intentions have been **incompletely achieved**." These two components (a sense that something is wrong in addition to a feeling that actions have been incompletely achieved) are found in all obsessive-compulsive spectrum disorders, so it is crucial to understand the mechanisms underlying each of them.

The first component (the inner sense of imperfection) is related to dysfunctional **error signals** that generate a distinct sense that *something is wrong*. To understand what is meant by an error signal better, take a look at the following picture:

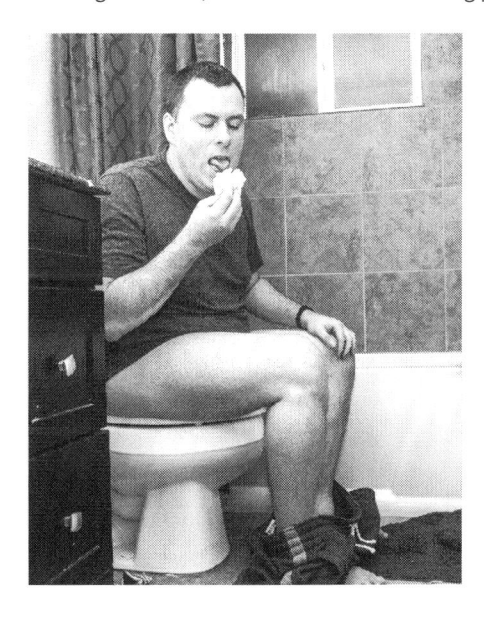

What do you feel? If you're like most people, your initial reaction is that this is disgusting, this is unacceptable, this is *wrong*. **Error signals** in response to situations like this are processed in a part of the brain known as the **anterior cingulate cortex** (ACC). The discrepancy between two situations that we know *should not go together* (such as "eating" and "toilet paper") makes the anterior cingulate cortex launch into action, creating a feeling of disgust and distress. This pattern is core to the idea of **obsessions**, with the sensitivity of the anterior cingulate cortex being linked to how likely someone is to recognize error signals. You can remember the function of the Anterior Cingulate Cortex by thinking that it's the part of the brain that yells, "**ACC**! That's so wrong!"

The distress we feel when our anterior cingulate cortex has recognized an error isn't there just to make us feel bad. Instead, its function is to put us into a state of **motivational arousal** that prompts us to act and fix the error. To understand this better, consider this image:

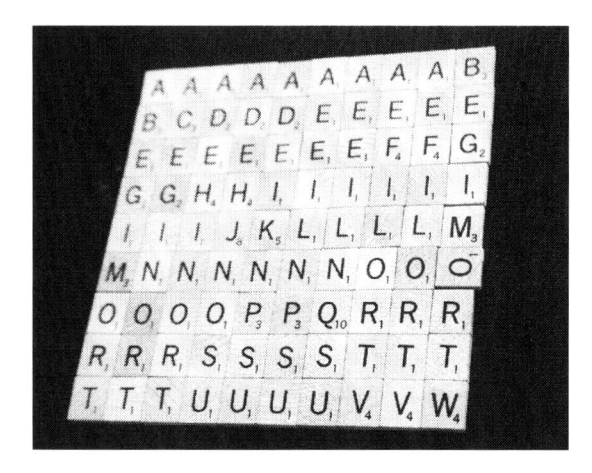

How do you feel when looking at this image? Some people feel upset by the perceived error in this image due to activation of their anterior cingulate cortex. This creates a state of motivational arousal that prompts them to want to turn the O tile 90° so it will fit with the rest of the tiles. However, other people will look at the image and not feel upset or bothered by it in any way. For them, this image does not generate an error signal or activate the anterior cingulate cortex. It is this spectrum of **sensitivity to error signaling** that appears to put people at higher or lower risk for obsessive-compulsive disorders. In some cases, the sensitivity to error signaling is so strong that people perceive errors even where none exist (as we will discuss further when talking about body dysmorphic disorder and hypochondriasis).

> The **anterior cingulate cortex** is involved in **error recognition** and is believed to be **hyperactive in obsessive-compulsive disorder**.
>
> The *Anterior Cingulate Cortex* makes you think, "*ACC! That's so wrong.*"

The relationship between error signaling and motivational arousal explains how obsessions give rise to compulsions, as recognition of an error signal practically *demands* action. However, there is nothing inherently pathological about either error signaling or motivational arousal, and we often use these processes to govern our behavior. For example, someone who is bothered by the O tile in the previous picture can simply turn it 90° and make it line up with all the other tiles. Upon completion of this task, they receive a "**feeling of knowing**" that the task has been completed which turns off the motivational arousal and allows them to return to an unbothered state. This "feeling of knowing" is registered in the **prefrontal cortex**, a region of the brain which (among many other things) links motivational arousal to a specific task. In this case, the link between the error signal and its associated behavior is **linear**: once the task is completed, the error signal goes away.

However, for patients with OCD, this pattern is not linear but rather occurs in a **loop**, with the error signal persisting *even once the task is completed*. People with OCD appear to have a deficient "feeling of knowing" and experience only a fraction of the relief from motivational arousal that most people receive upon completing a task (or even no relief at all). This leads to a distinct and unpleasant sensation that the behavior has not been not done even though they *know* intellectually that it has (this is the "perception that actions or intentions have been incompletely achieved" referenced earlier). This deficiency was demonstrated in a study in which two groups of people (one with OCD and one without) were asked to immerse their hands in a soiled diaper. Compared to people without OCD, people with OCD did not necessarily experience *more* motivational arousal when touching the dirty diaper (unsurprisingly, both groups wanted to wash their hands as soon as possible!). However, people with OCD differed from normal controls in that they were *less able to exit* this state of distress by washing their hands. The sense of being dirty and contaminated persisted much longer for people with OCD, leading to more hand washing. Because performing the compulsive behavior is only transiently effective at knocking out the sense of motivational anxiety driving the behavior (the "feeling of knowing" doesn't stick), the behavior continues over and over again in a loop.

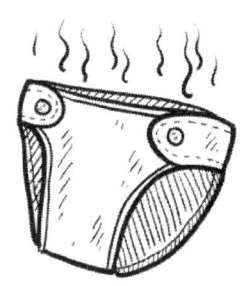

In this way, compulsions are revealed to result from a "**problem with stopping**" due to an ineffective "feeling of knowing" rather than a "problem with starting" as is seen in addiction and other disorders related to impulse control. People with OCD often report a conscious sense that they are unable to stop ("I can't move on because I can't convince myself that I've finished what I'm doing") and tend to engage in *few but extended* sessions of compulsive behavior (compared to people with addictions who tend towards *frequent but short* sessions of impulsive behavior).

This overall pattern (hypersensitive error signal → motivational arousal → compulsive behavior → lack of "feeing of knowing" → continuation of error signal) is key to understanding not only OCD but also the other disorders on the obsessive-compulsive spectrum, so keep it in mind while learning about each of the obsessive-compulsive disorders in the next section!

HOW TO DIAGNOSE OBSESSIVE-COMPULSIVE DISORDERS

While OCD is the most famous disorder involving both obsessions and compulsions, there are several other related conditions including **body dysmorphic disorder**, **hypochondriasis**, **tic disorders**, and **trichotillomania**. Like OCD, they all involve either an obsessional preoccupation with an idea (as in body dysmorphic disorder and hypochondriasis) or recurrent uncontrollable behaviors that appear more compulsive than impulsive (as in tic disorders or trichotillomania). These disorders also co-occur in the same person more often that would be predicted by chance and tend to respond to similar kinds of treatment, suggesting a shared mechanism. For these reasons, these conditions are considered to be sufficiently similar to OCD to warrant inclusion in an "obsessive-compulsive spectrum." We'll go over each one now in turn.

OBSESSIVE-COMPULSIVE DISORDER

OCD is defined by the presence of obsessions, compulsions, and a loop between the two. While obsessions are *required* for diagnosis, **compulsions are optional**. This is because compulsions are a **specific behavioral response** to obsessions which *often* (but do not *always*) develop. Because of this, everyone with clinically significant compulsions will have obsessions as well; however, not everyone with obsessions will develop compulsions. (This is similar to the development of agoraphobia in panic disorder or selective mutism in social anxiety disorder, as both are specific *behavioral* outcomes of core cognitive process.) Cases of obsessions without compulsions are sometimes known as **purely obsessional** (or "pure-O") OCD. The lack of compulsions does *not* mean that purely obsessional OCD is any less impairing; if anything, purely obsessional OCD is considered to be *more* impairing than "textbook" OCD and is significantly more difficult to treat.

BODY DYSMORPHIC DISORDER

Body dysmorphic disorder is an obsessive-compulsive spectrum disorder involving an obsessional preoccupation that **specific aspects of one's appearance are flawed or deformed**, such as a nose that is too big or a head that is too small. This is distressing, and people with body dysmorphic disorder fear that this will cause other people to reject or make fun of them. However, the key is that these flaws in appearance are entirely **imagined**, and no objective outside evaluator would find them deformed. (It's important to recognize that body dysmorphic disorder is not just vanity! People with body dysmorphic disorder want to *normalize* their appearance, as opposed to vanity where the goal is to make yourself look better than others.) Unlike obsessions in "textbook" OCD, preoccupations about appearance in body dysmorphic disorder are **ego-syntonic**, and the person does not admit that their fears are extreme or excessive in any way.

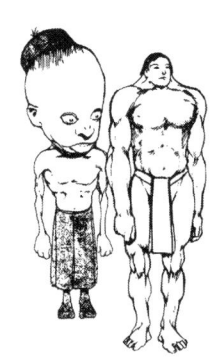

People with body dysmorphic disorder have a tendency to engage in specific **compulsive behaviors** such as body measuring, mirror checking, excessive grooming, and reassurance seeking that are aimed at hiding or fixing their perceived flaws. However, no amount of reassurance or covering up can convince the person that their features are not deformed: just like in OCD, the "feeling of knowing" that the defect has been fixed never comes. This sets up the potential for an endless loop between obsessions and compulsions. What makes this loop particularly troubling in body dysmorphic disorder is the fact that many people will go on to seek plastic surgery in an attempt to "definitively" correct the flaw. However, less than 5% of people with the disorder report feeling satisfied after surgery, making it a high-risk intervention with a low likelihood of benefit. In fact, some people with body dysmorphic disorder end up going under the knife dozens of times throughout their life without ever finding relief!

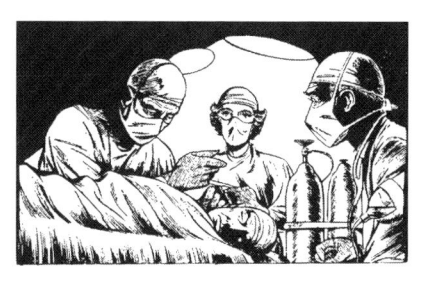

Body dysmorphic disorder is **relatively rare** and is found in only around 1-2% of the population. However, its prevalence may be much higher in certain settings (around 10% of patients in dermatology clinics and up to **one-third of patients seeking cosmetic surgery**). The disorder often begins during **adolescence** or early adulthood, with a mean age of onset of 16 years. However, many patients do not seek their first surgical consultation until later in life. Despite societal stereotypes, body dysmorphic disorder is equally common among both **men and women**. However, the content of dysmorphic beliefs tends to vary between the genders, with men being more likely to perceive parts of themselves as being *too small* (most often their muscles or genitals) while women are more likely to perceive body parts as being *too large or disfigured* (such as their nose or ears).

Without treatment, body dysmorphic disorder tends to remain and become **chronic**, with less than 10% of people experiencing remission within one year. However, with treatment, patients with this disorder can often do quite well and return to some semblance of normalcy. Treatment of body dysmorphic disorder is the same as for OCD, with a **very large effect size** for **CBT** (over 1.5) and a **large effect size** for **SRIs** (around 0.9).

You can remember the overall pattern of body dysmorphic disorder using the phrase **Fix ME DOC!** which should be easily linked to the concept of body dysmorphic disorder. This will help you to remember the **Fix**ation on a perceived flaw, the pattern of seeking **M**edical care, the **E**go-syntonic thought pattern, the **D**isabling nature of the disorder, the similarities to the **O**bsessive thought patterns found in OCD, and finally the **C**ompulsive grooming and checking behaviors that result.

Body dysmorphic disorder is an **obsessive-compulsive spectrum disorder** involving a **perceived flaw in physical appearance**.

"Fix ME DOC!":
Fixation on perceived flaw
Medical care-seeking
Ego-syntonic
Disabling
Obsessive thoughts
Compulsive behaviors

HYPOCHONDRIASIS

Hypochondriasis (called "illness anxiety disorder" in the DSM-5) involves an **obsessional preoccupation that one has a medical illness**. While everyone has physical symptoms at various points throughout the day (including random pains, aches, upset stomach, blurry vision, and ringing in the ears), people with hypochondriasis are likely to interpret these sensations as error signals of the most serious kind ("I've had this headache for a few hours now. This *must* mean that I have brain cancer!"). This leads them to spend lots of time and energy in **compulsive behaviors** such as researching possible causes of their symptoms on the internet or frequently going to the doctor for evaluation. However, just like in OCD, no amount of reassurance will lead to a "feeling of knowing" that they don't have an illness, and their obsessional preoccupation with the idea of having a medical condition will persist no matter how much evidence is presented to the contrary ("I don't *care* what all the doctors and labs and imaging reports say! I *know* that I have cancer!"). This leads to endless use of medical resources and puts the patient at risk of unnecessary medical harm (such as use of medications with side effects or high doses of ionizing radiation from repeated radiographic studies). This obsessional preoccupation can often begin to affect the patient's life as well, preventing them from engaging in normal activities, socializing with others, and remaining active due to the persistent belief that they are sick.

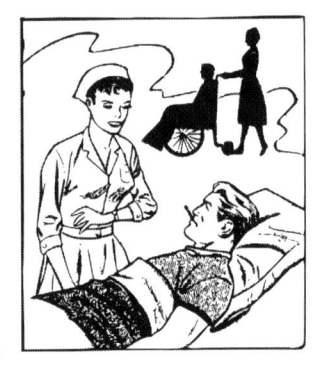

While certain forms of OCD involve fears of becoming sick or contaminated, in hypochondriasis the person isn't worried that they will *get* an illness, they are worried that they *have* an illness. In addition, the preoccupation with having a medical disease in hypochondriasis is **ego-syntonic**, and people with hypochondriasis have no conception that their interpretation of physical symptoms is in any way excessive or unreasonable (even though they often appear that way to an outside observer).

Clinically significant hypochondriasis appears to be **relatively uncommon**, with a prevalence of around 0.5% of the general population. Like other obsessive-compulsive disorders, hypochondriasis most commonly begins in **early adulthood** and is found equally among **men and women**. Clinical features that suggest hypochondriasis include a history of extensive work-ups for symptoms for which no medical cause is ever found (often involving consultation with multiple clinicians) as well as a pattern of the patient becoming *more* dissatisfied and anxious in response to negative findings (unlike for most people where news that nothing is wrong is received with elation and relief!).

Once diagnosed, treatment for hypochondriasis should consist of **CBT** as a first-line intervention, as it is associated with a **large effect size** (around 0.8 or 0.9). Use of **SRIs** appears to be helpful as well and can represent a reasonable treatment option. However, both of these treatments are limited by the fact that the patient needs to believe that there is something worth treating from a psychological perspective, leading to low rates of treatment adherence and engagement.

As a final note, a diagnosis of hypochondriasis should be given cautiously! Given its low base rate, it is more likely to be **overdiagnosed** than underdiagnosed. More importantly, diagnosing someone with hypochondriasis can be stigmatizing and can severely jeopardize the therapeutic relationship. There is also the risk of missing a medical condition that is actually present. For all these reasons, make sure that you have fully ruled out all other possibilities before diagnosing hypochondriasis, and always try to validate your patient's concerns while trying to point towards interventions that you believe will be the most likely to lead to positive outcomes.

> **Hypochondriasis** involves a **persistent belief** that one has a **physical illness despite reassurance** and **evidence to the contrary**.
>
> *In hypo-**conned**-riasis, the patient believes that the doctor is being **conned** by the normal signs and lab findings.*

TIC DISORDERS

Tics are **sudden contractions** of specific skeletal muscles or vocal muscle groups that tend to occur in **repetitive bouts**. Tics may involve simple movements (such as eye blinking, grunting, or throat clearing) or more complex actions (such as arm jerking, foot stomping, or forming a whole word or sentence). On a cognitive level, tics are preceded by a conscious sensation of **rising inner tension** (often described as an "urge") that is relieved by performing the tic. Tics are neither entirely voluntary nor entirely involuntary; instead, tics are best thought of as **irresistible** in the sense that they can be *delayed* with mental effort but not repressed entirely.

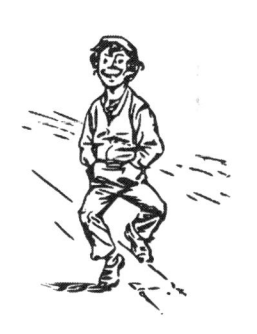

> **Tics** are **transient irresistible contractions** of specific **muscle groups** that occur **suddenly** in **repetitive bouts**.
>
> *A **TIC** is a **T**ransient **I**rresistible **C**ontraction.*

Tics are believed to be related to OCD in that they both follow a similar pattern (a state of increasing mental tension that must be discharged through performing a compulsive act). However, they differ from OCD in that they don't necessarily involve *conscious or verbal* thoughts and are instead experienced as vague urges.

Tics often begin in **childhood** between the ages of 3 and 8. Motor tics tend to appear first, followed by vocal tics. For the majority of people with this condition, tics occur in a waxing-and-waning course throughout childhood and adolescence, with bouts of tics occurring for a few months followed by periods of relative remission. There is often a gradual lessening of tics throughout adolescence such that by the age of 20 tics are significantly reduced, if not gone entirely. Tics are **relatively common**, with around 20% of school-age children experiencing transient tics and 5% experiencing chronic tics. However, it is only a minority (around 1%) of children who develop tics that are severe enough that they interfere with functioning and would therefore be said to have a **tic disorder**. A specific form variant of tic disorder known as **Tourette syndrome** involves a combination of multiple motor tics and at least one vocal tic. Despite popular media portrayals of Tourette syndrome often involving sudden shouts of profanity (known as *coprolalia*), this phenomenon occurs only in a minority of children with the disorder (around 10%).

> **Tourette syndrome** is characterized by **multiple motor tics** and at least one **vocal tic**.
>
> ***Two**-rette syndrome involves **two** forms of tics (both motor and vocal).*

Tics are not inherently pathological, and many people with tics do not need treatment. In cases where the tics are impairing or disruptive (such as someone whose tics interfere with their ability to go to school or play with others), treatment involves a specific type of CBT known as **habit reversal training**. This form of therapy involves learning to recognize when an urge is building up and then to voluntarily perform a "competing" action that physically cannot be done at the same time as the tic (such as someone with a shoulder shrug tic instead pushing their shoulders downward). The competing act should be held until the urge goes away. Habit reversal training is associated with a **large effect size** around 0.8 not only for tics but for several related conditions including stuttering, nail biting, and thumb sucking. Pharmacologically, **antipsychotics** are reasonably effective at reducing tics, with a **medium effect size** around 0.6. However, their high side effect burden means that their use should be limited to only severe or unusual cases.

TRICHOTILLOMANIA

Trichotillomania ("hair pulling madness") is a condition in which people **repeatedly pull out their hair**, leading to skin damage and hair loss. Many people with trichotillomania say they have no desire to lose their hair and wish that they could stop engaging in this unwanted repetitive behavior. However, just like tics, hair pulling is preceded by an urge that is **irresistible**. This places trichotillomania more in line with compulsive disorders than impulsive disorders (as the act of pulling hair out is not positively reinforcing). The link between trichotillomania and obsessive-compulsive disorders is further reinforced by the fact that this condition is found in higher rates in people with OCD or in relatives of those with OCD. Treatment involves **habit reversal training**. Medications like SRIs are only minimally effective at best and should generally not be used to treat trichotillomania.

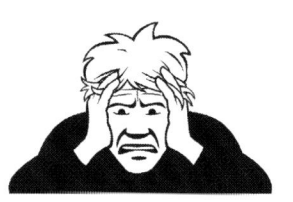

> **Obsessive-compulsive spectrum disorders** include **tic disorders, trichotillomania, hypochondriasis,** and **body dysmorphic disorder**.
>
> *Think of the **icks**: **tic**, **trich**, **sick**, and dysmor**phic**.*

A few other conditions (including dermatillomania and hoarding disorder) have previously been considered for inclusion in the OCD spectrum, but further research suggests that they are likely separate conditions. So that we are not tormented by an inner sense of incompleteness, we will briefly review them now.

DERMATILLOMANIA

Dermatillomania (also known as **pathologic skin picking** or excoriation disorder) is a condition in which people repeatedly pick at their skin, resulting in injury. It is similar to trichotillomania as both involve repetitive acts of damage to one's own body. However, evidence suggests that in most cases pathologic skin picking is driven more by *impulsivity* than compulsivity. Support for this comes from the facts that most people who engage in skin picking say they find it pleasurable (making it *positively* reinforcing), that there is no link between skin picking behaviors and obsessive thoughts, and that treatments for OCD are generally not very effective for dermatillomania. It's unclear why skin picking differs so much from hair pulling on a biological level (as they *seem* pretty similar at first glance), but at least for now we'll just have to accept that "they're just different."

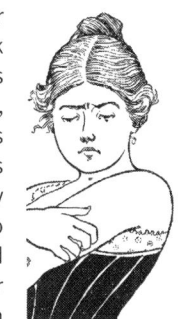

COMPULSIVE HOARDING

Hoarding, or the **continuous accumulation of possessions** to the point that it creates significant dysfunction in one's life, has a complex relationship to OCD. Like OCD, this behavior appears to be largely compulsive in nature and is driven by a sense of inner anxiety ("I can't throw this magazine away! I might need it later!"). However, unlike OCD, hoarding is **ego-syntonic**, as the person truly believes that hoarding these items is necessary and important.

For a long time, hoarding was simply seen as a type of OCD (similar to "contamination OCD" or "symmetry OCD"). However, hoarding is now considered to be a separate disorder. This distinction is based on the facts that hoarding and OCD have different prognoses (OCD tends to improve over time while hoarding generally worsens), different responses to treatment (with hoarding being poorly responsive to both CBT and serotonergic medications), and distinct neural mechanisms.

Just to add to the complexity, for a minority of people with OCD, hoarding can be a *manifestation* of OCD. In these people, hoarding is notably ego-*dystonic* and follows the pattern of OCD: an intrusive thought that can't be cleared away ("If you throw that book away, your mother will hate you!") leading to repeatedly engaging in a compulsive behavior (hoarding). This is rare, however, and in most cases hoarding should be considered a separate diagnosis from OCD.

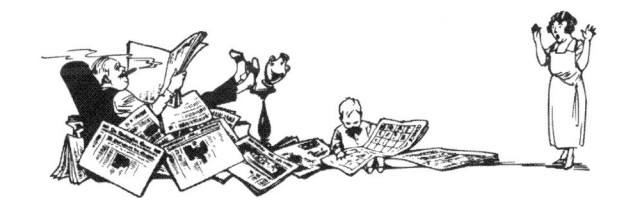

DIFFERENTIAL DIAGNOSIS OF OCD

OCD can resemble other psychiatric disorders that either feature distressing thoughts (such as anxiety) or involve rigid or repetitive behaviors (such autism). Having a clear grasp on the phenomenology of both obsessions and compulsions is the best way to protect against diagnostic confusion, so make sure that these concepts (as captured in the **I MURDER?** and **calm**-pulsion mnemonics) are straight in your head!

NORMALCY

As we talked about in the section on mechanisms of OCD, it is normal and adaptive to recognize errors, to experience motivational arousal, and to perform specific actions to reduce this arousal. However, the difference between normalcy and pathology lies in whether the connection between obsessions and compulsions is a *line* or a *loop*. It is only when the "feeling of knowing" breaks down and the compulsive actions start becoming repetitive and maladaptive that the disorder occurs. When trying to decide between normalcy and OCD, **look for the loop**!

The word "OCD" is often misused by people both inside and outside the medical community, leading to diagnostic confusion. Despite popular conceptions, OCD is *not* synonymous with being "clean" or "orderly" (although the concepts are not *entirely* unrelated). In addition, some degree of obsessiveness is likely adaptive, as people who maintain good hygiene are more likely to avoid illness, and a desire for cleanliness and order can be highly desired characteristics, especially in fields of work like engineering or healthcare where being detail-oriented is an asset. Because of this, avoid thinking that all people who are orderly or methodical have (or "are") OCD.

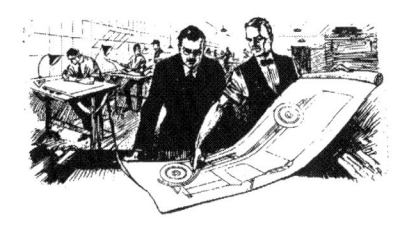

ANXIETY

OCD was previously classified as an anxiety disorder in the DSM, and while it has since been split off into its own section, several links between anxiety and OCD remain. For one, anxiety can often be the presenting symptom of OCD (remember that OCD is the **O** in the **O**NSTAGE mnemonic). In addition, OCD follows a very similar **A**larm—**B**eliefs—**C**oping pattern that characterizes other anxiety disorders.

However, there are also enough differences that make it so that OCD is best thought of as separate from anxiety. While anxiety is *sometimes* a prominent feature of this disorder, it is not the *core* pathology, and there are some cases of OCD that do not involve anxiety in any way. For example, someone with symmetry-related obsessions may be bothered when things are out of place, but they are not necessarily *worried* about anything bad happening because of it. In this way, the difference between the two disorders becomes apparent: OCD results from a dysfunctional *error* system while anxiety disorders result from a dysfunctional *alarm* system.

TRAUMA

PTSD and OCD share more than a few similarities. Both are characterized by recurrent, intrusive, and unwanted thoughts, and both were considered to be anxiety disorders before being split off into their own categories (with trauma being the **T** in the

ONSTAGE mnemonic). In addition, PTSD and OCD are frequently comorbid, and at least in some people, a traumatic event can sometimes "trigger" the development of OCD. Because of this, a history of trauma should be assessed in all patients presenting with obsessive-compulsive symptoms (and vice versa), as up to 30% of people who have one will end up having the other as well. In patients where only one disorder is suspected, one clinical feature that can help to differentiate between the two is **age of onset**, as OCD generally begins in adolescence whereas PTSD tends to begin later in life.

OBSESSIVE-COMPULSIVE PERSONALITY DISORDER
We have not talked about obsessive-compulsive personality disorder yet (it will be discussed more fully in Chapter 14), but it is characterized by extreme and inflexible traits of high conscientiousness and low openness to new experiences that manifests in **rigid and perfectionistic beliefs and behaviors**. Despite being named obsessive-compulsive personality disorder, this condition is not characterized by either obsessions or compulsions, making it one of the worst named disorders in the DSM. Don't let the words "obsessive" and "compulsive" in the name distract you! Obsessive-compulsive personality disorder is an entirely separate condition from OCD.

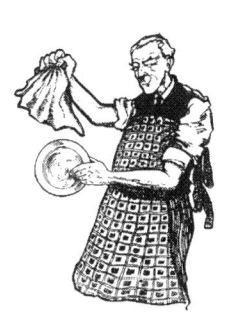

ADDICTION
Obsessive-compulsive disorders and addictive disorders both share a pattern of repeatedly engaging in specific behaviors despite negative repercussions. Because of this, it is easy to get the terminology wrong (you may hear someone say that a patient "uses cocaine compulsively" or is "addicted to washing their hands"). It's important to get this distinction right because the prognosis and treatment considerations for impulsive disorders like addiction differ significantly from those for compulsive disorders like OCD! Pay attention to whether the specific behaviors are **im**mediately **pos**itively reinforcing (in which case they would represent dysfunctions in **impos** control) or whether they serve to **calm** an internal sense of anxiety (in which case they would likely represent **calm**-pulsions).

PSYCHOSIS
Both OCD and primary psychotic disorders can include beliefs that others find odd or unreasonable. In some cases, it is impossible to tell whether a belief is related to OCD or psychosis just from the belief alone. A key differentiating feature between OCD and psychotic disorders is that bizarre beliefs in OCD are notably ego-*dystonic* while those in psychosis are ego-*syntonic*. Someone with obsessive thoughts *knows* that they are excessive, odd, or bizarre. In contrast, someone with a delusion does not necessarily see their thoughts as being strange and sincerely believes that they represent an accurate view of reality. In addition, the presence of other signs and symptoms of schizophrenia such as thought disorganization or auditory hallucinations would not be expected in OCD.

AUTISM
Obsessive-compulsive disorders and autism can both be characterized by repetitive or rigid behaviors, and just like with psychosis and OCD it is not always possible to tell from the behavior itself which disorder it belongs to. For example, someone who organizes all the items on their bathroom sink every single morning without fail may be diagnosed with either OCD, autism, or even plain old normalcy depending on the *reasons* why they do this behavior. If they engage in the behavior to neutralize obsessive beliefs, a diagnosis of OCD should be considered. If they do it out of a preference for sameness or to provide sensory stimulation, this is in line with an autism spectrum disorder. If they do it because they like to, it's probably just normal.

DEPRESSION
Depression and OCD are frequently comorbid. In addition, the ruminative thoughts in depression appear to share phenomenological and treatment similarities with OCD, suggesting at least some overlap in etiology. For this reason, it is helpful to rule out a diagnosis of depression when someone presents with OCD.

PUTTING IT ALL TOGETHER

Obsessive-compulsive disorders can be initially difficult to understand, as many of the conditions that fall within this group do not appear to have much in common ("What does hair pulling have to do with feeling that your nose is too big?"). However, by looking at the underlying pattern of these disorders (error signal → motivational arousal → compulsive behavior → lack of "feeling of knowing" → continuation of error signal), we can begin to see how the full spectrum of these disorders fits together.

Looking at OCD in particular, the **I MURDER?** and **calm**-pulsion mnemonics can help to remind you of the core phenomenology of this condition. For the other disorders in the obsessive-compulsive spectrum (remember **tic**, **trich**, **sick**, and dysmor**phic**!), try to think through how each of them fits this underlying pattern. In body dysmorphic disorder, the error signal is a persistent belief that some part of their body is disfigured which leads to excessive grooming and other behaviors intended to hide the perceived defect. In hypo-**conned**-riasis, the error signal is that the person believes they have a medical disease regardless of what the evidence says (they think that doctors are all **conned** by the negative work-up). In **TIC** disorder, these **T**ransient **I**rresistible **C**ontractions do not revolve around any specific thought pattern but still can be conceptualized as a compulsive behavior intended to reduce a state of inner tension. Finally, in trichotillomania, there is also a sense of motivational anxiety that is only transiently relieved by engaging in **compulsive hair pulling**. Do your best to view obsessive-compulsive spectrum disorders through the lens of this core underlying pattern, as this will help you to identify cases that are likely to respond well to appropriate forms of treatment (specifically, a robust effect from certain forms of **CBT** like exposure and response prevention, with **serotonergic medications** being used as an adjunctive or second-line treatment).

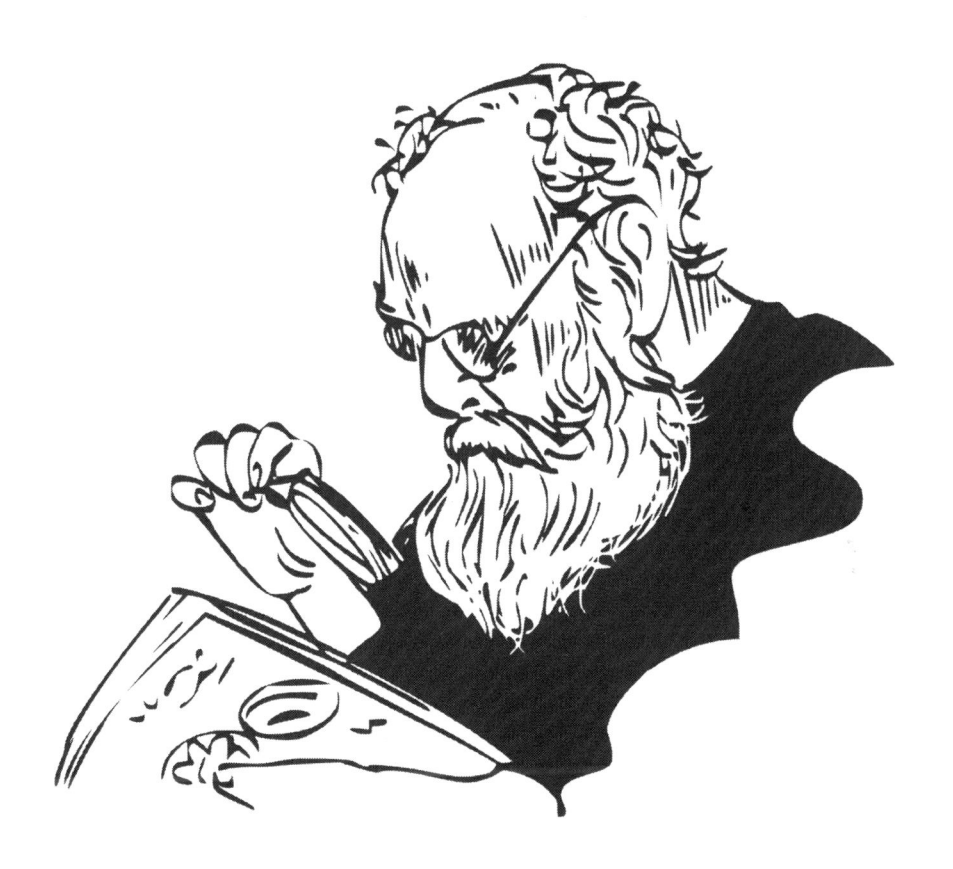

REVIEW QUESTIONS

1. A 23 y/o F presents to a psychiatrist's office for an initial evaluation. She was recently fired from her job after she arrived more than an hour late for the third time in a single week. When asked why she was late, she replies with some embarrassment that for the past year she has been spending several hours each morning cleaning her rectum using toothbrushes and enemas, as she feels "unclean" following a bowel movement. Recently she noticed that the amount of time that it takes for her to feel clean has been increasing. While she tried to accommodate this by both setting her alarm for 4:00 in the morning as well as reducing the amount of food she is eating to prevent bowel movements, she still finds that the process takes more time than she thought, resulting in her being late. The psychiatrist then asks the patient why she engages in this behavior. Which of the following responses is *least* consistent with a diagnosis of OCD?
   A. "I know it's weird, but I can't stop doing it."
   B. "I can't get these thoughts to go away."
   C. "If I don't spend hours cleaning, then God will view me as unworthy."
   D. "I don't understand what you're asking. This is completely normal."
   E. All of these responses are consistent with a diagnosis of OCD

2. (Continued from previous question.) Which of the following regions of the patient's central nervous system is most likely activated following a bowel movement?
   A. The anterior cingulate cortex
   B. The orbitofrontal cortex
   C. The prefrontal cortex
   D. The hypothalamus
   E. The ventral tegmental area

3. An 8 y/o M is brought into the pediatrician's office by his father who is concerned about his "weird movements." One month ago, the father noticed his son making sudden jerking movements of his neck while at soccer practice. The father says that his son "looks like a crazy person" and is worried that he will become the target of bullying by other children. When asked about the movements, the patient says that he feels that he has little control over them. He denies involuntary vocalizations. Which of the following statements is true?
   A. These movements would be diagnosed as Tourette syndrome
   B. It is rare for children to experience these types of movements
   C. These types of movements often decrease in frequency and severity in response to serotonergic medications
   D. These movements are often accompanied by an inner sense of tension or anxiety
   E. These types of movements are generally permanent once they begin
   F. None of these statements are true

4. A 23 y/o M makes an appointment with a plastic surgeon but does not write down the reason for his visit on the intake form. When the surgeon asks him why he is here, the patient looks down and embarrassedly says, "I would like for my penis to be bigger." He says that he has tried various methods of enlarging his penis, including using pumps, traction devices, and "jelqing." He has also bought and consumed pills claiming to increase penis size from various sources. However, none of these efforts have resulted in substantial increases in the size of his penis. Which of the following would argue most strongly *against* a diagnosis of body dysmorphic disorder in this patient?
   A. Low self-reported frequency of masturbation
   B. A penis that is 2 inches (5 cm) in length
   C. A belief that women will reject him because of his penis size
   D. A self-reported "high sex drive"
   E. Homosexual orientation

5. A 30 y/o M with a long history of untreated OCD comes to his psychiatrist's office for a follow-up appointment. At the last visit, the psychiatrist explained the various treatment options that were available to him, and the patient requested time to research each of these options and make a decision. At this visit, the patient says that he does not believe that he will have time to engage in CBT given his busy work schedule but is interested in starting a serotonin reuptake inhibitor. After discussing the risks and benefits, the patient and his psychiatrist decide on sertraline. Which of the following conditions would be *least* likely to respond well to sertraline if they were also comorbid in this patient?
   A. Body dysmorphic disorder
   B. Trichotillomania
   C. Dermatillomania
   D. Major depressive disorder
   E. Generalized anxiety disorder
   F. All of the above conditions would be expected to respond well to sertraline

1. **The best answer is D.** Obsessions in OCD are often ego-dystonic, meaning that the person who has these thoughts recognizes that they are excessive or unrealistic. This makes someone who responds by saying that they perceive their actions to be normal or reasonable less likely to have OCD. Obsessive thoughts are characteristically ego-dystonic (answer A) and recurrent (answer B). It is also not unusual for someone to have obsessions involving multiple themes, which in this case would be both cleanliness and religiously-oriented thoughts (answer C).

2. **The best answer is A.** The anterior cingulate cortex is involved in recognition of perceived errors and the generation of motivational arousal, which in this case takes the form of the patient believing that she is dirty following a bowel movement and feeling the urge to take steps to make herself feel clean again. The prefrontal cortex is involved in OCD, but its role appears most related to deficits in recognizing completion of tasks (the lack of any "feeling of knowing") rather than error recognition (answer C). The orbitofrontal cortex is implicated in mood disorders (answer B), while the hypothalamus is involved in anxiety disorders through its place in the hypothalamic–pituitary–adrenal axis (answer D). The ventral tegmental tract is part of the reward circuitry and is more related to addictive disorders than compulsive disorders (answer E).

3. **The best answer is D.** Tics are often accompanied by a sense of inner tension that is relieved by engaging in the movement. This case would not be diagnosed as Tourette syndrome, as Tourette syndrome specifically involves the combination of both motor and vocal tics (answer A). Tics are common, with around 20% of children experiencing them (answer B). For most children, they are transient and will resolve on their own (answer E). Medication treatment generally involves antipsychotics rather than SRIs (answer C).

4. **The best answer is B.** A diagnosis of body dysmorphic disorder is based on the presence of beliefs that certain aspects of one's body or appearance are flawed. However, an important point is that these flaws are imagined and are not reasonable by any objective standard. In contrast, a penis that is 2 inches in length is small by any objective standard and would likely meet common medical criteria for a diagnosis of a micropenis. For this reason, it cannot be said that he suffers from body dysmorphic disorder, as his perceived views are not necessarily imagined. None of the other factors listed has any bearing on a diagnosis of body dysmorphic disorder.

5. **The best answer is C.** Body dysmorphic disorder, trichotillomania, major depressive disorder, and generalized anxiety disorder (answers A, B, D, and E) are all expected to respond well to starting an SRI (although the size of the effect will differ between them). In contrast, dermatillomania is associated with a poor rate of response to SRIs and may be more related to impulse control disorders than compulsive disorders.

11 PTSD

In psychological terms, trauma is defined as an event that is **violent** or **life-threatening** to the extent that it evokes intense feelings of **fear, helplessness, and terror** in the people experiencing it. Common examples of trauma include war, combat, violence, assault, crime, terrorism, and accidents. Traumatic experiences are common, with the majority of people experiencing at least one major traumatic event in their lifetime. Experiencing trauma is not inherently pathological, and not everyone develops distressing or disabling symptoms after trauma. For some people, however, exposure to a traumatic event can provoke a characteristic syndrome of trauma-related signs and symptoms that can be incredibly impairing. These people are said to be suffering from a trauma or stressor related disorder, the prototype of which is **post-traumatic stress disorder** (PTSD).

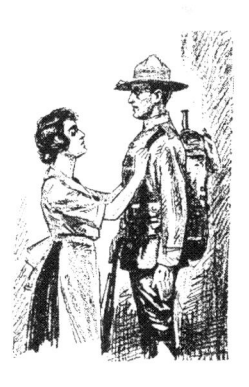

When discussing PTSD, we must make a choice between taking a broad view of the disorder or sticking to a narrow definition. The broad approach often takes the form of diagnosing PTSD in any patient in whom trauma has occurred and who is now presenting with any form of psychiatric symptoms. In contrast, the narrow approach restricts the diagnosis of PTSD to just those patients who have responded to trauma with the *specific* signs and symptoms that we will discuss shortly (re-experiencing, arousal, and avoidance). While there are pros and cons to each approach, it is best to begin with the narrow view as it is this strict definition that has been used to study PTSD for the past several decades. If we take too broad of an approach, we risk losing what we have learned about the prognosis of the disorder as well as our ability to link patients to the correct forms of treatment. For this reason, we will focus first on learning about the diagnosis of PTSD as it is presented in the DSM before moving on to talking about other forms of psychiatric pathology that can occur following a trauma in the next few chapters.

SIGNS AND SYMPTOMS OF PTSD

While not everyone develops a disorder following exposure to a traumatic event, those who do tend to experience a fairly consistent set of signs and symptoms. In fact, while the term "PTSD" was not used until the 1970s, this particular constellation of signs and symptoms has been referenced throughout history under various other names, including "railway spine" for victims of the frequent railroad collisions that occurred in the early 1800s, "shell shock" in World War I, and "combat stress reaction" in World War II. Handily for learning, the primary symptoms required for a diagnosis of PTSD can be captured in the acronym **TRAUMA**:

T is for Trauma. Exposure to a traumatic event is *required* for a diagnosis of PTSD, and the characteristic signs and symptoms of PTSD must not have been present prior to this event. Despite a general consensus that traumatic events exist, it has been much more difficult to define what exactly constitutes a traumatic event. Do we define trauma based on characteristics of the event itself, or is it defined based on a person's *reaction* to that event? Modern approaches attempt to take both into account. The event must either be **life-threatening** and/or involve actual or threatened **physical and/or sexual violence**, while the response must involve significant feelings of **fear, helplessness, and terror**. This means that other events (such as harassment, non-violent bullying, or having images of yourself posted online by an ex) do not "qualify" as trauma per the DSM-5 despite the fact that these experiences can often result in signs and symptoms indistinguishable from "textbook" PTSD. Secondary exposure to a traumatic event (such as hearing about a spouse or family member who was robbed at gunpoint) still qualifies per DSM-5 standards. The trauma can be a single event (as in a car crash) or it can be chronic (such as childhood abuse). The nature of the trauma has important considerations for the development of PTSD, as less than 10% of people experiencing a **non-intentional trauma** such as a car accident develop PTSD while nearly 50% of those experiencing **intentional trauma** such as rape or assault do.

R is for Re-experiencing. People with PTSD often re-experience their trauma in various ways. This primarily takes the form of **flashbacks** which are sudden and unexpected re-experiencing episodes of the trauma. Flashbacks can be either cued ("triggered" by certain stimuli that are reminiscent of the trauma, such as a Vietnam War veteran hearing a helicopter) or uncued (occurring seemingly at random or "out of the blue"). Flashbacks are not *thoughts* so much as *experiences*, and someone in the midst of a flashback tends to experience it in highly emotional and sensory ways (including specific images, sounds, or smells) rather than verbal or narrative memories ("I remember that one time in Vietnam..."). This appears to be related to how stress affects the ability to encode memories, with traumatic events often being encoded in a "flashbulb" manner rather than being stored in terms of a personal autobiographical narrative as most memories are. Flashbacks are experienced as occurring in the "here and now" and appear to be a form of **dissociation** (discussed more in Chapter 12).

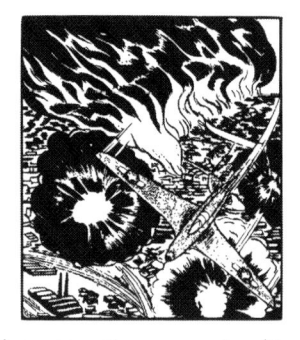

Re-experiencing can also occur in the form of **nightmares**, which are common in individuals diagnosed with PTSD (as over 70% of people with this condition reporting frequent nightmares compared to only 5% of the general population). The content of the nightmares is often, though not always, related to the trauma itself. Nightmares are impairing, as they can result in poor quality of sleep or even attempts to avoid sleep due to anxiety about having more nightmares.

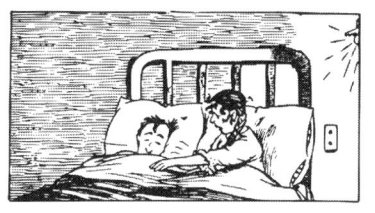

A is for Arousal. People with PTSD often develop a state of increased anxiety and awareness of their surroundings known as **hyperarousal**. This is similar to the state of arousal seen in fear that is mediated by the sympathetic nervous system (as discussed in Chapter 9). However, unlike adaptive fear, in PTSD this state of arousal becomes **persistent** and **generalized**, occurring most of the time and in multiple environments regardless of whether there is reason to be fearful or not. For example, someone who was robbed while traveling in another country may begin carrying forms of protection with them at all times and keeping these at their side before answering the doorbell at home. People in a state of hyperarousal often engage in constant scanning of their environment for possible clues to the presence of any danger (**hypervigilance**). Due to the involvement of the HPA axis, people with PTSD often experience the same symptoms that are seen in states of chronic anxiety as captured in the **MISERA**-ble mnemonic, including **M**uscle tension, **I**rritability, trouble with **S**leep, low **E**nergy, **R**estlessness, and inability to pay **A**ttention to non-trauma related stimuli.

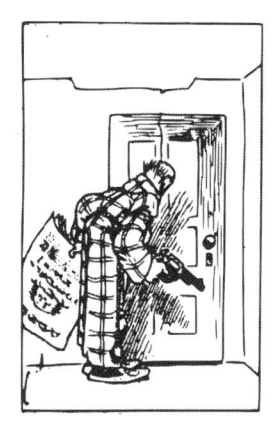

U is for Unable to function. The re-experiencing, hyperarousal, and avoidance patterns experienced by people with PTSD can be incredibly impairing for both social and occupational functioning. People with PTSD often find themselves unable to concentrate at work or have no interest in maintaining relationships with "normal people" who cannot understand the experiences that they have been through, leading to difficulty in maintaining a job and an adequate social support system.

M is for Month. By definition, PTSD is a **chronic** disorder, meaning that trauma-related symptoms must be present for a certain period of time. In the DSM-5, this period of time is defined as one month. (People showing signs and symptoms related to trauma for less than one month would be diagnosed as having acute stress disorder, discussed later in this chapter.) To be clear, this does not mean that symptoms have to be present in the *first* month after the trauma occurs! In fact, a **delayed onset** is most characteristic of PTSD, with nearly 80% of those who eventually receive this diagnosis not showing any symptoms within the first month after the trauma.

A is for Avoidance. People with PTSD will often go to great lengths to **avoid people, places, or things** associated with those memories so as to not trigger a flashback. For example, someone with PTSD from a construction-related accident may try to avoid tall buildings, while someone who was kidnapped while walking out of a friend's house at night may find it difficult to return to that part of town. Avoidance can go beyond *physical* avoidance to include a more *psychological* avoidance of emotions known as **numbing**. Emotional numbing helps to protect against strong negative emotions such as fear, helplessness, or anxiety, but it can also interfere with the ability to experience positive emotions such as joy, satisfaction, or love. This results in a **flattening of affect** which can impair one's ability to interact with other people and engage in meaningful relationships.

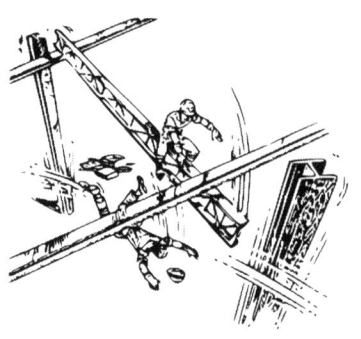

Post-traumatic stress disorder is characterized by exposure to a **life-threatening event** that results in **re-experiencing, hyperarousal, avoidance,** and **dysfunction.**

TRAUMA:
Traumatic event
Re-experiencing
Arousal
Unable to function
Month or more of symptoms
Avoidance

PTSD ACROSS THE LIFESPAN

EPIDEMIOLOGY
Approximately 3% of the population is affected by PTSD at any given time, with up to 10% experiencing symptoms during their lifetime. This makes it a **relatively common** syndrome. **Women** are affected twice as often as men even after accounting for significant differences in the nature of trauma experienced by each gender (such as sexual assault being more common in women). Unlike other psychiatric syndromes we have discussed so far, the age of onset of PTSD is quite variable. Logically, this makes sense, as traumatic events are generally unplanned and would be expected to occur on a seemingly random basis. However, there do appear to be upper and lower limits, with children **under the age of 10** being highly unlikely to develop PTSD (at least in the "textbook" sense) and adults **over the age of 55** also showing a dramatic decrease in rates of the diagnosis.

Exposure to trauma is common, and the majority of people will experience at least one traumatic event in their lifetime. However, not everyone exposed to trauma will develop PTSD. For example, while 20% of soldiers exposed to combat develop PTSD, the other 80% do not. In non-military populations, up to 60% of people experience at least one major trauma in their lives, but only 8% go on to develop PTSD. This can be confusing for someone learning about PTSD, as the medical model of illness often assumes a simple cause-and-effect explanation ("trauma → PTSD" just like "virus → infection"). However, the wide variation in human responses to trauma argues against this idea.

Traumatic disorders make much more sense when viewed through the lens of a core principle of psychodiagnostics: *it's never just one thing*. Like many psychiatric syndromes, PTSD requires both a **stress** and a **diathesis**. While most people would expect that the severity of PTSD symptoms would be most related to the nature of the traumatic event itself, research has found that *non*-trauma related factors (such as personality traits, psychological coping styles, presence of social support, and number of pre-trauma mental disorders) matter just as much as the details of the traumatic event. For someone who is particularly vulnerable to stress, even a relatively minor trauma (such as having their car broken into while at work) can be enough to induce PTSD. In contrast, someone who is relatively immune to the effects of stress may still develop PTSD provided that the event they experience is distressing enough (such as being the victim of a violent assault). Most cases fall somewhere in between these two extremes. Nevertheless, approaching PTSD from this perspective can provide more insight into the multifactorial nature of trauma's effects on the mind.

Other factors can also predict an increased risk of developing PTSD after trauma. In particular, people who are **younger** at the time of trauma, experience trauma **alone**, have **little time to process**, and have **low social support** tend to be at the highest risk for developing PTSD. These factors together help explain why soldiers who fought in the Vietnam War developed PTSD at much higher rates than those returning from World War II. Compared to World War II veterans, soldiers in the Vietnam War were younger (19 years compared to 26), served in variable timeframes which broke up social cohesion (as opposed to those in World War II who trained, fought, and returned home largely with the same group), had little time to process (a 16-hour flight from Vietnam to the United States compared to a 30-day boat ride home with your squad), and received little social support upon returning home (many were greeted with protestors rather than parades). These same risk factors also apply in non-military populations as well, highlighting the significant role that non-trauma factors play in who does and doesn't develop PTSD following a traumatic event.

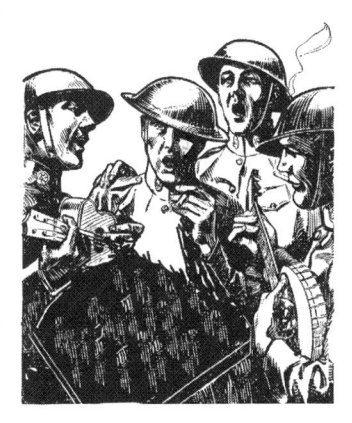

PROGNOSIS

Without treatment, PTSD is often **chronic** and **enduring**, with about 50% of cases showing continued symptoms and impairment over a 5 year period. In the other 50% of cases, the severity of PTSD symptoms appears to decrease over time. The distinction between intentional and non-intentional trauma appears to be important for the prognosis of PTSD, as symptoms related to non-intentional trauma appear to decrease over time while those associated with intentional trauma remain constant or even increase as time goes on. It's also important to realize that mental *dysfunction* is not the only possible outcome of trauma. In fact, around a third of people who experience a significant trauma go on to attribute that event to positive changes in their perspective on life (a phenomenon known as **post-traumatic growth**). However, post-traumatic growth appears to be more common following non-intentional trauma (such as a natural disaster or a diagnosis of cancer) compared to intentional trauma.

TREATMENT

Specific treatments for PTSD have been shown to be effective at reducing the distress and dysfunction related to trauma. The primary form of treatment for PTSD is **trauma-focused CBT**. In particular, a form of CBT known as **exposure therapy** helps to overcome avoidance by encouraging patients to intentionally come into contact with places and things that remind them of their traumatic experiences (such as driving a car in the area where an accident previously occurred) to re-encode these memories in a way that is less "flashbulb" and more "narrative," leading to fewer re-experiencing episodes. CBT for PTSD is very effective, with a **large effect size** over 1.0.

Medications (particularly **SRIs**) can be helpful as an adjunct to psychotherapy. However, they are generally not preferred as a first-line treatment given that they are not only less effective (with a smaller effect size around 0.5) but also produce effects that tend to disappear after treatment has ended (as opposed to the longer lasting beneficial effects associated with psychotherapy). In addition to SRIs, another drug known as **prazosin** (which works by blocking the sympathetic nervous system and its associated "fight or flight" response) has been shown to be helpful for preventing **PTSD-related nightmares** when taken before bed, with a large effect size of 1.0. Benzodiazepines rapidly reduce the anxiety and hyperarousal associated with PTSD, but they should generally be avoided as they appear to *worsen* many outcomes (including rates of depression, aggression, and substance abuse following a trauma).

Treatment for **PTSD** consists of **CBT**, with **SRIs** as an adjunctive treatment. **Prazosin** can be used to reduce **PTSD-related nightmares**.

Post Traumatic Stress? Try Prazosin, Therapy, and Serotonin.

While much is known about treatment of PTSD once it has occurred, recent research has focused on *preventing* PTSD following exposure to a trauma. Studies have shown that trauma-focused CBT can reduce the rate of developing PTSD, at least for "single exposure" traumas such as a car crash. In contrast, medications have not been shown to be helpful for preventing PTSD following exposure to a trauma.

MECHANISMS OF PTSD

PTSD is an incredibly complex and multifactorial disorder. One thing that complicates the matter significantly is the fact that many of the systems involved in PTSD are also implicated in other psychiatric syndromes as well. For example, people with PTSD display persistent overactivation of both the **sympathetic nervous system** and the **HPA axis** which can also be seen in anxiety and depression as well. (The involvement of these two systems explains why medications that interact with them, such as prazosin, appear to be effective in treating particular symptoms of PTSD.) In addition, **negative affective biases** (which you'll remember from the chapter on depression) appear to be present in PTSD as well, which could account not only for the persistently poor mood associated with the disorder but also for the benefits observed with CBT and SRIs. Finally, **dissociative mechanisms** (to be discussed in Chapter 12) appear to account for re-experiencing symptoms such as flashbacks and nightmares. Because the various symptom domains of PTSD each have their own mechanisms, it seems unlikely that there is going to ever be a single unifying mechanism for the disorder.

Nevertheless, despite this overlap in symptoms and mechanisms with other disorders, there do appear to be two consistent neurobiological findings that are both quite *specific* and *sensitive* for a diagnosis of PTSD, the first being *increased* activity in the **amygdala** and the second being *decreased* activity in the **medial prefrontal cortex**. Each of these plays a unique role in the fear response. The amygdala works to quickly generate **emotional responses to stimuli** (particularly those associated with fear), while the medial prefrontal cortex helps to police the amygdala's response by **integrating higher-level information** about the environment. For example, let's say that we suddenly hear the sound of a loud explosion. The amygdala immediately kicks in and suggests that "explosion = bad," activating the sympathetic nervous system's fight-or-flight response and inducing a state of fear. However, if we then notice that the sound of the explosion is happening on the Fourth of July, then the medial prefrontal cortex is able to take higher-level sensory information (such as visuals of American flags and the emotional context of smiling faces around us) and integrate them into a new reaction: "explosion = okay for now." The medial prefrontal cortex then steps in to tell the amygdala to back off, reducing the fear response and allowing us to enjoy the fireworks. In the picture to the right, the dad's medial prefrontal cortex has been able to integrate higher-level sensory information and tell the amygdala to turn off, while the boy is clearly disturbed by the experience (his amygdala has run rampant, unhindered by his medial prefrontal cortex). It is the boy's response that is most typical of PTSD: an *over*active amygdala that is insufficiently regulated by an *under*active medial prefrontal cortex.

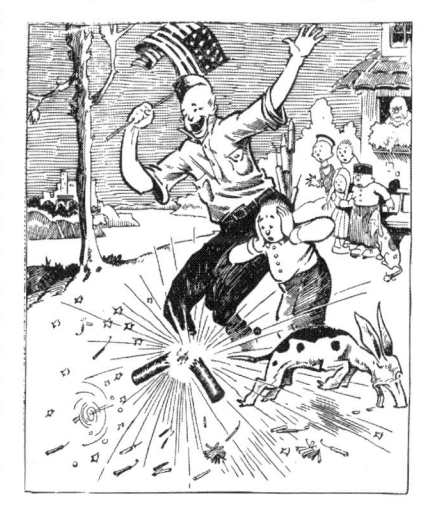

Another brain region known as the **hippocampus** also helps to regulate the amygdala, this time in response to **accumulated memories**. Using the same example of an explosion on the Fourth of July, someone may remember based on their memories of previous holidays that the sound of an explosion is not always bad, and this information can help to reign in the amygdala as well. This partly explains why the dad in the picture is having a much better time with the fireworks than the boy (who, due to his age, hasn't had the time to develop his hippocampus). An underdeveloped hippocampus is a risk factor for developing PTSD, even in people who have never experienced trauma (suggesting that it forms part of the *diathesis* for the disorder), as someone with an underdeveloped hippocampus would be less able to use memories of the past to control the fear response to the stimuli around them.

Someone with the trifecta of an overactive amygdala, an underactive medial prefrontal cortex, and an underdeveloped hippocampus is at high risk for developing PTSD, as they are more likely to react to trauma with fear and less able to use sensory information from the environment and memories of happier times in their lives to lessen the sting of a traumatic event. You can remember the association of these brain structures with PTSD by thinking of a girl named **Amy** who sees a **P**retty **F**rightening **C**amel and a **hippo**potamus while out at a park. Knowing that these animals can be aggressive (especially the hippo, which is considered one of the most dangerous large animals), her **fear response** is activated in response to this perceived life-threatening situation. However, the camel and the hippo try to calm her down by reminding her that she's in a private park with only tame animals (they are using contextual information to bring down her fear response). Use this situation to help you remember the relationship between the **Amy**gdala (which is prone to be frightened) and both the **P**re**F**rontal **C**ortex and the **hippo**campus (which try to calm the amygdala down using contextual information and prior memories).

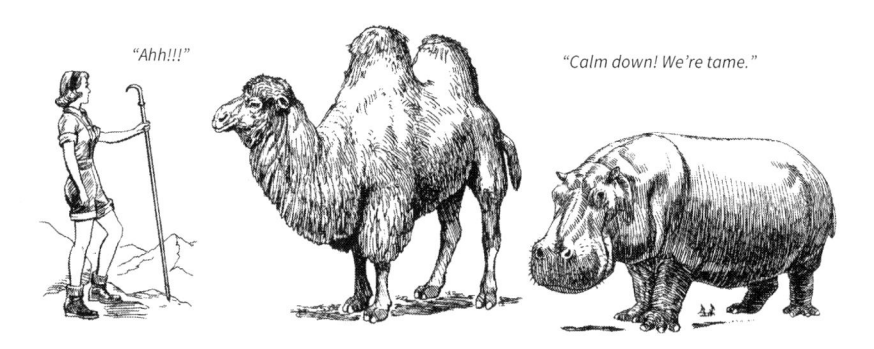

"Ahh!!!"   *"Calm down! We're tame."*

PTSD involves an **overactive amygdala** that is inadequately regulated by an **underactive medial prefrontal cortex** and an **underdeveloped hippocampus**.

*Remember **Amy**, the woman who encounters a*
***P**retty **F**rightening **C**amel and a **hippo**potamus while visiting the zoo.*

HOW TO DIAGNOSE TRAUMA-RELATED DISORDERS

Because the psychological impact of trauma depends not only on each patient's pre-existing vulnerabilities but also on the nature of the trauma itself, there was the possibility for endless complexity when it came to diagnosing trauma-related disorders. The DSM attempts to simplify things by offering only a **handful of diagnoses** that each encompass a wide range of possible experiences following a stressful event in its chapter on trauma- and stressor-related disorders. There are two disorders involving trauma (PTSD and acute stress disorder) that differ primarily on the basis of how long the symptoms have gone on. There is an additional disorder (adjustment disorder) that encompasses psychological distress following a major life event, albeit one that doesn't meet the standard required for it to be a traumatic event. Finally, there are two disorders that are diagnosed only in children (reactive attachment disorder disinhibited social engagement disorder) to reflect the fact that trauma often manifests very differently in children less than 10 years old. We'll talk about how to approach diagnosing each of these disorders now.

As a final note, when working with patients in clinical settings please remember that many people won't feel comfortable sharing their experiences of trauma, especially if it makes them feel vulnerable or ashamed (as can occur with domestic violence or sexual assault). Use the principles of trauma-informed care that were discussed back in the section on homelessness in Chapter 4, such as approaching sensitive issues in a nuanced way and being mindful of the patient's boundaries, to provide the highest quality of care for these patients!

POST-TRAUMATIC STRESS DISORDER

PTSD is the prototypical trauma-related disorder and is diagnosed based on a history of trauma as well as the characteristic signs, symptoms, and dysfunction that follow as captured in the **TRAUMA** mnemonic. From a diagnostic standpoint, simply asking two questions ("Have you experienced a life-threatening or violent event? If so, does the memory of this event interfere with your life?") can be a **very sensitive test for PTSD**. People who answer no to both of these questions are quite unlikely to have PTSD, while those who answer yes should be further evaluated to understand the nature of their dysfunction and whether they would qualify for a diagnosis of PTSD.

ACUTE STRESS DISORDER

Some people experience severe symptoms that begin almost immediately following a traumatic event. However, until the symptoms have been present for at least one month, you cannot diagnose PTSD. For cases where the core trauma-related symptoms (re-experiencing, arousal, and avoidance) have not yet reached a month in length, a diagnosis of **acute stress disorder** can be given. While one could assume that acute stress disorder is basically "pre-PTSD," this is not the case! Many people who are diagnosed with acute stress disorder will go on to develop PTSD after a month has passed, but not all of them do. In addition, the majority of people with PTSD did *not* qualify for a diagnosis of acute stress disorder within the first month, with many showing a **delayed onset** of symptoms. Therefore, the presence of acute stress disorder immediately following a traumatic event does *not* rule in later development of PTSD, nor does its absence rule it out!

ADJUSTMENT DISORDER
Because trauma is somewhat narrowly defined in the DSM as a *life-threatening* or *violent* event, a diagnosis of PTSD cannot be given to someone who is experiencing symptoms after other kinds of life experiences (such as losing a job or being cheated on by their spouse) that are still distressing but not necessarily life-threatening. In these cases, a diagnosis of **adjustment disorder** could be considered. It's important to point out that the symptoms seen in adjustment disorder, such as anxiety and depressed mood, are often broader in nature than the specific domains of re-experiencing, hyperarousal, and avoidance seen in PTSD.

REACTIVE ATTACHMENT DISORDER AND DISINHIBITED ATTACHMENT DISORDER
While "textbook" PTSD is rare in patients less than 10 years of age, children who have experienced trauma still can have distress and disability related to their experiences. To address this, there are a couple of diagnoses that are both related to severe neglect during early childhood and focus on the disordered interpersonal interactions that can result: **reactive attachment disorder** and **disinhibited attachment disorder** (the latter being known as "disinhibited social engagement disorder" in the DSM-5). In comparing the two disorders, reactive attachment disorder is characterized more by fearfulness and reluctance to accept comfort from parents or other caretakers, whereas disinhibited attachment disorder instead involves *overly* familiar patterns of interacting with adults such as wandering off with strangers without hesitation.

These disorders are fairly rare in the general population, so most psychiatrists will not diagnose them very often. However, they may be found more commonly in specific settings such as orphanages or group homes where opportunities for bonding are severely lacking. Both of these disorders occupy a strange place in the DSM, as no other disorders are diagnosed on the basis of attachment patterns alone.

COMPLEX PTSD
A growing body of research suggests that exposure to chronic trauma during childhood development (such as someone who endured years of child abuse) can lead to a set of signs and symptoms that overlaps with those found in "single exposure" traumas but also includes some distinct features. The term "**complex PTSD**" is increasingly being used to describe these cases. While there is no entry for complex PTSD in the DSM, it is listed in other diagnostic schemes such as the ICD where it is defined as encompassing all of the core signs and symptoms of PTSD (as captured in the **TRAUMA** mnemonic) in addition to three new criteria: **affect dysregulation**, a **negative self-concept**, and **disturbed relationships**. Notably, all three of these symptoms overlap with those seen in borderline personality disorder, raising questions about how complex PTSD fits in with that diagnosis. While more research is needed, from a practical perspective the concept of complex PTSD does highlight an important point: that differentiating between adult-onset "single exposure" PTSD and more prolonged developmental trauma is important and may increase not only the prognostic value of both diagnoses but also the likelihood of treatment success.

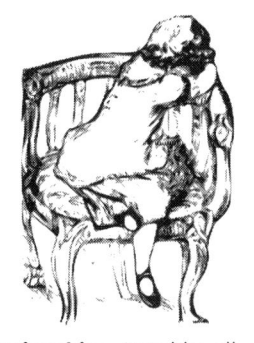

DIFFERENTIAL DIAGNOSIS OF TRAUMA-RELATED DISORDERS

PTSD is highly comorbid with other psychiatric disorders, as people with PTSD often meet criteria for several other diagnoses. Given this, PTSD is rarely a *mis*diagnosis, but it can be a *missed* diagnoses if care is not taken to do a thorough psychiatric interview!

Starting here and continuing over the next few chapters, we will talk about several types of disorders that are strongly related to trauma. While trauma increases the risk for nearly all types of mental disorders (including depression, anxiety, bipolar disorder, OCD, and schizophrenia), these disorders can and do occur in the absence of trauma. In contrast, there is a group of disorders consisting of PTSD, dissociative disorders, cluster B personality disorders, and somatoform disorders that tend to occur *almost exclusively* in the context of trauma (and, in the case of PTSD, cannot be diagnosed without it!). While only PTSD has "trauma" in the name, these other disorders can and should be on your differential when dealing with patients who have experienced trauma. We'll talk about each of them briefly here before revisiting them in more detail in subsequent chapters.

NORMALCY
Exposure to trauma and even experiencing some degree of distress as a result is not pathological in any way. Indeed, what *would* be strange is for someone to go through a life-threatening event and come out the other side exactly the same as before! This is a crucial distinction to make, as the term "PTSD" is sometimes used loosely to refer to anyone who experiences any sort of symptoms following a trauma. What is often missing from this discussion is a focus on the *disorder* part of "post-traumatic stress disorder," as we should be exceedingly careful not to medicalize ordinary responses to extraordinary events (even if they are experienced as painful or distressing). Make sure to look for **clear evidence of dysfunction** (the U in the TRAUMA mnemonic) before focusing on whether the symptoms themselves are present.

PERSONALITY DISORDERS
A history of trauma is associated with certain personality disorders, particularly those in cluster B. From a clinical standpoint, it is absolutely possible for someone to have PTSD and a personality disorder at the same time. The key is to make sure that the core patterns of both are present, which should be easy as the diagnostic criteria for PTSD and cluster B personality disorders do not share any overlapping signs or symptoms (despite their shared link to a history of trauma).

DISSOCIATION
Dissociation is common following exposure to trauma. Interestingly, it tends to appear more often in the initial period following a traumatic event (during the time when someone would be diagnosed with acute stress disorder) than in the months or years following (when they would be diagnosed instead with PTSD). Nevertheless, for some people, dissociation can become chronic and disabling, turning into a dissociative disorder. The boundary between dissociative disorders and PTSD is not always clear, especially when it comes to knowing whether to diagnose both instead of just saying that dissociation is a specific symptom of PTSD. We will revisit this more in Chapter 12, but for now it is enough to know that dissociation can either be a symptom of PTSD or a disorder all on its own.

SOMATIZATION
While somatization is universal, it happens more often (and causes more distress) in people who have experienced trauma. Out of all the somatoform disorders, the one most associated with a history of trauma is conversion disorder, in which patients experience a sudden loss of neurologic function (such as the sudden inability to move their legs). People with conversion disorder score highly on tests of dissociation, suggesting a shared mechanism between it and other disorders that are characterized by trauma exposure.

DEPRESSION
PTSD is frequently comorbid with depression, with approximately half of all patients with PTSD also having depression. Despite this, depression should *not* be seen as a "natural consequence" of having PTSD, as people with both PTSD and depression are characterized by greater symptom severity, lower levels of functioning, worse response to treatments, and less symptom remission compared to patients with either disorder alone. While there are some symptoms that overlap between the two disorders (including anhedonia, insomnia, and reduced range of affect), try to focus on the **non-overlapping symptom domains** such as re-experiencing, hyperarousal, and avoidance in PTSD and episodic changes in mood and neurovegetative functioning in depression to differentiate between mere diagnostic overlap and true comorbidity.

ANXIETY
Like OCD, PTSD was once considered to be an anxiety disorder, as symptoms of anxiety are often prominent ("I'm scared to sleep in the same bed as my wife for fear that I'll have another nightmare and attack her again!") and the same neurobiological systems (including the sympathetic nervous system and HPA axis) are implicated in both. However, while anxiety is often found in the disorder, it is not *always* seen. Instead, the core symptoms of PTSD are (once again) re-experiencing, hyperarousal, and avoidance. While for some people these symptoms can lead to anxiety, this is not always true, making it difficult to consider a disorder that doesn't always feature anxiety to be an *anxiety disorder*. Despite now being considered its own diagnostic category, PTSD remains highly comorbid with anxiety disorders, making it essential to screen for possible comorbid diagnoses.

PSYCHOSIS
While they are not included in the diagnostic criteria for PTSD, psychotic symptoms (including paranoia, delusions, and auditory hallucinations) are not uncommon in people with PTSD and are reported by around one-third of patients with the condition. On closer evaluation, the details of these symptoms differ significantly from "classic" primary psychosis: paranoid delusions tend to be non-bizarre ("Everyone is trying to screw me over all the time!") while voices are often directly related to the trauma and are recognized as coming from *inside* one's head ("I hear my dead husband asking me why I didn't take a different route home that night..."). Pay attention to **differences in phenomenology** to avoid diagnosing schizophrenia in patients who have psychotic symptoms only related to PTSD.

ADDICTION
Use of substances is common in PTSD. Due to its anxiety-relieving effects and wide availability, **alcohol** is the most commonly used substance (with around 35% of people with PTSD meeting criteria for an alcohol use disorder), although it is definitely not the only one. For this reason, it is essential to screen everyone with a trauma-related disorder for addiction and vice versa. In cases where both are present, treatment of addiction must often take priority, as frequent intoxication tends to interfere with meaningful efforts to engage in therapy and other treatments for PTSD.

OBSESSIVE-COMPULSIVE DISORDERS
The relationship between trauma and obsessive-compulsive disorders was explored in more depth in the previous chapter. As a reminder, OCD occurs more commonly in people who have experienced trauma (and in some cases may even be "brought out" by a traumatic event in someone who never had symptoms of OCD before).

MALINGERING
One of the main benefits of diagnosis is that it validates distress on not only a personal level but also societally as well, resulting in special privileges (such as time off work or disability payments) being given to those *with* a diagnosis but not to those without. PTSD is particularly vulnerable to malingering for several reasons. For one, as with any psychiatric syndrome the primary symptoms are *subjective* and are therefore both easy to mimic and difficult to verify (as no objective signs are required). In addition, a diagnosis of PTSD is relatively non-stigmatizing, as most people view it as a blameless diagnosis ("I didn't do anything wrong! I'm the victim here!"). Finally, there can often be a clear secondary gain from receiving the diagnosis (such as higher damages being awarded in workers' compensation lawsuits when symptoms of PTSD are present). Therefore, it is imperative to keep malingering on the differential for anyone presenting with symptoms of PTSD, as malingered PTSD diminishes both the tangible and intangible benefits that people who truly suffer from PTSD receive from society.

Your suspicion for malingering should be increased whenever there is clear evidence of potential secondary gain (such as someone currently involved in legal proceedings), whenever someone eagerly volunteers their symptoms from the beginning of your evaluation but then is unwilling to cooperate with further exams or treatment, or whenever symptoms are vague, nebulous, or do not match what is known about the phenomenology of this condition. When evaluating PTSD, make sure to ask **open-ended questions** as much as possible ("How has the trauma affected your life?") rather than unintentionally educating the patient on what symptoms to report ("Do you ever have times when you suddenly re-experience the trauma out of nowhere? This is often a sign of PTSD."). In difficult cases, formal assessment using psychodiagnostic testing in a clinic that specializes in compensation evaluations may be warranted.

PUTTING IT ALL TOGETHER

Trauma is painful and unsettling for those who are unfortunate enough to experience it. However, for some people, trauma can become a gift that keeps on giving, leading to distressing and disabling symptoms for months or even years after the event itself.

When evaluating patients with a history of trauma, consider taking different approaches as the situation demands. Some patients will require a "**top-down**" approach (evaluating *symptoms* from a *known trauma*) where the history of trauma is clear from the beginning, such as someone coming in for medical treatment after an assault. For other patients, your tactic will need to be more "**bottom-up**" approach (evaluating *trauma* from *known symptoms*) where it is unknown if there is a history of trauma *but* the symptoms present are telling you that there is a possible chance of traumatic exposure in the past, such as someone who comes in with affective flattening, frequent nightmares, and a hyperactive startle response. In both of these cases, your task is to determine whether their traumatic exposure has resulted in clinically significant signs and symptoms that warrant diagnosis with a *disorder* (rather than representing a normal and expected response to a tragic event). You can use the **TRAUMA** mnemonic to provide a systemic framework for recognizing the signs, symptoms, and timeframe seen in PTSD.

In all cases of trauma, it is essential to keep in mind that PTSD is **just one possible manifestation of trauma**. It is absolutely incorrect to say that everyone who has been exposed to trauma has PTSD (or even that everyone who has problems as a result of trauma has PTSD). Instead, do your best to maintain a narrow definition of PTSD as a disorder of **re-experiencing**, **hyperarousal**, and **avoidance** related to differences in emotional processing in the amygdala, medial prefrontal cortex, and hippocampus. By taking a narrow approach, we are not saying that other people who have experienced trauma but don't have these specific symptoms are any less deserving of the positive benefits of diagnosis! Someone who has experienced trauma but instead expresses their distress through feelings of unreality or depersonalization (as in a dissociative disorder), medically unexplained symptoms (as in a somatoform disorder), or hypersensitivity to interpersonal rejection and abandonment (as in a cluster B personality disorder) deserves just as much empathy, validation, and treatment as someone who experiences "textbook" PTSD. Try your best to strike a balance between keeping a strict definition of PTSD (in order to increase the reliability and validity of the diagnosis as much as possible) while also having compassion and empathy for people who manifest trauma in other ways.

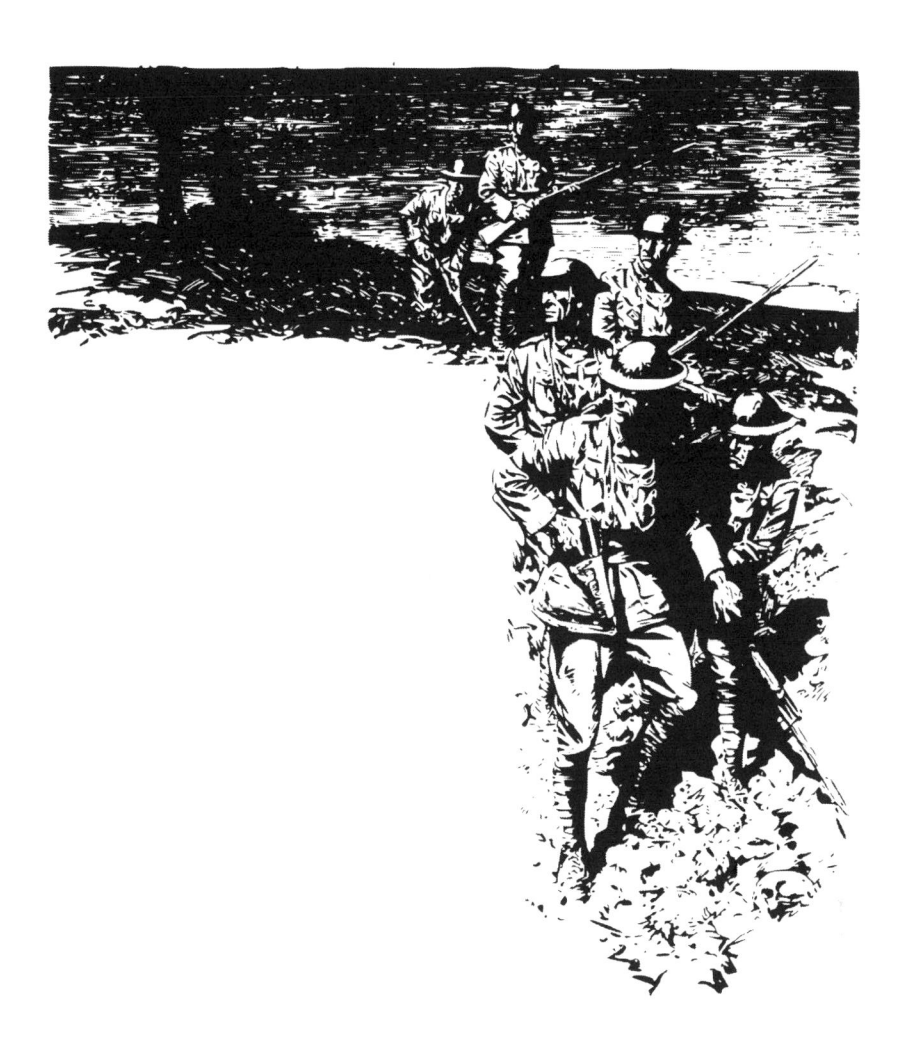

REVIEW QUESTIONS

1. A 33 y/o F is seen for a workers' compensation evaluation. Two months ago, she was working at a tire repair shop when a tire exploded and sent a piece of the rim flying at high velocity. The object lodged in the patient's left thigh, and she was rushed to the hospital. She has since had to undergo four separate surgeries. She currently is unable to walk and uses a wheelchair to get around. Upon evaluation, she reports thinking frequently about the incident, saying that the event "replays" in her mind "all the time." She denies nightmares or any changes in mood. She denies anhedonia, feelings of hopelessness, or thoughts of suicide. She does endorse feeling fatigued but attributes this to "those painkillers they have me on." Her affect is reactive with a full range. She is accompanied by her partner who, when interviewed separately, says that the patient is handling the trauma "overall fairly well, there are good days and bad days." What is the most appropriate diagnosis at this time?
   A. Post-traumatic stress disorder
   B. Acute stress disorder
   C. Major depressive disorder
   D. Specific phobia
   E. None of the above

2. (Continued from previous question.) Six months after the incident, the patient has recovered enough to return to work. Her mood has remained stable, and her episodes of re-experiencing have diminished. As the patient's partner is driving her to her first day back at work, the patient experiences a sudden flashback to the trauma and feels her heart begin to race. Hyperventilating, she yells, "Turn around! Turn around!" She begins to feel lightheaded and dizzy. Which of the following structures is most likely overactivated in this patient's brain?
   A. The amygdala
   B. The anterior cingulate cortex
   C. The medial prefrontal cortex
   D. The hypothalamus
   E. The hippocampus

3. An 18 y/o M graduates from high school and moves across the country to attend a prestigious college. He does not know any other people at this college but decided to go after being offered a full scholarship. On the weekend before school starts, he goes to a welcome party at a local fraternity and is sexually assaulted by another student there in a private room. In the days following the assault, he misses all of his classes as he feels afraid to leave his room. He frequently experiences a sensation that he does not know who he is or whether or not he is in a dream. His sleep is disturbed by nightmares every night. One week after the incident, the college's student life center contacts him to inquire about his having missed so many days of school. Two days later, he is in the school psychologist's office. He endorses a lack of appetite, inability to concentrate, lack of enjoyment of any activities, and feelings of restlessness, anger, and irritability. He reports that he was diagnosed with social anxiety disorder during his teenage

years and underwent therapy two years ago. Which of the following is the most appropriate diagnosis at this time?
   A. Post-traumatic stress disorder
   B. Acute stress disorder
   C. Major depressive disorder
   D. Adjustment disorder
   E. Panic disorder
   F. None of the above

4. (Continued from previous question.) Which of the following features of this case does *not* predict a higher chance of having PTSD one year from the incident?
   A. The intentional nature of the assault
   B. Experiencing the trauma alone
   C. Lack of social support network since moving across the country
   D. Presence of at least one pre-trauma psychiatric diagnosis
   E. Presence of symptoms soon after the onset of the traumatic event
   F. All of the following predict a higher chance of PTSD one year from the incident

5. (Continued from previous question.) One month after the initial traumatic event, the patient continues to experience daytime flashbacks and severe nightmares. Which of the following medications would be the best option for addressing his sleep concerns?
   A. Fluoxetine (a serotonin reuptake inhibitor)
   B. Ziprasidone (an antipsychotic)
   C. Prazosin (a sympatholytic)
   D. Lorazepam (a benzodiazepine)
   E. All of the above would be equally effective
   F. None of the above would be effective

1. **The best answer is E.** This patient has definitely experienced a traumatic event as defined in the DSM, and she currently exhibits signs and symptoms consistent with PTSD (such as frequent re-experiencing). However, by definition PTSD cannot be diagnosed unless there is evidence of dysfunction as a result, and in this case her reaction to her circumstances appears to be appropriate (answer A). This also rules out acute stress disorder, as does the length of time that has passed since the trauma (answer B). There is no evidence of major depressive disorder (answer C) or a specific phobia (answer D). It is possible that this patient may meet criteria for an adjustment disorder, although this would still be considered within the realm of normalcy.

2. **The best answer is A.** This patient is experiencing significant distress while returning to her first day back at the place where she experienced a traumatic event. Her fear response likely represents overactivation of the amygdala, which generates emotional reactions to stimuli. In contrast, the medial prefrontal cortex and the hippocampus appear to be *under*active in PTSD (answers C and E). While the hypothalamus is associated with PTSD through the hypothalamic–pituitary–adrenal axis, it plays a larger role in chronic responses to trauma rather than the immediate fear reaction that this patient is experiencing (answer D). The anterior cingulate cortex is more strongly linked to OCD than PTSD (answer B).

3. **The best answer is B.** The patient's history is consistent with an acute stress disorder given the onset of signs and symptoms of psychological distress following exposure to a trauma. Given that it has been less than one month since the trauma, a diagnosis of PTSD should not be given (answer A). While the patient has many symptoms of depression, the timing of their onset strongly suggests that they should be attributed to the trauma rather than an entirely separate diagnosis (answer C). The patient's distress is also constant rather than episodic, arguing against a diagnosis of panic disorder (answer E). Finally, the presence of significant distress and functional impairment as well as the traumatic nature of the inciting event all argue against a diagnosis of adjustment disorder (answer D).

4. **The best answer is E.** Acute stress disorder does not predict a higher rate of PTSD in the months or years following the traumatic event, and the majority of people diagnosed with PTSD do *not* meet criteria for acute stress disorder in the first month after the trauma occurred. Intentional violence, experiencing trauma alone, having a poor social support network, and having a pre-trauma psychiatric diagnosis are all associated with an increased risk of developing PTSD (answers A through D).

5. **The best answer is C.** Prazosin is a helpful medication for reducing the severity and frequency of nightmares related to PTSD. While benzodiazepines are effective at reducing anxiety and inducing sleep, they are associated with overall worse outcomes in PTSD and should generally be avoided (answer D). SRIs like fluoxetine can improve overall outcomes in PTSD but are not helpful specifically for either sleep or nightmares (answer A). Finally, antipsychotics like ziprasidone have no role in treating PTSD (answer B).

12 DISSOCIATION

Dissociation refers to a subjective feeling of being **detached from one's sense of reality**. It is particularly common following **traumatic experiences**. Similar to anxiety, dissociation is both a *state* and a *trait* as the term can be used to describe both a transient phenomenon ("She dissociated for several minutes following the car crash") as well as a long-term predisposition towards these experiences ("He is highly prone to dissociating when under stress"). Dissociation can be experienced in two primary ways: **derealization**, or a feeling that one's experience of reality is fake or "unreal," and **depersonalization**, or a feeling that one has become separated from their sense of self and identity.

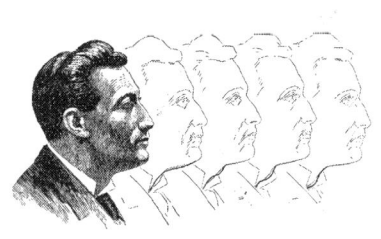

While dissociation can often be experienced as confusing, bewildering, or shocking, it is not an inherently pathological state. In fact, up to 20% of people have experienced depersonalization or derealization in the past year. However, for some people, dissociative experiences can become frequent or severe enough to form the basis of a **dissociative disorder**. Dissociative disorders that are recognized in the DSM include the trio of dissociative amnesia, depersonalization-derealization disorder, and dissociative identity disorder. Each of these conditions features dissociation in some form, but they differ from each other in terms of their cause, severity, and prognosis.

As mentioned previously, dissociative disorders are highly correlated with a history of trauma (especially when it occurred chronically during early development), placing them alongside PTSD, cluster B personality disorders, and somatoform disorders. Dissociative states are also believed to play a role in the pathophysiology of each of these other conditions, so learning about dissociation will be helpful in understanding the effects of trauma as a whole (even when working with someone who is not formally diagnosed with a dissociative disorder).

SIGNS AND SYMPTOMS OF DISSOCIATION

Dissociative experiences involve a variety of signs and symptoms. These can roughly be divided into three categories: **subjective experiences** (depersonalization and derealization), **memory abnormalities** (retrograde amnesia and memory errors of commission), and **hypnotic phenomena** (absorption, motor automaticity, and suggestibility). To help keep these straight, use the mnemonic **DDREAMS**:

D is for Depersonalization. Depersonalization is the feeling of having become mentally detached from one's sense of self. People experiencing depersonalization may look at their body and think, "I'm not myself," or look in the mirror and say to themselves, "That isn't me." This can be experienced as a sense that one's body is out of their control or that one is observing their body from an outside perspective.

D is for Derealization. Derealization is a sudden and profound sense that one's current experience of the world is illusory or fake. People often describe derealization as a mental "fog" or "veil" that suddenly descends and makes their surroundings seem alien or dream-like (even if they are in a familiar place like their own home). People in a state of derealization also report that they often feel unsteady or uneasy ("It's like I am walking on shifting ground"). Notably, depersonalization and derealization are not in any way mutually exclusive states, and people will often feel both at the same time!

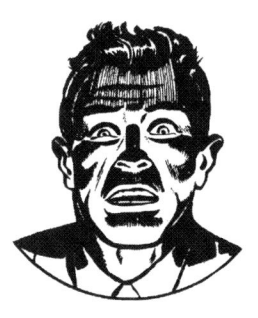

R is for Retrograde amnesia. While derealization and depersonalization are the two primary ways in which dissociation is subjectively experienced, there are often other signs as well. Most prominently, lapses in memory are a key clinical symptom of dissociation. Memory loss during dissociation is characterized by **retrograde amnesia** which is the loss of *previously* encoded memories (as opposed to anterograde amnesia where *new* memories cannot be encoded). For example, someone diagnosed with dissociative amnesia may be unable to remember any significant events in the month-long period after the death of their son but would be able to encode and memorize new information, such as a list of items to buy from the store, that she is given.

E is for Errors of commission. Memory lapses in dissociation are also characterized by the presence of both omission and commission errors. **Omission errors** are things that happened that you cannot remember (you have *omitted* the information from your mind) whereas **commission errors** are false memories of things that didn't actually happen (you remember yourself *committing* an act that hasn't actually been committed). Human memory is far from perfect, and omission errors are incredibly common (can you remember what you ate for dinner exactly one year ago?). In contrast, *commission* errors appear to be related to the capacity to dissociate, and evidence suggests that people who score high on measures of dissociation differ from most people primarily in the increased number of commission errors (rather than omission errors) that they make. This is not to say that "normal" people don't make commission errors of memory as well (they absolutely do!). However, people with a high degree of trait dissociation appear to remember false or suggested memories with a much higher frequency than most and with an intensity similar to their memories of actual events.

A is for Absorption. The last three signs and symptoms of dissociation all overlap with phenomena observed during a state of **hypnosis**. In fact, there is evidence to suggest that dissociation may be similar to or even the same thing as hypnotic states, with the main difference being that it occurs spontaneously rather than being induced by others. The first of these symptoms is **absorption** which is a state of being highly engaged in or entranced by mental imagery to the exclusion of everything else going on. Think of someone who is taking a walk in the woods while reading a gripping fantasy novel! This person is absorbed in their imagination to the point where they are not consciously aware of everything going on around them.

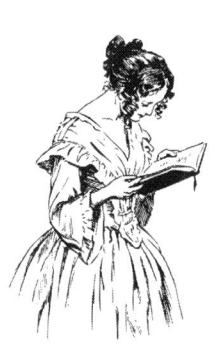

M is for Motor automaticity. Automaticity refers to behaviors that a patient does automatically without conscious awareness or effort. Consider the example of walking while reading from before: for someone who is absorbed in the story, the process of walking is done without conscious effort, including more complex tasks such as staying on the path or avoiding walking into a tree! In more extreme cases of automaticity, someone may not even be aware that they are doing the behavior and, when asked, may report no desire to do it.

S is for Suggestibility. Finally, **suggestibility** is a trait of being inclined to accept and act on the ideas of others. People who are highly suggestible may believe information without critically examining it or may do as someone tells them without considering whether it is the right thing to do. For example, let's say someone goes on a roller coaster for the first time and has a great time while on it. However, after getting off the ride their friend tells them, "You looked so terrified!" If the person is highly suggestible, they may now remember being terrified on the ride rather than excited. Suggestibility can also take more subtle forms, such as a lawyer asking leading questions in an attempt to get an eyewitness to remember something differently.

> **Dissociative episodes** involve feelings of **depersonalization and derealization**, specific types of **memory errors**, and **hypnosis-like phenomena**.
>
> *DDREAMS:*
> **D**epersonalization
> **D**erealization
> **R**etrograde amnesia
> **E**rrors of commission
> **A**bsorption
> **M**otor automaticity
> **S**uggestibility

If you're feeling confused at this point, that's okay! Dissociation is notoriously difficult to explain, even with a mnemonic. (In fact, one of the most common words that people who have dissociated use to describe the experience is "indescribable.") Much of this difficulty comes from the fact that most people have not had the experience of dissociating. Only 20% of all people have the capacity to spontaneously dissociate, which makes the concept of dissociation difficult to grasp for the other 80% who haven't had this experience. This difficulty is increased further by the fact that dissociation is not an severe variant of a common state (in contrast to something like depression which can be understood as an extreme version of sadness even by someone who has not personally had a depressive episode during their lifetime).

Nevertheless, there are clues that can help anyone to better understand the experience of dissociating. The closest experience that most people have had to dissociation is the transient "head rush" lightheadedness that occurs upon standing up too quickly. When this happens, there is often a distinct but ineffable sensation of unreality that is similar to what is described by people in a state of derealization or depersonalization. Like lightheadedness, the onset of dissociative experiences is often sudden, startling, and somewhat unsettling. Interestingly, symptoms of dissociation—including both depersonalization and derealization—can also be experimentally induced in healthy volunteers by injecting warm or cold water directly into the external auditory canal (please don't try this at home!). In addition, drugs known as dissociative hallucinogens (such as ketamine, dextromethorphan, and phencyclidine) can also induce a state of dissociation in most people who take them, suggesting that all people have the *ability* to dissociate even if only a few do so *spontaneously*.

DISSOCIATION ACROSS THE LIFESPAN

Dissociative disorders have not benefitted from the same level of research that has been done on other psychiatric disorders, resulting in little being known about the epidemiology, prognosis, and treatment of these disorders. Nevertheless, based on what data are available, a few themes have emerged.

EPIDEMIOLOGY

As mentioned before, dissociation is experienced by around 20% of the population, making it a relatively common experience (at least as far as psychiatric conditions go). However, dissociative *disorders* are much more rare, with estimates placing the prevalence at around **1-3%** of the population. They are most commonly diagnosed in **early adulthood**, with very few cases beginning after one's 20s or 30s.

Non-pathological dissociation occurs with approximately the same frequency in both women and men. However, *pathological* dissociation appears to be much more common in **women**, with diagnoses such as dissociative identity disorder being found up to 10 times more frequently in women than men. This discrepancy is believed to be at least partially related to higher rates of abuse histories in women compared to men, as a **history of trauma** (especially during early childhood) is a major risk factor for developing a dissociative disorder. In fact, more than 90% of people diagnosed with a dissociative disorder report a history of childhood trauma.

PROGNOSIS

Dissociative disorders are generally associated with high levels of **disability and dysfunction**, including psychiatric symptoms in multiple domains (such as mood, anxiety, sleep, and cognition), unstable interpersonal relationships, increased rates of physical illness, frequent substance abuse, and an elevated risk for suicide. Dissociative disorders also appear to be some of the most **disabling** conditions, with studies consistently finding low rates of employment and high utilization of welfare. Interestingly, the prognosis for the *dissociative disorders* themselves is often better than it is for the *patient* as a whole. One study found that a decade after diagnosis only a quarter of patients still met criteria for a dissociative disorder whereas over 80% still met criteria for *any* psychiatric disorder, with anxiety, dissociative, somatoform, and personality disorders (especially borderline personality disorder) being common.

TREATMENT

Like other aspects of dissociative disorders, treatment for these conditions is severely under-researched. Part of the problem is that it is not always clear what the specific targeted outcomes of treatment should be ("Are we trying to eliminate all episodes of dissociation or simply trying to reduce the distress and dysfunction related to them?"). Treatment studies on dissociative disorders also have an unfortunate tendency to refer to "treatment" in a general sense and rarely clarify the exact type of interventions used. Because of this, there is a **lack of clearly defined treatment strategies** for dissociative disorders, with most studies referencing a grab-bag of therapies in different forms (such CBT, dialectical behavior therapy, supportive therapy, hypnosis, art therapy, experiential therapy, and psychoeducation) in both group and individual formats. Interestingly, therapy appears to be only somewhat effective at addressing dissociation itself; instead, the most robust effects of therapy tend to involve reducing comorbid depression, anxiety, suicidality, trauma-related symptoms, and symptoms of borderline personality disorder. Studies have suggested that effective therapy for dissociative disorders typically requires **long-term treatment** in the order of years rather than weeks or months. However, given what we know about the natural lessening of dissociative pathology even without treatment, it remains unclear whether the beneficial effects observed with therapy over time are a direct result of therapy or simply the natural course of the disorder. This demonstrates a clear need for more rigorously designed and controlled trials.

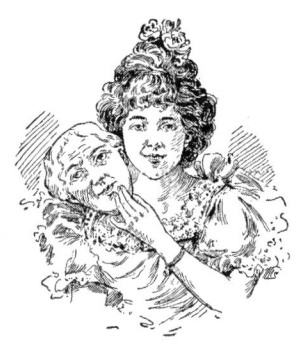

Medication treatment has *not* been found to be helpful at improving functional outcomes for dissociative disorders. When medications are used, they are generally focused at alleviating specific symptoms rather than targeting the underlying process of dissociation directly.

MECHANISMS OF DISSOCIATION

We learned earlier using the **DDREAMS** mnemonic that the phenomenology of dissociation involves three things: subjectively experienced **feelings of unreality**, objectively observed **deficits in memory**, and **hypnotic phenomena**. However, it is not immediately obvious what ties these three domains together, nor is it clear why they tend to happen most around the time of traumatic events.

Current research suggests that dissociation results from an unstable sleep-wake cycle that causes **intrusions of the dreaming state into waking life**. When we are awake, we are generally responsive to external stimuli and have the ability to remember our experiences in a durable way. During dreaming, however, the brain enters a unique state in which vivid images and experiences are generated *in the absence* of any external stimuli. In contrast to waking, the memories from our dreams tend to be quite *fragile* and are forgotten quickly upon awakening.

People in a state of dissociation show signs of activation of the neural networks responsible for state during normal waking life. This leads to a sort of **halfway point between dreaming and wakefulness** in which overall consciousness and awareness are preserved (as in the awake state) while also having an ability to generate and react emotionally to internally generated imagery (as in dreaming). These "**dream attacks**" are involuntary and often occur quite suddenly (similar to the sudden episodes of re-experiencing seen in PTSD, which are believed to be related to dissociation, if not the same thing in many cases). Just like we can occasionally become conscious that we are dreaming, someone in a state of dissociation can recognize that they are having an unusual experience which is reflected in the feelings of **derealization** and **unreality** that accompany dissociation episodes.

The activation of dream-related neural networks during waking consciousness also presents a mechanism that can account for the two different types of memory errors seen: **retrograde amnesia** and **memory errors of commission**. To understand this, consider your own experiences with dreams. Upon awaking from a particularly vivid dream, you have in your mind a memory of events that did not actually happen (a memory error of commission). However, this memory rapidly fades over the next few minutes or hours, even if you tried to hold onto it (retrograde amnesia). Memories created during a dissociative state appear to have these features as well. The co-occurrence of both retrograde amnesia and memory errors of commission is *highly specific* for both dreaming and dissociation, suggesting a shared mechanism.

Finally, the involvement of dream-like consciousness in dissociation explains each of the three hypnotic phenomena (absorption, automaticity, and suggestibility) that are seen in dissociation. **Absorption** is highly correlated with imagination, so it makes sense that dreaming (an inherently imaginative act) would be involved. In addition, **automatic behaviors** can be done while asleep or dreaming. Sleepwalking is the most known example, but other behaviors (even very complex ones like walking, cooking, or driving) can be seen as well. Of note, parasomnias like these are notably more common in patients with dissociative disorders than the general population. Finally, people who are tired or sleep deprived are much more likely to accept false information as true, demonstrating not only a tendency towards memory errors of commission but also the **suggestibility** that is another core sign of dissociation.

If there now exists a solid foundation of evidence suggesting the involvement of dreamlike consciousness in dissociation, how then do we explain the fact that these experiences are much more common in people who have experienced trauma? For many people, the stress of a traumatic experience directly impairs their ability to get quality sleep. Disrupted sleep following a traumatic event appears to be the **first link in a chain** leading to dissociative experiences. Indeed, studies on healthy subjects have found that even a single night of sleeplessness led to a variety of patterns associated with dissociation, including all of the symptom types captured in the **DDREAMS** mnemonic.

Importantly, sleeplessness also appeared to have effects not only on whether memories were encoded but also *how* they were encoded. Sleep deprived people were more likely to **retain negative memories** over positive ones (a pattern mediated largely by a strengthening of the amygdala as well as decreased connection to the medial prefrontal cortex, a similar pattern to PTSD) as well as to remember events in **isolated sensory fragments** rather than in cohesive narratives ("On the day he was shot, I remember the smell of the flowers, the breeze from the ocean, the sound of the birds calling…"). Together, this leads to a pattern of remembering events in so-called "**flashbulb memories**" which are incredibly vivid snapshots of particular moments in time when something disruptive occurred. The emotion associated with the memory enhances one's ability to recall particular details, but it also makes it more difficult to store memories in the usual narrative format, leading to memories being stored instead as **strong but isolated sensory fragments** which is exactly the pattern that is seen in the re-experiencing of PTSD as well.

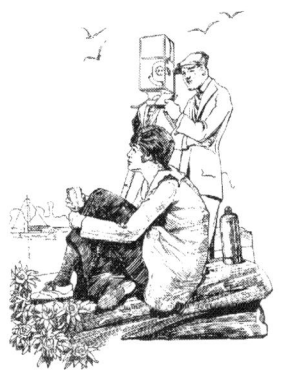

The involvement of a dream-like state during dissociation and its associated impact on memory both have important implications for treatment. One study found that a program focusing exclusively on sleep hygiene can improve dissociative symptoms significantly, suggesting that sleep patterns are a key aspect of evaluating and treating dissociative disorders.

To summarize, dissociation appears to be related to a disrupted sleep-wake cycle in which the dreaming state overlaps with waking life, resulting in the highly characteristic combination of feelings of unreality, specific forms of memory errors, and hypnotic phenomena. To remember this, use the same **DDREAMS** mnemonic from earlier to link dream-like consciousness to dissociative experiences. (As a final note, while daydreaming and imagination are both likely related to dissociation, they are completely normal parts of life and should not be considered pathologic in any way!)

Dissociative episodes involve sudden **intrusions of dreamlike consciousness** into waking life caused by an **unstable sleep-wake cycle**.

Dissociation involves DDREAMS that happen during waking consciousness!

HOW TO DIAGNOSE DISSOCIATIVE DISORDERS

There are three dissociative disorders listed in the DSM: **dissociative amnesia**, **depersonalization-derealization disorder**, and **dissociative identity disorder**. In comparison to other chapters, we won't be using a lot of mnemonics for dissociative disorders. This is because the DSM criteria for these disorders are more like *definitions* than lists (with only one or two key features), making mnemonics rather pointless. Focus instead on understanding the nuances that make these states unique!

When assessing for the presence of a dissociative disorder in clinical settings, keep in mind that some patients have a tendency towards suggestibility. For this reason, do your best to avoid suggesting responses either implicitly or explicitly. Instead of leading questions ("When people have been abused, they often experience strange pains in their genitals. Does this happen to you?"), ask **open-ended questions** ("Tell me about any physical pains, discomforts, or ailments that you have"). This will help you get a more accurate picture to diagnose the presence (or absence!) of each dissociative disorder.

DISSOCIATIVE AMNESIA

Dissociative amnesia refers to **episodes of retrograde amnesia** that lead to gaps in one's autobiographical memory. These gaps often occur around the time of traumatic events and tend to have **well-defined borders** (everything before and after a specific time period is remembered, just not that period itself). The amnesia can be brief (only a few minutes or hours), but it usually only becomes a disorder when it lasts for a while (months or even years for some patients). In severe cases, the amnesia can be so profound that people forget their own name and identity, leading to a **fugue state** in which they will wander around with no knowledge of who they are or where they are from. Dissociative amnesia is a **diagnosis of exclusion**, and other causes for memory loss must be ruled out. The prognosis for dissociative amnesia is good in that most people will recover their memories even without treatment. However, the overall level of functioning for these patients is often poor, although this is more likely related to various comorbidities (such as PTSD or depression) than from the dissociative amnesia itself.

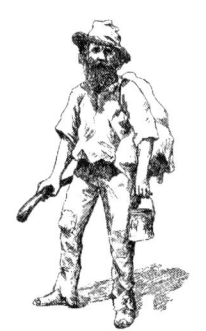

DEPERSONALIZATION-DEREALIZATION DISORDER

Depersonalization-derealization disorder is characterized by depersonalization and/or derealization symptoms that are severe and persistent enough to result in significant distress and impairment. This diagnosis is broad enough to capture a **wide range** of pathology related to dissociative experiences. For most people with the disorder, depersonalization and derealization are **chronic**, although for a minority they occur in transient episodes. The onset of symptoms can either be **spontaneous** or linked to specific **triggers** (with common ones being stress, depression, or use of drugs like cannabis or hallucinogens). Age of onset is typically in the **teenage years**, although some people describe experiencing depersonalization and/or derealization as far back as they can remember. It affects **men and women** equally. In studies, patients are generally well-educated and employed, but often they feel that their life functioning is below where it should be (such as having employment that is below their training).

DISSOCIATIVE IDENTITY DISORDER

While dissociative identity disorder is the rarest of the dissociative disorders (affecting only 1% of the population, in contrast to dissociative amnesia and depersonalization-derealization disorder which each affect around 5 or 10%), it is considered to be the most impairing of the three. Dissociative identity disorder is characterized by a consistent pattern of derealization, depersonalization, and memory lapses that are severe enough that someone experiences them as **completely separate identity states**, leading to a **fragmentation of identity** and a sensation that they are a completely different person from one moment to the next.

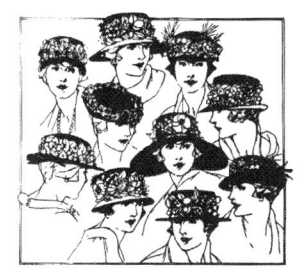

Because the core phenomenology of dissociative identity disorder is nebulous and based on abstractions rather than concretely observable signs, misconceptions about the disorder abound. For this reason, it can be just as helpful to know what the disorder is *not* as to know what it is. Contrary to popular media depictions (ranging from "The Strange Case of Dr. Jekyll and Mr. Hyde" in the 19th century and "The Three Faces of Eve" in the 20th all the way to *Split* in the 21st), dissociative identity disorder does *not* involve multiple different people, each with their own names, personalities, and backstories, all living in the same body and switching back and forth between one another in a sudden or dramatic way. (Media is not the only thing to blame here: the DSM previously called this disorder "multiple personality disorder" which only further contributed to this inaccurate conception of the syndrome.)

Instead, dissociative identity disorder is best described as involving a *sensation* of different identities rather than their literal *presence*. This fragmentation of identity can lead to observable changes in mannerisms, behavior, and speech patterns between the different identities (sometimes called "alters"). A patient's identity at any given time appears to correspond most with their **emotional state**, such as feeling like one identity when angry, another when scared, another when sad, and another when elated. The sense of identity fragmentation is compounded further by the fact that patients with dissociative identity disorder often have **affective lability**, or the tendency to switch quickly from one emotion to another. A tendency toward memory errors also makes it harder for patients to hold onto a consistent sense of self.

To understand how affective lability and memory errors can lead to a sensation of changing identity, ask yourself: how do you know that you are the same person from one moment to the next? It may surprise you to realize that things like physical appearance don't seem to matter too much. Instead, most of us will say that we know ourselves based on two things: a consistent set of **memories** and a consistent pattern of **thoughts, behavior, and emotions**. We know, based on our memories of the past, how we feel and act in various situations, and recognizing these patterns in ourselves helps to build a consistent sense of identity. However, if your memories were shaky and your thoughts, behaviors, and emotions were constantly changing in response to new emotional states, it can be difficult to feel like the same person at 5 o'clock (when you are calmly sitting in a chair reading a book) than you did at 4 o'clock (when you were angrily shouting and throwing things around the room). This is how dissociative identity disorder feels for a patient experiencing it, and this is the pattern you should look for (rather than anything involving multiple people living inside the same body).

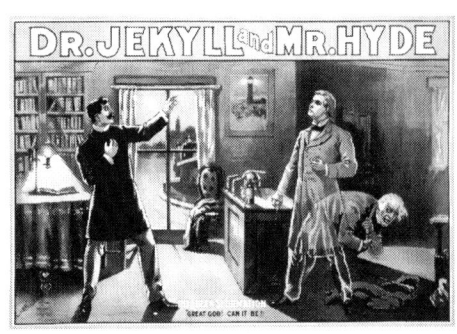

Not quite.

If this is what dissociative identity disorder *really* is, how do we square that with the fact that some patients still present in a way that fits the "dramatic" picture of the disorder? It appears most likely that people who present with "dramatic" dissociative identity disorder are using media depictions as an **idiom of distress** to demonstrate a severe level of pathology that will be validated and taken seriously by others. The fact that clinical presentations tend to follow media depictions of the disorder (rather than the other way around) helps to support this notion. For example, movies and TV shows featuring characters with dissociative identity disorder in the United States tend to depict the shifts between personalities as instantaneous, while in India the transitions between different identities is shown as happening during sleep. Patients in each of these countries behaved accordingly in clinical settings. (While cultural factors do play a large role in how patients experience these disorders, the tendency to reflect media depictions in dissociative identity disorder far exceeds what is seen with other disorders like bipolar disorder and schizophrenia.) **Suggestibility** appears to play a large role as well, as these patients may be inclined to act out provider expectations of what dissociative identity disorder looks like. The fact that this disorder is studied and diagnosed almost exclusively by a small number of clinics and clinicians rather than being commonly recognized among all practitioners supports this notion as well. It is possible that the "dramatic" form of dissociative identity disorder doesn't even *exist* but rather is an **iatrogenic diagnosis** (a disorder that is *caused* by medical treatment rather than cured by it). The clearest evidence for this comes from the fact that dissociative identity disorder was at the center of a diagnostic "fad" that happened in the 1980s across the United States, when multiple personality disorder was being diagnosed in nearly 10% of all patients which is significantly greater than the **1% prevalence** for dissociative identity disorder that has been observed before and since. Taking all of this into account, it is likely that "dramatic" dissociative identity disorder is less of a consistent psychiatric *syndrome* than it is a false diagnostic *construct* that has been perpetuated by overzealous clinicians and imposed upon patients with a high capacity for suggestibility.

Nevertheless, while rates of the diagnosis have never reached the same levels as in its 1980s heyday, they haven't gone away completely. In addition, cases consistent with dissociative identity disorder have been described for hundreds of years across multiple cultures (even those that do not prominently feature media depictions of the disorder). In light of this, it is reasonable to conclude that dissociative identity disorder *does* exist but only in the form described earlier: as a sensation of different personalities owing to affective lability, memory errors, and fragmentation of identity. For patients who are diagnosed with this form of dissociative identity disorder, the prognosis is often poor. Research suggests that most people with this condition experience ongoing distress and disability, although (like other dissociative disorders) this may be due as much to comorbidity with other psychiatric conditions as it is to the dissociative experiences themselves. Evidence about effective forms of treatment is lacking, with no clear guidelines. The research that does exist suggests that most patients with dissociative identity disorder do not feel that any form of treatment meets their goals, and many drop out of treatment entirely. Most of this may be due to a mismatch between patient and provider goals. Some clinicians focus so much on the idea of trying to "re-integrate" the various identities back into one that they neglect to focus on other symptoms, such as depression, anxiety, somatization, and substance use, which may be significantly more treatable than the dissociative pathology itself.

When working with patients presenting with dissociative identity disorder, always take a supportive and validating stance, and keep in mind that *taking someone seriously does not always mean taking them literally* (especially for patients presenting with the "dramatic" form). In addition, make sure to be have a discussion about the patient's goals of care as well as what they can expect to happen with treatment ("I can't promise that we will be able to fully re-integrate your sense of various identities, but I *can* work with you to improve your ability to cope with fragmentation of identity as well as the panic attacks and depressive episodes you described").

DIFFERENTIAL DIAGNOSIS OF DISSOCIATIVE DISORDERS

Dissociative disorders are almost always comorbid with other conditions, including depression, anxiety, PTSD, and cluster B personality disorders. However, they can also be easily misdiagnosed as other disorders due to common misconceptions about each disorder and the abstract nature of symptoms. In this section, we will review some common misdiagnoses and missed diagnoses in patients with dissociative disorders.

NORMALCY

Dissociation is not inherently pathological, as up to a quarter of all people experience dissociative symptoms but are not particularly troubled by them. Even within medical settings, dissociation is rarely the primary reason that someone seeks mental health care. For this reason, don't let the mere *presence* of dissociative symptoms form the basis for a diagnosis. Instead, a dissociative disorder should only be diagnosed when there is clear evidence that the episodes of derealization and depersonalization are frequent or severe enough that they are causing dysfunction in and of themselves.

While dissociative disorders can often present with memory loss, care should be taken to avoid diagnosing a dissociative disorder in everyone who believes that they have lost their memory for certain events in their life. Certain forms of memory loss are normal, as most adults are unable to remember most memories for events that happened when they were **pre-verbal** (before the age of five or six), that occurred **long ago** (with memories of events diminishing with time), or were experienced during **sleep or dreaming**.

Finally, care should be taken not to pathologize patients who say that they act like a "different person" in different situations. The normal range of personality is large enough to encompass even major differences in emotions and behavior between various settings (such as someone who is quiet and reserved with their parents yet outspoken and disinhibited when with friends), and this type of compartmentalization should not be seen as pathological in any way.

PSYCHOSIS

Dissociation is commonly confused for psychosis. In fact, up to half of all patients with dissociative identity disorder had been diagnosed with or treated for schizophrenia. This has to do with the fact that the words used to describe dissociation ("feelings of unreality") is often quite similar to those used to describe psychosis ("loss of contact with reality"). While both psychosis and dissociation involve alterations in someone's subjective experience of reality, they are ultimately quite different. A person in a state of dissociation is generally able to distinguish between their own internal experiences and the objective reality of the outside world (their experiences don't *feel* real even though they recognize that they *are* real). In contrast, someone in a state of psychosis is *genuinely unable* to tell that their subjective experiences do not form a shared reality, and their **reality testing ability** (or the capacity to tell what is real from what is fake) is distinctly impaired. Other symptoms, such as thought disorganization and negative symptoms, can also help to differentiate psychosis from dissociative disorders (although some symptoms, such as paranoia and auditory hallucinations, can be found in both, especially if there is comorbid borderline personality disorder).

BORDERLINE PERSONALITY DISORDER

Dissociation is a core symptom of borderline personality disorder, making these two diagnoses **highly comorbid**. In fact, some studies have found rates of comorbidity between borderline personality disorder and dissociative identity disorder above 80%. Many symptoms (such as identity disturbance and affective lability) are central to both disorders, leading some researchers to propose that dissociative identity disorder is in fact an "epiphenomenon" of severe borderline personality disorder (similar to how agoraphobia can be an "epiphenomenon" of panic disorder). At the very least, the overlap in patterns between the two disorders should put borderline personality disorder on the differential for all patients presenting with dissociative disorders.

TRAUMA

The relationship of dissociative disorders to trauma is well established. While dissociation is often a transient state in response to trauma, for some people these dissociative symptoms can become persistent, especially when the trauma is prolonged or occurred during early childhood development. This is consistent with studies showing that around 95% of people with dissociative identity disorder report chronic childhood trauma often beginning before the age of 6. (In contrast, the rate of child abuse in the general population is around 5-15%.) Abuse histories in patients with dissociative identity disorder cannot be attributed entirely to memory errors of commission, as studies have found outside evidence corroborating histories of abuse in the majority of cases (although in some cases the memory of abuse does appear to exceed what was prospectively recorded in both nature and extent).

Given that dissociation is a symptom of both acute stress disorder and PTSD, the line between when you consider dissociation to be a symptom of those disorders and when it is a diagnosis in and of itself is unclear. This confusion is likely the result of a messy diagnostic scheme more than it reflects a genuine separation between these clinical entities. As a practical rule of thumb, consider diagnosing a separate dissociative disorder in individuals for whom the dissociative episodes exceed the flashbacks and nightmares seen in "textbook" PTSD, who have specific forms of dissociative experiences that match these disorders (such as someone in a clear fugue state), or who experience significant distress as a direct result of feelings of depersonalization or derealization rather than only from the trauma itself.

SOMATIZATION
Somatization is frequently comorbid with dissociative disorders, with up to 80% of patients with dissociative identity disorder meeting criteria for a somatoform disorder as well. In particular, conversion disorder is a common co-occurrence and is actually believed to be dissociative in nature (as we will talk about more in the next chapter). Keep somatization high on your differential when evaluating someone with both medically unexplained symptoms and a tendency towards dissociation.

DEPRESSION
Feelings of unreality and depersonalization have been associated with a state of depression for as long as this disorder has been described, even if they are not in the DSM criteria themselves. Dissociative experiences that occur exclusively during an episode of depression and disappear when the episode resolves should be thought of as a symptom of depression rather than necessitating a diagnosis of a separate dissociative disorder.

BIPOLAR DISORDER
People with bipolar disorder can appear to be very different people depending on whether they are depressed, manic, or euthymic. However, these switches between mood states happen over weeks or months (as opposed to over minutes or hours in dissociative identity disorder). In addition, people with bipolar disorder rarely report feelings of derealization or depersonalization, even during mood episodes (in fact, people with bipolar disorder report some of the lowest rates of dissociative experiences of any psychiatric diagnosis!).

PANIC ATTACKS
Dissociative symptoms are common during a panic attack, with over two-thirds of all patients with panic disorder reporting depersonalization or derealization during an episode. However, for people with panic disorder, dissociative experiences outside the context of a panic attack are no more common than in the general population. For this reason, a dissociative disorder should only be diagnosed in someone with panic disorder if there is a clear history of episodes *outside* the context of a panic attack.

DEMENTIA
Dissociative disorders and dementia both share memory loss as a core clinical feature, but there are enough differences that these two conditions should rarely be confused. Of note, people with dissociative amnesia show a distinct **awareness** of (and distress about) their lapses in memory whereas people with dementia are generally oblivious to the fact that their memory is fading. In addition, dissociative disorders rarely present with actual deficits on the **cognitive tests** that are used to diagnose dementia. However, the easiest way to differentiate between the diagnoses is to remember that most people with dissociative disorders are diagnosed in their late teens or early adult years (as opposed to the older ages seen in dementia).

ELECTROCONVULSIVE THERAPY
Amnesia is a common side effect of ECT and occurs to some degree in most patients who undergo the procedure. Do not confuse the amnesia seen in dissociation with this unfortunate but expected effect of ECT.

PUTTING IT ALL TOGETHER
Dissociative disorders can be confusing. Rather than face this complexity, clinicians often have a tendency to avoid these diagnoses completely. Given that patients rarely present with dissociation as their *primary* concern, it is actually possible to do so, and as a result dissociative disorders tend to be **underdiagnosed**. However, this does a disservice to the many patients who struggle with dissociation as it deprives them of evidence-based treatment and further perpetuates stigma. In response to this situation, some clinicians instead go the *opposite* direction and attempt to champion these disorders by searching for evidence of dissociation everywhere they look. While this is intended to be a helpful counterpoint to the status quo, it has the potential to make dissociative disorders **overdiagnosed** by certain clinicians, further muddying the waters.

Try to strike a balance between these two extremes by understanding that **dissociation exists**, that it often **results from trauma**, and that for some people it can become **severe, persistent, and impairing**. In addition to focusing on the subjective symptoms of **D**epersonalization and **D**erealization, use the presence or absence of objective abnormalities in memory (**R**etrograde amnesia and memory **E**rrors of commission) and specific psychological traits (**A**bsorption, **M**otor automaticity, and **S**uggestibility) to establish the diagnosis with more certainty. (Handily, all of these are captured in the **DDREAMS** mnemonic!) Remembering that dissociative disorders mechanistically involve a **disrupted sleep-wake cycle** can also help to not only confirm the diagnosis but also provide targets for treatment (which remains very poorly understood). Finally, keep in mind that dissociation itself is not inherently bad! Indeed, dissociative mechanisms appear to be related to things like imagination which form the basis of art and creativity—things that most people would agree are the exact opposite of pathology.

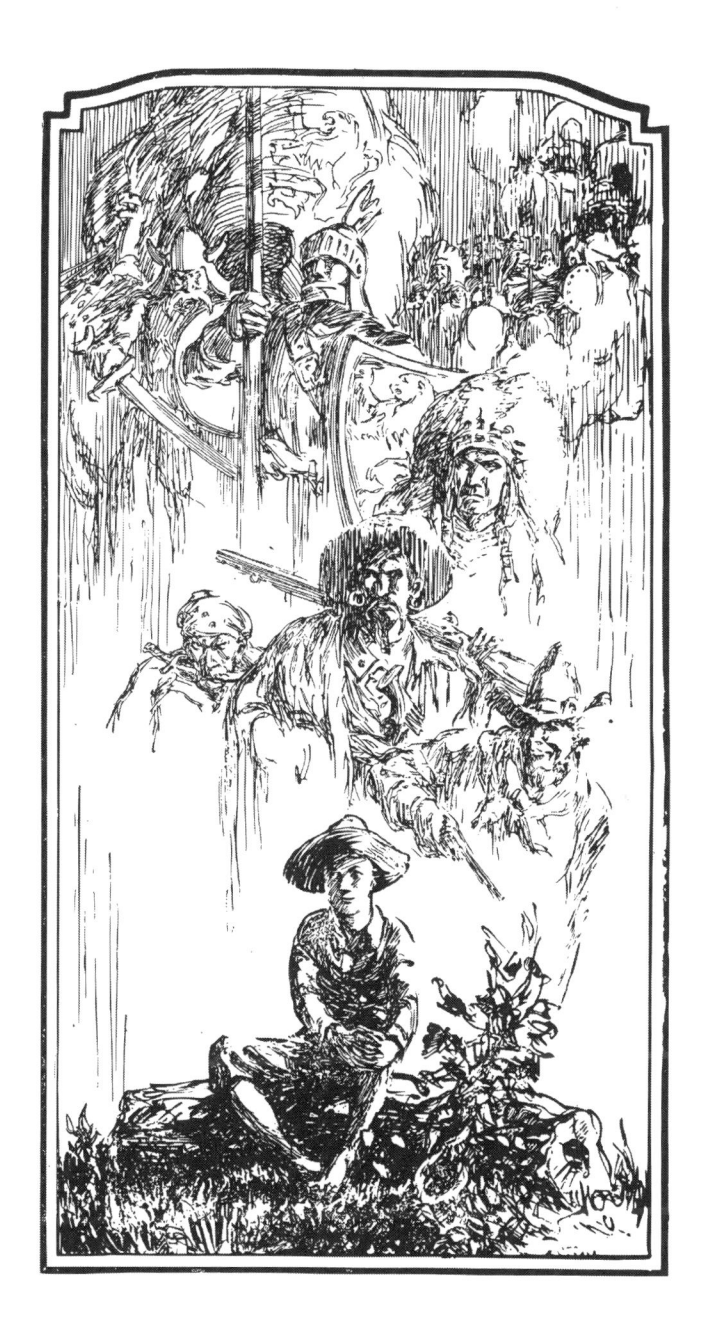

REVIEW QUESTIONS

1. A 21 y/o M is brought to the emergency department by his parents. They became concerned when they called him two days ago and he appeared to have no knowledge of who they were. They immediately drove to his university to pick him up and bring him in for evaluation. On interview, the patient says that he is here because "I've lost my memory." He says, "People tell me that I was very into a girl who broke my heart. I wish I could remember her so I could tell her not to do it. But I can't even remember her name. It's completely gone." He denies feeling depressed and says, "No, I feel completely fine. Everyone else seems to be concerned, but I am fine." Physical and neurologic examination is normal. He is able to perform a 10-minute recall of 5 words given to him by the psychiatrist. What term best describes the type of memory error that he is experiencing?
    A. Anterograde amnesia
    B. Retrograde amnesia
    C. Global amnesia
    D. Memory errors of commission
    E. Aphasia

2. (Continued from previous question.) When interviewed, the patient's parents report that he was diagnosed with ADHD as a child but later "outgrew" it. They also report that he was hospitalized for one week at the age of 16 after he became suicidal following a break-up with his high school girlfriend. To their knowledge, he currently takes no medications other than a few doses of alprazolam (a benzodiazepine) each month for a diagnosis of panic disorder. During the interview, his father begins crying and says, "I just hate that he can't remember who we are. We raised him. We're his parents. Will he ever know who we are again?" What is the best response to his father?
    A. "Yes, it is an absolute certainty that he will regain his memories."
    B. "You don't have to worry. It is very likely that he will."
    C. "It's tough to say at the moment. There's around a 50% chance."
    D. "It's unlikely that he will regain his lost memories, but we will do our best to work with him and with you both during this process."
    E. "This is a hard thing for me to say, but those memories are gone."

3. A 23 y/o F is admitted to the hospital following a suicide attempt in which she attempted to overdose on 10 pills of lamotrigine (a mood stabilizer which she has been prescribed). This is her third hospitalization in the past year. She normally sees her therapist two times a week but has not been attending sessions for the past month. During her interview with the hospital psychiatrist, she initially comes across as lighthearted and flirtatious in a way that seems at odds with the circumstances. When asked about the suicide attempt, her affect immediately switches to a brooding, serious expression. She responds by saying, "I don't talk about that. I don't want to talk to you anymore," and asks the psychiatrist to leave. Later, when talking with the nurses, she says that she has "no clue" why she is in the hospital but she is "glad to be back." Which of the following disorders is this patient *least* likely to have?

A. Post-traumatic stress disorder
B. Major depressive disorder
C. Bipolar disorder
D. A substance use disorder
E. A personality disorder
F. A somatoform disorder

4. (Continued from previous question.) The patient is discharged from the hospital three days later and begins seeing a new therapist who has extensive experience working with dissociative disorders and offers trauma-focused psychotherapy. The patient remains in treatment for two years and is noted to have significant improvements in interpersonal and occupational functioning. Which of the following symptoms is most likely to still be present at the end of two years?
    A. Episodes of dissociation
    B. Depressed mood
    C. Feelings of anxiety
    D. Frequent suicide attempts
    E. Frequent non-suicidal self-harm
    F. All of the above are equally likely to be present at the end of treatment

5. A 22 y/o F is robbed at gunpoint on her way home from work. Following this incident, she begins to feel very depressed and frequently has trouble sleeping. Normally outgoing and vivacious, she begins to come across as pessimistic and isolated to the point that her friends have commented to each other that she looks "like a different person." She does not seek psychiatric care, nor does she tell anyone else about the incident. Three months later, her friends receive an invitation to attend a stand-up comedy gala that she is hosting. At this event, she is gregarious and warm, laughing and telling jokes as she introduces each new comedian. While most of the audience is having a wonderful time, her friends feel uneasy about this "transformation" and worry about her mental health. What is the most likely diagnosis at this time?
    A. Dissociative amnesia
    B. Depersonalization-derealization disorder
    C. Dissociative identity disorder
    D. Bipolar I disorder
    E. Bipolar II disorder
    F. None of the above

1. **The best answer is B.** The patient's inability to recall details from his past suggests a retrograde amnesia, while his ability to recall new information (such as the 5 words given to him by the interviewer) rule out anterograde amnesia (answer A). Global amnesia is a combination of both anterograde and retrograde amnesia, but this patient is only suffering from retrograde amnesia (answer C). Memory errors of commission involve remembering events that did not happen, and there is no evidence of that in this case (answer D). Aphasia involves impairments in comprehending and generating language, both of which are intact in this case (answer E).

2. **The best answer is B.** This patient appears to be suffering from dissociative amnesia which is characterized by loss of memories in a retrograde fashion. The usual prognosis for dissociative amnesia is for a spontaneous recovery of lost memories, although it cannot be said with complete certainty that the memories will return (answer A).

3. **The best answer is C.** This patient shows signs consistent with dissociative identity disorder which is strongly correlated with a history of childhood abuse. Accordingly, this disorder is highly comorbid with other disorders related to abuse, including PTSD, depression, substance abuse, personality disorders, and somatoform disorders (answers A, B, D, E, and F). In contrast, while bipolar disorder is related to stress, it is not associated with childhood trauma in the same way as the other disorders listed. The mere fact that this patient is taking lamotrigine (a mood stabilizer) is not enough to confirm that she has bipolar disorder, as she may have been prescribed lamotrigine to treat another condition such as epilepsy (not to mention that bipolar disorder itself is frequently overdiagnosed and overtreated).

4. **The best answer is A.** While the optimum treatment strategies for dissociative identity disorder remain poorly defined, evidence suggests that trauma-focused psychotherapy is effective at improving outcomes in the disorder. However, episodes of dissociation themselves appear to be the least responsive to therapy, while other outcomes including depressive symptoms, anxiety, and frequency of suicide attempts and self-harm appear to respond much better (answers B through E).

5. **The best answer is F.** Despite a history of trauma, there is no indication of either dissociative or bipolar pathology in this clinical vignette. The changes in affect and behavior described in this case occur from one setting to another (as opposed to being inflexible across various settings) and are adaptive and appropriate to the context of the situation. There is no evidence to suggest amnesia (answer A), feelings of depersonalization or derealization (answer B), or fragmentation of a sense of identity (answer C). No form of bipolar disorder is diagnosed based on the presence of a single evening of different behavior (answers D and E). While it is possible that this patient is suffering from another disorder (such as PTSD or depression), these are not available as answer choices.

13 SOMATIZATION

Somatization is the process by which *mental* distress is subjectively experienced as *bodily* (or "somatic") symptoms like pain, nausea, shortness of breath, or neurologic deficits. Mental disorders that have somatization as a prominent feature are known as **somatoform disorders** because they resemble (or take the "form" of) body-based illnesses like infection, heart disease, stroke, or cancer without actually involving the core pathology of these diseases. Historically, the starting point for somatoform disorders was the mere presence of **medically unexplained symptoms**. However, because grounding a diagnosis on the *absence* of an explanation is a fundamentally problematic notion, attempts have been made to revise the diagnostic criteria to include a greater focus on **maladaptive thoughts, feelings, and behaviors** related to the symptoms, including frequent thoughts about the seriousness of the symptoms, excessive anxiety about what they might mean, and lots of time, energy, and effort spent on activities related to the symptoms.

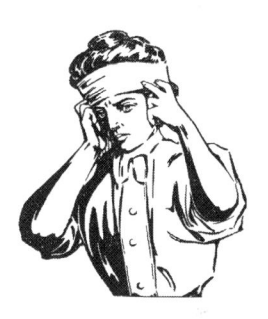

Somatoform disorders are among the most controversial psychiatric diagnoses, for several reasons. For one, diagnosing a somatoform disorder has a high chance of producing the negative aspects of diagnosis (such as being highly stigmatizing) without delivering much in the way of benefits (it doesn't validate distress). When done incorrectly, telling a patient about a diagnosis of a somatoform disorder can significantly **damage the doctor-patient relationship**, especially if it's implied that the problem is "all in your head." In addition, interpreting a particular symptom as somatoform in nature is often a **diagnosis of exclusion**: it assumes that, once medical explanations have been ruled out, the only remaining explanation is that the person's symptoms are psychological rather than physical. This can lead to a premature sense of closure, especially for conditions that are poorly understood. (Consider that asthma was considered to be a "psychosomatic" disorder up until the 1960s, resulting in some cases being treated with psychoanalysis rather than medications!) It is possible that further research will discover the roots of other medical syndromes that currently do not have a biological explanation, including conditions such as fibromyalgia, chronic fatigue syndrome, and irritable bowel syndrome.

Nevertheless, there is a reason that the concept of a somatoform disorder has existed for so long and continues to be used in modern medicine. Nearly every medical specialty sees at least one biologically unexplained syndrome that often seems to be accompanied by **maladaptive cognitive and behavioral patterns**, including fibromyalgia (rheumatology), non-cardiac chest pain (cardiology), irritable bowel syndrome (gastroenterology), chronic pelvic pain (gynecology), chronic fatigue syndrome (primary care), tension headaches (neurology), hyperventilation syndrome (pulmonology), multiple chemical sensitivity (allergy), and chronic Lyme disease (infectious disease). In addition, to completely dismiss any link between physical and mental health would be to ignore a wealth of research and clinical experience that has built up over centuries. People with medically unexplained symptoms tend to have a high rate of other mental conditions, including depression, anxiety, and trauma-related disorders (including not only PTSD but dissociative and cluster B personality disorders as well). In addition, treatment of medically unexplained symptoms often involves the **same treatments as for anxiety and depression** (medications and psychotherapy) which results in improvement in the physical symptoms themselves (not just the distress related to them). With all this in mind, it seems reasonable to conclude that a relationship *does exist* between medically unexplained symptoms and mental health, even if there are many potential pitfalls to diagnosing this pattern too easily or often.

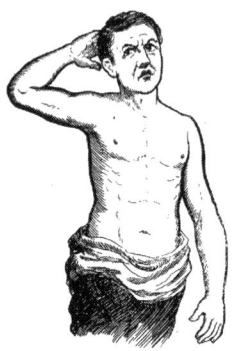

As with dissociative disorders, a balanced perspective on somatoform disorders appears warranted. First, do not be led into thinking that if particular symptoms are psychological or psychiatric in origin then they are somehow feigned, imaginary, or non-existent! Instead, patients prone to somatization appear to **genuinely experience** the symptoms that cause them so much discomfort and distress. Therefore, if we apply what we have learned so far and remember that *taking a patient seriously does not always mean taking them literally*, we can still provide good care for our patients without exposing them to the risks of physical harm and unnecessary medicalization that would occur by treating all medical *symptoms* as medical *illnesses*.

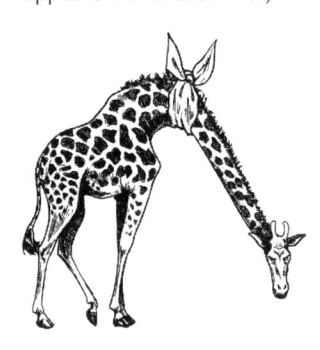

SIGNS AND SYMPTOMS OF SOMATIZATION

The specific symptoms involved in somatization can involve **every organ system in the body** (including fatigue, fever, headaches, dizziness, visual problems, stiffness, weakness, itching, chest pain, palpitations, wheezing, shortness of breath, nausea, diarrhea, constipation, and urinary pain) and can range from mild to severe. The **gastrointestinal tract** is the most common location for somatic symptoms, with over 95% of persistent somatizers experiencing unexplained symptoms related to this organ system. In women, gynecologic complaints (including pelvic pain and menstrual irregularity) are the second most common symptom and are experienced by over 90% of women with somatoform disorders. Next most common are symptoms of the central nervous system, musculoskeletal system, and urinary tract. The vast majority of patients with persistent somatization experience symptoms in **multiple organs** of the body throughout their life. However, it is also common for each person to have one or two "preferred" organs that are most commonly involved.

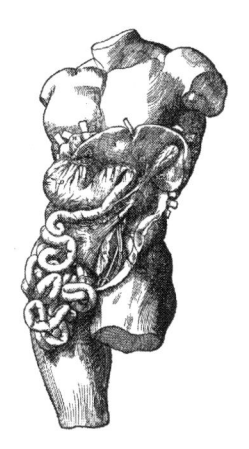

As mentioned before, symptoms in somatization are **genuinely experienced**. This contrasts with other conditions (such as factitious disorder or malingering, discussed later in this chapter) where signs and symptoms are feigned or intentionally induced. However, the line between "real" and "fake" symptoms is not always clear cut, and around 20% of people who experience somatization have intentionally self-induced a disease state on at least one occasion.

Behaviorally, people with medically unexplained symptoms often persist in seeking treatment despite repeated negative examinations and tests. For this reason, people who experience persistent somatization can incur healthcare costs up to *ten times higher* than people who do not, including more primary care appointments, more specialist consultations, more emergency department visits, and more hospital admissions. These patients are also much more likely to be prescribed unnecessary medications and be subjected to invasive tests, procedures, and even surgical operations. People with frequent and severe somatization undergo a median of eight surgical procedures over their lifetime, with procedures on the uterus and gastrointestinal tract being the most common. These surgeries are much more likely to be diagnostically and therapeutically unhelpful, with over 60% of surgeries in persistent somatizers showing no abnormal findings (compared to 20% for non-somatizers). Because of this, people with persistent somatization are at high risk for **iatrogenic injuries** including surgical accidents, complications from anesthesia, medication side effects, and radiation exposure. This makes understanding, preventing, and treating somatization a major personal and public health concern.

SOMATIZATION ACROSS THE LIFESPAN

Somatization is **universal**. Every person alive has experienced distressing medical symptoms for which no cause was ever found. Somatization is frequently a reason for seeking medical care. In fact, it is believed that up to a third of all primary care visits are for medically unexplained symptoms. For the majority of patients, these symptoms are transient and resolve on their own. For a significant minority of these patients, however, somatization becomes persistent and leads to distress and dysfunction. These people are said to be suffering from **somatoform disorders**.

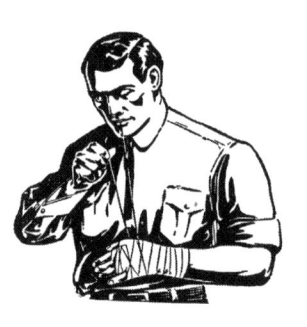

EPIDEMIOLOGY
The prevalence of somatoform disorders in the general population is **about 5%**, making it neither as common as disorders like depression and anxiety nor as rare as disorders like bipolar disorder and schizophrenia. **Women** are affected vastly more often than men, with some estimates placing the gender ratio as high as 10 to 1. Persistent somatization begins as early as childhood, and for people with chronic somatoform complaints, this pattern almost always begins **before the age of 30**.

PROGNOSIS
For some people, somatization is a transient phenomenon which tends to increase around times of stress. However, for around 25% of people with somatoform symptoms that are severe enough to go to a doctor's office, somatization becomes **chronic and enduring**. For those with persistent somatization, the vast majority improve during follow-up, even without treatment. However, for around 20% of persistent somatizers, the clinical course is characterized by worsening symptoms and increasing anxiety.

TREATMENT
Because people presenting with somatoform disorders are often seen in primary care clinics or other non-psychiatric settings, treatment is frequently given by providers who have not received specific training in these disorders. In addition, patients with somatoform disorders are often quite hesitant to see mental health providers out of concern that their symptoms will be dismissed as "psychosomatic" or otherwise not taken seriously. Because of this, somatoform disorders are often trapped in a "no man's land" between primary care, neurologists, and other specialists (who are asked to see these patients but do not believe that they can help) and psychiatrists (who may feel more able to help but often won't be seen by the patients). Because of this, treating somatization requires a fundamentally different approach. Use the mnemonic **I Do CARE** to remember the necessary ingredients for successful treatment of somatoform disorders:

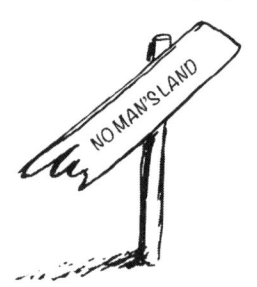

I is for Interface. Patients who somatize tend to have many healthcare providers, including multiple specialists in various areas of medicine. Work closely to interface with all the medical providers on the patient's team, and integrate your findings so that none of you are working in isolation.

Do is for "Do no harm." Patients who somatize are at high risk for injury, disability, or even death as a result of frequent tests and treatments. Because of this, keep the dictum "do no harm" closely held in your mind, and always weigh the potential risks of treatment against the benefits to avoid doing more harm than good.

C is for CBT. CBT is the best studied treatment for somatization, with a **small to moderate effect size** and benefits that are durable (lasting years after treatment has stopped). **Mindfulness-based therapies** have also been shown to be helpful, with a similar effect size. However, getting patients to buy into the idea that they need these treatments is difficult, leading to high drop-out rates.

A is for Antidepressants. Antidepressants are the best studied medication treatment for somatization, and evidence suggests that they can be effective (though with a **smaller effect size** compared to CBT). However, their potential benefits must be weighed against the possibility that the medications themselves can cause side effects which may further trigger or exacerbate somatization.

R is for Regular visits. For someone suffering from severe anxiety about physical symptoms, a visit to the doctor can be very comforting. However, this can have the effect of inadvertently providing *negative reinforcement* for having experienced severe symptoms in the first place, as it is easy for the patient to think (even unconsciously) that "I get to go to the doctor *only when I'm sick.*" You can reduce this association by scheduling visits on a regular basis rather than only seeing the patient when they have a physical complaint.

E is for Empathy. Try to spend most of your time during the appointment listening to the patient, empathizing with their distress, and educating them on the overall good prognosis for symptoms that they are concerned about ("In similar cases I've worked on, these symptoms went away on their own without the need for potentially harmful treatments, and I'm hopeful that this will happen for you too!").

Treatment of somatization involves **therapy, antidepressants,** scheduling **regular appointments,** and **avoiding iatrogenic harm.**

I Do CARE:
Interface
"Do no harm"
CBT
Antidepressants
Regular visits
Empathy

MECHANISMS OF SOMATIZATION

If people who somatize genuinely experience the pain and other bodily sensations that cause them so much distress, then the next question naturally is: *why*? There are two possible explanations. One is that people who somatize receive more pain signals than people who do not, making it a *peripheral* problem of too many nerve signals being generated. The other explanation is that people who somatize generate the same number of pain signals but are excessively focused on them, making it a *central* problem of hypersensitivity to noxious stimuli.

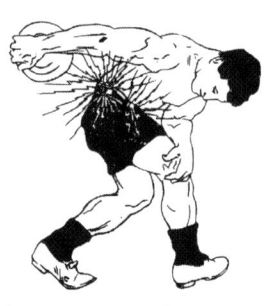

Between these two views, the overwhelming amount of evidence supports the central problem hypothesis. In studies that have been performed, people with somatoform disorders who were given the exact same stimulus (a painful but ultimately harmless electric shock) were significantly more likely to react to this with distress, anxiety, and other negative emotions than people who did not have a somatoform disorder.

The key to understanding this process is the concept of **interoception**, or the ability to sense one's *internal* bodily state (as opposed to exteroception, which is the ability to focus on stimuli *outside* of the body). People differ in their interoceptive abilities. (For example, some people are more able to sense their own heartbeat than others.) A brain region known as the **insula** appears to be the key player involved in interoception, with the activity of this region correlating to the degree of pain that is reported. People who experience persistent somatization appear to have hyperactive signaling pathways connected to the insula which manifests as a heightened awareness of, and a tendency to overfocus on, signals from one's own body.

However, this is only half of the story. Someone with a hyperactive insula may be more prone to pay attention to somatic sensations, but this doesn't necessarily need to be distressing or impairing. In people who somatize, however, the increased perception of somatic signals is accompanied by a tendency to overinterpret these bodily signals as being "bad." For example, someone who is resting and notices that they can hear the sound of their heartbeat may simply think, "Oh that's interesting," or they could respond by thinking, "Oh no, what does this mean? Am I having a heart attack?!" It is the latter response that is typical of somatization. On a biological level, the **anterior cingulate cortex** is believed to be involved in this process. As you'll recall from the chapter on obsessive-compulsive disorders, the anterior cingulate cortex is responsible for recognizing *error* signals. When the insula passes along interoceptive information to the anterior cingulate cortex, the anterior cingulate cortex interprets that signal as representing an error ("something bad is happening") and generates alarm signals. This creates a state of motivational arousal that prompts the person to take action (such as seeing a doctor or asking a friend for reassurance).

In this way, somatization is revealed to be a two-step process between increased **IN**teroception in the **IN**sula along with a tendency for the **A**nterior **C**ingulate **C**ortex to overinterpret these signals as representing a problem and then take **ACC**-tion on them. You can remember this by thinking that these abnormalities together cause someone to generate **IN-ACC**-urate self-diagnoses.

> **Somatization** involves hyperactivity of the **insula**, which mediates **interoception**, and the **anterior cingulate cortex**, which interprets the signal as an **error**.
>
> *When someone's self-diagnosis is repeatedly **IN-ACC**-urate, consider abnormalities in the **IN**sula and **A**nterior **C**ingulate **C**ortex.*

On a behavioral level, somatization is believed to be at least partially a **learned behavior**. Much of this has to do with the specific actions that signal to others that one is sick (known as illness behavior) as well as the actions that others do in response, including gifts and favors (bringing chicken soup), increased leniency with responsibilities (giving a day off of school or work), and increased care, attention, and affection from friends and family. Many children can relate to feeling a bit of jealousy when a schoolmate comes to school in a cast due to having broken a bone. The increase in attention and affection given to these individuals is enviable (even if the pain of having a broken bone is not).

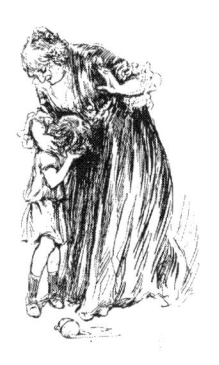

Somatization appears to be a mechanism by which some people have learned to obtain specific needs in their life. Evidence for this comes from the fact that many people with persistent somatization have had family members with severe illnesses during their childhood, which increases exposure to the social dynamics of (and benefits associated with) being in the sick role. An increased need for social support is frequently found in persistent somatizers and is a consistent predictor of ongoing somatization. In contrast, for people experiencing acute stress, *more* social support is associated with *less* reporting of medical symptoms.

In this way, somatization provides **both positive and negative reinforcement** for illness behavior: the increased affection from others is powerfully rewarding, while being excused from unwanted responsibilities can be negatively reinforcing. Doctors and other healthcare providers can unwittingly play into this dynamic just by trying to be empathic and provide a high quality of care. By seeing people only when they have an illness, doctors reinforce the idea that symptoms are required for their attention. This underscores why scheduling regular visits is so important when working with someone who experiences persistent somatization: it helps to break the positive reinforcement of somatization by providing the patient with attention even when no symptoms are present.

In summary, somatization is a complex phenomenon that involves both biological and behavioral processes. While the neurobiological findings have yet to play a significant role in finding treatments for somatoform conditions, understanding the behavioral dynamics of somatization can help to inform treatment on a day-to-day clinical level.

HOW TO DIAGNOSE SOMATOFORM DISORDERS

The DSM lists several conditions in its section on somatic symptom and related disorders, including somatic symptom disorder, conversion disorder, and factitious disorder. Illness anxiety disorder (or hypochondriasis) is also listed in this chapter, although we established back in Chapter 10 that this is more accurately conceived of as an obsessive-compulsive spectrum disorder. Finally, malingering (or the intentional feigning of symptoms for some kind of secondary gain) is *not* considered to be a medical or psychiatric diagnosis, but we will discuss it here as it can present similarly to other disorders involving somatization.

SOMATIC SYMPTOM DISORDER

Somatic symptom disorder is the prototype somatoform disorder and is characterized by **persistent and impairing somatization**. As with all forms of somatization, these symptoms are genuinely experienced by the patient. To remember the diagnostic criteria for somatic symptom disorder, use the mnemonic **SOME ATTIC**. This should remind you of the somatic **S**ymptoms that are at the heart of the disorder. Most people with this disorder have multiple symptoms, but ultimately only **O**ne is required. The symptoms are often either **M**edically unexplained or so clearly in **E**xcess of what would be expected from any given disease process that it suggests a large psychological component. The symptoms must be accompanied by maladaptive thoughts, feelings, and behaviors such as **A**nxiety about what the symptom could mean, frequently **T**hinking about the symptom, and lots of **T**ime and energy being spent in activities related to the symptom such as researching things online for hours each day. The patient must be clearly **I**mpaired or distressed by the disorder. Finally, somatic symptom disorder is **C**hronic, lasting months or years at a time.

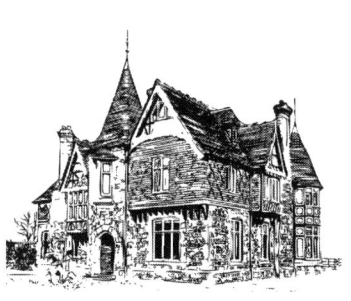

> **Somatic symptom disorder** involves **persistent somatic symptoms** that are **excessive** and **lead to impairment**.
>
> *SOME ATTIC:*
> **S**ymptoms
> **O**ne or more
> **M**edically unexplained
> **E**xcessive
> **A**nxiety about the symptom
> **T**hinking about the symptom
> **T**ime and energy consumed by the symptom
> **I**mpaired or distressed
> **C**hronic (months or years)

CONVERSION DISORDER

Conversion disorder is when a patient presents with **neurologic abnormalities** with no evidence of an observable neurologic cause. These abnormalities can be either subjectively reported *symptoms* such as blindness, blurry vision, and loss of sensation or objectively observed *signs* such as weakness, imbalance, or shaking. Notably, conversion disorder can involve either the *absence of function* (as in motor paralysis) or the *presence of dysfunction* (as in convulsions). Historically, the DSM required that there be a **recent stressor** (the stressor being the thing that is "converted" into the neurologic abnormality) such as a patient developing leg weakness and becoming unable to walk after their parents are killed in a car crash. However, this requirement was dropped in the DSM-5, and the more neutral name "functional neurological symptom disorder" is increasingly being used.

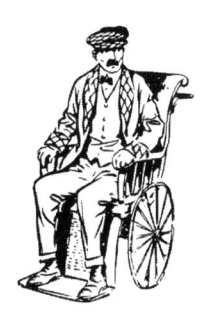

Given that the majority of neurologic deficits involve areas that people have voluntary control over, it is easy to come to the conclusion that people with conversion disorder are either "faking it" or not trying hard enough. However, clinical experience tells us that most people with conversion disorder are not manufacturing their symptoms, and recent research even suggests that conversion disorder (and in particular cases involving the presence of abnormal movements such as seizure-like fits) is a specific manifestation of the **automaticity seen in dissociation**.

You can remember the core features of conversion disorder by thinking of it as **CAN'T**-version disorder which should help you remember that it involves a **C**linically unexplained **A**bnormality specifically involving the **N**ervous system that is sometimes, but not always, brought on by a stressful **T**rigger. The CAN'T will help you remember as well that these patients aren't faking it: they genuinely *can't* do the things they say they can't, even in the absence of observable evidence.

Conversion disorder involves **clinically unexplained neurologic signs or symptoms** that are often, but not always, brought on by a **stressful event**.

CAN'T-version disorder:
Clinically unexplained
Abnormality
Neurologic
Trigger (sometimes)
(Can't = genuinely unable)

Conversion disorder has a **decent prognosis**, although it does vary depending on the presentation. Cases of conversion disorder that involve the absence of function have a better prognosis than those that involve the presence of dysfunction. The majority of cases resolve by the time of discharge from the hospital, although around 25% relapse within a year. Treatment consists of educating the patient and their family about the nature of conversion disorder. When doing so, it is important not to "confront" the patient or in any way imply that they are lying or not trying hard enough, as this can be counterproductive. Instead, emphasize that a lack of objective medical lab or imaging results is *good news*, and be optimistic that their condition will improve with time. In some cases, **physical and/or occupational therapy** has been shown to improve functional outcomes. It's worth pointing out that typical treatments for somatization, such as CBT and antidepressants, are not helpful here (underscoring the idea that conversion disorder is closer to *dissociation* than it is to *somatization*, despite being listed in the same DSM chapter as other somatoform disorders).

As with all somatoform disorders, don't allow a diagnosis of conversion disorder to lead you into a premature sense of closure! Studies on conversion disorder have revealed that a medical or neurologic cause is ultimately found in up to 30% of all cases, so always keep your mind open to alternative explanations.

FACTITIOUS DISORDER

Unlike somatic symptom disorder and conversion disorder (in which the unexplained symptoms are genuinely experienced by the patient), in factitious disorder the medically unexplained symptoms are intentionally feigned or exaggerated. Why would someone fake being sick? In cases of the factitious disorder, the goal is **primary gain**, a term used to refer to all of the intangible benefits associated with being sick such as sympathy and nurturance. For example, someone with factitious disorder may complain of severe abdominal pain that they aren't actually experiencing in order to be admitted to the hospital and receive medical attention. In some cases, people with factitious disorder will even permit significant disfigurement and disability (such as undergoing multiple surgeries) because they desire to remain in the "sick role" over and above preserving their own bodily integrity. Frequent visits to the hospital can also result in a financial toll, as can overuse of medical treatments.

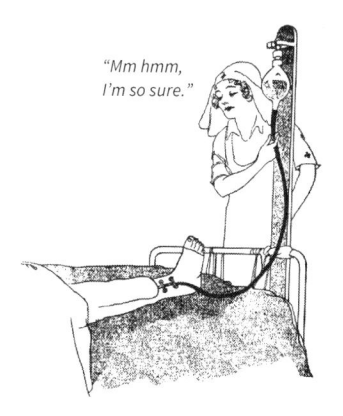

In extreme cases, people with factitious disorder may even intentionally harm themselves to provide evidence that they are truly sick. For example, someone in the hospital *claiming* symptoms of an infection may begin injecting feces into their bloodstream to *actually* give themselves an infection. This is known as **Munchausen syndrome** (or "factitious disorder imposed on self" in the DSM-5). At other times, someone may harm their children or other dependents for similar purposes, as they strongly desire the sympathy and attention that accompanies having a sick child. This is known as **Munchausen syndrome by proxy** (or "factitious disorder imposed on another" in the DSM-5) and is one of the **deadliest forms of child abuse** that exists. As in other cases of abuse, immediate steps to protect the child should be taken once a diagnosis is suspected.

It's difficult to study factitious disorder directly because a true diagnosis requires clear evidence (whether by verbal admission or directly witnessed injurious behavior) that the patient is intentionally fabricating their symptoms, which cannot always be found. Nevertheless, some patterns of epidemiology and prognosis have been found. People who engage in factitious behavior are more often **female** (with a gender ratio of 2 to 1) and typically in their 30s. Interestingly, more than 50% of people with factitious disorder **work in a medical field** (with nursing being the most common occupation), suggesting that exposure to the dynamics of the sick role plays a part in the development of the disorder. Cases of factitious disorder are usually diagnosed based upon an unsubstantiated presentation, although other patterns (including a pattern of excessive healthcare utilization, atypical symptoms, recurrent failure of medical treatments, and questionable behaviors) can provide clues as well.

Factitious disorder is a syndrome with a relatively **poor prognosis**, in large part because people with factitious disorder tend to have many other mental disorders as well (predominantly personality, trauma-related, mood, and anxiety disorders). The presence of suicidal thoughts or a history of suicide attempts in people with factitious disorder is high (around 15%), placing it on par with the mood disorders. Treatment for factitious disorder is difficult, as **neither medications nor psychotherapy** have been shown to be effective in any large study. In addition, it is unclear whether confronting the patient about known or suspected factitious behavior is helpful or harmful, as studies have shown no difference between confrontational and non-confrontational approaches. Nevertheless, it seems reasonable to try to approach patients with factitious disorder from the perspective of trying to create a safe and therapeutic relationship while acknowledging that allowing the patient to continue their unsafe behavior is likely to result in harm.

MALINGERING

Like factitious disorder, malingering involves the *intentional* production or exaggeration of medical or psychiatric symptoms. However, malingering differs from factitious disorder in the reasons for producing the symptoms. In contrast to factitious disorder (where the main draw is all the benefits *intrinsic* to being in the sick role), in malingering the goal is **secondary gain** or an *extrinsic* benefit that someone is getting from the sick role, including obtaining disability payments, an excuse from work or military service, a lighter sentence in a criminal case, financial compensation for a fake injury, or admission to a hospital with its associated food and shelter. It's important to note that malingering does not always involve complete fabrication of symptoms. Often, at least some of the symptoms do exist but are significantly played up or exaggerated (known as **partial malingering**). For example, someone involved in a workplace accident may indeed have back pain related to the injury; however, if they intentionally exaggerate their back pain and say that it prevents them from moving at all (when they are actually able to move), this would be partial malingering.

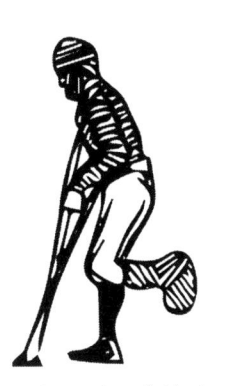

Malingering is *not* considered to be a mental disorder, as people will exaggerate, fabricate, or lie for various reasons (not all of them related to mental health). For this reason, there are **no clear patterns of epidemiology, prognosis, or treatment** associated with malingering. Several tests have also been developed to help identify malingering such as the Structured Inventory of Malingered Symptomatology (SIMS), although these are used more often in forensic settings than clinical ones.

To distinguish between **MAL**ingering and **FAC**titious disorder, look at the pattern of behavior once the patient's need has been met. Someone who is **M**alingering **A**lways **L**eaves once their need has been met (for example, if disability payments have been approved) because there is no longer a reason for them to seek medical care. In contrast, someone with **F**actitious disorder **A**lways **C**omes back for more treatment because their primary motivation is in the medical care itself.

> **Factitious disorder** and **malingering** both involve **intentional production** of medically unexplained symptoms but differ in regards to the **reason why**.
>
> *Malingering **A**lways **L**eaves once their need has been met whereas*
> *Factitious disorder **A**lways **C**omes back for more.*

DIFFERENTIAL DIAGNOSIS OF SOMATOFORM DISORDERS

By their very nature, somatoform disorders are highly liable to misdiagnosis. The best defense against misdiagnosis is for healthcare providers to have a firm grasp of the disorders that they are treating so they can quickly recognize when a pattern is (or isn't) typical. For example, a neurologist should know the features that are commonly associated with a generalized tonic-clonic seizure (such as biting the inside of the mouth, urinary incontinence, the presence of automatisms during the seizure, and a distinct postictal period) and use this knowledge to be able to pick up on cases where enough atypical features (such as seizures involving side-to-side head movements, closing of the eyes, or a duration of more than 2 minutes) are present to suggest a somatoform diagnosis.

While we have largely talked about somatization in terms of bodily symptoms, some of the conditions we have mentioned can involve psychiatric symptoms as well (such as someone who feigns hearing voices in an attempt to be admitted to the psychiatric hospital). As with any specialty, the key to picking up on these cases remains a solid foundation of knowledge about each of the syndromes that we treat (such as being able to assess auditory hallucinations using the **Vague AWD LIARS** mnemonic from Chapter 7).

While misdiagnoses are the biggest problem surrounding somatoform disorders, missed diagnoses are a very real issue as well. In fact, one study found that 99% of all people diagnosed with a somatoform disorder had at least one additional psychiatric diagnosis, with over 90% having depression and 60% having a personality disorder. Be mindful not to prematurely conclude that someone with a somatoform disorder does not have other types of pathology that you could potentially help with.

NORMALCY
Like all psychiatric disorders, somatization exists on a spectrum. Everyone has experienced medically unexplained symptoms from time to time, and many people have intentionally produced or exaggerated symptoms at least once in their life so they could stay in bed all day eating saltine crackers and chicken soup. However,

consistent with the idea that *at extremes the quantitative becomes qualitative*, some people have such severe or recurrent somatization that it leaves no doubt that there is a disorder. One notable case of factitious disorder reported in the literature involved a single patient who underwent more than 40 surgical procedures over the course of 850 admissions at 650 different hospitals, leading to disability and disfigurement but (amazingly!) not death. While the line between normalcy and somatization is never clear, look for **clear evidence of dysfunction** to make this distinction.

TRAUMA
Somatoform disorders are often found in people with a history of trauma. A diagnosis of PTSD also appears to increase the risk for developing a somatoform disorder even after controlling for comorbidities such as depression and anxiety. In fact, of all the psychiatric disorders, PTSD is perhaps the one with the strongest relationship to somatization and medically unexplained pain. Always remain vigilant to assess for histories of abuse so you can provide meaningful interventions (such as referring someone to trauma-focused CBT or dialectical behavior therapy when appropriate).

DEPRESSION
The majority of people who experience persistent somatization are either currently depressed or have been at some point in their lives. However, this "depression" more closely resembles the **chronic dysphoria** found in borderline personality disorder (as discussed in Chapter 15) than episodic major depressive disorder, resulting in higher rates of treatment failure. On a clinical level, it may make sense to generally consider depressive symptoms in somatoform disorders to represent chronic dysphoria (rather than "textbook" major depressive disorder) unless it becomes evident that there is a clear episodic pattern to the mood states.

PSYCHOSIS
Due to stigma, many people (including medical professionals) tend to take psychosis more seriously than disorders like depression or anxiety. This makes schizophrenia an attractive condition to be feigned, and the data suggest that it is one of the most commonly malingered mental disorders. Schizophrenia can be distinguished from malingering or factitious disorder through a good understanding of its typical phenomenology. In particular, people with schizophrenia have a **tendency to hide their symptoms** whereas people who are feigning psychosis want to make sure that you are aware of their symptoms.

OBSESSIVE-COMPULSIVE DISORDERS
The DSM chapter on somatoform disorders previously included hypochondriasis, as it seemed logical that a disorder based on an excessive fear of illness would be closely related to other conditions involving concern about somatic symptoms. However, this resemblance is only superficial, and the phenomenology of hypochondriasis (involving obsessional and intrusive thoughts about having an illness) as well as its treatment requirements more closely resembles an obsessive-compulsive disorder. For this reason, distinguishing between somatization and hypochondriasis is crucial. In somatization, the focus is on the *symptoms themselves* along with anxiety about what these symptoms might represent ("*Why* do I feel tired all the time?"). In contrast,

hypochondriasis is characterized by the **obsessive belief** that one *has* a disorder even when presented with conflicting evidence ("Feeling tired all the time is a sure sign that I have a colon cancer! I don't care what the colonoscopy report says!"). While there is some overlap between the two (including abnormalities in the anterior cingulate cortex), they should ultimately be conceptualized as separate conditions.

DEMENTIA
While it's rare for someone to feign dementia *per se*, evaluating memory impairments following an injury is a common task in certain settings (such as when doing disability evaluations). People who are feigning memory deficits are likely to overplay their hand by reporting symptoms that are **vastly in excess** of what people with genuine disability report. For example, many people will have *some* memory deficits following a car crash (such as being unable to remember new items on a shopping list). However, someone trying to feign memory deficits may say that the car crash caused *complete and total amnesia* to the point where they forget their own name and are unable to recognize family and friends, a level of disability that isn't seen even in severe injuries. As with many somatoform disorders, try to put on your detective hat whenever a patient eagerly volunteers a number of disabling symptoms during an evaluation.

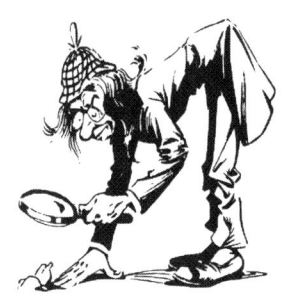

PUTTING IT ALL TOGETHER

Somatization is a complex phenomenon involving multiple biological, psychological, and social factors that result in someone having a greater sensitivity to pain and other bodily signals which manifests clinically as medically unexplained symptoms. While these symptoms must be present for a somatoform disorder to be diagnosed, the symptoms must also be accompanied by maladaptive patterns of thought, feeling, and behavior as well.

When evaluating someone with medically unexplained symptoms, it is not a priority to give an *exact* diagnosis based on strict adherence to diagnostic criteria. In fact, studies done on somatoform disorders have found that the vast majority of people who have medically unexplained symptoms do not meet criteria for a specific disorder in the DSM chapter on somatic symptom and related disorders. Instead, it may be more helpful to think of these separate diagnostic categories as **descriptions of behavior** with an **assumption about cause**.

In many cases, your ability to know the "why" is (at best) a wild stab in the dark. Nobody can read minds, so providing an explanation for someone's behavior is always going to be an inexact science. For this reason, somatoform disorders can (and very often do) overlap. For example, someone may have a history of epileptic seizures (a genuine medical condition) but then have an increase in both epileptic and non-epileptic seizures following a traumatic incident (conversion disorder). Due to the worsening of their condition, they end up spending more time in the hospital and find that they have learned to appreciate being cared for by the doctors and staff in the hospital (which could lead to factitious disorder), especially as it provides them with some time away from their dysfunctional family. In addition, they are in the process of applying for disability so that they do not have to return to their stressful job and believe that they cannot stop having seizures if they are to be successful in this (which could lead to malingering). To accomplish this goal, they have been purposefully vomiting up their antiepileptic medications in an attempt to lower their seizure threshold (which now adds the diagnosis of Munchausen syndrome). This is just one example, but it illustrates how fluid the diagnostic boundaries between somatoform disorders are and how many people will not fit neatly into one category or another.

Treatment of patients with somatoform disorders can be difficult, especially considering that patients are rarely motivated to engage in treatment. Nevertheless, you can use the mnemonic **I Do CARE** to remember the specific steps you can take to avoid causing unnecessary iatrogenic harm and to maximize your patient's chances of recovery and wellness.

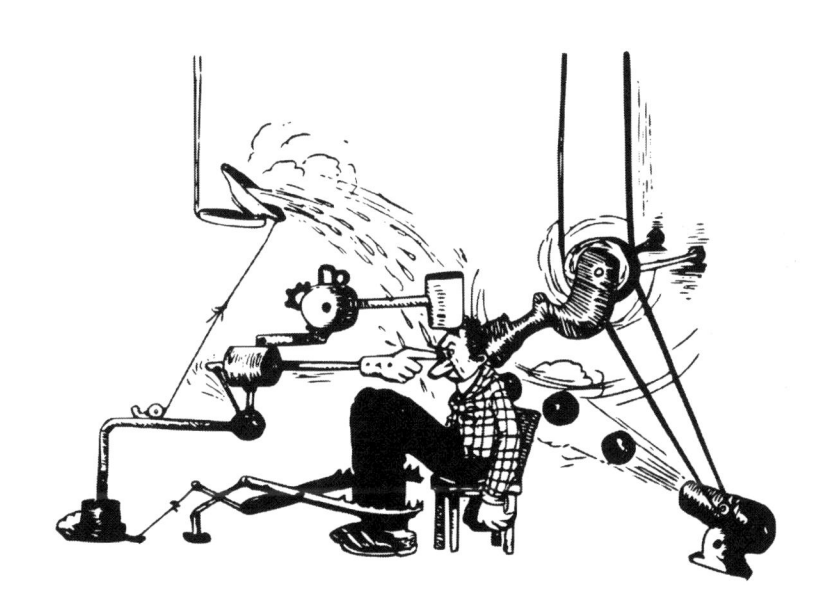

REVIEW QUESTIONS

1. A 38 y/o F comes to see her primary care doctor complaining of "constant watery diarrhea" for the past 3 days. She is concerned that she has a "stomach flu" and desires a colonoscopy. Vital signs (including orthostatics) and physical exam are both completely normal. She was seen last week by the same doctor for a headache and the week before for a "sharp stabbing pain" in her lower abdomen. She has been diagnosed with fibromyalgia, irritable bowel syndrome, and chronic fatigue syndrome. These complaints have resulted in multiple referrals to specialists; however, all work-ups have returned without significant findings. The staff at the clinic are frustrated when they see her name on the schedule because they feel powerless to help her. Which of the following brain regions is most likely involved in overinterpreting bodily sensations as being symptoms of an illness?
    A. The ventral tegmental area
    B. The insula
    C. The anterior cingulate cortex
    D. The orbitofrontal cortex
    E. The hypothalamus

2. (Continued from previous question.) Which of the following interventions is *least* likely to be effective at reducing the level of distress related to her symptoms?
    A. Initiating a work-up for diarrhea including a colonoscopy
    B. Referring to a therapist who specializes in CBT
    C. Scheduling regular visits
    D. Prescribing an antidepressant
    E. All of the above are likely to be effective

3. A 41 y/o M sees his primary care provider complaining of a persistent headache. He is concerned that this headache is a sign of a brain tumor. Family history is notable for a father who died from glioblastoma multiforme at the age of 66. A full physical and neurologic exam are normal, as is a complete set of blood tests. He has undergone both a CT scan and an MRI within the past 3 months, neither of which showed any signs of pathology. As soon as the doctor walks into the room, he says, "I know the CT and MRI are normal. You've told me before. But I think we're missing something! We only did a standard MRI. I've been reading about perfusion MRI and MR spectroscopy which are supposed to be more accurate than standard MRIs. Do you think we could do that next?" The doctor reviews his chart and sees that he has been to multiple healthcare providers in the area over the past 2 years with similar concerns despite over a dozen negative head scans and one brain biopsy. What is the most likely diagnosis at this time?
    A. Glioblastoma multiforme
    B. Somatic symptom disorder
    C. Conversion disorder
    D. Factitious disorder
    E. Malingering
    F. None of the above

4. A 4 m/o girl is brought to the emergency department by her mother. The mother says that the girl has had "rectal bleeding" for the past two days and provides several diapers from her bag that contain streaks of blood. The girl is admitted to the hospital and undergoes several diagnostic procedures including a physical exam, a complete set of blood tests, and endoscopic examination under general anesthesia. None of these studies reveal any abnormalities, and a plan is made to discharge the patient for outpatient follow-up. After being told of this plan, the mother becomes incredibly angry and yells, "How dare you try to kick my kid out of the hospital! She's bleeding and she's going to die! You don't care about anyone except yourselves. This is malpractice. I'm going to report you to the medical board." Intimidated, the pediatrician agrees to keep the girl in the hospital for further testing. That night, a nurse walks in on the mother making a cut on her thigh and using her finger to insert the blood into the infant's rectum. What is the best next step?
   A. Avoid a confrontational approach and continue the hospitalization
   B. Discharge the patient from the hospital to return home with her mother
   C. Contact social and legal services
   D. Consult psychiatry to evaluate the mother
   E. Prescribe an antidepressant to the mother

1. **The best answer is C.** While the insula is involved in the process of interoception (or the ability to sense one's internal bodily state), it is not directly involved in interpreting these sensations as being representative of a serious medical condition (answer B). Instead, the anterior cingulate cortex appears to be the region of the brain that is most implicated in overinterpreting bodily sensations as medical symptoms. While abnormalities in the hypothalamic–pituitary–adrenal axis have been observed for people who experience frequent or severe somatization, this region does not appear to be directly responsible for overinterpretation of symptoms (answer E). The ventral tegmental area is involved in addictive disorders (answer A), while the orbitofrontal cortex is involved in mood disorders (answer D).

2. **The best answer is A.** Repeated work-ups for somatoform symptoms are unlikely to relieve the distress associated with the symptoms and may put the patient at greater risk of iatrogenic harm. For this reason, medical work-ups should generally be avoided when there is a clear pattern of somatoform complaints and no evidence of abnormalities (such as vital sign instability or other concerning findings). All of the other answer choices have been shown to be at least partially effective for reducing somatoform symptoms.

3. **The best answer is F.** This patient is likely suffering from hypochondriasis which is an obsessive-compulsive disorder characterized by excessive alarm about medical symptoms that results in a conviction that they either have a serious illness or will acquire one soon. It differs from somatic symptom disorder in that the concern is not about the symptoms themselves but rather an obsessional belief that they have a disorder even in the face of evidence to the contrary (answer B). The lack of any specific neurologic deficits rules out conversion disorder (answer C). It is possible that the patient is feigning this illness either for primary or secondary gain; however, there is no evidence of this, and his insistent belief that he has a medical disease (as opposed to seeking the attention or benefits associated with the sick role) argues more strongly in favor of hypochondriasis (answers D and E). Finally, the negative work-up thus far argues against a diagnosis of a brain tumor (answer A).

4. **The best answer is C.** This is an example of Munchausen syndrome by proxy. As with any form of child abuse, the immediate priority is to ensure that the child is safe. Therefore, either continuing hospitalization (answer A) or discharging the patient to stay with the mother (answer B) would both be inappropriate, as either option leaves the girl in the care of her mother. Instead, social and legal services should be contacted immediately to ensure that the girl is safe. While people with Munchausen syndrome by proxy often have comorbid psychiatric conditions that may warrant evaluation and treatment, this is not the priority right now (answers D and E).

14 PERSONALITY

Personality is defined as a **consistent and enduring pattern of behavior, thought, and emotion** that a person demonstrates throughout their life. While there is often considerable stability in these patterns, most people also show a certain degree of range and flexibility when interacting with the world. For some people, however, this pattern of interacting with the world has become **inflexible and maladaptive**, resulting in distress, disability, and dysfunction. These people are said to have **personality disorders**. Personality disorders are incredibly complex. More than any of the conditions that we have discussed so far, personality disorders exist on a continuum with normalcy without a clear line demarcating what is "abnormal." In addition, most personality disorders involve multiple domains of mental health that often overlap with or are easily mistaken for other syndromes. For example, borderline personality disorder involves persistent feelings of emptiness and dysphoria (which can resemble depression), extreme swings of emotion (which can resemble mania), stress-induced paranoia (which can resemble psychosis), frequent worrying (which can resemble anxiety), impulsivity (which can lead to addiction), a history of trauma (which can overlap with PTSD), and so on. Because personality disorders lie at the boundary not only of normalcy but also of nearly every other psychiatric syndrome as well, they are among the **most frequently misdiagnosed** forms of mental pathology. Therefore, a thorough understanding of personality disorders (and their associated personality traits) will improve your diagnostic skills in every area of psychiatry and enable you to provide help to some of your most troubled patients.

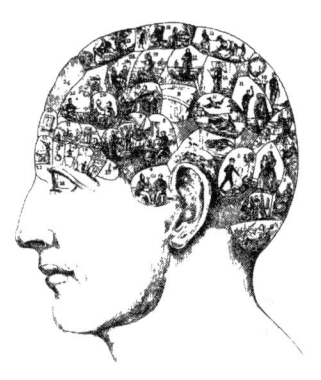

PERSONALITY TRAITS

To recognize what happens when personality becomes disordered, we must first have an understanding of what is meant by "normal" personality. There have been many attempts to describe patterns of personality going back thousands of years. The majority of schemes have attempted to divide people into distinct **personality types**. For example, the Greek physician Hippocrates tried to describe personality in terms of four "humors," including sanguine (social, extroverted, and fun-loving), choleric (hot-tempered, quick-thinking, and strong-willed), melancholic (artistic, introverted, and private), and phlegmatic (calm, easy-going, and conflict-averse). More recent personality typing schemes, including the well-known Myers–Briggs Type Indicator, similarly attempt to group people into distinct categories.

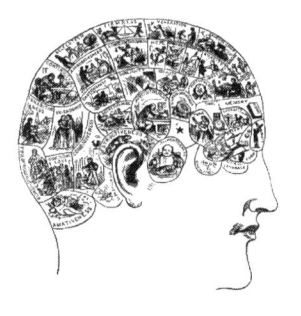

However, personality is best viewed through the lens of **personality traits** rather than types. This is because personality characteristics (like basically everything else in psychiatry) are not binary but rather exist on a spectrum. While *qualitative* personality types may do a good job of explaining the extremes of personality, they do a poor job of capturing the majority of people who are somewhere in the middle. For these people, more *quantitative* personality traits (which better capture the nuances seen in real life) are preferred. For example, someone who is extremely withdrawn socially and prefers to spend most of their time alone could be called "an introvert" while someone else who is more outgoing and tends to be the life of the party could be called "an extrovert." However, most people fall somewhere in between by spending some of their time with others and some time alone. For these people, dimensional descriptions of personality do a much better job than discrete categories.

There are five core personality traits (known as **the Big Five personality traits**, the **five factor model**, or the **OCEAN model**) that have been shown to be **both reliable and valid**. They are remarkably stable over time, staying consistent from childhood through adulthood and even into old age. In addition, someone's self-assessment of their scores on these traits generally agrees with ratings by significant others, family, and friends. These traits have each been observed in different cultures across the world, suggesting that they reflect patterns inherent to humanity and not just one particular society. These traits can be represented by the acronym **OCEAN**:

O is for Openness to experience. People who rate highly on measures of openness to experience are generally **imaginative** and tend to be interested in **novelty**, whether that involves the arts, travel, or innovative ideas. Conversely, those who score low on this trait tend to be more conventional in their outlook, valuing perseverance and pragmatism than novelty.

C is for Conscientiousness. Conscientiousness is the tendency to act in accordance with both **personal and societal expectations**, including following rules, working to meet goals, and keeping things orderly. People who are highly conscientious tend towards **planned behaviors** (though they perhaps risk being overly rigid) while those who are less conscientious are more often spontaneous and free-spirited (though they may risk being impulsive or unreliable).

E is for Extroversion. Extroversion refers to a tendency to engage with one's external environment and, in particular, with **other people**. It exists on a continuum with introversion, or a tendency to focus on one's inner mental and emotional state. At its core, extroversion means that you *gain* mental energy from interacting with others, while introversion means that being with others *depletes* your mental energy. Because of this, extroverts tend to spend more time with others while introverts need some time away from others to "recharge." That doesn't mean that introverts don't like being around other people! They do, but they tend to prefer a few deep relationships over having many acquaintances.

A is for Agreeableness. Agreeableness refers to the priority that one places on **getting along** with other people. Those with high agreeableness tend to place others' interests ahead of their own and are seen as helpful, kind, and trustworthy (though they may be more prone to peer pressure and groupthink as a result). In contrast, those who score low on agreeableness tend to be less willing to expend effort to help others and may view other people's motives with skepticism or suspiciousness.

N is for Neuroticism. Finally, neuroticism refers to the tendency to **experience negative emotions** such as anger, sadness, and anxiety over positive emotions such as happiness, joy, and contentment. People with high neuroticism tend to spend more time focusing on negative stimuli in the present, thinking of mistakes from the past, and worrying about bad things happening in the future. Because of this, people with high neuroticism are much more vulnerable to disorders like depression. On the other hand, those who score low on neuroticism are less emotionally reactive and tend to become upset less often. It's important to note that low neuroticism does *not* mean a perpetually positive mood! Rather, it implies *freedom* from persistent *negative* moods.

From a clinical perspective, assessing the Big Five personality traits is not a standard part of the psychiatric interview. However, when there is a need for additional diagnostic clarity, formal personality assessments can be done as part of a more thorough evaluation known as **neuropsychological testing**. While personality testing isn't done for every patient, having an understanding of these personality traits can still help to provide a better perspective on your patient.

The **five factor model** is a **reliable and valid** model of **personality traits** that has been validated in multiple societies and cultures.

OCEAN:
Openness to experience
Conscientiousness
Extroversion
Agreeableness
Neuroticism

SIGNS AND SYMPTOMS OF PERSONALITY DISORDERS

Personality disorders are a **heterogeneous group** of conditions that are almost more different than they are alike. Because personality disorders differ significantly from one to the next, we will wait until we discuss each personality disorder individually to talk about the specific signs and symptoms associated with each. For now, we will focus primarily on the core features shared by *all* personality disorders. To remember these characteristics, think of an **OCEAN** that has been disrupted by a violent **TIDE**. This will remind you that a personality disorder is defined by one or more **T**raits that are **I**nflexible, **D**isabling, and **E**xtreme. Like the 3 Reapers of addiction, you need all three to make a disorder!

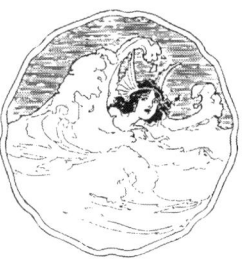

No personality traits are inherently "good" or "bad." As we will see soon, any personality trait can become dysfunctional when taken to an **extreme** degree. Even traits that appear generally positive on the surface (such as conscientiousness or agreeableness) can lead to severe dysfunction when taken to an extreme.

The problems associated with extremely high or low personality traits become compounded when the trait is **inflexible**. Most people have personality traits that, while generally consistent, are malleable depending on the situation. For example, someone who is spontaneous and free-spirited may bring joy to their group of friends with their exciting and fast-paced lifestyle. However, they still need to be able to reign in their impulsive side in situations where this is necessary, such as being at work or giving testimony in a court case. In contrast, if this person had a maladaptively inflexible level of impulsivity, they would be spontaneous and careless in all areas of their life, which could make it difficult for them to maintain relationships or hold a job.

The extreme and inflexible nature of the traits seen in personality disorders are not only **distressing** to the individual but also aggravating to the people around them, resulting in significant social and occupational **dysfunction**. Because these traits are a core part of one's personality (they are ego-*syntonic*), patients rarely seek medical attention saying, "There's something wrong with my personality." Rather, most people with personality disorders come in reporting depression, anxiety, or stress due the *effects* of their personality (such as conflicts at work or a lack of close friends due to an inability to hold relationships).

Disordered personality traits are those that are **inflexible, extreme,** and **disabling**.

TIDE: Traits that are Inflexible, Disabling, and Extreme.

PERSONALITY DISORDERS ACROSS THE LIFESPAN

EPIDEMIOLOGY
Personality disorders are **common**, with a relatively high base rate in the population around 10 or 15%. However, in certain settings the prevalence is even higher, with up to 25% of people in primary care clinics and up to 50% of those in outpatient psychiatric settings meeting criteria for a personality disorder. Personality disorders as a whole are also found with roughly the same frequency in both **men and women**, although the gender ratio varies significantly from one personality disorder to another (such as narcissistic personality disorder being more common in men while histrionic personality disorder is more common in women).

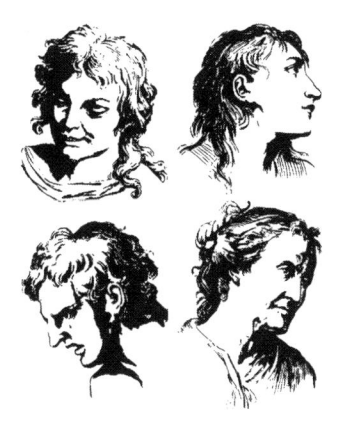

PROGNOSIS
As with all things related to personality, the dysfunction seen in personality disorders is **chronic and enduring** (rather than transient or episodic). The characteristic patterns of disordered personality tend to develop **early in life**, with most people showing signs by their teenage years if not earlier. Without treatment, personality disorders tend to persist, although for some personality disorders (particularly those in cluster B) there is a natural leveling off of symptom severity that occurs as one enters later adulthood and old age.

People with personality disorders tend to have higher rates of illness, disease, and even death compared to their peers, with some estimates placing the decrease in life expectancy as high as 20 years. Like with schizophrenia, the reasons for this gap in expected lifespan are not clear, although higher rates of suicide and substance abuse, the deleterious effects of chronic stress on one's physical health, and the frequent lack of social support all likely play a role.

TREATMENT
Available evidence on effective treatment of personality disorders is severely **lacking**, as personality disorders remain one of the most understudied groups of disorders in psychiatry. The problem is compounded further by the fact that effective treatment tends to differ significantly from one personality disorder to the next. However, what evidence exists tends to suggest that personality disorders are **difficult to treat**. When treatment is used, it appears that **psychotherapy** as a whole is significantly more effective than medications and should be the primary form of treatment.

Because personality disorders are chronic and pervasive, treatment should be aimed at improving the specific aspects of the personality disorder that create the most distress and dysfunction (such as thoughts or behaviors that prevent meaningful work or social relationships from forming). If medications are used, they should generally be seen as symptomatic (rather than curative) treatments.

HOW TO DIAGNOSE PERSONALITY DISORDERS

Correctly diagnosing a personality disorder is one of the most challenging tasks in psychiatry. Many personality disorders also have aspects of both a **trait** and a **state** which strongly influence each other (for example, someone with a personality *trait* of high neuroticism is more likely to find themselves in a *state* of depression).

This complexity is compounded further by the fact that the current diagnostic scheme for personality disorders in the DSM-5 is, frankly, **kind of a mess**. The DSM does not base its diagnoses on any specific framework of personality like the OCEAN personality traits. Instead, the theoretical framework for personality disorders in the DSM is based largely on old and outdated psychological theories. Like a broken clock that happens to be right several times a day, at times the DSM's diagnostic scheme works, with some personality disorders mapping neatly onto extremes of specific traits. For other personality disorders, however, the relationship with OCEAN traits or any other validated theoretical framework is tenuous if not non-existent.

The DSM's focus on symptoms (rather than the patterns underlying those symptoms) also leads to personality disorder diagnoses that are **highly comorbid** with each other. In fact, the majority of people diagnosed with one personality disorder will meet criteria for another, with many meeting criteria for even more than that. This likely reflects a shared tendency towards extreme and inflexible personality traits rather than truly distinct pathologies (even though the DSM treats them as separate disorders). The problem of comorbidity is further compounded by the fact that personality disorders are highly comorbid with other mental disorders, including depression, bipolar disorder, anxiety disorders, addiction, PTSD, and ADHD.

To further add to the challenge, personality disorders are **highly stigmatizing**, making many clinicians reluctant to diagnose them. For a long time, it was believed that by the age of 30 one's personality had set "like plaster" and would never soften again. This made giving a patient a diagnosis of a personality disorder akin to sentencing them to a lifetime of an incurable and untreatable disease. However, recent evidence suggests that, while changes are *slower* to happen after a certain age, personality remains malleable over the entire lifespan. This means that personality disorders are no longer a "life sentence," and for certain conditions like borderline personality disorder, remission is the norm rather than the exception.

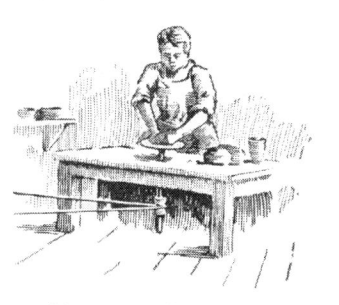

The outdated notion that personality is completely *rigid* during adulthood is often accompanied by the equally incorrect idea that personality is completely *fluid* during childhood. This idea makes some clinicians similarly reluctant to diagnose personality disorders before the age of 18, as they want to avoid diagnosing such a "permanent and unchanging disorder" at a time when personality is thought to be entirely malleable. However, we now know that just as personality isn't completely "hard" in adulthood, it also isn't completely "soft" in childhood. While it is important to allow for variations in personality during childhood and adolescence, it does a disservice to our patients to ignore clear signs of a personality disorder (which would generally begin in childhood and adolescence) when they are present.

Finally, many clinicians avoid diagnosing personality disorders because people with personality disorders can be **difficult to work with**. It is challenging for clinicians to set aside their own feelings when working with patients who are often perceived as being extremely self-centered (narcissistic personality disorder), manipulative (antisocial personality disorder), rigid (obsessive-compulsive personality disorder), or clingy (dependent personality disorder). Accordingly, many clinicians prefer not to work with these patients or, if they do, to focus on specific symptoms (such as insomnia or depressed mood) that are seen as "treatable." However, this can lead to a cycle of ineffective treatment, as the presence of a comorbid personality disorder is a major risk factor for treatment failure when trying to treat other conditions. Because of this, it is helpful to conceptualize the negative feelings you may have towards a patient with a personality disorder (such as frustration, rage, or annoyance) as being a *direct result of their disorder*. If the patient is making you feel this way during a 30-minute appointment, it is likely that they are making everyone else in their life feel this way as well, leading to fractured relationships and social isolation.

Due to all of these challenges, personality disorders are often **underdiagnosed** compared to other mental disorders such as depression, bipolar disorder, and schizophrenia. While some people believe that they are doing patients a service by avoiding the potentially stigmatizing diagnosis of a personality disorder, the fact of the matter is that doing so also deprives them of the benefits of diagnosis, including providing information about their prognosis, predicting their response to treatment, allowing for referrals to evidence-based forms of therapy, and relieving distress through psychoeducation. For personality disorders in particular, a diagnosis often provides a helpful **unifying framework** for why someone is experiencing multiple different types of symptoms at once.

PERSONALITY DISORDER CLUSTERS

Traditionally, the DSM has categorized personality disorders into three distinct groups: **cluster A** (the "weird" cluster of paranoid, schizoid, and schizotypal personality disorders), **cluster B** (the "wild" cluster of borderline, antisocial, narcissistic, and histrionic personality disorders), and **cluster C** (the "worried" cluster of dependent, avoidant, and obsessive-compulsive personality disorders). It's important to note that these clusters are based more on **superficial resemblances** between the disorders than on actual shared pathological processes. For example, cluster A personality disorders are grouped together because they are most likely to resemble psychotic disorders such as schizophrenia. However, analysis of the personality traits and genetic factors related to each has shown that they all have distinct causes and etiologies despite the superficial resemblance each has to certain aspects of psychotic disorders. This is a terrible way to categorize mental pathology, and when learning about personality disorder clusters, you should not assume that these clusters reflect any sort of shared genetic, symptomatic, or prognostic factors between the disorders within them. Nevertheless, you may be asked to identify disorders from each cluster, so having a mnemonic to group them can be helpful.

You can remember the specific disorders that fall into each cluster by thinking of what happens when you invite people from each cluster to a party. Cluster A (**P**aranoid, **S**chizoid, and **S**chizotypal) will want to Pa**SS** on the invitation as people with these disorders tend to shy away from social interaction. Cluster B (**B**orderline,

Antisocial, Histrionic, and Narcissistic) will come to the party but run the risk of being **BAHN**ed from future parties for engaging in overly emotional, self-centered, manipulative, or even downright antisocial behavior. Finally, cluster C (**D**ependent, **O**bsessive-compulsive, and **A**voidant) will join, but the party will be **DOA** (Dead On Arrival) given their tendency to be highly neurotic, which will drag down the spirit of the party.

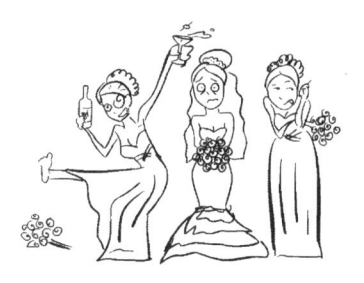

Personality disorders are grouped into **3 clusters** based on superficial similarities.

*Think of what would happen if each cluster were **invited to a party**:*
***Cluster A**: PaSS on the party (Paranoid, Schizoid, Schizotypal)*
***Cluster B**: BAHNed from the party (Borderline, Antisocial, Histrionic, Narcissistic)*
***Cluster C**: Party will be Dead On Arrival (Dependent, Obsessive-compulsive, Avoidant)*

With that framework in mind, we will now examine each of the individual personality disorders in more depth.

CLUSTER A PERSONALITY DISORDERS

Cluster A personality disorders include **paranoid**, **schizoid**, and **schizotypal** personality disorders. As you might infer from their names, these disorders have the highest chance of being misdiagnosed as **psychotic** disorders like schizophrenia due to some overlap in their symptoms (at least on a superficial level) and their tendency to cause *restrictions* in affect rather than the wild swings of emotion seen in cluster B personality disorders. In actual practice, cluster A disorders **rarely** come to clinical attention as many of the disorders have features that make people less likely to seek clinical care (such as pervasive distrust in paranoid personality disorder, a preference for being alone in schizoid personality disorder, and fear of social ostracism in schizotypal personality disorder).

PARANOID PERSONALITY DISORDER
Paranoid personality disorder is characterized by a persistent pattern of **fear, mistrust, and suspiciousness** of other people. The level of paranoia is often excessive and is directed towards most, if not all, of the people in their lives. The predominant personality trait in people with paranoid personality disorder is extremely and inflexibly **low agreeableness**. People with paranoid

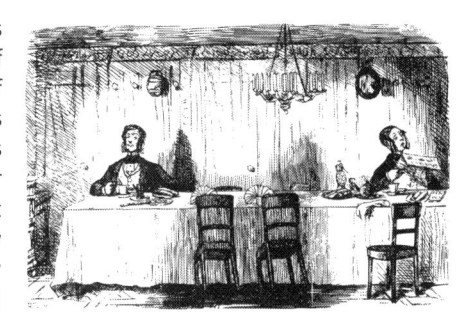

personality disorder tend to become quite socially isolated, although given that they think that everyone else is only out to get them, they say they don't mind too much (even if they also commonly report a sense of loneliness). In contrast to the paranoid delusions seen in primary psychosis, paranoid personality disorder tends not to involve a single complex delusional belief system. Instead, people with paranoid personality disorder are constantly jumping around between multiple paranoid ideas without sticking to any one belief for too long, suggesting a stable pattern of paranoia (even if the beliefs change too frequently to be considered a stable delusion).

SCHIZOID PERSONALITY DISORDER

Schizoid personality disorder is characterized by a consistent **lack of interest in social relationships**, which maps to the OCEAN trait of extremely and inflexibly **low extroversion**. People with schizoid personality disorder commonly lead solitary lives and are aloof or detached from others. Unlike in avoidant personality disorder (a cluster C personality disorder), this lack of social contact doesn't appear to bother them. This isn't to say that people with schizoid personality disorder don't get lonely—sometimes they do, but they generally find that being alone is preferable to the constant demands for connection and intimacy that others put upon them. Schizoid personality disorder is often accompanied by other symptoms, including emotional coldness, restricted affect, anhedonia, and apathy. You can remember the key pattern of schizoid personality disorder by thinking that schi**zoid** a**void**s.

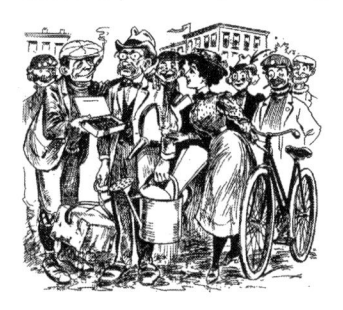

> People with **schizoid** personality disorder tend to **avoid social relationships** and do not often seek out the presence of others.
>
> *Schizoid avoids.*

SCHIZOTYPAL PERSONALITY DISORDER

Schizotypal personality disorder is defined by the presence of **odd beliefs** and **difficulty relating to other people** that strongly resembles, though is not quite as impairing as, schizophrenia. Like other cluster A personality disorders, schizotypal personality disorder tends to lead to loneliness and isolation, although in this disorder the avoidance is often out of fear that others will judge them for their odd beliefs, strange mannerisms, or unconventional manner of dress. Despite its classification in the DSM as a personality disorder, in reality schizotypal personality disorder is **not really a personality disorder**. For one, it doesn't map to extremes of any specific personality traits in the same way that paranoid and schizoid personality disorders do. In addition, studies have shown that schizotypal personality disorder is **linked to**

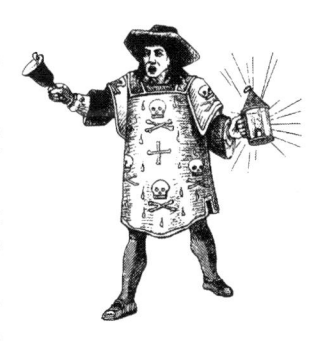

schizophrenia both phenomenologically and genetically (unlike the other cluster A disorders which have only a superficial resemblance to schizophrenia). Further reinforcing the idea of a link between those two disorders is the fact that about a third of patients with schizotypal personality disorder "progress" to a diagnosis of schizophrenia (whereas rates of progression to schizophrenia from paranoid or schizoid personality disorder are no higher than the general population). Based on these studies, it may be more accurate to think of schizotypal personality disorder as a low-grade schizophrenia that, at least in some cases, has not yet "declared itself." You can remember this by thinking that **schiz-o-typal** is a **type-o'-schizo** that has clear links to schizophrenia.

> Schizotypal personality disorder is genetically and phenomenologically **related to schizophrenia**.
>
> *Schiz-o-typal is a type-o'-schizo(phrenia).*

CLUSTER B PERSONALITY DISORDERS

Cluster B personality disorders include **borderline, antisocial, narcissistic**, and **histrionic** personality disorders. This cluster is sometimes known as the "wild" group due to the **emotional instability** associated with each. Indeed, one of the core factors linking all cluster B personality disorders together is a sense that one's emotions are unbalanced. The involvement of extreme emotional states makes these disorders commonly misdiagnosed as mood disorders like depression and bipolar disorder. However, it's important to realize that cluster B personality disorders are not defined by any particular mood *state* in the same way as depression or bipolar disorder but rather by a *tendency* towards negative emotions of all kinds (which maps to the OCEAN trait of extremely and inflexibly **high neuroticism**). This tendency manifests in chronic feelings of dissatisfaction, anger, irritability, and sadness. Accordingly, people with cluster B personality disorders often suffer from low self-esteem and an unstable sense of identity, which is less surprising when you consider that all cluster B disorders (with the exception of histrionic personality disorder) have strong statistical associations with histories of **childhood abuse or neglect**.

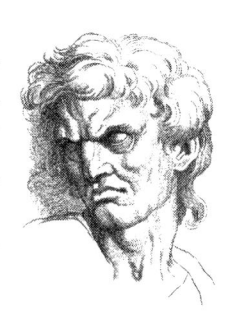

All personality disorders are not created equal, and those in cluster B deserve a greater level of attention than those in either cluster A or C as they are the group that is most likely to come to clinical attention as a **primary diagnosis** (rather than an ancillary diagnosis given by diligent clinicians taking a thorough history). Because of this, we will cover these disorders in a greater level of detail, including devoting the entirety of the next chapter to borderline personality disorder and then the following two chapters to both forms of antisocial personality disorder.

BORDERLINE PERSONALITY DISORDER

Borderline personality disorder is a syndrome of **chronic instability** in multiple areas of life, including an insecure sense of identity, chronic negative emotions, emotional instability, suicidal acts, psychotic and/or dissociative phenomena, anger, impulsivity, and unstable relationships. In many ways, it is the **prototypical cluster B personality disorder**, and learning more about this condition (as we will in the next chapter) will enable a deeper understanding of the other cluster B disorders.

ANTISOCIAL PERSONALITY DISORDER

Antisocial personality disorder is characterized by a persistent pattern of behavior that **infringes on the rights of others**, including breaking the law, deceitfulness, impulsivity, aggressiveness, disregarding the safety of others, irresponsibility, and/or lack of remorse. Viewed through the lens of the OCEAN personality traits, antisocial personality disorder is defined by a combination of both **low agreeableness** and **low conscientiousness**. As we will discover in Chapters 16 and 17, antisocial personality disorder is really two different disorders masquerading as one! Stay tuned.

NARCISSISTIC PERSONALITY DISORDER

Narcissistic personality disorder is characterized by a sense of **inflated self-importance** along with associated behaviors intended to draw attention to one's self or to make one's self appear superior to others. These behaviors are often accompanied by an **inability to empathize** with other people's feelings, leading to trampling upon the *emotions* of others (although not to the same extent as the reckless disregard for the *rights* of others seen in antisocial personality disorder).

While people with narcissistic personality disorder act or speak in a way that suggests that they see themselves as the greatest person ever, this is merely an illusion, as just below the surface lurks a pervasive **sense of insecurity** and a **debilitating fear that they are unloved**. Accordingly, people with narcissistic personality disorder often have **difficulty tolerating criticism** or not constantly being the center of attention. In this way, narcissistic personality disorder is revealed to be a maladaptive way of artificially inflating a sense of self-worth to mask an inner insecurity. It is almost twice as common in **men** as in women.

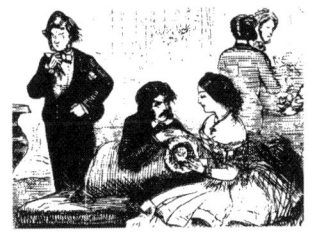

HISTRIONIC PERSONALITY DISORDER

Histrionic personality disorder is defined as a pattern of **excessive or exaggerated behaviors** intended to draw attention to one's self or to gain the approval of others. Specific behaviors include being very **dramatic, flirtatious, or sexually provocative** as a way of commanding attention. These gestures, which can come across as shallow or manipulative to people around them, appear to stem from an intense desire to be loved which is itself related to poor self-esteem and an unstable sense of self. It is four times as common in **women** as men.

If this sounds familiar after reading about narcissistic personality disorder, you are not far off! In a lot of ways, the core pattern of narcissistic personality disorder is very similar to histrionic personality disorder in that both are characterized by a sense of inner insecurity for which they engage in **compensatory behaviors to gain attention or approval**. In histrionic personality disorder this takes the form of dramatic, flirtatious, or provocative behaviors, while in narcissistic personality disorder it involves repeatedly boasting about one's accomplishments or self-worth. Based on this, some have hypothesized that histrionic personality disorder and narcissistic personality disorder are essentially **different expressions of the same core disorder**, with differences in expression largely being mediated by societal expectations for each gender (such as Western cultures finding it more acceptable for women to engage in flirtatious behaviors while men are encouraged to brag or boast).

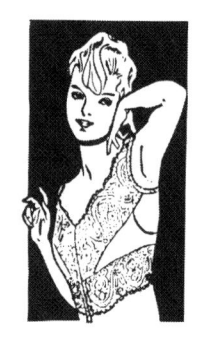

Histrionic personality disorder is the only cluster B disorder that does *not* have a clear relationship to a history of childhood abuse. It is likely that people with histrionic personality disorder share a similar *diathesis* to other cluster B disorders (including the same underlying need for approval and desire to avoid rejection) but take a different path in life due to a lack of environmental *stressors* like child abuse during development. Because of this, histrionic personality disorder lacks the anger, destructiveness, and inability to empathize seen in the other cluster B disorders. Overall, the behavior of people with histrionic personality disorder can come across as obnoxious to others, but it is seldom associated with severe impairment in the same way that the other cluster B disorders are. For this reason, histrionic personality disorder is rarely given as a primary diagnosis.

CLUSTER C PERSONALITY DISORDERS

Finally, we arrive at cluster C of the personality disorders which includes **dependent**, **obsessive-compulsive**, and **avoidant** personality disorders. If cluster A disorders resemble psychosis and cluster B disorders resemble mood states, then cluster C disorders resemble **anxiety**. Because of this, the cluster C personality disorders are sometimes called the "worried" group. However, just like in cluster A the similarities between the disorders in this group are ultimately superficial, and their inclusion together should not make you think that there is any shared genetic or phenotypic diathesis between them. In contrast to cluster B disorders (which *often* come to clinical attention) and cluster A disorders (which *rarely* come to clinical attention), cluster C disorders *sometimes* come to clinical attention.

DEPENDENT PERSONALITY DISORDER

Dependent personality disorder is characterized by an **overreliance upon other people** in multiple areas of life. People with dependent personality disorder often feel unable to live life on their own and instead rely on others for any number of things, including making decisions (both large and small), having a sense of purpose, or believing in their own self-worth. They will often be **extremely deferential** in most of their relationships in order to avoid even the slightest possibility of conflict. In the OCEAN model, dependent personality disorder is conceptualized as an extreme and inflexible trait of **high agreeableness**. While at first it may seem odd that high agreeableness could be *pathological*, in reality even agreeableness can become maladaptive when present in extreme forms, as trust becomes gullibility, cooperation becomes subservience, and thoughtfulness becomes capitulation. Treatment of dependent personality disorder is very poorly studied but should generally be focused on addressing the cognitive biases that are found in the disorder (including automatic thoughts like "I am weak and ineffectual"), addressing relationship dynamics that contribute towards this pattern, and working towards promoting independence and self-efficacy.

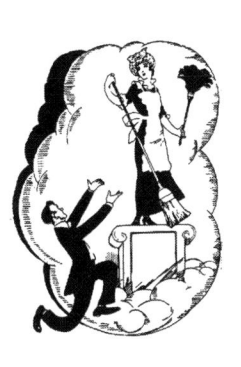

> **Dependent** personality disorder is caused by pathologically **high agreeableness**.
>
> *Think of someone who fake-laughs at all of your lame jokes (**HA-HA-HA**) to avoid conflict. This person has extremely **H**igh **A**greeableness.*

OBSESSIVE-COMPULSIVE PERSONALITY DISORDER

Obsessive-compulsive personality disorder (OCPD) is characterized by **emotional and behavioral rigidity**, resulting in a need for things to be controlled and orderly at all times. Viewed through the lens of the OCEAN personality traits, this involves an extreme and inflexible trait of **high conscientiousness** with a side of **low openness to new experiences**. This combination of traits manifests itself in an overreliance on structure (such as rigidly adhering to a checklist to complete a task without ever questioning if the task needs to be done in the first place).

Despite having "obsessive-compulsive" in the name, this disorder does *not* involve either obsessions or compulsions as they were defined in Chapter 10. Instead, the rigid and repetitive tasks that people with this disorder engage in are distinctly **ego-syntonic**. People with obsessive-compulsive personality disorder truly feel that the way they are doing things is the "right" or "correct" way to do them. (In contrast, people with OCD have ego-*dystonic* rituals that tend to cause feelings of *distress* rather than satisfaction.) In this way, obsessive-compulsive personality disorder more closely resembles anorexia nervosa (which we will discuss more in Chapter 18), and some studies have found that over 50% of people with anorexia meet criteria for this disorder. Don't let yourself get confused: OCD and obsessive-compulsive personality disorder are not the same thing, as obsessive-compulsive personality disorder does not feature either obsessions or compulsions!

> **Obsessive-compulsive personality** involves **emotional and behavioral rigidity** related to **high conscientiousness and low openness to experience**.
>
> *OCPD = **O**verly **C**onscientious **P**ersonality **D**isorder.*

AVOIDANT PERSONALITY DISORDER

Like schiz*oid* personality disorder, people with avoidant personality disorder are characterized by their **chronic avoidance** of other people. However, what sets them apart is that people with avoidant personality disorder still desire human contact whereas in schizoid personality disorder the interest is not even there in the first place. What holds people with avoidant personality disorder back from seeking companionship is a severe and crippling sense of **self-doubt and inadequacy** which is often related to extreme sensitivity to rejection.

Like schizo*typal* personality disorder, avoidant personality disorder is **not really a personality disorder**. For one, it does not map clearly to extremes of any particular personality traits. More telling, however, is the fact that the diagnosis is **redundant**, as the core symptoms of the disorder are almost exactly the same as those of social anxiety disorder. In fact, studies have suggested that comorbidity between social anxiety disorder and avoidant personality disorder is over 90% (and may even reach 100%). Shared genetic vulnerabilities between the two disorders as well as significant overlap in treatment (SRIs and CBT) further support the hypothesis that avoidant personality disorder is best conceptualized as a **severe and chronic form of social anxiety disorder** rather than as a personality disorder.

DIFFERENTIAL DIAGNOSIS OF PERSONALITY DISORDERS

Personality disorders involve patterns that **resemble nearly every other mental disorder**. This makes them among the most chronically misdiagnosed disorders in all of psychiatry. However, this also means that if you have a good grasp of personality disorders, your diagnostic abilities in nearly every area of psychiatry will improve. Because of this, pay careful attention to personality disorders when learning about the differential diagnosis of each major class of mental disorders.

NORMALCY

All personality traits exist on a spectrum with normalcy, so normalcy should always be on the differential when evaluating for a personality disorder. The key is to avoid fixating on the *presence* of any specific personality traits and instead focus on the *process* by which those traits manifest (such as being particularly extreme or inflexible). Indeed, even supposedly "good" personality traits like agreeableness and conscientiousness can go awry when present to a severe degree (as in dependent and obsessive-compulsive personality disorders, respectively). Use the presence of **clear dysfunction** as a benchmark to determine whether personality pathology is actually present, and avoid using any of these diagnoses pejoratively to refer to people whose personalities you might find distasteful but are not actually dysfunctional.

DEPRESSION AND MANIA

Mood disorders are most often confused for cluster B personality disorders due to the involvement of emotional extremes. However, many people with cluster A or C personality disorders also experience depression as a result of the impairment present in their conditions (including social isolation or chronic worry). Mood disorders can easily be differentiated from personality disorders in that they are **episodic** rather than chronic. In addition, affect in personality disorders is often **reactive** to external events (versus being non-reactive in depression or mania). Finally, it's wise to be cautious with diagnosing narcissistic personality disorder when someone is in an acute mania episode. While the grandiosity seen during a manic episode can resemble narcissism, these characteristics will go away once the episode resolves.

PSYCHOSIS
While it makes sense that cluster A personality disorders would easily be confused for psychotic disorders, it is not uncommon for cluster B personality disorders to be confused as well. The aggressive behavior seen in antisocial personality disorder can at times be mistaken for the agitated or paranoid states seen in schizophrenia, while the dissociative and paranoid symptoms of borderline personality disorder can resemble psychosis as well. The lack of other symptoms of psychosis (such as thought disorganization or negative symptoms) can help to clarify, as can the *increased* range of affect seen in cluster B personality disorders (compared to the *restricted* range seen in schizophrenia).

ANXIETY
The personality disorders in cluster C are most often confused for anxiety disorders, though anxiousness and worry are also found frequently in cluster B as well given their general tendency towards negative emotions. Therefore, careful assessments for symptoms of anxiety is warranted in most people who have a personality disorder.

OBSESSIVE-COMPULSIVE DISORDERS
As discussed previously, obsessive-compulsive personality disorder should be carefully distinguished from OCD and its related disorders, as they differ significantly in phenomenology, prognosis, and treatment response despite having a similar name. Determining whether rigid behavior (which is seen in both conditions) results from ego-*syntonic* or ego-*dystonic* thoughts can be illuminating (with the former being seen in obsessive-compulsive personality disorder and the latter being seen in OCD).

TRAUMA
A history of trauma is associated with most personality disorders, although the presence of extended abuse or neglect (especially in early childhood) is most strongly associated with cluster B personality disorders. For this reason, keep personality disorders on the differential when evaluating someone with a trauma history or other related conditions such as dissociation or somatization.

ATTENTION DEFICIT HYPERACTIVITY DISORDER
Cluster B personality disorders share a high degree of impulsivity with ADHD, making it easy to confuse them. Diagnostically, the boundaries between the two disorders are not entirely clear, and rates of comorbidity are high. In general, you should avoid giving a comorbid diagnosis of ADHD unless there is clear evidence that the dysfunction started in childhood, and a diagnosis of a personality disorder should be avoided in someone who is merely impulsive unless the other signs and symptoms characteristic of personality pathology are present.

ADDICTION
Most personality disorders are associated with higher rates of substance use, so keep this on your differential to avoid addiction becoming a "missed diagnosis" that is interfering with effective treatment.

EATING DISORDERS
Both of the major forms of eating disorders (anorexia nervosa and bulimia nervosa) are linked to specific personality disorders. Anorexia shares phenomenological and genetic links to obsessive-compulsive personality disorder, while bulimia is associated with cluster B personality disorders in the majority of cases.

PUTTING IT ALL TOGETHER
Personality disorders are one of the most challenging groups of disorders to study. No other chapter of the DSM attempts to lump so many disparate and unrelated conditions into a single category. Even past attempts to draw some connections between the disorders (including the "cluster" system used by the DSM) seem to introduce more problems than they solve. The best unifying framework appears to be the **OCEAN model** of personality traits which provides an explanatory framework for some personality disorders such as low agreeableness in paranoid personality disorder or high agreeableness in dependent personality disorder. However, this model doesn't capture every personality disorder, such as schizotypal or avoidant personality disorder which instead appear to be related to other existing psychiatric conditions (schizophrenia and social anxiety disorder, respectively).

Because of the high variability between each personality disorder, it hasn't been possible to delve deeply into each condition the same way we have with the other disorders we have discussed so far (though we will examine borderline and antisocial personality disorder in this level of detail in the next few chapters). However, there is some comfort in knowing that with most personality disorders it is not so important that you remember each and every individual symptom of the disorder. You'll notice that there aren't a lot of mnemonics in the style of SIGECAPS or DIG FAST in this chapter, and that is because using a "cookbook" approach for personality disorders is largely a waste of time. Rather, focus on the underlying *process* of **extreme, inflexible, and disabling personality traits** seen in each disorder, and the other pieces will fall into place.

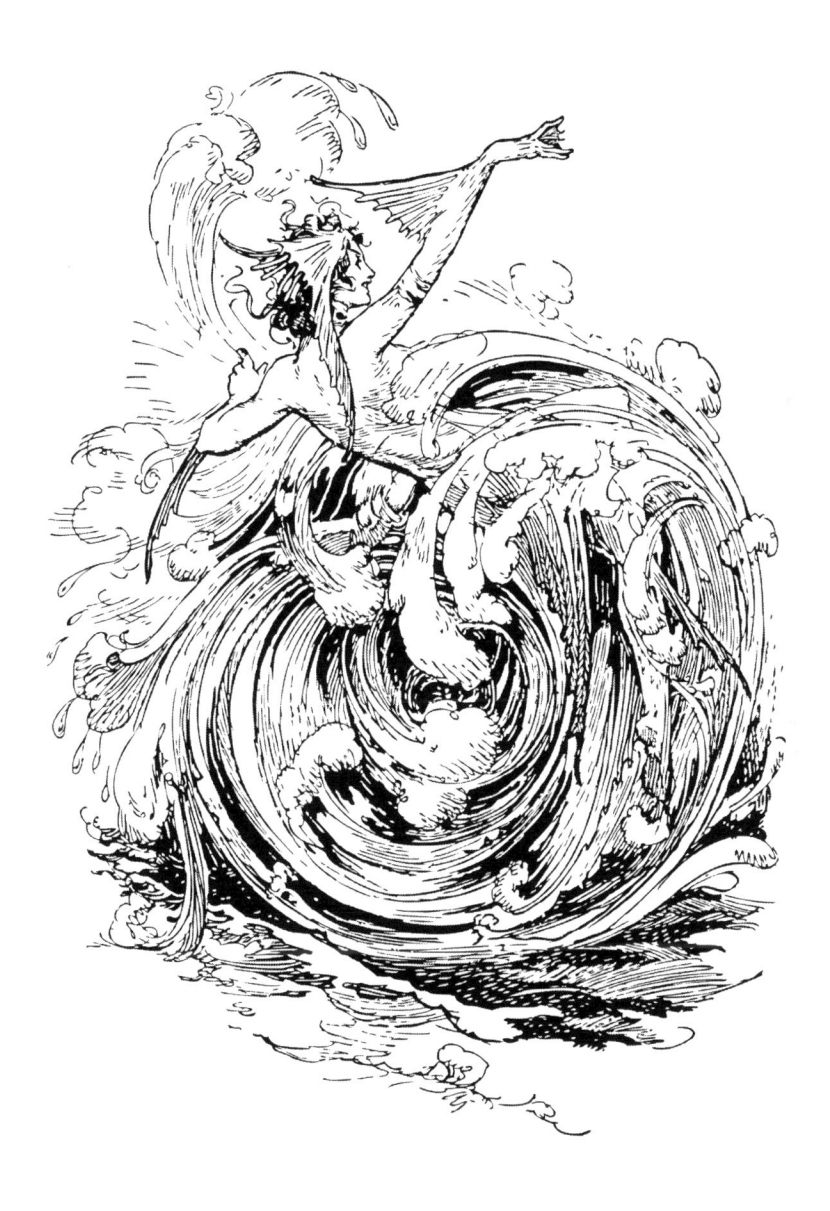

REVIEW QUESTIONS

1. A 45 y/o M comes to see a psychotherapist specializing in relationship issues. He tells the therapist at the beginning of the appointment, "I've read a lot about you and believe that you are the most qualified person to help me right now." He works as an entrepreneur and has been very successful in various aspects of his life, including winning several marathons in the past few years. He is financially well-off and is able to afford the $500 hourly rate that the therapist charges. He describes himself as an "incredibly competent" person who has "many, many friends" ("If you can't tell already, people like to be around me!"). His company is "one of the best, I'm sure you've heard of it. We're constantly making headlines." His primary concern right now is his relationship with his wife whom he says "doesn't appreciate me for who I am." They have been married for 12 years. Early in their relationship, his wife was "very subservient and demure," but recently she has begun "talking back to me and belittling me all the time" which infuriates him. They have not had sex in over 3 years, and he has had "literally dozens" of sexual partners over this time period without his wife's knowledge or consent. He describes his wife's current behavior as being similar to his mother who was frequently critical of him throughout his childhood. He asks the therapist, "I feel like I can do better than my wife. I am used to having the best at work. Why can't I have the best in my marriage?" As the 90-minute time slot is running out, the therapist attempts to interject and bring the session to a close; however, the patient continually interrupts, leading to the session running 30 minutes over and making the therapist late for his next session. As the therapist is ending the session, he asks the patient to bring in his wife to the next appointment. The patient replies by saying, "Why? Don't you trust what I am telling you? If you can't take me at face value, then you're not the therapist I thought you were, and I will be going elsewhere." The therapist watches the patient leave the office and return to his car to discover a parking ticket on the window. He immediately rips it up and throws it on the ground. As he backs his sports car out of the parking spot, he hits another car's bumper and leaves a dent; however, he then drives off without getting out to inspect the damage or leaving a note. Which of the following statements is most likely to be true of this patient's case?
    A. He is likely to meet criteria for more than one personality disorder
    B. He was almost certainly abused as a child
    C. His company is unlikely to be as successful as he claims
    D. His wife likely believes that their relationship is "fine"
    E. None of the above statements are likely to be true

2. (Continued from previous question.) Which of the following would most argue for a diagnosis of bipolar disorder in this case?
    A. Being arrested for a hit-and-run
    B. Going from laughing one minute to crying the next
    C. A history of having seen a therapist for a year in high school
    D. Coming in 3 months later with none of the same signs
    E. Reporting current symptoms of depression

3. A 38 y/o F presents to her therapist complaining of "stress" and a desire to "fix my husband." She is a stay-at-home mother and says that she tries to be the "best mom I can be for my kids." She spends several hours a day researching the nutritional information for all food she packages for her children and ensures that the meals not only follow the age-specific recommended ratios for fat, carbohydrates, and protein but also are arranged in a variety of shapes. She sometimes stays up until 2:00 or 3:00 in the morning working on making sure that each lunch is perfect, saying, "It's how I show my love to my children." Despite her children's requests, she does not permit them to eat candy or dessert at any time, saying, "That stuff is grade A garbage." In regards to her husband, she says that "he needs help" as he has called off work three times over the past year "when he's not even sick!" She has extensively researched this behavior online and has concluded that he is "a malingerer" and that he "needs to seek psychiatric help but won't do it, so I'm coming in on his behalf." When asked, she says that neither she nor her husband have taken a vacation since they had children 10 years ago, as "it's best for children to be raised in a consistent environment." She says, "Sometimes I feel like I'm the only one holding this ship afloat, and if I stop for even one second then everything will fall apart." She describes constant muscle tension and says that she often feels like yelling at other people, although she will only yell at her husband because "he made a vow saying that I could." She denies that she needs psychiatric help of any kind, saying, "I told you, there's nothing wrong with me. I'm just here on behalf of my husband who is too lazy to help himself." Which of the following quotes from the vignette most argues for a diagnosis of obsessive-compulsive personality disorder over an anxiety or obsessive-compulsive disorder?
    A. "Sometimes I feel like I'm the only one holding this ship afloat, and if I stop for even one second then everything will fall apart."
    B. "[Candy and desserts are] grade A garbage."
    C. "[Making perfect lunches] is how I show my love to my children."
    D. "I told you, there's nothing wrong with me. I'm just here on behalf of my husband who is too lazy to help himself."
    E. "It's best for children to be raised in a consistent environment."

4. Which of the following personality disorders is *incorrectly* paired with its corresponding personality trait?
    A. Dependent personality disorder – High agreeableness
    B. Avoidant personality disorder – Low extroversion
    C. Borderline personality disorder – High neuroticism
    D. Paranoid personality disorder – Low agreeableness
    E. Histrionic personality disorder – High extroversion
    F. All of the above are correctly paired

1. **The best answer is A.** This patient shows signs of narcissistic personality disorder including excessive self-praise, grandiose statements, and interpersonal exploitation. People with one personality disorder often meet criteria for another, and narcissistic personality disorder is no exception. While a history of child abuse is more common in cluster B disorders, it is by no means almost certain (answer B). In addition, while many people with narcissistic personality disorder will exaggerate their claims, the disorder does not preclude them from being highly successful, and it should not be assumed that he is making up or embellishing the success of his company (answer C). People with narcissistic personality disorder often have dysfunctional interpersonal relationships, and it is likely that his wife believes there is a problem in their relationship, possibly even mores than the patient does (answer D).

2. **The best answer is D.** Narcissistic personality disorder can occasionally be confused for bipolar disorder, as some of the same signs can be found in both. However, the key is to look at the timing of the signs and symptoms as these will be enduring in narcissistic personality disorder but episodic in bipolar disorder. Therefore, for the patient to return in 3 months with none of the same symptoms would strongly suggest bipolar disorder. Reckless behavior (answer A), onset of symptoms during adolescence (answer C), and comorbid depressive symptoms (answer E) can all be found across both disorders, while affective lability is more characteristic of cluster B personality disorders than bipolar disorder (answer B).

3. **The best answer is D.** This patient is likely suffering from obsessive-compulsive personality disorder as evidenced by her high degree of conscientiousness in combination with her rigid and controlling behavior. Obsessive-compulsive personality disorder is notably ego-syntonic, so her continued insistence that there is nothing wrong with her is most consistent with this diagnosis. Feeling like the only person holding everything together can be seen in cases of obsessive-compulsive personality disorder but can also be found in anxiety disorders as well (answer A). Inflexibility in choosing food for others can sometimes be found in anorexia nervosa, which is frequently comorbid with obsessive-compulsive personality disorder; however, it is not inherently suggestive of the disorder (answer B). Neither showing love for children through spending extra effort on making school lunches nor wanting children to be raised in a consistent environment are inherently pathological, and neither argue for a diagnosis of obsessive-compulsive personality disorder (answers C and E); however, in the context of inflexible and rigid behavior (such as staying up late each night making the lunches or desiring consistency to the extent that the children are never exposed to new experiences such as a vacation) these can be signs of pathology.

4. **The best answer is B.** Avoidant personality disorder does not map neatly to an extreme or inflexible personality trait and is best conceptualized as a severe manifestation of social anxiety disorder. Instead, low extroversion is most characteristic of schizoid personality disorder. All of the other personality disorders are correctly paired with their corresponding traits.

15 BORDERLINE

Borderline personality disorder is a complex syndrome of specific signs, symptoms, and behaviors that result in **chronic instability** in multiple parts of one's life, including **emotions**, **identity**, and **relationships**. In many ways, it can be seen as the **prototypical cluster B personality disorder**, and you may often hear the term "cluster B" used synonymously with borderline personality disorder, as the **persistent and enduring** forms of dysfunction seen in this condition epitomize the difficulties faced by people with other cluster B diagnoses like narcissistic or histrionic personality disorder.

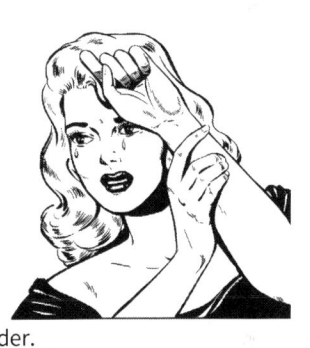

Borderline personality disorder is among the most challenging conditions in all of psychiatry, both in terms of diagnosis and treatment. The signs and symptoms of the disorder cover a vast array of symptoms and can easily be confused for just about every other psychiatric diagnosis, making it the **great imitator of mental health**. In addition, working with people who have borderline personality disorder can be emotionally demanding, as the core features of the disorder (such as hostility, destructiveness, and impulsivity) can make maintaining a therapeutic relationship a major challenge. However, it is helpful to keep in mind that these difficulties in the patient-provider relationship are a core feature of the disorder itself. Just as it would be ludicrous to give up on working with a person who has schizophrenia because they "kept hearing voices," so too is it ridiculous for clinicians to avoid patients with borderline personality disorder because of their persistent difficulties in interpersonal relationships. At the end of the day, people with this condition deserve the same level of compassionate and evidence-based care as anyone else despite the challenges that the disorder presents. To help prepare you as much as possible to approach this condition with clarity and compassion, we will spend quite some time understanding borderline personality disorder.

SIGNS AND SYMPTOMS OF BORDERLINE PERSONALITY

The range of signs and symptoms that are associated with borderline personality disorder is vast. In fact, the word "borderline" was initially linked to this syndrome because it was considered to be at the "border" between psychotic disorders like schizophrenia and neurotic disorders such as depression by encompassing aspects of each. Because of this, the signs and symptoms of borderline personality disorder can seem overwhelming at first compared to the other disorders we have studied so far.

The DSM boils these signs and symptoms down into 9 key criteria that can be encapsulated in the mnemonic **I DESPAIR**. We'll go over each of these domains one by one. These symptom domains are highly interrelated, and we will make frequent references between them as we go through each one.

I is for Identity. People with borderline personality disorder often have an unstable identity that manifests as an **inconsistent sense of self and purpose**. While everyone has aspects of their personality that change depending on the time and circumstances, most people are able to see these seemingly contradictory states as still being rooted in the same core identity. In contrast, people with borderline personality disorder have difficulty seeing themselves as the same consistent person throughout their lives. Instead, their sense of identity may change entirely depending on whom they are around, such as appearing to like particular hobbies when they are with one group of friends but then showing no interest in those same activities on their own. This manifests in a lack of long-term goals which leads to an agonizing sense of purposelessness or "drifting" over time known as **painful incoherence**. This symptom is similar in nature to, if not the same thing as, the feelings of depersonalization and fragmentation of identity seen in dissociative states which explains the strong association between dissociative disorders and borderline personality disorder.

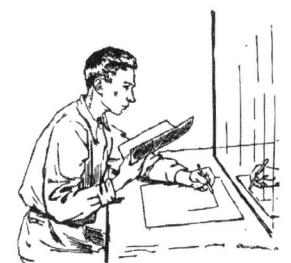

D is for Dysphoria. Dysphoria is a pattern of **experiencing primarily negative emotions** that results in a sensation of profound internal pain or emotional aching. It is found in basically all people with borderline personality disorder, with some studies estimating a frequency of nearly 100%. Chronic dysphoria is often described as persistent feelings of depression, anxiety, or emptiness. This sensation is typically accompanied by a sense of boredom, apathy, despair, anhedonia, and alienation ("I feel like I don't belong anywhere on the earth"). Dysphoria differs from depression and dysthymia in that it is a **reactive state** whereas depression and dysthymia are generally non-reactive to circumstances. Dysphoria is often **quite stable** and is found across the lifespan (in contrast to other symptoms of borderline personality disorder, such as impulsivity and self-harm, that tend to "burn out" as time goes on). Because of this, chronic dysphoria can be seen as an enduring hallmark of the disorder, making it a sensitive marker of the diagnosis.

E is for Emotional instability. The emotional state of individuals with borderline personality disorder is characterized by sudden and drastic swings between extremes of emotion known as **affective lability**. People with borderline personality disorder can easily "fly off the handle" and quickly go from laughing to crying to yelling to pacing and then back to laughing again. These shifts tend to happen within **seconds or minutes**, which helps to differentiate them from the mood changes in depression and mania which occur over weeks or months.

People with borderline personality disorder also **feel emotions very strongly** and have been said to experience "grief instead of sadness, humiliation instead of embarrassment, rage instead of annoyance, and panic instead of nervousness." (This is not to suggest that people with borderline personality disorder cannot experience positive emotions as well—they absolutely do and will feel those just as strongly, such as elation instead of happiness or pride instead of contentment.) Changes in affect are often **precipitated by interpersonal events**, either positive (such as being thrown a surprise birthday party) or negative (like being stood up for a date). These emotional responses can often come across as wildly out of proportion to the actual events that prompted them, at least to an outside observer. For this reason, living with affective lability can be disorienting not only for the person experiencing these emotional shifts but also for those around them, leading to unstable relationships.

S is for Suicide and self-harm. People with borderline personality disorder often engage in self-harm, with **non-suicidal self-injury** (such as repeatedly making shallow cuts on one's skin with no clear intention of wanting to die) being common. The question of why people with borderline personality disorder hurt themselves can seem like a difficult one to answer. After all, it seems counterintuitive that anyone would intentionally behave in a way that would cause pain. Research suggests that people with the disorder self-inflict *physical* pain as a way of managing *psychological* pain. For some patients with borderline personality disorder, cutting appears to *relieve* suffering rather than exacerbate it. Interestingly, rates of cutting correlate strongly with the tendency to dissociate, suggesting that self-injurious behavior may allow someone to mentally distance themselves from emotional pain. While self-harm is neither perfectly sensitive nor specific for borderline personality disorder, a history of non-suicidal self-harm should put this disorder high on your differential.

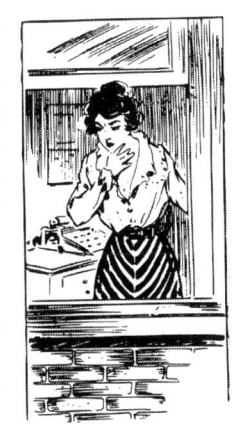

In addition to *non*-suicidal self-injury, people with borderline personality disorder also experience frequent **suicidal thoughts, intentions, or attempts** (such as overdosing on medications). In fact, it is estimated that the majority of patients presenting to emergency departments with recurrent suicidality have borderline personality disorder. In contrast to the *episodic* suicidality seen in mood disorders, most people with borderline personality disorder are **chronically suicidal**. This makes the decision to hospitalize someone more difficult than with depression or bipolar disorder, as suicidality in borderline personality disorder tends to be more of a *constant* rather than a modifiable risk factor.

P is for Psychosis-like and dissociative symptoms. Up to half of all people with borderline personality disorder will experience symptoms that appear psychotic in nature at some point in their lives, including auditory hallucinations, paranoia, and delusions. However, while these symptoms superficially resemble those seen in schizophrenia, they do not fit the phenomenology of primary psychosis. For example, people with borderline personality disorder who experience auditory hallucinations will say that the voices are *inside* their heads or that they are vague. The psychosis-like symptoms experienced by people with borderline personality disorder are often *transient* and tend to occur primarily in **times of severe interpersonal stress**, and when the stress decreases (often in several hours or days), the symptoms will remit as well. Paranoid ideation does not typically involve complex delusional belief systems as in schizophrenia but rather is related to extreme interpersonal sensitivity ("I think my classmates are spying on me just to laugh at what a failure I am"). Dissociative experiences including all of the signs and symptoms from the **DDREAMS** mnemonic are common as well, with many patients with borderline personality disorder showing high levels of dissociative traits.

A is for Anger. Anger, antagonism, and hostility are hallmark emotions of borderline personality disorder. People with borderline personality disorder have a strong tendency towards negative emotions which makes anger and irritability among the most common emotions experienced by people with the disorder on a daily basis ("I hate you! I wish you had never come into my life, you asshole!"). However, it's also important to point out that not all people with borderline personality disorder show overt or obvious expressions of anger and hostility. While some people with the condition frequently yell or engage in aggressive behavior, "quiet borderlines" instead hold these emotions inside and do not express them, though they will still report having frequent angry thoughts when asked.

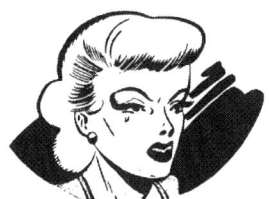

I is for Impulsivity. Emotions drive behavior, so it is no surprise that someone with extreme and erratic emotions would also engage in extreme and erratic behavior. People with borderline personality disorder have a tendency to **act quickly without fully considering the consequences** of their actions, leading to substance abuse, unsafe sex, reckless driving, job loss, running away from home, lashing out at others, and self-harm. While some of the behaviors that patients with borderline personality disorder engage in involve pleasure (such as drugs or sex), there is often an element of compulsivity as well, as many of these actions help to temporarily relieve the chronic state of dysphoria. This is manifested in a high degree of **negative urgency** which is a measure of how quickly someone feels that they must act when they experience negative emotions, such as cutting to relieve distress. However, the repercussions of impulsive behaviors often end up exacerbating the underlying dysphoria even further, leading to a vicious cycle. Impulsivity is frequently seen in teenagers and young adults with borderline personality disorder but tends to "burn out" as people get older, so the absence of impulsivity should not rule out this diagnosis.

R is for Relationships. Relationships are difficult for people with borderline personality disorder. They often show a pattern of **short-lived and unstable relationships** with most or all of the people in their lives. Difficulty in relationships involves not only romantic relationships but also other types as well, including family, friends, and co-workers. There are several patterns that help to explain why people with borderline personality disorder tend to have unstable relationships. For one, like in other cluster B disorders people with borderline personality disorder are extraordinarily **sensitive to interpersonal rejection**. While being rejected, dumped, or abandoned doesn't feel good for anyone, people with borderline personality disorder often react to these circumstances in an extreme way and may lash out with angry or violent behavior by threatening suicide, engaging in self-harm, or asking to be hospitalized in order to feel safe. Because being rejected is such an aversive feeling for people with borderline personality disorder, they will often engage in frantic **efforts to avoid abandonment** ("If you leave me, I will take this knife and kill myself!"). Much of the interpersonal rejection sensitivity that people with borderline personality disorder experience is likely related to a fundamental **intolerance of being alone**, as these individuals often rely upon others to feel a sense of identity and to lessen feelings of chronic dysphoria. Relationships for people with borderline personality disorder are also complicated by their tendency to see the world in extreme or black-and-white terms, known as **splitting**. Friends, relatives, and healthcare providers interacting with people with borderline personality disorder often find themselves on one side or the other of a split: they are either "the best person ever" or "the cruelest person ever to walk the face of the earth." This overall pattern of unstable relationships involving extremes of idealization and devaluation is both **highly sensitive and highly specific** for the disorder, with a sensitivity of 75% and a specificity over 85%. (For clarity, it's worth pointing out that the DSM splits relationship difficulties into two separate criteria: unstable and intense relationships characterized by splitting and frantic efforts to avoid real or imagined abandonment. As these two domains are so closely related, we will consider them as a single symptom domain.)

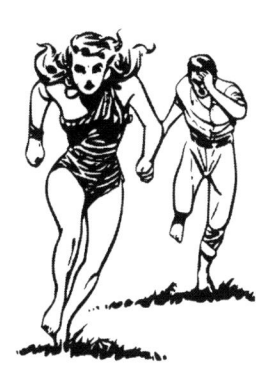

Borderline personality disorder is characterized by **chronic instability** in the domains of **mood, affect, behavior, relationships**, and **identity**.

I DESPAIR:
Identity disturbance
Dysphoria
Emotional instability
Suicide and self-harm
Psychosis-like and dissociative
Anger
Impulsivity
Relationships

BORDERLINE PERSONALITY ACROSS THE LIFESPAN

While all personality disorders require an understanding of the illness across the lifespan, borderline personality disorder is significantly more complicated because its symptoms can present clinically not only as a *trait* but also as a *state*. For example, you may see someone coming into the hospital in a *state* of extreme distress after cutting themselves following a break-up. However, if you saw them several months later, these state-specific behaviors would not necessarily be present. At that time, they may instead present with feelings of emptiness and dysphoria (the chronic *traits* of the disorder). Perhaps the best analogy with another condition can be drawn with schizophrenia, which is similarly characterized by **chronic deficits with occasional exacerbations**. Also like schizophrenia, the most well-known symptoms of borderline personality disorder (including impulsivity, hostility, and dramatic suicidal gestures) are very *specific* for the disorder but tend to be present primarily in the early stages of life such as adolescence or young adulthood. In contrast, the chronic and enduring features of the syndrome are often present throughout life and are associated with significant and lasting dysfunction, making them *sensitive* markers of borderline personality disorder no matter what stage of the disorder the patient is in (similar to negative symptoms in schizophrenia).

EPIDEMIOLOGY

Borderline personality disorder is **common**, with up to 10% of the population showing signs and symptoms that are severe enough to cause dysfunction. In clinical settings, borderline personality disorder is significantly more common and may account for up to one-third of all patients in any given general psychiatry clinic. This prevalence gives it a **high base rate** and makes it liable to **underdiagnosis** rather than overdiagnosis.

Borderline personality disorder is historically associated with women, and in clinical settings it tends to be diagnosed in women three times as often as men. However, research suggests that when structured evaluations are used, borderline personality disorder is found **equally in men and women**. The historical association of borderline personality disorder with women appears to be related to the fact that women are more likely to seek medical and psychiatric care in general, leading to higher rates of *clinical* diagnosis. However, when men have borderline personality disorder, they are more likely to come to attention for substance abuse or reckless behavior which are more often treated in *legal* settings. There is also reason to believe that the diagnostic criteria for borderline personality disorder themselves may be biased towards a greater rate of diagnosis in women, with nearly all features of the disorder (with the exception of anger and hostility) being seen as more common in women than men. Because of this, the patient's gender should *not* play a large role in evaluating the likelihood of a diagnosis of borderline personality disorder despite the long-standing and outdated associations with women.

Like other personality disorders, signs and symptoms of borderline personality disorder most often **begin in adolescence** (although onset either earlier in childhood or later in young adulthood is not uncommon). It is a common misconception that you cannot diagnose borderline personality disorder in patients under the age of 18. This is entirely untrue! The only caveat to diagnosing borderline personality disorder in children and adolescents is that the dysfunction must be **persistent** (typically at least one year or more) to reflect the more malleable nature of personality in youth.

PROGNOSIS

Conventional wisdom has long held that borderline personality disorder is a chronic and unchanging diagnosis. This makes clinicians quite reluctant to diagnose it, as it was felt that assigning the diagnosis would "doom" the patient to a lifetime of misery and distress. However, systematic studies that have followed people with borderline personality disorder over decades have revealed that the condition is not persistent and unchanging. In fact, 50% of people who initially meet criteria for the diagnosis no longer do by 2 years, with 85% being in remission by 10 years (even without treatment!). The fact that **the majority of people enter remission** from the disorder strongly argues against the idea that it is an unchangeable condition.

Looking more closely at the data, however, it appears that *complete* remission from symptoms is quite rare. The more intense and dramatic symptoms (including impulsivity, self-harm, and overt hostility) tend to remit, but others (such as affective lability, dysphoria, difficult relationships, and issues with self-image) remain. Because of this, even if most patients no longer *technically* meet DSM criteria for borderline personality disorder, this does not mean that they are completely "free" from the disorder, a fact which is reflected in lower than average rates of employment and life satisfaction even after remission. While the prognosis for borderline personality disorder is not as bad as it was once thought to be, there is often some level of **persistent dysfunction** even after active symptoms have disappeared.

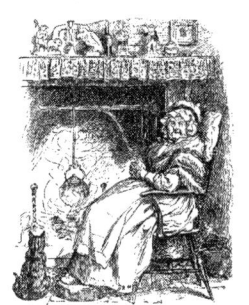

TREATMENT

Borderline personality disorder is a **treatable condition**, with psychotherapy being by far the most effective modality of treatment. Studies have shown that specific forms of psychotherapy that are geared towards patients with borderline personality disorder appear to be the most helpful. The most well-studied of these is **dialectical behavior therapy** (DBT) which teaches specific skills including **mindfulness**, **distress tolerance**, **emotion regulation**, and **interpersonal effectiveness** each of which is targeted towards specific things that patients with borderline personality disorder tend to struggle with. Dialectical behavior therapy has been shown to improve patient outcomes by decreasing rates of self-harm, suicide attempts, and hospitalizations.

While dialectical behavior therapy is the most famous treatment for borderline personality disorder, other forms of therapy (such as mentalization-based treatment) have been shown to work as well. In general, patients with borderline personality disorder should be encouraged to engage in dialectical behavior therapy or another evidence-based form of psychotherapy if possible!

> A variety of **evidence-based treatments for borderline personality disorder** exist, with **dialectical behavior therapy** (DBT) being the most well-studied.
>
> ***DBT = De-Borderline Therapy.***

While specialized forms of treatment like dialectical behavior therapy can be incredibly helpful, the downside of these treatments is that they tend to be costly and time-consuming, often requiring one to two years in specialized treatment before meaningful and sustained effects are observed. In addition, many patients are unable to access these treatments due to lack of insurance coverage, long waiting lists, or geographic distance from the treatment centers, leading to the vast majority of people with borderline personality disorder being seen in general psychiatric or medical settings. For this reason, it is it essential for *all clinicians* to be able to treat borderline personality disorder in any setting. A model of treatment known as **Good Psychiatric Management** (GPM) has been found to be just as effective as dialectical behavior therapy at improving outcomes and, importantly, can be practiced by *any* healthcare provider! The mnemonic **DELAPSE** can help you to remember the core principles of Good Psychiatric Management:

D is for Diagnose. Many providers initially try to avoid giving a diagnosis of borderline personality disorder and instead focus on specific symptoms (like depression or anxiety) that are seen as "more treatable" or "less stigmatizing." Do not give into this impulse. Telling your patient about the diagnosis and the reasons why you believe they likely have it is one of the most helpful things you can do, as it provides a **unifying framework** for the multiple concerns (like depression, difficulty holding a job, and unstable relationships) that the patient may have. It also helps both you and the patient to avoid spending years trying treatments that work for other people (such as antidepressants) but are ineffective for people with borderline personality disorder.

E is for Educate. Don't just diagnose, take time to teach as well! Educating a patient about borderline personality disorder and its relationship to extreme **interpersonal sensitivity** provides a helpful explanatory model that allows them to place their symptoms in context when they experience them. In addition, patients shown be informed about the **underlying causes** of borderline personality disorder (including its high heritability) as well as the overall **good prognosis** for the disorder. Many patients report feeling more hopeful after learning about the disorder, and education is a key component of that!

L is for Life outside of treatment. Because the effects of borderline personality disorder can often extend into every area of someone's life, you can and should provide guidance on things besides just therapy and medications. Inquire about the patient's life outside of treatment and try to enhance **social functioning** by encouraging the patient to work or volunteer in activities that they find meaningful and to develop healthy interpersonal relationships. The phrase "**work before love**" can be a helpful guiding principle, as employment tends to provide a more consistent and stabilizing structure to a patient's life than romantic relationships.

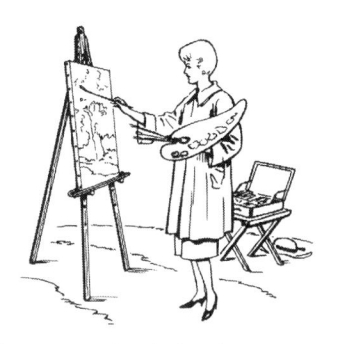

A is for Avoid medications. Medications should generally be avoided for patients with borderline personality disorder, as a higher number of medications is associated with a *lower* chance of clinical improvement. If medications must be used, they should only be for *symptomatic* treatment of specific symptoms (such as insomnia or impulsivity) rather than being seen as something that will fundamentally alter the trajectory of the condition. **Anticonvulsants** and **antipsychotics** are the most frequently used medications, with anticonvulsants helping to reduce anger and impulsivity and antipsychotics helping to alleviate paranoid or dissociative symptoms.

P is for Prioritize. The majority of people with borderline personality disorder meet criteria for multiple other conditions as well, including depression, anxiety, PTSD, and more. Because of this, it is essential to prioritize all of their conditions and triage which ones should receive treatment first. As a general rule of thumb, **treatment of borderline personality disorder should come first**. Attempting to treat other disorders (like depression) without addressing borderline personality disorder is often futile, whereas treating the personality disorder tends to improve related symptoms in and of itself! There are only a few exceptions to this rule, including active substance abuse, acute mania, and severe eating disorders (all of which would be an immediate threat to health or would interfere with the ability of the patient to engage in therapy).

S is for Safety plan. Given the high rates of suicidality, self-harm, and reckless behavior seen in borderline personality disorder, coming up with a good safety plan is essential. Determine the patient's current level of safety, then make plans for what to do if the patient develops an acute crisis, including explaining when it is (and is not) appropriate to go to the hospital or call 911.

E is for Expect change. Finally, make it clear to the patient that you are committed to helping them change whatever they are most concerned about (whether that is their mood, persistent anxiety, frequent self-harm, or repeated suicide attempts). However, it is essential to clarify each of your roles. Many providers like to view themselves as the agent of change ("*I* will be the one to fix the patient!"). However, this paradigm simply does not work for patients with borderline personality disorder. Your role instead is provide education about the disorder as well as guidance about treatment options in exchange for their commitment to working towards change.

Borderline personality disorder is treatable by all mental health providers using a Good Psychiatric Management approach.

DELAPSE:
Diagnose
Educate
Life outside of treatment
Avoid medications
Prioritize
Safety plan
Expect change

MECHANISMS OF BORDERLINE PERSONALITY

Many of the signs and symptoms of borderline personality disorder are found across other psychiatric conditions as well (including impulsivity in addiction, affective extremes in mood disorders, and a tendency towards negative emotions in anxiety). Therefore, in order to truly understand the mechanisms underlying the disorder, we need to look at the characteristics that are most *unique*. The one pattern that is most specific to borderline personality disorder and other cluster B disorders is **extreme interpersonal sensitivity**, as the symptoms of the disorder can almost always be traced back to interpersonal sensitivity (such as abrupt changes in affect often being triggered by social conflict). In addition, this pattern tends to persist throughout life (in contrast to the symptoms mentioned before that tend to "burn out" with time), suggesting that it is directly linked to the underlying pathophysiology of the disorder.

To gain a better understanding of what is meant by "extreme interpersonal sensitivity," think back to the first experience you ever had with **heartbreak**. Perhaps a cute new boy or girl joins your class after their family moves from across state. You think constantly about going up to them to say hi, but your stomach gets tied up in knots every time you do, so you hold back. Later that day during class, your eyes meet during one of your nervous glances. They smile and blush, but you aren't sure whether they are responding to your looks or are creeped out by them. Days and weeks pass. Desperate for their affection but too scared to make a move, you cozy up to their best friend in an attempt to get closer. After a while, you can't take the uncertainty anymore and you ask their friend point-blank if they like you. (And not just like but, like, *like* you.) Their friend embarrassedly looks down and says, "They actually just started dating someone else."

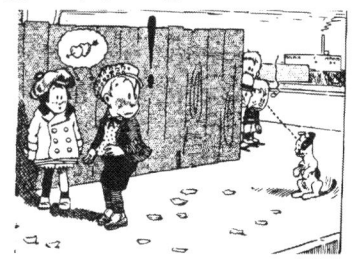

Take the emotion you were feeling at that exact moment and put it in a bottle labeled "**dysphoria**" (you can place that bottle on the same shelf as the one labeled "pro-salient state"). While most people feel this sort of dysphoria for a few days or weeks following rejection or a major break-up, this is the mental state in which people with borderline personality disorder live *chronically*. Having this dysphoric state as their baseline makes it so that when someone with borderline personality disorder experiences *further* rejection, it hurts twice as bad. This leads to levels of emotional pain and turmoil that people without the disorder will not be able to understand. It also explains why people with borderline personality disorder go to such extreme lengths to avoid abandonment or other circumstances that make them feel this way. However, to understand why the *specific* behaviors that are often seen in a "borderline crisis" (including self-harm, suicidal threats, attention-seeking, and dissociation) are used, we need to look at the underlying neurobiology of the disorder.

On a biochemical level, the **endogenous opioid system** appears to be involved in borderline personality disorder. The endogenous opioid system is responsible for releasing peptides in response to physical strain. These morphine-like substances (such as **endorphins** or "**endo**genous m**orphin**e") act as natural painkillers to help reduce the perception of pain. For example, long distance runners often report feeling the most pain at the beginning of a marathon. However, as they continue their run, endorphins and other endogenous opioids are released and result in reduced pain perception and a pleasant, almost euphoric feeling (the "runner's high"). In this way, runners are able to engage in a specific activity (exercise) that boosts signaling in the endogenous opioid system as a way of off-setting incoming pain signals.

While the link between the endogenous opioid system and *physical* pain is well-known, this system appears to play a central role in **social pain** as well. Social pain describes the aversive emotional state that someone experiences in response to rejection (such as being excluded from a group or feeling devalued by another person). It is no coincidence that the words used to describe social pain (including "broken-hearted," "burned," "slapped in the face," or "wounded") are the same used to describe physical pain in a more literal sense (a pattern that remains true across many different cultures and languages worldwide). Studies suggest that social pain causes an immediate *decrease* in the release of endogenous opioids, leading to feelings of *dys*phoria (rather than the *eu*phoria caused by the *in*crease in endogenous opioid release that occurs during a runner's high).

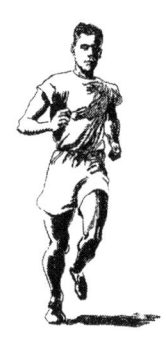

People with borderline personality disorder are believed to have an endogenous opioid system that is **chronically underperforming**, leading to feelings of chronic dysphoria and emptiness at baseline (two symptoms that are reported by almost everyone with the disorder). However, this baseline level of hypoactivation makes it so that when someone with borderline personality disorder experiences social rejection, their release of endogenous opioids plummets even *further*, prompting an immediate emotional crisis state. This explains why a "borderline crisis" is almost always precipitated by threats of social exclusion or rejection and often appear to be extremely out of proportion to the circumstances to most outside observers.

To help offset this state of endogenous opioid depletion during a crisis, people with borderline personality disorder often engage in a variety of behaviors to **stimulate release of endogenous opioids** in an attempt to restore balance and bring some relief from the intense dysphoria. These behaviors include:

Seeking comfort from others. Neuroimaging studies show that endogenous opioids are released in higher amounts during hugs, talking about your problems, or even just *thinking* about being loved and supported. For most people, this is an essential part of feeling better after social exclusion. For people with borderline personality disorder, however, this need for social connection is so extreme that it can almost resemble an addictive disorder. This explains the great lengths to which people with borderline personality disorder will go (such as making an exaggerated show of threatening to kill themselves if their partner doesn't stick around) in order to obtain this feeling from their partners, families, and friends.

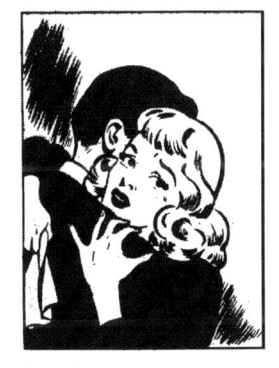

Engaging in self-harm. Non-suicidal self-injurious behavior like cutting is common in borderline personality disorder. As mentioned before, people with the disorder tend to report that it *relieves* pain rather than causes it. Neuroimaging studies have shown that self-harm induces the release of endogenous opioids in response to physical pain (similar to how the strain of running also causes endogenous opioid release). Inflicting *physical* pain upon one's self to cause the release of endogenous opioids is an effective method of relieving *social* pain, and people who self-harm often report that it makes them feel "normal" or "forget about their pain" at least for a few minutes.

Dissociating. Dissociative symptoms in people with borderline personality disorder are often immediately precipitated by traumatic events or threats of social exclusion. Interestingly, endogenous opioids appear to be involved in generating feelings of both derealization and depersonalization, as specific medications that block the opioid receptor (such as naltrexone or naloxone) have been shown to reduce dissociative symptoms in people with these disorders.

Using drugs or other substances. Perhaps the most direct way to activate one's opioid receptors is through substances like prescription painkillers, illicit opiates, or other drugs (such as alcohol) that all appear to help someone in a dysphoric state feel "normal" again. This explains the high rates of substance use and addiction in people with borderline personality disorder, as use of these drugs is not only *positively* reinforcing but also quite *negatively* reinforcing by providing immediate relief from the feelings of dysphoria and emptiness that these individuals experience chronically.

If the signs and symptoms of borderline personality disorder can be traced back to dysregulation of the endogenous opioid system, the next question then becomes, "Where does this dysregulation come from in the first place?" As with many things in psychiatry, *it's never just one thing*, and there are likely both biological and environmental factors at play. Research has shown that differences in opioid receptor activity appear to be heritable, with genetic differences appearing to correlate with specific behaviors (such as infants showing higher reward system activation during parental contact and greater distress upon separation) that mirror the interpersonal patterns seen in adults with borderline personality disorder. On the other hand, common environmental precipitants of the disorder, such as a history of trauma and abuse, may exacerbate these underlying vulnerabilities to the point where they become clinically significant. The release of endogenous opioids appears to mitigate perception of both physical and emotional pain in response to trauma. However, this is only a short-term fix, and if the pain of the trauma goes on for too long (such as under conditions of abuse and neglect), long term changes can occur in the opioid system, leading to receptors that become persistently unresponsive.

The concept of high interpersonal sensitivity and its rooting in a dysregulated endogenous opioid system explain much of what we see in borderline personality disorder, including its lasting *traits* (such as chronic dysphoria, affective instability, and sensitivity to abandonment), its crisis *states* (such as self-harm, dissociation, and attention-seeking behaviors), and its relationship to histories of chronic trauma. By tying together these seemingly disparate traits and patterns, you will be better able to recognize borderline personality characteristics when they occur in your patients.

HOW TO DIAGNOSE BORDERLINE PERSONALITY DISORDER

When diagnosing borderline personality disorder, use the mnemonic **I DESPAIR** to remember the 9 core signs and symptoms of this condition. (As mentioned before, the DSM splits **R**elationships into the two domains of "unstable relationships" and "sensitivity to abandonment" which is why there are only 8 letters in the mnemonic but 9 criteria in the DSM.) **At least 5** of these 9 criteria must be met for a diagnosis.

As a *personality* disorder, this diagnosis should not be based on a "snapshot" view of the patient's presentation at a particular moment in time but instead on the presence of **extreme and inflexible** patterns of personality across the lifespan. There should also be evidence that the dysfunctional traits are **persistent and enduring** across years or decades. (After all, almost everyone becomes "a little bit borderline" at various times in their lives, such as after experiencing social rejection.)

Borderline personality disorder **can be diagnosed in children and adolescents**. Because of what we know about the malleability of personality across the lifespan, a diagnosis of borderline personality disorder should not be avoided simply because someone is less than the age of 18 when the specific signs, symptoms, and patterns are clearly present and are not better accounted for by other explanations.

Finally, a word of caution: avoid using a diagnosis of borderline personality disorder as a shorthand for people who can come across as infuriating, manipulative, entitled, demanding, or frustrating. While these characteristics can sometimes be found in people with borderline personality disorder, they fail to differentiate patients with borderline personality disorder from people who have these characteristics for other reasons. Therefore, consider this diagnosis in people for whom these traits appear to directly stem from a pattern of *extreme interpersonal sensitivity*, but avoid adding to the stigma by using the diagnosis pejoratively.

DIFFERENTIAL DIAGNOSIS OF BORDERLINE PERSONALITY

The differential diagnosis for borderline personality disorder is **broad**. Because the disorder is pervasive and touches on every aspect of one's life, it frequently overlaps with nearly every other psychiatric syndrome, making it the "great imitator" of mental health. For that reason, consider borderline personality disorder when assessing patients, especially if there are atypical signs, symptoms, or patterns that suggest something other than the "textbook" variety of the disorder is present!

NORMALCY

The traits of borderline personality disorder are on a spectrum with normalcy, as feeling emotions strongly, valuing relationships, and having one's identity be at least partially dependent upon the people around you are not inherently negative traits. Indeed, these traits often make people with borderline personality disorder quite passionate about things or people that they love, and it is not uncommon to find people with these traits excelling in creative fields like the arts because of their greater ability to feel emotion. As it so often does, the key here involves looking at the **level of dysfunction** in someone's life that can be attributed to these traits as well as a pattern of **inflexibility** that causes these same traits to be maladaptive rather than helpful. In cases where someone has borderline traits but hasn't quite reached the point where these have caused problems, you can always recommend specific readings or techniques from dialectical behavior therapy (such as learning about emotion regulation or mindfulness) that can be helpful for just about anyone regardless of whether they technically meet criteria for the disorder or not.

DEPRESSION

Depressed mood is incredibly common in people with borderline personality disorder, and some estimates place the rate of comorbid depression at over 90%. However, it's not always clear that people with borderline personality disorder have depression in the "textbook" sense of an episodic mood disorder. Rather, in the vast majority of cases comorbid depression is more likely to be a manifestation of **chronic dysphoria** than it is a truly separate depressive disorder. This has important implications for treatment, as conventional treatments for depression (such as SRIs and CBT) are generally *not* effective at relieving depressive symptoms in people with this disorder. Therefore, avoid diagnosing a comorbid depressive disorder in someone with borderline personality disorder unless if it is clear that their particular presentation cannot be entirely explained by chronic dysphoria (such as a clear episodic pattern to symptoms with pronounced mood non-reactivity). In addition, the longstanding belief that you should not diagnose borderline personality disorder during a depressive episode does not appear to hold water, as personality assessments performed both during and after depressive episodes show considerable stability within the same person. Therefore, you should not avoid diagnosing borderline personality disorder during a depressive episode when there are highly specific and sensitive features present (such as extreme interpersonal sensitivity).

ATYPICAL DEPRESSION

Recall from Chapter 5 that interpersonal rejection sensitivity is also a core feature of atypical depression, suggesting at least some degree of diagnostic overlap. Indeed, up to half of all people with atypical depression also meet criteria for borderline personality disorder, making it unclear whether the two are separate disorders with overlapping features or just two ways of describing the same thing.

MANIA

Cases of borderline personality disorder have been misdiagnosed as bipolar disorder for as long as both disorders have been around. Much of the confusion stems from the fact that the word "bipolar" is often used to refer to someone who is **affectively labile** rather than someone who experiences long-lasting mood episodes, especially in popular media. Differentiating between borderline personality disorder and bipolar disorder should be done on the basis of their **underlying mechanisms** (such as looking for patterns of extreme interpersonal sensitivity in the former or increased goal-directed activity in the latter). In addition, the **timing** of symptoms is crucial, as affective changes occur over minutes or hours in borderline personality disorder but weeks or months in bipolar disorder (even in the rapid-cycling subtype).

PSYCHOSIS
Psychosis-like symptoms are common in borderline personality disorder and occur in up to half of all people with the diagnosis. The phenomenology of psychotic symptoms in borderline personality disorder differs significantly from schizophrenia. In addition, "micropsychotic" phenomena are often **transient** (rather than ongoing) and tend to occur primarily in times of interpersonal stress.

ADDICTION
Rates of comorbid addictions are high in patients with borderline personality disorder, with over half of patients developing a substance use disorder at some point in their lifetime. Make sure to screen patients with borderline personality disorder for the presence of comorbid addictions and to have a frank discussion about a higher risk of dependence when prescribing controlled medications like benzodiazepines.

ANXIETY
Anxiety is incredibly common and occurs in nearly 90% of those with borderline personality disorder. Social anxiety disorder is particularly common, with nearly half of all people with the disorder meeting criteria for this comorbidity (which makes sense given the interpersonal hypersensitivity that is at the core of the condition).

TRAUMA
PTSD is common in patients with borderline personality disorder, with over half meeting criteria for a diagnosis of PTSD. Other conditions related to trauma, including dissociative and somatoform disorders, are quite common as well. Despite their shared links to trauma, borderline personality disorder is not the same thing as PTSD, and there are no overlapping symptoms between the disorders (review the **TRAUMA** and **I DESPAIR** mnemonics if you need to remind yourself of this). Complex PTSD *does* have some overlapping features (unstable relationships, an unstable sense of self, and affective lability), leading to as-yet-unanswered questions about how these two disorders relate to each other.

EATING DISORDERS
Comorbidity between borderline personality disorder and eating disorders is high. **Bulimia nervosa** is much more commonly associated with borderline personality disorder compared to anorexia nervosa (which is itself more often associated with obsessive-compulsive personality disorder).

AUTISM
You may think that borderline personality disorder and autism would rarely be confused since the former is associated with *increased* affect and desire for the affection of others while the latter is characterized by *decreased* affect and a generally low desire to socialize. However, both borderline personality disorder and autism are linked by **deficits in mentalization**, or an inability to correctly determine the mental state of others. For example, people with borderline personality disorder or autism can both have difficulty correctly guessing someone's emotions based on their facial expression. However, the reasons for this differ significantly. Individuals with autism tend to *hypo*mentalize by failing to accurately read facial expressions, neglecting non-

verbal communication, and showing a lack of consideration for situational context. In contrast, people with borderline personality disorder tend to *hyper*mentalize by overinterpreting facial expressions or making overly complex assumptions based on context and social cues. (To get a better sense of this, think about your thought process when you've sent a message to someone you've liked and they don't respond immediately. Did they not get the text? What if they don't like me? Are they taking time to craft a response because they don't want to hurt my feelings? All of these would be examples of hypermentalization.) While both conditions have the same result (decreased ability to accurately read the emotions of others), the underlying reason is different, making differentiation between hypomentalization and hypermentalization crucial to avoid diagnosing autism in people who struggle with social communication for other reasons.

PSEUDOBULBAR AFFECT
Pseudobulbar affect is a neurologic condition in which one experiences uncontrollable and inappropriate outbursts of emotion such as suddenly crying or laughing. These episodes of "emotional incontinence" can resemble the affective instability that is a core trait of borderline personality disorder. However, they differ in a few key ways. For one, changes in expression in pseudobulbar affect are **incongruent** with the underlying emotional state (even though someone is laughing or crying, that doesn't mean that they are happy or sad). In addition, changes of affect in pseudobulbar affect are not precipitated by environmental triggers (unlike the affective lability seen in borderline personality disorder). Using these clues to accurately recognize pseudobulbar affect is important as it can often be a sign of an underlying neurologic disorder such as amyotrophic lateral sclerosis or stroke (so misdiagnosing it as borderline personality disorder could mean missing a potentially serious neurologic condition).

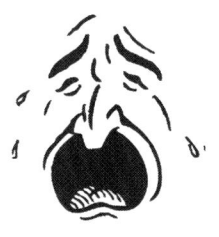

PUTTING IT ALL TOGETHER

Borderline personality disorder doesn't enjoy the same amount of attention or public awareness as the "big ones" in psychiatry like depression, schizophrenia, or bipolar disorder. However, this does not make it any less impairing, and people with the disorder often suffer persistent dysfunction across their lifespan. Because of the mismatch between the seriousness of the condition and the low level of interest in it, borderline personality disorder has been described as a **disorder in search of advocacy**. Clinicians are reluctant to talk about it, patients are averse to hearing about it, and insurance companies often do their best to avoid covering effective treatments. There is also an unfortunate tendency to try and diagnose these patients with just about any other disorder, with bipolar disorder and PTSD being particularly common. Yet ignoring borderline personality disorder does a disservice not only to patients but to society as a whole, as the majority of research seems to indicate that it is a treatable condition with a much better prognosis than originally thought.

Being educated about this disorder helps to prevent diagnostic reluctance and allows you to provide patients with an accurate view of their condition. To remember what you have learned about borderline personality disorder, keep the **I DESPAIR** and **DELAPSE** mnemonics in mind, as even just understanding both of these frameworks will put you miles ahead of most providers when it comes to diagnosing and treating patients with this disorder. Understanding the key role that extreme interpersonal sensitivity plays in the phenomenology of the disorder can also help you to be sure of your diagnosis and to educate your patients on the nature and timing of their symptoms. By doing this, you can avoid the cycle of failed treatments and unmet expectations that occurs when people try to call borderline personality disorder by any other name.

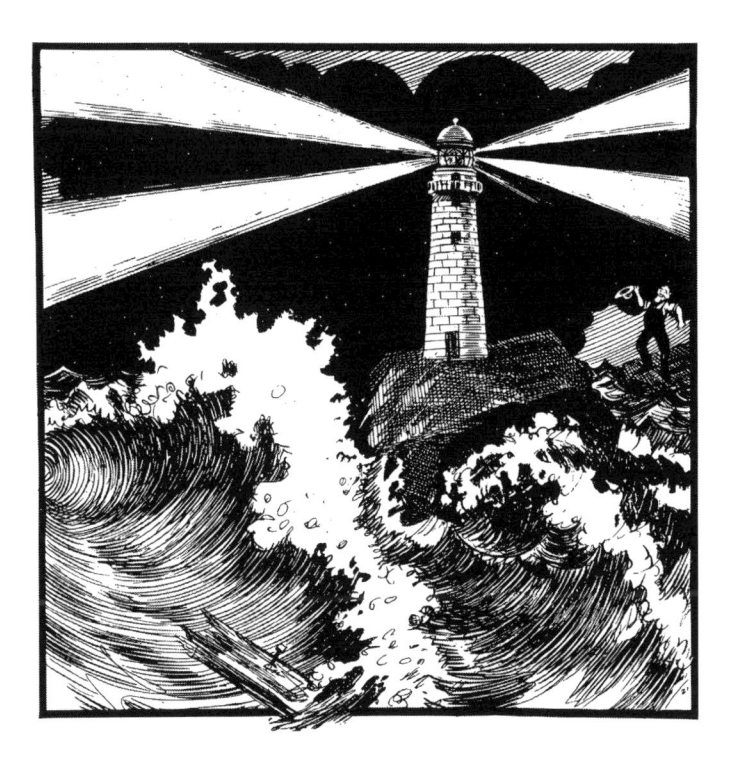

REVIEW QUESTIONS

1. A 28 y/o F suddenly moves across the country after meeting "the man of my dreams" at a music festival. She moves in with him, and they enjoy several weeks of passionate romance. However, after one month of living together, she begins to suspect that he is cheating on her. He works at a consulting firm and often has to stay at the office until 10:00 or 11:00 at night which leaves her at home by herself. During her time alone, she constantly thinks about other women that he might be sleeping with and imagines them making love. She develops narratives about each of these women and even names them. She cries frequently when he works late and accuses him of infidelity every night when he walks through the door. However, upon being hugged and reassured that he has been faithful, she instantly begins smiling and laughing. One night, her partner returns home to find the words "LOVE ME" written in red lipstick on the bathroom mirror and her in the bathtub with multiple superficial cuts on her arms as seen below:

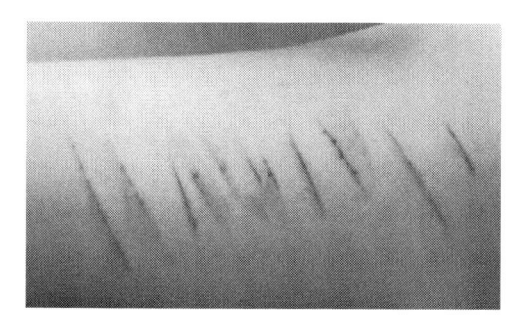

   Which of the following is the *least* likely purpose of this patient's self-injurious behavior?
   A. Attempting to distract from emotional pain
   B. Fulfilling a desire to be dead
   C. Demanding that her partner provide reassurance and comfort
   D. Making the current situation feel less real
   E. Stimulating the release of endogenous opioids

2. (Continued from previous question.) Her partner calls 911, and she is soon admitted to a local psychiatric hospital. During the initial evaluation, the treating psychiatrist asks her, "Do you sometimes hear voices of people who aren't there or see things that other people don't?" The patient responds by saying that she hears voices inside her head belonging to "all the people that he's cheating on me with telling me what a stupid ugly whore I am." She denies ever having heard voices before in her life. What is the best interpretation of this symptom?
   A. Evidence of schizoaffective disorder
   B. Evidence of a primary psychotic disorder
   C. Evidence of a comorbid psychotic disorder
   D. Evidence of malingering
   E. None of the above

3. (Continued from previous question.) With the patient's consent, the treating psychiatrist calls her mother to obtain collateral information. During their conversation, the psychiatrist asks when the patient first began to show signs of a psychiatric condition. What is the mother's likely response?
   A. "She's been like this as long as I can remember."
   B. "It probably started when she was in elementary school."
   C. "Things took a turn for the worse when she was in high school."
   D. "I only really noticed anything different in the past few years."
   E. "She has never been this way before."

4. (Continued from previous question.) On the first morning of her admission, the patient meets with her treatment team to discuss goals of hospitalization. Upon sitting down, she immediately says, "Look, I've been through this song and dance before. You're going to tell me I'm depressed and then medicate me and send me to a therapist, but nothing's going to help and I'll end up back here again in a few weeks. You all seem nice but let's face it, it's not like you're doing me any favors by keeping me here in this hideous hospital gown eating shitty hospital food." She laughs sarcastically and then looks up at the ceiling in the room for a few seconds before tears start coming down her face. Which of the following is most likely to reduce her chances of hospital readmission?
   A. Taking a thorough medication history and prescribing a medication that has not been tried before
   B. Telling the patient of her diagnosis of borderline personality disorder
   C. Working with a social worker to find local therapists who specialize in dialectical behavior therapy
   D. Discharging the patient from the hospital as soon as possible
   E. None of the above are likely to reduce her chances of readmission

5. (Continued from previous question.) The patient is treated in the hospital, and soon both the inpatient team and the patient feel that she is ready for discharge. On her last day in the hospital, she asks the team if she is going to "be this way forever." What is the most appropriate response?
   A. "Yes, this is an unchangeable part of your personality."
   B. "Yes, most likely. If you had gotten the right help earlier it might have been different, but given your age it is unlikely to change."
   C. "No, you are suffering from an episode of this disorder. It will likely pass soon, but there is always the possibility of future episodes."
   D. "No, you are likely to get better, but only if you stay in treatment."
   E. "No, you are likely to get better, but it will likely take a few years."

1. **The best answer is B.** This patient is likely suffering from borderline personality disorder given the presence of self-harm, hostility, affective instability, unstable relationships, and impulsivity. While the functions of self-harm are complex, it appears to serve multiple purposes including distracting from emotional pain (answer A), forcing others to provide comfort (answer C), and inducing a state of dissociation (answer D). Each of these purposes is mediated at least in part through the increased release of endogenous opioids (answer E). In contrast, it is only a minority of people who engage in this form of self-harm who have a genuine desire to commit suicide at that time.

2. **The best answer is E.** The patient's reported auditory hallucinations are not phenomenologically consistent with a primary psychotic disorder and are most likely a representation of the transient, stress-induced micropsychotic symptoms that are common in borderline personality disorder. Therefore, a diagnosis of a diagnosis of schizoaffective disorder or either a primary or comorbid psychotic disorder appears unwarranted in the absence of other symptoms (answers A, B, and C). It is unclear that these symptoms represent malingering, and the severity of her self-harming behaviors suggests a level of distress that argues against her primarily seeking some form of secondary gain (answer D).

3. **The best answer is C.** As with most personality disorders, the age of onset for borderline personality disorder is generally during adolescence. While cases of borderline personality disorder beginning in childhood or later adulthood are not unheard of, the most common pattern is onset during one's teenage years.

4. **The best answer is C.** Out of the listed options, only dialectical behavior therapy has been demonstrated to reduce rates of hospitalization in people with borderline personality disorder. While educating the patient on the nature of borderline personality disorder can be helpful, it has not been shown to make a clinically significant impact on readmission rates in and of itself (answer B). Prolonged admissions are generally advised against in borderline personality disorder to avoid creating behavioral dependency on the structured setting of a hospital, but early discharge has not been shown to reduce rates of hospitalization (answer D). Medications on the whole are unlikely to significantly alter the clinical trajectory of someone with borderline personality disorder (answer A).

5. **The best answer is E.** Borderline personality disorder is characterized by chronic deficits with occasional exacerbations. However, it is not considered to be an episodic disorder given that signs and symptoms often remain across the lifespan (answer C). Contrary to previous conceptions of the disorder, longitudinal studies have found that the majority of people with borderline personality disorder enter remission from the disorder during their lifetime (answers A and B) and that this pattern is seen even in people who do not receive evidence-based treatments for the disorder (answer D). Therefore, it is most accurate to say that the patient will likely enter remission but that this will take a period of several years.

16 ANTISOCIAL

Antisocial personality disorder is characterized by a persistent pattern of **behavior that infringes on the rights of others**, including purposeful deception, aggression, violence, and theft. In an attempt to make the diagnosis as *reliable* as possible, the DSM has placed the diagnostic focus for antisocial personality disorder exclusively on the supposedly objective presence of frequent "bad behavior" without making reference to the less objective (though more relevant) question of *why* someone is engaging in this behavior. After all, people commit bad behavior for any number of reasons. For example, think of a man who frequently steals from his work. Conceivably he does it because he lives in poverty and has a hungry family, or perhaps he comes from a privileged background and steals for the "thrill" of it? Maybe he suffers from an addiction and needs money to fuel his habit, or possibly he never developed an inner sense of morality and can't tell right from wrong? Because the reasons for "bad behavior" are so numerous, it seems ludicrous to attempt to lump all of them together under a single diagnosis. Yet that is exactly what the DSM attempts to do, and the results are telling: antisocial personality disorder as a diagnosis has **very poor validity** and **little prognostic value**.

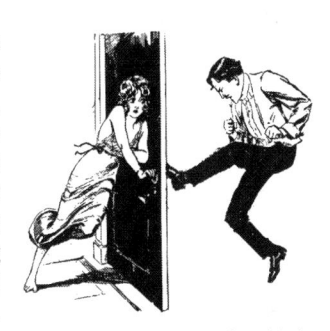

It is only when you break down the *causes* of antisocial behavior that clear patterns begin to emerge. For people who consistently and repeatedly engage in antisocial behaviors, two consistent patterns are seen. While the terminology is varied and inconsistent, in this book we will refer to one pattern as **psychopathy** (or the "psychopathic form" of antisocial personality disorder), with **antisocial personality disorder** on its own used to describe specifically the *non*-psychopathic form. Psychopathy will be discussed in the next chapter, so for this chapter we will focus primarily on *non*-psychopathic antisocial personality disorder as well as various related disorders, including those seen primarily in childhood.

SIGNS AND SYMPTOMS OF ANTISOCIAL BEHAVIOR

The DSM criteria for antisocial personality disorder can be encapsulated in the mnemonic **ACID LIAR**, with 3 or more of the last 7 items being required:

A is for Adult. By definition, antisocial personality disorder cannot be diagnosed before the age of 18. However, the pattern of antisocial behavior must have started by the age of 15, if not earlier.

C is for Criminality. The actions of people with antisocial personality disorder often fall outside of the law, and many are arrested or spend time in jail due to their actions.

I is for Impulsivity. As would be expected in a personality disorder that is associated with low conscientiousness, people with antisocial personality disorder tend to be highly impulsive and often neglect or fail to plan.

D is for Disregard for safety. People with antisocial personality disorder routinely ignore, disregard, or show outright disdain for the safety of not only themselves but others as well. They may act in ways that are dangerous, such as speeding through a residential street where children are playing.

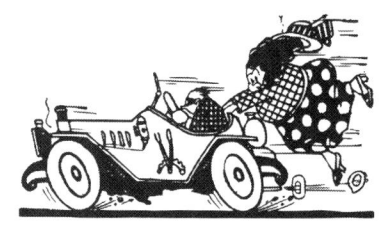

L is for Lying. People with antisocial personality disorder frequently lie, cheat, and deceive others. This can be done for some kind of secondary gain (such as stealing someone's credit card information) or simply for the thrill of it.

I is for Irresponsibility. Another manifestation of low conscientiousness is a chronic failure to honor both personal and societal obligations, such as failures to repay debts, an inability or unwillingness to work, and neglecting to care for dependents.

A is for Aggression. Mental irritability can turn into physical aggression. Notably, this is not purposeless agitation as is seen in other psychiatric conditions like delirium or intoxication. Instead, people with antisocial personality disorder tend to attack others in a purposeful or targeted way.

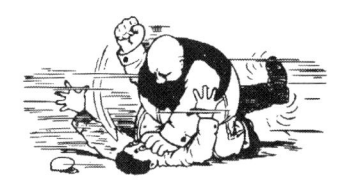

R is for Remorselessness. Finally, people with antisocial personality disorder often show a lack of remorse for their actions. They will try to rationalize their behavior by saying that the other person deserved it or that they had no choice but to act that way. However, this is not necessarily diagnostic, and some patients do show remorse.

These actions are typically done with some degree of **intention to cause frustration or harm**. This distinguishes antisocial personality disorder from the disruptive behaviors found in other disorders such as ADHD, in which the patient does not intend to upset others but is unable to control their impulsivity.

Antisocial personality disorder involves a pattern of **intentional aggression and hostility** that is **persistent and pervasive**.

ACID LIAR:
Adult (18+)
Criminality
Impulsivity
Disregard for safety
Lying
Irresponsibility
Aggression
Remorselessness

While the diagnostic criteria for antisocial personality disorder primarily involve behaviors, this condition features consistent signs and symptoms as well. People with antisocial personality disorder tend to engage in bad behavior as a result of **emotional instability**, with a propensity towards affective lability and strong reactions to interpersonal triggers such as being rejected, devalued, or humiliated. Most commonly, this takes the form of intense feelings of **anger, sadness, or irritability** that immediately precede the impulsive acts. These emotions are experienced quite strongly and often seem to be significantly **out of proportion** to the circumstances that provoked them. For some people, episodes of aggression are followed by an emotional "thrill" or feeling of power that provides immediate positive reinforcement. The emotional swings that accompany aggressive acts are often in addition to a long-lasting **tendency towards negative emotions**, including feelings of emptiness, boredom, meaninglessness, and alienation. In this way, antisocial personality disorder is revealed to have the same core "cluster B-ness" as other disorders in its class, resulting in similar **difficulties in relationships** due to a need for attention and a fear of abandonment.

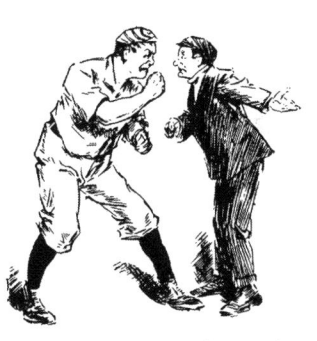

On a psychological level, most people with antisocial personality disorder do not go around *trying* to be "bad people." Instead, people with antisocial personality disorder engage in antagonistic behavior as a way of **externalizing negative emotions** by projecting them outwardly. (This is in contrast to *internalizing* which is the process of directing negative emotions *inward* towards the self, which instead results in disorders like anxiety or depression.)

While **impulsive aggression** is the primary pattern seen in antisocial personality disorder, it does not account for the whole picture. In fact, many people with antisocial personality disorder also commit **premeditated** acts such as stealing or defrauding others. These acts are normally justified on the basis of saying that "I need to look after myself because no one else will," a rationalization that makes more sense when you consider the history of both parental and societal neglect that typifies the backgrounds of many people with antisocial personality disorder.

While behavioral *excesses* of antisocial personality disorder are the most noticeable, patients with this disorder often have specific *deficits* as well including profoundly poor social skills, lack of executive function, and difficulty understanding rule-based structures. This often leads them to have few acquaintances and no close friends, resulting in a persistent sense of **loneliness and isolation** that further drives the negative emotions underlying the aggressive behavior.

ANTISOCIAL BEHAVIOR ACROSS THE LIFESPAN

While we know that antisocial personality disorder cannot be diagnosed before the age of 18, we also know that in nearly all cases the initial pattern of disruptive behavior *began* during **childhood and adolescence**. Younger patients with recurrent aggression are instead diagnosed using one or more **externalizing disorders** (known formally as "disruptive, impulse-control, and conduct disorders" in the DSM). This arbitrary age cut-off makes antisocial personality disorder an incredibly difficult condition to study across the lifespan, as what is likely the same core condition will go by different names based on what stage of life the patient is in. Nevertheless, we will do our best to make sense out of the confusion and try to establish some clear patterns between externalizing disorders and antisocial personality disorder.

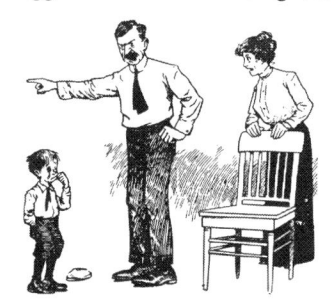

EPIDEMIOLOGY

Antisocial personality disorder is **common**, with as many as **5%** of people having it. However, it is even higher in certain populations such as prisons or jails, with up to 60% of criminal inmates meeting criteria for the diagnosis. It is up to 5 times more common in **men** than in women.

Antisocial behaviors are even more common in children than adults, with up to 10% of youth showing a consistent pattern of disruptive behavior. The prevalence is significantly higher in certain areas such as the child welfare system where up to 25% of children living in orphanages or foster care show signs of an externalizing disorder. Externalization is far more common in **boys**, with a gender ratio of 10 to 1.

PROGNOSIS

Similar to other cluster B personality disorders like borderline personality disorder, antisocial personality disorder has a **tendency to peak in adolescence and early adulthood**, with a natural lessening to severity by one's 30s and 40s. Around 25% improve and another 25% remit completely, although that leaves around 50% who continue to struggle with ongoing antisocial behavior. Even among people who improve, antisocial personality disorder can still be conceptualized as a **life-long disorder**, as most patients still struggle with negative mood states, poor functioning, ongoing substance use, and inability to sustain relationships even into older age.

For children and adolescents with externalizing behaviors, the prognosis varies based on the age at which the behaviors first emerged. People whose externalizing behaviors were apparent earlier in life (during early childhood and school-age) are characterized by a significantly more severe and persistent prognosis. These so-called **life-course externalizers** are often diagnosed with antisocial personality disorder as adults, and many end up incarcerated or institutionalized with limited social support.

In contrast to life-course externalizers, **adolescence-limited externalizers** begin demonstrating disruptive behaviors only during their teenage years, with no earlier signs of aggression during childhood. Externalizing behaviors in this group are often disruptive (such as throwing tantrums, disobeying instructions, and vandalizing property) but rarely reach the levels of overt violence and aggression that are seen in life-course externalizers. Reassuringly, these behaviors often remit within a few years and do not necessarily predict worse psychological or social outcomes as an adult. Interestingly, the gender ratio for adolescence-limited externalization is more even (with 2 females for every 3 males) than it is for life-course externalization.

TREATMENT

Antisocial personality disorder is considered to be a **difficult disorder to treat**, as no medications or psychotherapies have consistently been shown to be effective at reducing rates of reoffending, increasing life satisfaction, or improving one's level of social or occupational functioning. Treatment is limited further by the fact that people with antisocial personality disorder often show very **little motivation for treatment**. Incarceration is often used as a legal rather than clinical intervention. Data suggests that **short periods of incarceration** (less than a year) may be associated with lower rates of reoffending, but longer periods were not.

There is a lack of high-quality studies on how to treat children and adolescents with externalizing disorders. Most evidence seems to suggest that the best outcomes are seen with use of specific forms of therapy, such as various forms of **behavior modification** (including applied behavior analysis) and **parent-child interaction therapy**. These treatments teach specific skills to *both* the child and their family unit with the goal of reducing the emotional dysregulation that leads to disruptive behavior as well as providing alternatives to acting out (like screaming into a pillow instead of punching a sibling). As a rule, medications have *not* been shown to be effective at treating externalizing disorders. Nevertheless, they are frequently used, especially in under-resourced settings such as group homes where money and time to appropriately address externalizing disorders are lacking. **Stimulants** are commonly used, although it is unclear whether they have any effect in the absence of comorbid ADHD. **Antipsychotics** are often used as well, with variable efficacy. However, this must be balanced against the clear evidence of long-term risks associated with antipsychotic use (including weight gain and extrapyramidal symptoms). A number of small studies have suggested that SRIs may be helpful if there is an underlying negative mood state, but few of these studies have been replicated enough times to be considered high-quality evidence. In situations where there is a lack of resources available for either behavioral or family therapy, it is likely that medications will continue to be used despite a lack of evidence.

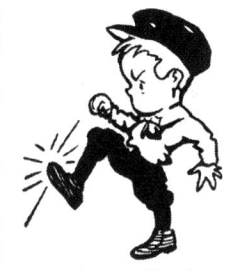

MECHANISMS OF ANTISOCIAL BEHAVIOR

Antisocial behavior is a complex phenomenon for which no single explanation is likely to be found. This is because the core characteristics of antisocial personality disorder (misbehavior and emotional dysregulation) are both **multifactorial phenomena** that can each be related to many different things. Despite the wide range of pathology captured in these terms, however, some patterns have begun to emerge. Decades of research on childhood development have found that **neglect** (particularly in the early years of life) produces a characteristic syndrome of impairments in attention, impulse control, and social ability that accounts for many adults diagnosed with antisocial personality disorder as well as the majority of children and adolescents diagnosed with externalizing disorders. While it is true that neglect increases the risk of developing *most* mental disorders, its association with externalizing disorders is particularly strong. Indeed, while disorders like depression and anxiety are 2 to 3 times more common in impoverished settings, severe externalizing disorders like conduct disorder are over 10 times as frequent.

The association of neglect to antisocial behaviors appears to be fairly *specific* as well. For example, in children who were *neglected* but *not abused*, there *is* an increased prevalence of externalizing disorders while there does not appear to be a significant increase in rates of trauma-related disorders like PTSD. Whether someone who experienced childhood maltreatment ends up developing an externalizing disorder, an internalizing disorder, or both appears to depend largely upon a few key factors, including the **type of maltreatment** (with sexual abuse appearing to cause internalizing disorders while neglect and physical violence cause more externalizing disorders), **age** (with externalizing disorders being more common with maltreatment in early childhood while internalizing disorders are more common in older children), and **gender** (with boys more likely to develop externalizing disorders than girls).

To understand why neglect is associated specifically with the development of antisocial behavior, consider the role that someone's caretaker normally provides. Infants and toddlers have a need for **reciprocal interactions** where the child and caregiver are each engaged in both giving and receiving social interaction. The game peekaboo is a perfect example of this, and tellingly it is found in nearly every society and culture across the world! These sorts of interactions play a key role in forming a child's concept of how their actions affect the feelings and emotions of others. For example, while playing peekaboo it is common for the infant to laugh when the caretaker's face is revealed which in turn causes the caretaker to laugh. By engaging in this behavior, the infant can see that their actions have effects on others and that interacting with others can be incredibly rewarding. In contrast, if the infant does not have opportunities to engage in this kind of behavior, they will likely not be able to intuitively understand the effects of misbehavior on others later in life. This likely explains why **social neglect** is correlated with antisocial behavior much more than other forms of neglect such as physical or medical neglect.

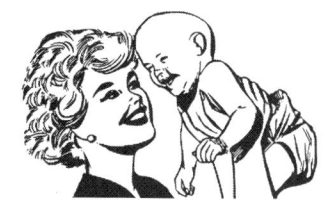

This lack of opportunity to engage in reciprocal interactions appears to directly affect the development of the central nervous system. In fact, studies have found that specific areas of the brain (in particular the **prefrontal cortex**) are noticeably smaller in people with a history of early childhood neglect. These brain regions are involved in attention, impulse control, emotional regulation, and responses to stress—the *exact* cognitive domains that are most dysregulated in antisocial personality disorder. Deficits in these domains are noticeable as early as childhood but persist throughout life, which mirrors the chronic life course associated with antisocial behavior.

The environment outside of just the parent-child relationship can play a large role as well. Unstable living arrangements, lack of access to appropriate medical care, food insecurity, and exposure to violence in the community are all known to be additional risk factors for externalizing behaviors in children. Indeed, you should not walk away thinking that all children with externalizing disorders have "bad parents." Neglect comes in many forms, and not all of them are voluntary. Most parents truly want to take good care of their children, but some are unable to due to factors outside of their control. Discrimination, mass incarceration, and socio-economic disadvantage all intersect here, creating a **vicious cycle** in which exposure to poverty and parental institutionalization lead to externalizing behaviors on the part of the child, resulting in *their* becoming institutionalized and impoverished which continues the cycle further.

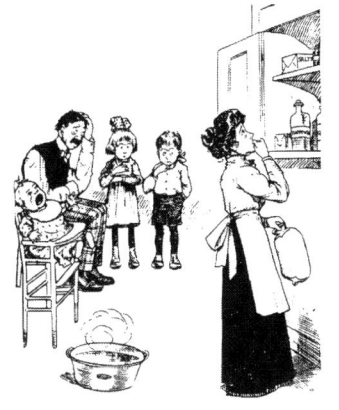

Despite the strong association between antisocial behavior and a history of neglect, it is neither sufficiently sensitive nor specific to be able to work backwards. (In other words, you can never be sure that someone with antisocial personality disorder was neglected, nor can you be sure that someone who was neglected will develop antisocial personality disorder.) In addition, some children who were neglected develop internalizing disorders (either instead of or in addition to externalizing disorders) while others are remarkably resilient and develop no mental disorders at all. Consistent with the idea that *it's never just one thing*, you should never think that a history of neglect explains everything about antisocial behavior. There is likely a substantial genetic contribution present, as parents who neglect their children often have their own externalizing patterns as well.

Overall, the association between neglect and antisocial behavior is a robust one that provides an explanatory framework when working with patients whose behaviors we can have difficulty understanding. It can be frustrating and emotionally draining to work with patients who repeatedly hurt or deceive other people, especially when they seem to have no desire to stop. However, by understanding that these patients often were not afforded the same kinds of developmental opportunities that are given to most people, we can be better equipped to approach their care from a position of empathy and humility.

HOW TO DIAGNOSE DISORDERS OF ANTISOCIAL BEHAVIOR

Up until now, we have largely treated externalizing disorders as a group rather than focusing on the differences between them. We will now turn our attention to teasing out the key distinctions between **oppositional defiant disorder**, **conduct disorder**, **intermittent explosive disorder**, and **disruptive mood dysregulation disorder**, all of which are generally diagnosed in children and adolescents. For children diagnosed with externalizing disorders, many (but not all) will go on to "graduate" to antisocial personality disorder when they turn 18. The precise graduation rate depends on the specific diagnosis but is highest with conduct disorder (at a little over 40%).

We will also talk about two other disorders (**kleptomania** and **pyromania**) in the DSM chapter on "disruptive, impulse-control, and conduct disorders" which are also typically diagnosed in adulthood.

ANTISOCIAL PERSONALITY DISORDER
Antisocial personality disorder is a broad diagnosis capturing many forms of recurrent "bad behavior" in adults. The **ACID LIAR** mnemonic can help you remember the core pattern. While patients must be over the age of 18 to receive the diagnosis, the DSM's diagnostic criteria do specify that the behavior must have started before the age of 15, reinforcing the notion that an early onset is associated with a more life-long course. Notably, antisocial behavior must be persistent and pervasive, and it cannot occur exclusively in the context of another disorder like schizophrenia or bipolar disorder.

OPPOSITIONAL DEFIANT DISORDER
Oppositional defiant disorder (ODD, an unfortunate abbreviation) is an externalizing disorder defined by a consistent pattern of **argumentativeness, vindictiveness, and defiance** of authority figures that is excessive, destructive, and maladaptive to the point where it causes harm to both the patient and those around them. Children and adolescents diagnosed with oppositional defiant disorder frequently argue, ignore rules, and purposefully do things to upset others. However, these behaviors do not cross the line into violation of others' rights and stop short of overt violence, aggression, or theft (which would instead be conduct disorder).

These patterns of disruptive behavior must be in excess of what is normally expected for a child and must occur for at least 6 months. As with other externalizing disorders, there is a significant mood component to oppositional defiant disorder, with **persistent anger and irritability** being enduring emotional states. Treatment involves working with the family both as a unit (as in family therapy) and individually (with psychotherapy and behavioral training for the child and education on behavioral principles for the caregivers). Despite being frequently used, there is little evidence that medications are effective for treating oppositional defiant disorder.

INTERMITTENT EXPLOSIVE DISODER
Intermittent explosive disorder (IED, another unfortunate abbreviation) is defined by a consistent pattern of disruptive behaviors, including screaming, hitting, kicking, or throwing tantrums. However, as highlighted by the word "intermittent" in the name, these behaviors tend to happen in **discrete episodes** each lasting no more than an hour (which is distinct from the persistent oppositionality seen in oppositional defiant disorder). These episodes often occur **in response to external events** (such as being

told "no") and are accompanied by intense feelings of anger or irritability that appear to be significantly **out of proportion** to how most children would react. In between episodes, mood returns to normal (in contrast to the *persistent* negative mood state seen in oppositional defiant disorder and disruptive mood dysregulation disorder).

Intermittent explosive disorder can be conceptualized as a disorder of *both* **emotion regulation** and **impulse control**, as the patient not only has difficulty regulating their emotions in response to external stressors but also has trouble *not* acting out in a way that is counterproductive and harmful towards others. Indeed, many children diagnosed with intermittent explosive disorder express **remorse** about their actions once they have calmed emotionally (in contrast to people with oppositional defiant disorder or conduct disorder who are more likely to continue believing that they were justified in their actions). Like other externalizing disorders, treatment involves behavioral interventions aimed at improving distress tolerance and impulse control. **Family and behavioral therapy** can be helpful as well. Medications play more of a role in treating intermittent explosive disorder compared to oppositional defiant disorder or conduct disorder, with most evidence favoring use of **SRIs**. However, the effect of medication is overall quite limited, so behavioral and family therapy should be offered as first-line options whenever possible.

DISRUPTIVE MOOD DYSREGULATION DISORDER

Disruptive mood dysregulation disorder (DMDD) is similar to intermittent explosive disorder in that the disruptive behaviors occur in **intermittent episodes**. However, it differs from intermittent explosive disorder in that there is **chronic irritability, sadness, or anger** even *between* outbursts. It further differs from oppositional defiant disorder and conduct disorder in that patients with this disorder show **remorse** for their actions. As disruptive mood dysregulation disorder is a relatively new diagnosis, data are not available on its prognosis in relation to other externalizing disorders. Most children who meet criteria for disruptive mood dysregulation disorder will also meet criteria for oppositional defiant disorder, although the reverse is not true.

CONDUCT DISORDER

More than the other externalizing disorders, conduct disorder is the "child version" of antisocial personality disorder, as it involves a **flagrant disregard for the rights of others** (including violence, aggression, and theft) that is not seen in oppositional defiant disorder, intermittent explosive disorder, or disruptive mood dysregulation disorder. In many cases, a diagnosis of conduct disorder is preceded by oppositional defiant disorder (although it's worth pointing out that *most* children diagnosed with oppositional defiant disorder do *not* progress to conduct disorder). Conduct disorder is itself conceptualized as a **precursor to antisocial personality disorder**, with half of all children and adolescents diagnosed with conduct disorder ultimately meeting criteria for antisocial personality disorder as adults. Even people who don't technically meet criteria for a formal diagnosis as adults often still struggle with work functioning and social relationships, suggesting an overall poor prognosis for this condition.

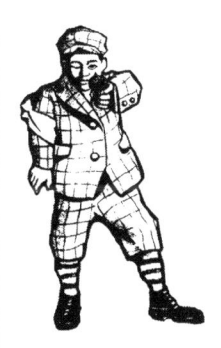

KLEPTOMANIA

Kleptomania is a condition in which people regularly steal items that do not belong to them. Unlike "normal" theft, these items are not stolen for personal or financial gain. Rather, for someone with kleptomania the act of stealing is experienced as **intensely pleasurable** (often described as a "thrill" or an "adrenaline rush") resulting in positive reinforcement. For this reason, kleptomania is considered a disorder of **impulse control**, placing it closer to addictive disorders than compulsive disorders. Indeed, many of the treatments that are successful for kleptomania resemble those used for treating addiction, including naltrexone. Kleptomania also appears to be associated with other externalizing disorders that also feature a high degree of impulsivity such as intermittent explosive disorder and disruptive mood dysregulation disorder.

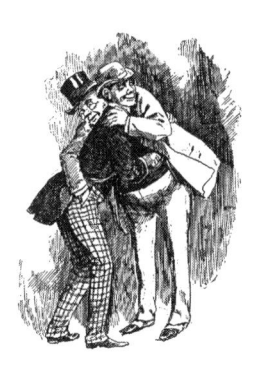

PYROMANIA

Pyromania is a relatively rare condition characterized by **recurrent fire setting** leading to destruction of property. Similar to kleptomania, fire setting in pyromania is done not for any sort of external gain (in which case it would be arson). Rather, for someone with pyromania the act of fire setting is experienced as being euphorically pleasurable. In contrast to kleptomania, people with pyromania often describe a **build-up of mental tension** that can only be relieved by starting fires, making it appear that compulsivity likely plays as large of a role in this disorder as impulsivity.

DIFFERENTIAL DIAGNOSIS OF ANTISOCIAL BEHAVIOR

Antisocial behaviors sit at a strange nexus of many different psychiatric diagnoses, having elements of cluster B personality disorders, mood disorders, addictive disorders, trauma-related disorders, and neurodevelopmental disorders like ADHD. In this section, we'll go over some of the most common areas of diagnostic confusion when working with patients with recurrent antisocial behavior.

NORMALCY

Diagnosing either antisocial personality disorder or an externalizing disorder must be done with **significant caution**, as it usually involves someone *other* than the identified patient saying that there is a problem (it's usually "*He's* acting out again!" rather than "*I'm* acting out again!"). This is in contrast to something like depression where it is typically the identified patient who decides to seek clinical attention because they *themselves* feel that something is wrong. In addition, the tendency to characterize all disruptive or challenging behaviors as being indicative of psychiatric pathology is concerning as it minimizes the contribution from other factors. Indeed, disruptive behaviors have many possible sources, not the least of which is being a logical (though not necessarily adaptive) response to **stresses and injustices** in one's home, school, or society as a whole. For example, many children living in foster care or residential group homes end up being diagnosed with oppositional defiant disorder, yet many of these cases resolve when the child is placed in a more stable living arrangement. By assigning a diagnosis, it is easy for someone to get the impression that the "problem" lies entirely within the patient when in reality they may simply be the **most vulnerable person** in a complex system of inequality and dysfunction. For both of these reasons, there is a higher risk of unjustly "labeling" or pathologizing behavior when diagnosing antisocial behavior compared to most psychiatric conditions. Therefore, it is best to approach antisocial behavior from a place of clinical humility by always keeping normalcy on the differential.

ATTENTION DEFICIT HYPERACTIVITY DISORDER
Given that externalizing disorders and ADHD (specifically its hyperactive or combined subtypes) both begin in childhood and are characterized by persistent misbehavior, it is no wonder that there is frequent confusion between the two. A key way to differentiate between these diagnostic categories is to look at the **intentionality** of the behavior, as disruptive behaviors in ADHD are rarely done with the intention of frustrating others (even if they end up having that effect). The course of each disorder is important as well, as the hyperactivity from ADHD tends to *improve* during the transition from childhood to adolescence in many cases while the disruptive behaviors found in externalizing disorders often *worsen* as a teenager. (Fortunately, disruptive behaviors related to ADHD and externalizing disorders both tend to improve as one enters adulthood.)

However, even when careful diagnostic assessments are made, there are many cases where people appear to have *both* ADHD and an externalizing disorder. Indeed, the comorbidity of externalizing disorders with ADHD may be as high as 40% even after conducting a thorough differential diagnosis. The presence of both externalizing behavior and inattention predicts significantly poorer outcomes than with either disorder alone. In addition, treatment using stimulants for children with externalizing disorders appears to result in positive improvements in behavior only when there is comorbid ADHD, further strengthening the concept that these are two separate disorders with separate treatment considerations.

INTERNALIZING DISORDERS
Externalizing disorders stand in contrast to **internalizing disorders** (like anxiety or depression) which involve negative thoughts and emotions that are directed *inward* towards the self, leading to feelings of worthlessness and low self-esteem. Externalization and internalization are not mutually exclusive, and most people with an externalizing disorder will also have an internalizing disorder (although the reverse is not true, with only a minority of people with internalizing disorders also having an externalizing disorder). Some disorders have both internalizing and externalizing dimensions (such as borderline personality disorder which features not only internalizing symptoms like chronic dysphoria but also externalizing behaviors such as anger and impulsivity).

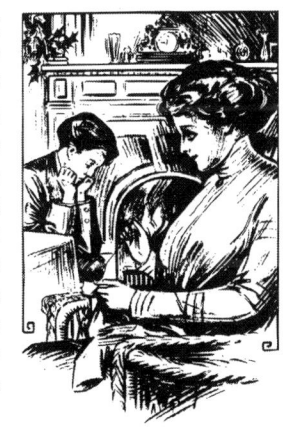

While externalizing behaviors are often the most pressing concern for the *family*, it is the internalizing symptoms that are more likely to be distressing to the *patient*. Therefore, never let the presence of externalizing behaviors distract you from looking for internalizing symptoms as well when working with children. Patients who struggle with depression and anxiety can occasionally externalize their frustrations as well (such as yelling or punching a wall when they are upset). However, a diagnosis of an externalizing disorder should be based upon disruptive behavior that is **frequent and persistent** and not just a single episode of externalization.

BIPOLAR DISORDER

The diagnostic criteria for antisocial personality disorder specifically mention that the behavior must not occur exclusively in the context of bipolar disorder. If antisocial behavior is accompanied by mood changes and presents in a way that is clearly different than one's usual baseline, a diagnosis of a mood disorder is more likely.

In children, there is a tendency to diagnose bipolar disorder in children with misbehavior, particularly if there is any element of mood symptoms. However, there is significant controversy about this, as the primary symptoms of pediatric bipolar disorder (such as irritability, rapid speech, distractibility, and high energy) are all **incredibly non-specific** and are found in a variety of other disorders, including externalizing disorders and ADHD. In addition, longitudinal studies have shown that pediatric cases of bipolar disorder rarely "graduate" to bipolar disorder as adults, suggesting that the syndrome that is called "bipolar disorder" in children is *not* the same as the one that is called "bipolar disorder" in adults. There is reason to be cautious, as incorrectly ascribing misbehavior to bipolar disorder has been shown to increase use of powerful and often harmful medications like mood stabilizers and antipsychotics. As a general rule of thumb, avoid diagnosing pediatric bipolar disorder unless there are *specific* signs of mania (such as increased goal-directed activity) and a high-degree of certainty that the symptoms cannot be attributed to any other cause.

PSYCHOSIS

As with bipolar disorder, the DSM specifies that the misbehavior seen in antisocial personality disorder cannot occur exclusively during schizophrenia. While some patients with schizophrenia do act violently, this is more often due to disorganized agitation than it is due to aggression. When aggression is involved, it tends to be **related to paranoia** or the content of the patient's delusional belief systems. Overall, patients with schizophrenia are more likely to be *victims* of violence than perpetrators.

TRAUMA

Many children with externalizing disorders have a history of trauma, with neglect and exposure to violence being particularly common. However, because various types of maltreatment tend to occur together, it is worthwhile to be on the lookout for signs and symptoms of the "abuse cluster" for anyone diagnosed with a disorder from the "neglect cluster." Interestingly, "textbook" PTSD appears to be fairly rare following exposure to trauma during childhood (with rates of less than 5% in children living in foster care or residential group homes). Instead, cluster B personality disorders, somatization, and dissociation appear to be much more common, especially in later adulthood.

OBSESSIVE-COMPULSIVE DISORDER
While some people with obsessive-compulsive disorder do struggle with intrusive thoughts of violence, these thoughts are notably **ego-dystonic**. In fact, studies suggest that patients with OCD are actually at *lower* risk of violence than the average person on the street, making actual antisocial behavior rare in this (often highly conscientious) population.

PERSONALITY DISORDERS
Most people with a personality disorder meet criteria for more than one, so it should not come as any surprise that people with antisocial personality disorder often shown signs of other personality disorders as well, particularly those in cluster B. This likely reflects that the different disorders listed are simply different expressions of the same core pathology, though still with a few key differences. Patients with borderline or narcissistic personality disorder can also be impulsive and manipulative, but this is generally to gain the affection or approval of others and tends not to cross the line into overt violence.

ADDICTION
Substance use disorders are highly comorbid with antisocial personality disorder. In fact, out of all the personality disorders, antisocial personality disorder appears to have the highest rate of comorbidity with addiction, which is not too surprising given that lawlessness, impulsivity, irresponsibility, and lack of concern for safety are all key themes of this disorder.

AUTISM
Children with autism may engage in violent behavior or otherwise act out due to the core features of their disorder. For example, they may throw a tantrum when someone interferes with their engaging in a restricted interest, or they may become upset if they are unable to express their needs due to their communication deficits. Take time to determine if either of these are present when assessing children who are engaging in problematic behavior, and look for other signs of autism (such as delays in meeting speech-related milestones) to help solidify the diagnosis.

DELIRIUM
While delirium can involve disorganized agitation (particularly in cases of hyperactive delirium), this tends to present very differently from the purposeful aggression that is seen in antisocial personality disorder.

PSYCHOPATHY
We will talk more about psychopathy in the next chapter, but hopefully it is not too much of a spoiler to say that people with psychopathy tend to engage in misbehavior not as a way of *expressing* negative emotions but rather due to a temperamental *lack* of empathy that blinds them to the pain and suffering that their behavior causes.

PUTTING IT ALL TOGETHER

Antisocial behavior is a tragically common finding in clinical settings, yet psychiatry as a profession has little to offer in the way of explanation or treatment. This is because our understanding of these disorders is incredibly limited and our diagnostic schemes for them are a bit of a mess. While the **ACID LIAR** mnemonic can make it seem like diagnosing antisocial personality disorder is relatively straightforward, the fact is that these criteria have sacrificed *validity* for the sake of *reliability*. For the disorder to truly reflect the pathology that it is intending to capture, it would need to make a distinction between psychopathic and non-psychopathic forms of antisocial behavior (which it currently lumps together into a single diagnosis) and would need to erase the arbitrary distinction that it makes between cases that occur in patients above or below the age of 18 (after all, nature doesn't care one bit whether the patient is 17 ½ or 18 years old!).

While there are definitely problems with the current diagnostic system, there are also some silver linings. The classification scheme for antisocial behavior in children and adolescents at least *attempts* to provide some boundaries between different conditions (unlike antisocial personality disorder, which places all adults with recurrent bad behavior into the same diagnostic box). When approaching patients with recurrent antisocial behavior, it can be helpful to have a structured framework for diagnosing the likely origin. The mnemonic **PIRATES** can help you take a systematic approach to this:

P is for Purpose. What is the purpose of the behavior? Reactive violence involving a specific emotional trigger is more suggestive of antisocial personality disorder or an externalizing disorder, while instrumental violence involving an extrinsic reward is more associated with psychopathy (as we will discuss in the next chapter).

I is for Intention. How intentional is the behavior? A high degree of intentionality argues for psychopathy, oppositional defiant disorder, or conduct disorder while a more impulsive pattern suggests non-psychopathic antisocial personality disorder, intermittent explosive disorder, or disruptive mood dysregulation disorder.

R is for Remorse. Whether the patient shows remorse for their actions can be a helpful clue into whether the behavior is impulsive or not. Individuals with impulsive disorders like intermittent explosive disorder or disruptive mood dysregulation disorder often say that they regret having acted out while those with oppositional defiant disorder and conduct disorder usually stick to their guns (so to speak). The presence or absence of remorse is less diagnostically helpful in adults, as patients with antisocial personality disorder will sometimes express remorse but will also often try to rationalize or justify their behavior. Notably, patients with psychopathy almost never express remorse of any kind.

A is for Activity. Disruptive behavior occurring in the context of elevated levels of activity can be a helpful diagnostic clue. Persistent hyperactivity suggests ADHD while a sudden change in level of activity would be more characteristic of mania. For this reason, knowing the patient's baseline level of activity and whether the disruptive behavior represents a significant change from it is crucial.

T is for Timing. The timing of antisocial behaviors across the lifespan is important. Misbehavior that begins at a younger age is more likely to suggest ADHD, psychopathy, or life-course externalization. In contrast, bad behavior that is seen only during certain periods of life (such as adolescence-limited externalization) is likely to have a much better prognosis.

E is for Emotion. The nature of the emotions that a patient experiences around the time of disruptive behavior contains important diagnostic clues. A high degree of intense negative emotion is more consistent with an externalizing disorder or antisocial personality disorder, while a *lack* of emotion instead suggests psychopathy. Within externalizing disorders, you can separate intermittent explosive disorder and disruptive mood dysregulation disorder by the presence of a persistent negative mood state in disruptive mood dysregulation disorder (as opposed to the generally normal mood state punctuated by episodes of intense negative affect seen in intermittent explosive disorder).

S is for Severity. Conduct disorder is separated from other externalizing disorders primarily by the severity of misbehavior (which escalates to involve overt violence and abuse only in conduct disorder).

Antisocial behavior can be characterized by its **purpose, intention, remorse, timing,** and associated levels of **activity** and **emotion.**

PIRATES:
Purpose
Intention
Remorse
Activity
Timing
Emotion
Severity

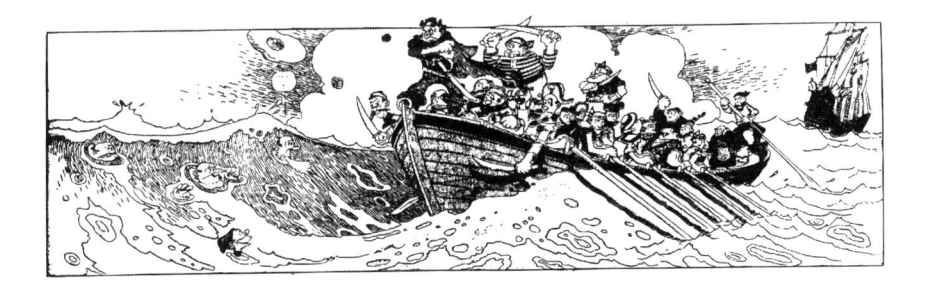

REVIEW QUESTIONS

1. A 25 y/o M is brought to the hospital after he is found smashing car windows with a brick. His urine drug screen is positive for methamphetamines. He is admitted to the hospital on an involuntary hold. He has a history of multiple incarcerations for assaulting police and stealing a car. He has previously been tried on an SRI and a mood stabilizer, with poor results. He grew up as a ward of the state after his mother overdosed on heroin shortly after his birth while he was in the next room. Which of the following would most argue *against* a diagnosis of antisocial personality disorder for this patient?
    A. Onset of antisocial behavior before the age of 10
    B. Persistent negative emotions including dysphoria and emptiness
    C. Presence of narcissistic statements ("I'm smarter than all of you!")
    D. Rapid swings in emotional state from one moment to the next
    E. Expressions of remorse for past actions

2. A 7 y/o M is brought into a psychiatrist's office by his adoptive mother who says that she is "completely fed up." He has been suspended from school for the third time this year after he punched one of his classmates during an argument over whose turn it was to use the handball court. In the past, he has gotten in trouble for hitting the classroom rat after it bit him and throwing a classmate's birthday cake onto the floor after she refused to give him a piece before everyone else. Which of the following questions could the psychiatrist ask the mother to best distinguish between intermittent explosive disorder and disruptive mood dysregulation disorder?
    A. "Has he ever done anything more violent like trying to rob someone or attacking them with a weapon?"
    B. "Has he ever hurt other people without being upset about something first?"
    C. "What is his mood like most of the time?"
    D. "Is he like this at home as well or only at school?"
    E. "How does he feel about these actions after he has calmed down?"

3. A 13 y/o F living in a group home meets with a psychiatrist for an appointment. A complete psychiatric evaluation reveals that the patient meets diagnostic criteria for panic disorder, kleptomania, the hyperactive subtype of ADHD, oppositional defiant disorder, and a history of inhalant abuse. Which of these disorders should the psychiatrist address first in order to most improve the therapeutic relationship?
    A. Panic disorder
    B. Kleptomania
    C. Attention deficit hyperactivity disorder
    D. Oppositional defiant disorder
    E. A history of inhalant use disorder

4. A 16 y/o F is brought to a psychiatrist's office by her father who says that "she is acting like a little shit these days." Over the past year, she has begun skipping school on multiple occasions and has seen her academic performance decline. She has been arrested on two separate occasions: one for smoking cannabis in a public place and another for spray-painting a billboard. Prior to one year ago, she was a straight-A student and had plans to go to college on a softball scholarship. She lives at home with her parents and younger sister. Although her parents are married, they argue frequently and have threatened to divorce each other on multiple occasions. The patient herself participates in the interview only minimally, saying, "You're just one of my dad's lackeys. Why should I tell you anything?" What is the most likely outcome for this patient's behavior?
   A. This behavior will only get worse, and she will likely be incarcerated during her lifetime for a violent crime
   B. This behavior will remain at the same level throughout her adult years
   C. This behavior will partially improve on its own, but she will continue to engage in frequent disruptive behaviors throughout her life
   D. This behavior will improve on its own within several years
   E. The psychiatrist will be able to intervene immediately and resolve the behavior today

5. A 17 y/o M drops out of school to support his mother who has recently been diagnosed with metastatic breast cancer. His mother lacks health insurance, and they have depleted their bank accounts paying for medical bills. He works over 14 hours per day between three different jobs in order to bring in enough income to afford rent. On the way home from work one night, he fails to come to a complete stop at a stop sign and is pulled over by a policeman. The policeman orders him to step out of the car and put his hands above his head. Frustrated and angry, he yells, "I'm not fucking doing that! I've had it! I've fucking had it!" and proceeds to honk his car horn repeatedly. He is detained and taken to a local psychiatric emergency room. During his initial assessment, the patient reports that he is "constantly angry," and he has yelled at both members of his family and several customers at work in the past few weeks. He has one prior arrest for possession of cannabis but says that he was selling drugs to "make ends meet." At one point, he breaks down crying in front of the psychiatrist and says that he wants to punch the face of "every single person I see." What is the most likely diagnosis?
   A. Oppositional defiant disorder
   B. Conduct disorder
   C. Intermittent explosive disorder
   D. Disruptive mood dysregulation disorder
   E. Antisocial personality disorder
   F. None of the above

1. **The best answer is E.** While most patients with antisocial personality disorder lack remorse, the presence of remorse does not rule out the diagnosis. Onset of antisocial behavior during childhood is the rule rather than the exception (answer A). Most cases of antisocial personality disorder involve persistent negative emotions (answer B) and/or affective instability (answer D). Antisocial personality disorder is highly comorbid with other personality disorders, especially those in cluster B like narcissistic personality disorder (answer C).

2. **The best answer is C.** While all of these questions would provide helpful information about this patient's case, the key difference between intermittent explosive disorder and disruptive mood dysregulation disorder involves whether there are persistent mood symptoms between episodes of acting out. Assessing the severity of aggression can differentiate between oppositional defiant disorder and conduct disorder (answer A), while asking about violence in the absence of emotional dysregulation can help to evaluate intentionality (answer B). Assessing remorse would distinguish intermittent explosive disorder and disruptive mood dysregulation disorder from oppositional defiant disorder and conduct disorder (answer E). Finally, knowing whether the behaviors are present in multiple settings is helpful diagnostically but does not distinguish between intermittent explosive disorder and disruptive mood dysregulation disorder (answer D).

3. **The best answer is A.** Out of all the disorders listed, only panic disorder is considered to be purely an internalizing disorder rather than an externalizing or impulse control disorder. While externalizing disorders are often concerning to others (such as parents, teachers, and supervisors), patients themselves most often want help with internalizing problems. Therefore, prioritizing treatment of internalizing disorders is likely to result in a better therapeutic relationship.

4. **The best answer is D.** This case describes a pattern of adolescence-limited externalization. In contrast to life-course externalization, adolescence-limited externalization generally resolves on its own within several years and does not necessarily predict worse psychological or social outcomes as an adult (answers A, B, and C). It is unlikely that a psychiatrist will be able to change externalizing behavior during a single visit (answer E).

5. **The best answer is F.** This patient appears to be having a normal response to extraordinarily abnormal circumstances. While there are some elements of externalization present in how he is acting, a key feature of externalization is that emotions and behaviors are considered to be significantly out of proportion to the situation that provoked them. While the line between externalization and normalcy is often ambiguous, there is at least some element of reasonableness to how he is reacting, making a diagnosis of an externalizing disorder much less likely (answers A through D). Based on the presentation, this patient is much more likely to be suffering from an internalizing disorder such as depression or PTSD, or to have no disorder at all. As a reminder, antisocial personality disorder cannot officially be diagnosed in people less than 18 years of age (answer E).

17 PSYCHOPATHY

Psychopathy is a persistent and pervasive disorder resulting in **recurrent antisocial behavior**. Unlike non-psychopathic antisocial personality disorder and the externalizing disorders of childhood (such as intermittent explosive disorder and disruptive mood dysregulation disorder) which are all characterized by *over*emotionality, psychopathy is characterized instead by a distinct *lack* of emotion and *absence* of empathy. These so-called **callous-unemotional traits** form a very reliable diagnostic construct which carries important implications for both prognosis and treatment. For this reason, it is essential to understand the concept of psychopathy when evaluating individuals with antisocial behavior.

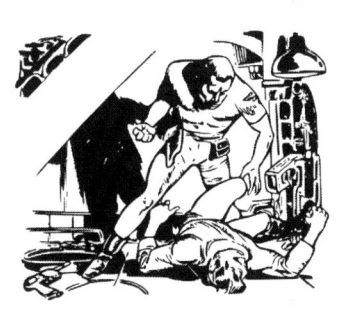

The terms **psychopathy** or **sociopathy** are often used interchangeably as an easy shorthand to describe the presence of callous-unemotional traits in adults diagnosed with antisocial personality disorder. However, just like with antisocial personality disorder, these terms are not used to describe someone under the age of 18 to avoid assigning a diagnosis viewed as "unchangeable" and "untreatable" to someone who is still in the process of developing. Nevertheless, most individuals with callous-unemotional traits begin to show signs during childhood which is highly predictive of later development of psychopathy as an adult. Because "callous-unemotional traits" and "psychopathy" refer to the same thing (except that the former can be used to refer to children and adolescents while the latter can not), for the most part we will use them interchangeably throughout this book. As a quick reminder, please remember that the term antisocial personality disorder, when used without a qualifier, should be assumed to mean *non-psychopathic* forms of the disorder (even though, strictly per DSM standards, psychopathic individuals would still be diagnosed with "antisocial personality disorder").

SIGNS AND SYMPTOMS OF PSYCHOPATHY

Despite the fact that psychopathy appears to be a separate condition from antisocial personality disorder, the DSM does feature any diagnostic criteria for it. Instead, most of what we know about psychopathy comes from other psychological assessment tools, with the most commonly used one being the Psychopathy Check List Revised (PCL-R). The signs and symptoms of psychopathy can generally be broken down into four distinct areas which you can remember using the mnemonic **BDSM**. (Please note that this is not intended to kink shame or imply that consensual erotic practices have anything to do with psychopathy! It is just a convenient, evocative, and not entirely unrelated mnemonic...)

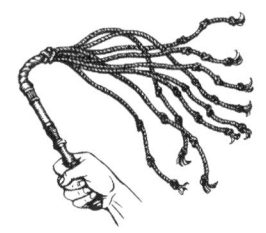

B is for Boldness. People with psychopathy often have a characteristic pattern of cognitive traits involving **boldness** or a high level of self-confidence, an above-average tolerance of danger, and a general fearlessness in many areas of life. Many people with psychopathy will put themselves into situations that would overwhelm most people with fear, such as breaking into someone else's house. They also appear to rebound quickly from even major punishments such as being arrested or thrown into jail. This fearlessness is involved in the recurrent nature of criminal acts in psychopathy, as the fear of being caught does not deter these people in the same way it does for most.

D is for Disinhibition. Psychopathy features a high degree of **disinhibition** as manifested in poor impulse control and difficulty with planning (a characteristic that it shares with non-psychopathic antisocial personality disorder as well). However, the specific behaviors seen in psychopathy differ significantly from "cluster B" antisocial personality disorder in both their **severity** and **purpose**. Psychopathic individuals tend to engage in more overtly violent behaviors such as assault, robbery, fraud, rape, and murder compared to the threats, petty theft, and fights that are more common in non-psychopathic forms of antisocial personality disorder. In addition, people with psychopathy often show a pattern of **criminal versatility** involving multiple types of offenses committed by the same person. In contrast to the emotion-driven reactive violence seen in antisocial personality disorder (such as coming home to find one's wife in bed with another man and proceeding to shoot both of them), people with psychopathy are more likely to engage in acts of predatory or "cold-blooded" **instrumental violence** involving some form of secondary gain (such as murdering a wealthy-looking stranger walking home on the street just to steal their purse). In fact, over 90% of homicides committed by psychopathic individuals are instrumental in nature compared to less than 50% for non-psychopathic offenders.

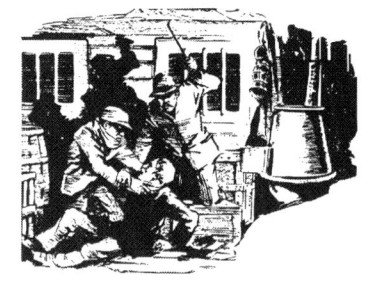

S is for Shallowness. The shallowness of the patient's emotional range is the biggest and most reliable difference between "garden variety" antisocial personality disorder and psychopathy. In contrast to the affective lability and chronic dysphoria seen in the former, people with psychopathy instead present with a highly restricted ability to feel emotions leading to **callousness** and **lack of empathy**. The lack of empathy is notable and profound, and many people with psychopathy appear unwilling or unable to understand the feelings of others. In particular, psychopathy appears to prevent someone from feeling the pain that they cause others, which explains why many of the most notorious serial killers in history often have psychopathy rather than "just" antisocial personality disorder (Ted Bundy, for example, scored 39/40 on the Psychopathy Check List). The callousness seen in psychopathy is also associated with a higher prevalence of **sadism**, as evidenced by the fact that over 80% of psychopathic individuals with a history of sexual homicide have engaged in some degree of sadistic behavior during the crime. Many psychopathic individuals also struggle with perpetual feelings of **boredom** and may engage in aggressive or unscrupulous acts simply to entertain themselves, such as manipulating someone into falling in love with them just to show that they can. The boredom that people with psychopathy experience is exacerbated by routine, which often leads to a pattern of **irresponsibility** and a **lack of long-term goals** like having a family or career. This frequently results in **parasitic behavior**, such as cheating and stealing from others, rather than providing for one's self in the usual ways.

M is for Meanness. While **meanness** doesn't *sound* like a clinical term, the word can accurately be used to describe the **interpersonal and social patterns** of people with psychopathy. When psychopathic individuals actually interact with other people (as opposed to, say, anonymously robbing them on the street), a host of distinct patterns are seen. Psychopathic individuals are often noted to be **superficially charming** and will engage in pleasantries when it suits them, such as flirting with or even beginning a relationship with someone in order to cheat them out of their money. Pathological **lying and deceit** are, unsurprisingly, quite common. Psychopathic individuals are generally very **manipulative** and can be highly skilled at influencing the emotions of others in order to maneuver themselves into an advantageous position. This *behavioral* pattern of aggressive resource-seeking goes hand in hand with a *cognitive* pattern of **self-importance** and outright narcissism that they use to justify their behaviors ("Someone's got to teach her the importance of not being so goddamn naïve, why not me?").

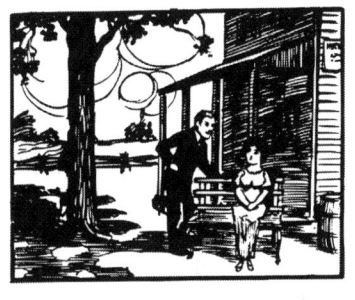

> **Psychopathy** involves a combination of **boldness, disinhibition, shallowness, and meanness** that leads to antisocial behavior.
>
> *BDSM:*
> *Boldness*
> *Disinhibition*
> *Shallowness*
> *Meanness*

PSYCHOPATHY ACROSS THE LIFESPAN

EPIDEMIOLOGY

Psychopathy is **rare** (thank goodness!), with estimates placing the prevalence at around 0.5% of the population. However, it is much more common in incarceral settings, with around 15% of all prisoners and 30% of violent prisoners showing signs of psychopathy. As with other disorders featuring aggressive behavior, psychopathy is significantly more common in **men** than women, with an even higher gender ratio (around 20 to 1) compared to non-psychopathic antisocial personality disorder.

Psychopathy is a **highly heritable** condition (possibly the *most* heritable in all of psychiatry, in fact!), with over 90% of the variance in psychopathic traits between individuals being attributable to genetic factors. This is even more pronounced than for non-psychopathic antisocial personality disorder (which is around 60% heritable) and the adolescent-limited form of externalization (which has very low heritability). However, even with a higher contribution from "nature" over "nurture," environment still matters a great deal, as the biological children of parents with psychopathy have lower rates of developing antisocial behavior themselves when the adoptive parents have provided appropriate behavioral reinforcement patterns.

Psychopathy is similar to antisocial personality disorder in that it cannot be diagnosed before the age of 18. However, the presence of callous-unemotional traits is noticeable **as early as childhood or even infancy**! In fact, people with callous-unemotional traits were often described as having a **difficult temperament** as babies, with incessant crying, irritability, lack of a social smile, and persistent hyperactivity. The nature of antisocial behavior often "evolves" as the child ages, with mild physical aggression such as biting and hitting seen during early childhood; stealing small objects, setting fires, and torturing animals during school age; bullying others and stealing larger objects such as cars during adolescence; and progressing to robbery, fraud, assault, and rape as an adult.

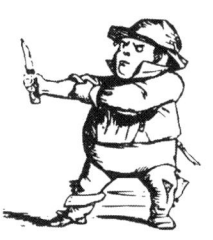

PROGNOSIS

Psychopathy has a **worse prognosis** than non-psychopathic antisocial personality disorder, with a higher severity of aggressive acts and higher rates of recidivism after punishment. Callous-unemotional traits show **considerable stability** over years and decades, even when assessed during childhood. Diagnostically, once someone is on the callous-unemotional trait "train," it is exceptionally hard to get off.

TREATMENT

Psychopathy is considered **very difficult to treat** using conventional psychiatric treatment approaches (even more so than non-psychopathic forms of antisocial personality disorder). There are **no medications** that have proven effective at changing the core personality traits associated with psychopathy or at reducing the frequency or severity of antisocial acts. While some medications (like anticonvulsants) are used to reduce reactive violence in non-psychopathic antisocial personality disorder, they rarely work here, as violent acts related to psychopathy are typically *instrumental* in nature rather than reactive.

Traditional **psychological therapies** are also quite limited in their efficacy, as patients with psychopathy tend to be less engaged in treatment, show little motivation for ongoing therapy, and demonstrate more limited improvement in almost all outcomes compared to non-psychopathic antisocial personality disorder. A large part of this may be attributed to **poor compliance with treatment**, as many people with psychopathic traits do not believe that they have a problem (their actions are ego-syntonic) and are often compelled to engage in treatment by the legal system rather than being intrinsically motivated to change on their own. Alarmingly, people with psychopathic traits who appear to be the *most* engaged in treatment are actually more likely to commit crimes again in the future (particularly violent or sexual crimes), suggesting that the *appearance* of treatment success may in and of itself be a marker of a worse prognosis (possibly as it suggests a greater degree of deceitfulness and manipulation). Despite incarceration and other legal punishments being used frequently in this population, it is unclear whether any forms of punishment are effective at treating psychopathy or reducing rates of violence in this population, particularly when you consider the boldness and fearlessness that are intrinsic traits of psychopathy.

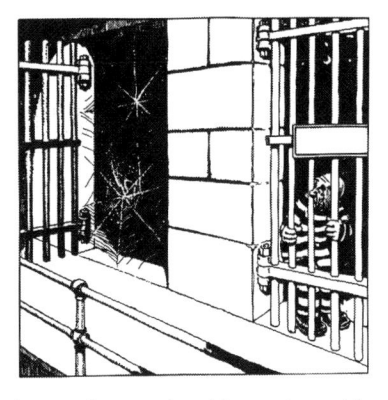

MECHANISMS OF PSYCHOPATHY

On a mechanistic level, a couple of neurobiological differences have been found in cases of psychopathy. Research has consistently found that psychopathic individuals **lack intrinsic empathic ability** and do not experience the same aversive reactions to the pain and distress of others that most people do. Consider the following image:

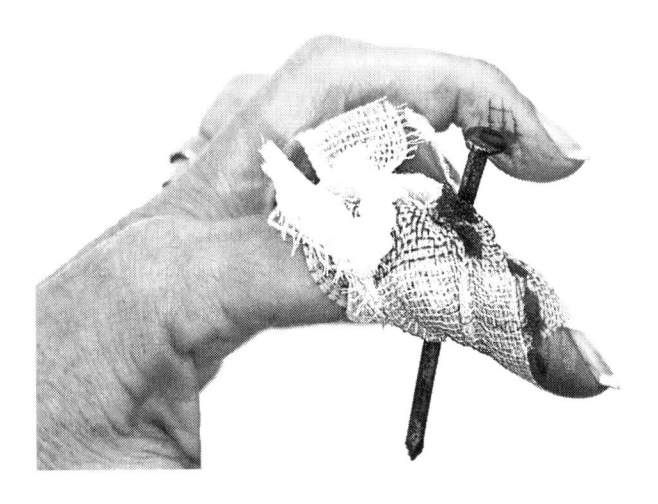

For most people, even just looking at the picture will provoke an automatic emotional reaction that is experienced as painful (it is even processed in the same parts of the brain that register pain signals even though no actual injury has occurred!). Someone with psychopathy, however, will not automatically experience a negative emotional reaction to seeing someone else in pain, and these parts of the brain stay turned "off" when watching other people in distress. This insensitivity appears to be related to structural and functional differences in how the **amygdala** processes fear and facial expressions. Interestingly, people with psychopathic traits are not necessarily *unable* to empathize with the feelings of others, as the regions of the brain associated with empathy did turn "on" when they were specifically asked to consider how others felt. Instead, it appears that the empathic networks of the brain are **"off" by default**, even if they can be activated with effort. This explains why people with psychopathic tendencies have the ability to be very charming and manipulative even while engaging in acts of destruction or violence, as they can turn on their "empathic switch" when it suits them and leave it off the rest of the time.

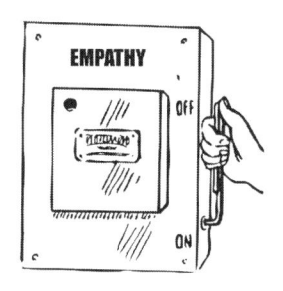

The other characteristic neurobiological difference that is seen in psychopathy is an inherent trait of **fearlessness** which appears to separate psychopathy from "cluster B" antisocial personality disorder as reliably as an "off by default" empathic switch. Individuals with psychopathy do not experience fear in the same way that most people do, with some evidence even suggesting that there is *reduced* activity of the sympathetic nervous system and HPA axis in these people (which stands in stark contrast to the usual pattern seen in anxiety, depression, and other internalizing disorders). This fearlessness accounts for the boldness and tolerance of unfamiliarity that is a core feature of psychopathy. Fearlessness makes psychopathy a particular challenge for the legal system, as most societies try to prevent antisocial behavior through the fear of punishment (such as the threat of imprisonment or death). If psychopaths lack fear, however, then these punishments would not work, and that is exactly what we see: imprisonment and other punishments appear to have little effect on preventing future crimes. This has led to the widespread belief that psychopaths do not respond to rewards and punishments. However, this is not true, as psychopaths clearly make decisions based on the relative rewards available to them. Where they differ is in *how* they respond to rewards and punishments.

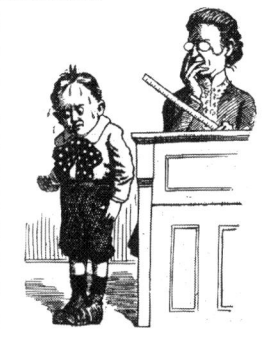

Let's return to the example of the cookie jar that we first brought up in the chapter on addiction. The cookie serves as a positive reinforcer that most children would find pleasurable to eat. To prevent spoiling their appetite, however, a parent will threaten some kind of punishment (like a swift *wap!* on the hand with a ruler) to anyone who eats it early. Under this sort of threat, a child with a normal reward processing system will experience significant anxiety and autonomic arousal while approaching the cookie jar. The level of anxiety gets higher and higher as they approach the cookie jar, and for many children this anxiety reaches a critical point where it becomes aversive enough *in and of itself* to make them walk away. For these children, the *threat itself* is enough of a positive punishment to modify their behavior. In addition, by walking away from the cookie jar, this anxiety rapidly dissipates (a negative reinforcement for the "good behavior" of not taking a cookie).

In contrast, someone with psychopathy-related fearlessness would *not* experience any sort of anxiety as they approach the cookie jar, so there is no built-in positive punishment just for thinking about it. In fact, for these children walking *away* from the cookie jar is associated with *more* anxiety than walking towards it due to the feeling that they have lost out on the opportunity to get the cookie. This makes "doing the right thing" for these children associated with *positive punishment* rather than negative reinforcement! In contrast, if they actually go through with it and take a cookie, then they are both *positively* reinforced by the taste of the cookie as well as *negatively* reinforced by avoidance of "lost opportunity anxiety." In this way, trait-based fearlessness sets up the decisional calculus in such a way that following the rules is actually *punished* while acting selfishly is rewarded. This **differential response to rewards and punishments** can be seen at a very early age and is predictive of future conduct problems as an adolescent and adult.

To use a real-world example, a "normal" adult without psychopathic traits who is experiencing hard times may get the idea that they could hold someone at gunpoint to steal their wallet. However, in deciding whether or not to do this, they would balance the reward (money) against the punishment (including not only anxiety about going to jail but also the extremely unpleasant physiologic and psychological distress of seeing someone else in pain that would occur whether they got caught or not). Based on these factors, this person would likely decide *against* robbing someone at gunpoint, as the money is not worth the possibility of punishment or the guaranteed aversive emotional reaction. In contrast, someone with psychopathy would be more likely to choose to go ahead with it as they are not aversively affected by the pain and distress of others. For them, the only thing offsetting the prospect of a financial reward is the chance of getting caught (which is itself reduced or even negated by the trait-based fearlessness). With these two physiological and psychological differences in play, it makes some sense why people with psychopathic traits decide to engage in antisocial behavior.

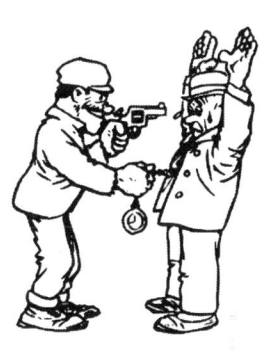

This specific cognitive profile of both an **"off by default" empathic switch** and an underlying trait of **fearlessness** results in the insensitivity to traditional punishments that is seen in people with psychopathy which often prevents efforts at rehabilitating them to live by the rules of society. This combination also provides a diagnostic focus that differentiates people with psychopathy from other forms of misbehavior like non-psychopathic antisocial personality disorder as well as the childhood-onset externalizing disorders like intermittent explosive disorder.

HOW TO DIAGNOSE PSYCHOPATHY

Psychopathy is not recognized as a diagnosis in the DSM. Instead, all patients with psychopathic traits would get a diagnosis of antisocial personality disorder (provided they are over the age of 18). In reality, only around 10% of those who meet criteria for antisocial personality disorder have psychopathic traits. In the absence of discrete DSM criteria, specific **diagnostic assessments** for psychopathy (like the Psychopathy Checklist mentioned earlier) can be used to more formally evaluate the presence of psychopathic traits.

DIFFERENTIAL DIAGNOSIS OF PSYCHOPATHY

Misdiagnoses for psychopathy are generally limited to the other diagnostic categories characterized by bad behavior: externalizing disorders and ADHD. Missed diagnoses are relatively rare, as the fearlessness seen in psychopathy appears to actually *protect* against many common mental disorders like depression and anxiety.

NORMALCY

It's difficult to imagine how a disorder characterized by violent acts and a lack of empathy could be on the spectrum of normalcy. This is because most people with psychopathic traits who come to clinical attention do so through the legal system, which by definition only captures those who have gotten in trouble with the law. However, studies have found that a significant minority of people have callous-unemotional traits but do *not* engage in violent or criminal behavior. These people generally have the same abnormalities in brain regions linked to empathy, moral decision-making, and impulse control seen in psychopathic criminals, yet many spend their days raising a family and holding a job. Through this, we see once again that *it's never just one thing*. Even for someone with a genetic vulnerability towards callous-unemotional traits, a stable and nurturing can mitigate the potential for damage and allow them to be funneled into more pro-social activities. If anything, some degree of fearlessness may actually be adaptive in risky or competitive fields such as business and finance where boldness can give one a competitive advantage!

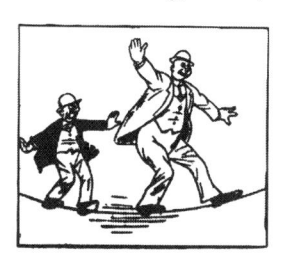

ANTISOCIAL PERSONALITY DISORDER

We've gone over the differences between psychopathy and "garden variety" antisocial personality disorder many times in this chapter already, so we won't rehash those details here. Using the **PIRATES** mnemonic, psychopathy is distinguished primarily by its **P**urpose (more frequent use of instrumental violence), **R**emorse (generally lacking), **E**motion (a shallow range of emotion rather than affective lability), and **S**everity (more frequent and violent antisocial behavior).

ATTENTION DEFICIT HYPERACTIVITY DISORDER
ADHD can also present with disruptive behavior beginning in childhood. In contrast to psychopathy, however, misbehavior in ADHD is **unintentional**.

ADDICTION
Addiction is the main exception to the rule that missed diagnoses are rare in psychopathy, as up to two-thirds of all people with psychopathy have an addictive disorder. It is likely that the fearlessness of psychopathy is directly responsible for this finding, as the anxiety about legal consequences or other negative repercussions that holds many people back from using substances is not effective here.

PSYCHOSIS
While people with schizophrenia are more likely to be victims of violence than perpetrators, a small minority of people with schizophrenia do engage in violence. This can occasionally be confused with psychopathy, as these violent acts can be premeditated and planned (in contrast to the reactive aggression seen in non-psychopathic antisocial personality disorder). The key difference is that premeditated violence in schizophrenia is almost always related to a **delusional belief system**, whereas in psychopathy the primary objective is more often instrumental in nature.

TRAUMA
Histories of mistreatment during early childhood (including both abuse and neglect) are frequently found in adults with psychopathic traits. However, this does not necessarily result in higher rates of trauma-related disorders like PTSD in this population. In fact, the boldness and fearlessness that are core traits of this disorder (combined with *hypo*reactivity of the HPA axis) may make comorbidity with PTSD, which is often characterized by an *over*active fear response and *hyper*reactivity of the HPA axis, much less likely. Nevertheless, while PTSD in its narrowly defined form may be rare, it can still be helpful to take a trauma history in patients presenting with psychopathy, if for no other reason than to try and understand better where they have come from in life (although be cautious as this can inadvertently provide the patient with an easy way to deceive or manipulate you!).

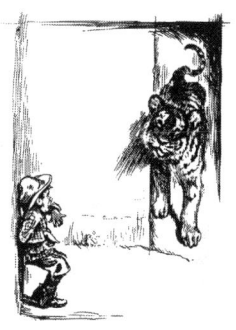

OBSESSIVE-COMPULSIVE DISORDERS
Intrusive thoughts related to obsessive-compulsive disorder can often be of an intensely aggressive nature (including thoughts of murder or sexual violence). However, it's important to point out that (consistent with the I MURDER? mnemonic) these thoughts are distinctly **ego-dystonic**, and people with OCD rarely if ever actually act on the thoughts. (Many will even go to great lengths to avoid situations that could possibly lead to this behavior such as removing all knives or other sharp objects from their home.) People with violent thoughts related to OCD often are quite motivated to seek help as well, which contrasts with the poor treatment motivation seen in psychopathy.

MANIA
People in a manic state may act in a way that harms others or infringes on their rights either through impulsive recklessness (such as driving while under the influence) or by seeing other people as acceptable collateral damage in the service of a goal-oriented activity. However, this behavior will be limited to the time of a mood episode (in contrast to psychopathic traits which are relatively stable across the lifespan).

PUTTING IT ALL TOGETHER

Despite not being recognized as its own disorder in the DSM, psychopathy is a **consistent and enduring diagnostic construct** with important implications for prognosis and treatment. Use the **BDSM** mnemonic to remember the pattern of **B**oldness, behavioral **D**isinhibition, emotional **S**hallowness, and interpersonal **M**eanness that characterizes patients with psychopathy. When evaluating anyone presenting with concerns about disruptive or antisocial behavior, use the **PIRATES** mnemonic to systematically describe the nature of their behavior. While the presence of callous-unemotional traits is associated with an incredibly poor prognosis, that does not mean that you should ever "give up" on a patient with this condition. Indeed, the fact that some people with psychopathic traits appear to function well in society suggests that there is always hope.

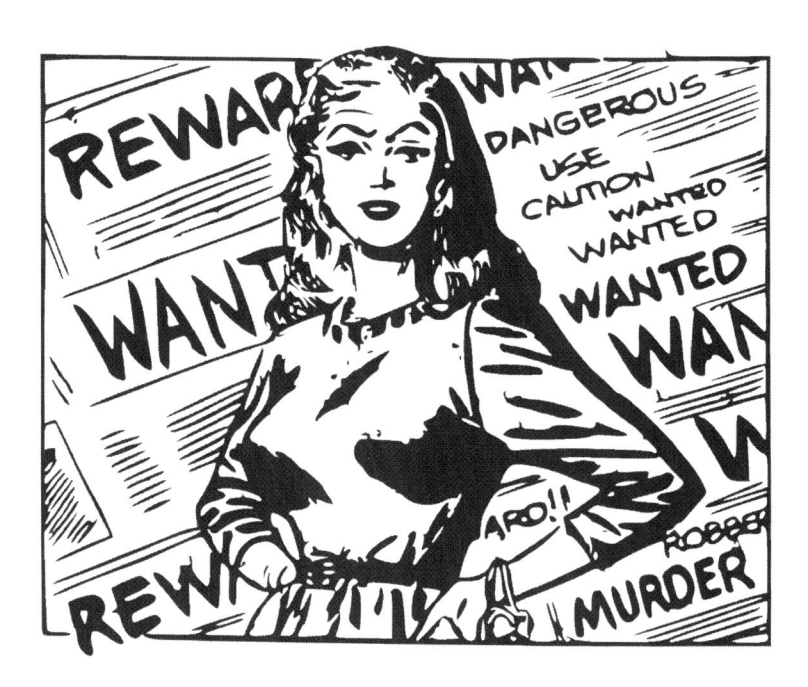

REVIEW QUESTIONS

1. A 25 y/o M is interviewed by a forensic psychiatrist in a maximum security prison. He was sentenced to life in prison after DNA evidence linked him to the rapes and murders of 5 women over a 7 year period. During the interview, the patient gives simple and straightforward answers to the questions he is asked with no perceptible change in affect even when describing details of his victims' murders. Electrophysiologic testing reveals a lack of perspiration when exposed to an anxiety-provoking situation. Which of the following behaviors is this patient *least* likely to have participated in?
   A. Hitting a stranger in the head and stealing their hand bag
   B. Losing control and slapping a significant other during a tense argument
   C. Using a knife to intentionally inflict pain upon his victims
   D. Memorizing a stranger's credit card number to make a large purchase
   E. All of the above are equally likely

2. (Continued from previous question.) Which of the following most likely describes this patient's pattern of neuroanatomical activity in response to situations involving the pain and distress of others?
   A. Decreased in both the amygdala and HPA axis
   B. Decreased in the amygdala but increased in the HPA axis
   C. Increased in the amygdala but decreased in the HPA axis
   D. Increased in both the amygdala and HPA axis
   E. None of the above

3. (Continued from previous question.) Which of the following statements about this patient's childhood is most likely true?
   A. He exhibited no interpersonal or behavioral problems until the age of 18
   B. He exhibited no interpersonal or behavioral problems until the age of 13
   C. He exhibited no interpersonal or behavioral problems until the age of 8
   D. At least one parent likely had callous-unemotional traits
   E. None of the above are true

4. A 39 y/o M works as a stock trader at a large financial investment company. He has a reputation as a fearless trader who "never breaks a sweat" even when making multi-million dollar transactions. He was orphaned as an infant and was raised by adoptive parents from the age of 3. However, he has not seen them in over 20 years since moving to the city and reports no feelings of closeness to them. He is single and lives alone. He reports no interest in pursuing friendships or romantic relationships. Hobbies include base jumping and playing poker. Which of the following is the most likely diagnosis?
   A. Psychopathic antisocial personality disorder
   B. Non-psychopathic antisocial personality disorder
   C. Narcissistic personality disorder
   D. Avoidant personality disorder
   E. None of the above

1. **The best answer is B.** People with psychopathy are more likely to engage in antisocial behaviors characterized by instrumental violence with a clear secondary gain (answers A and D). They are also more likely than average to engage in sadistic acts (answer C). In contrast, due to their lower emotional range they are less likely to engage in reactive violence such as striking a partner during an emotional argument.

2. **The best answer is A.** Studies on people with psychopathic traits have revealed key differences in two functional areas of the brain: the amygdala, which is less responsive to the pain and distress of others, and the hypothalamic–pituitary–adrenal axis, which is less likely to activate in response to fear-inducing or stressful situations. The combination of these differences leads to the boldness and meanness that are commonly seen in people with this condition.

3. **The best answer is D.** Callous-unemotional traits are often apparent even from early childhood although the nature and degree of antisocial behavior tends to increase in severity as one ages (answers A, B, and C). These traits are among the most heritable of all traits seen in mental health settings, with over 90% of the variance between individuals being explained by genetic differences. Therefore, it is likely that one or more parents showed evidence of having callous-unemotional traits even if they did not necessarily meet criteria for a disorder.

4. **The best answer is E.** This person may have some degree of callous-unemotional traits as evidenced by his fearlessness and boldness in both his work and his hobbies. However, there is no indication of antisocial behavior of any kind, ruling out a diagnosis of antisocial personality disorder even if callous-unemotional traits are present (answers A and B). It is possible that he has narcissistic traits as well, but this is not clear from the vignette (answer C). It is unlikely for him to have avoidant personality disorder as people with this condition generally *desire* to have relationships with others (answer D).

18 EATING DISORDERS

An eating disorder is a pattern of **dysfunctional food intake** that has the potential to jeopardize one's physical and/or mental health. Classically, this term has been used primarily to refer to **anorexia nervosa** and **bulimia nervosa**, although there are other patterns of disordered eating (such as binge eating) that are now recognized in the DSM as well. Because they directly impact the ability of the body to maintain physical health, eating disorders are among the most harmful and destructive of all mental disorders.

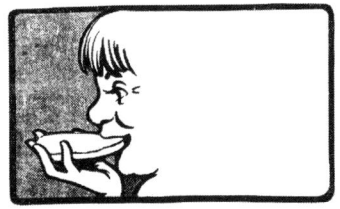

Both anorexia and bulimia follow a similar pattern involving two things: **overvalued beliefs about weight** ("I am fat") as well as the **maladaptive behaviors** that follow (such as restricting food intake or vomiting after eating). From there, however, the similarities between the two disorders quickly end. In fact, while anorexia and bulimia are often lumped together in the general category of eating disorders, in practice there are so many differences between the two that it is helpful to conceive of them as **entirely separate disorders** despite the fact that they both involve eating habits. What is crucial to understand is that the line separating these two disorders does not lie in the specifics of the behavior involved. While popular conceptions generally hold that "restricting = anorexia" and "vomiting = bulimia," the fact of the matter is that neither of these behaviors is diagnostic of either condition (as some cases of anorexia involve purging and some cases of bulimia involve restricting). Instead, what differs between these disorders is not the *content* of the behavior but rather the *context* by which those behaviors come about, as we will find out over the following chapter.

ANOREXIA NERVOSA

Anorexia nervosa is a condition in which people **perceive themselves to be overweight** even when they are **severely underweight** by any objective standard. This perception causes them to make changes to their eating habits such as restricting food intake to include only "healthy" or low calorie foods ("Did you know that eating celery actually *burns* more calories than it gives?"). In severe cases, food intake can be eliminated altogether. These restrictions in diet are often accompanied by other **weight loss behaviors** including excessive exercise, self-induced vomiting, and/or abuse of laxatives. Even when these measures are successful at inducing weight loss, however, someone with anorexia *still* perceives themselves as being overweight and will continue their efforts, leading to further weight loss, malnutrition, and eventually even starvation. The key to understanding anorexia (as opposed to normal efforts at losing weight) is that the patient's **self-perception is distorted**, and no amount of weight loss ever convinces the person that they are at an appropriate weight. This leads to an endless loop between thoughts about appearance and attempts to lose weight. You can remember the core patterns of anorexia by thinking of it as **UNDER**-rexia which stands for the patient being **U**nderweight (which is a required part of the diagnosis), being abnormally **N**ervous or fearful about gaining weight, having **D**istorted perceptions about their weight and their health, engaging in **E**xercise, purging, or other behaviors to interfere with weight gain, and finally **R**estricting caloric intake through food avoidance or other means.

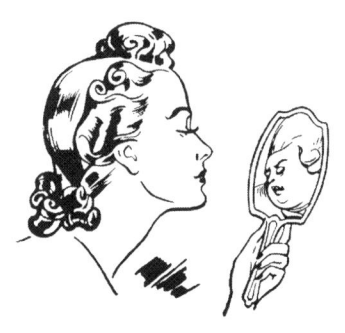

> **Anorexia nervosa** is defined by a pattern of **distorted perception of weight** leading to **food restriction and avoidance** in a significantly **underweight** patient.
>
> *UNDER-rexia:*
> *Underweight*
> *Nervous/fearful about gaining weight*
> *Distorted perceptions about weight*
> *Exercise, purging, or other behaviors*
> *Restricting caloric intake*

Anorexia is a **relatively rare** condition that is found in less than 0.5% of the population. **Women** are affected by anorexia 10 times as often as men. Anorexia often begins around the time of **puberty and young adulthood**, with a median age of onset of 18 years. Social circumstances that can produce extreme pressure to be thin (such as participating in modeling or dancing) are associated with higher rates of anorexia, suggesting that environmental and social factors play a large role in the pathogenesis of the disorder.

The prognosis for anorexia is variable, with some people only engaging in transient episodes of food restriction while others avoid food entirely for weeks or months at a time. Complete elimination of food intake can lead to a state of severe malnutrition which can negatively impact every organ system in the body. People with anorexia often develop various medical problems including fatigue, amenorrhea, infertility, osteoporosis, electrolyte abnormalities, and cardiac arrhythmias, and it is not uncommon for someone with severe anorexia to end up in the hospital due to medical complications from persistent malnutrition. Even when this happens, however, people with anorexia will often deny that anything is wrong and will continue to refuse food, leading to a state of total starvation in which damage to essential organ systems begins to occur. Because of the associated medical complications (as well as a not-insignificant risk of suicide), anorexia is the **single most deadly mental illness**, with up 20% of people dying as a result of the disorder (with 5% dying within a decade of the initial diagnosis).

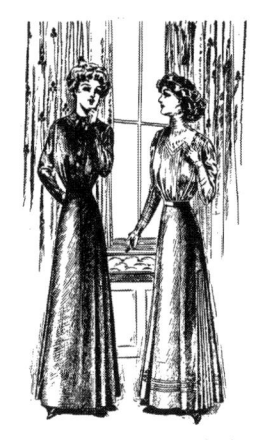

Treatment of anorexia involves **nutritional rehabilitation**, **monitoring for medical complications** of malnutrition, and engaging in **psychotherapy** (with no specific form of therapy having been shown to be more or less helpful than any other). Medications play a very limited role in treatment of anorexia, as none have been shown to improve any clinically significant outcomes. Even with full effort on the part of the clinician, however, anorexia is considered to be a particularly **difficult disorder to treat**, as the ego-syntonic nature of the condition frequently makes patients reluctant to engage in treatment ("Why should I go to therapy? *I'm* fine, it's everyone else in this corn-addicted country who's got an issue!").

Treating malnutrition related to anorexia is not as simple as sending someone to the nearest all-you-can-eat buffet. While you might think that the goal would be to get someone who is severely malnourished back to their normal weight as fast as possible, in practice this is a terrible idea, as people in a state of starvation are at high risk of severe complications related to re-initation of nutrition, a condition known as **refeeding syndrome**. Re**ph**eeding syndrome is a potentially **ph**atal condition that occurs in up to 20% of patients hospitalized for anorexia in which reinitiation of food provokes severe complications, including hypokalemia, vitamin deficiencies, swelling, muscle breakdown, seizures, hemolysis, heart failure, and even death. The hallmark of re**ph**eeding syndrome is hypo**ph**osphatemia which is the direct cause of most of the ensuing abnormalities. In someone with chronic malnutrition, phosphate stores are already low. When they are suddenly fed again, insulin is released which causes further uptake of phosphate into cells and leads to even greater hypophosphatemia. The low availability of phosphate prevents metabolic intermediates from being produced, leading to hypoxia and muscle dysfunction. This is particularly bad for the myocardium and the dia**ph**ragm, and death can rapidly occur when these organs shut down. Given the potential for serious adverse outcomes, re**ph**eeding should be done with serious **ph**orethought!

In someone with **severe malnutrition** as a result of anorexia nervosa, always **reinitiate feeding slowly** to avoid **refeeding syndrome**.

*Re**ph**eeding syndrome is a potentially **ph**atal condition caused by hypo**ph**osphatemia.*

Because of the potentially deadly nature of both severe malnutrition and the complications of refeeding, inpatient medical hospitalization may be required in some cases of anorexia. While there are no consistently agreed upon guidelines for when to admit someone, the mnemonic **CRAVE** can help you to remember specific signs that should make you at least consider hospitalization, including **C**ardiac complications such as breakdown of the heart muscle and slowed electrical conduction; **R**enal injury from dehydration related to excessive exercise or abuse of laxatives; **A**rrhythmias such as an abnormally slow or fast heart rate; **V**ital sign instability such hypotension or hypothermia; and **E**lectrolyte imbalances such as hypokalemia or hypoglycemia.

Consider **hospitalizing patients with anorexia** who develop **cardiac** complications, **renal** insufficiency, or **electrolyte abnormalities**.

*Remember the **CRAVE** criteria for considering medical hospitalization in anorexia:*
***C**ardiac*
***R**enal*
***A**rrhythmias*
***V**ital signs*
***E**lectrolytes*

Mechanistically, anorexia is best understood through the lens of **obsessive-compulsive disorders** as it involves obsessive thoughts about appearance that lead to specific compulsive behaviors (such as food restriction and excessive exercise) intended to help calm these thoughts. Just like in obsessive-compulsive disorders, however, no amount of weight loss ever leads to that "feeling of knowing" that one is finally thin enough. Neurobiological studies have shown that anorexia and OCD both are associated with structural and functional abnormalities in the anterior cingulate cortex. Despite these similarities, however, anorexia differs from OCD in a few key ways. Most prominently, the obsession with weight is distinctly **ego-syntonic** rather than ego-dystonic, as the person does not view their attempts at losing weight as being in any way excessive or dysfunctional. From this perspective, anorexia may actually be closer to obsessive-compulsive *personality* disorder than OCD itself, which is reflected in higher rates of comorbidity with obsessive-compulsive personality disorder than "textbook" OCD. Anorexia also shares with obsessive-compulsive personality disorder a characteristic **rigidity of behavior** (patients will often eat the same thing at the same time every day with little variation) and a **high level of conscientiousness** that plays directly into the distorted beliefs at the heart of the condition ("I am fat, and it is *wrong* to be fat").

BULIMIA NERVOSA

Bulimia nervosa is a pattern of disordered eating that involves episodes of impulsive **binge eating** (or consuming large amounts of food in a short amount of time) over which the patient feels like they have very little control. These binges are followed by **purging** (or compensatory behaviors intended to prevent the food that has just been binged from being absorbed into the body as calories). While self-induced vomiting is the most common form of purging, it is not the only one, and people with bulimia will often engage in other behaviors that serve the same purpose (such as frequent use of laxatives). In between binge eating episodes, almost all people with bulimia engage in dieting and food restriction (although this is not required for a diagnosis of bulimia in the DSM). Like anorexia, the disordered eating behaviors are accompanied by distress about feeling overweight. For someone with bulimia, however, concerns about being overweight are often rooted in **extreme interpersonal rejection sensitivity** ("If I am fat, then other people will not like me").

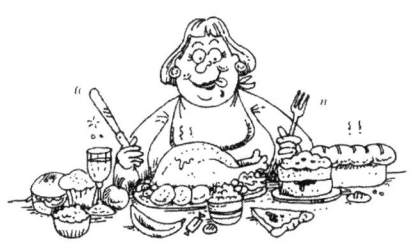

You can remember the overall pattern here by picturing a **BOWL** of ice cream and thinking of the name as **BOWL**-imia which should remind you of impulsive and out of control **B**inges where the patient eats lots of food at once and then engages in **O**ffsetting behaviors where they try to purge the food and its associated calories through vomiting, laxatives, or other means. Per DSM criteria, these episodes must have happened at least **W**eekly for a period of 3 months. Unlike anorexia which is linked to distorted *perceptions* of weight, in bulimia the core psychological pattern is that the patient has **L**inked their *self-esteem* to their weight and worries that being overweight will lead to them being rejected or alone.

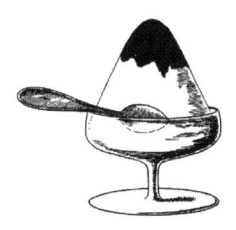

Bulimia nervosa is characterized by **impulsive binge eating** followed by **compulsive purging** to remove the food.

BOWL-imia:
Binges (impulsive, out of control)
Offsetting behaviors (purging)
Weekly for at least 3 months
Linked to self-esteem

The prevalence of bulimia in the general population is around 1%, making it **relatively rare** (though still twice as common as anorexia). Like anorexia, bulimia is diagnosed more than 10 times as often in **women** compared to men. The age of onset is roughly the same, with the patterns of bulimia beginning in **adolescence or early adulthood**. In contrast to anorexia (where someone must be underweight to be diagnosed), in bulimia most people have a **normal weight or are even slightly** overweight. A variety of findings from the physical exam can argue for the presence of active purging, including erosion of dental enamel, swollen salivary glands, and injuries on the back of the knuckles from scraping against the teeth during self-induced vomiting.

Bulimia has a variable prognosis, with some people being able to stop bingeing and purging on their own while others require intensive treatment. Ten years after their initial diagnosis, about half of people with bulimia will have recovered fully, one third will have made a partial recovery, and 10 to 20% will still have disordered eating habits. Medically, self-induced vomiting is associated with significant health problems, including dehydration (leading to tachycardia and hypotension), electrolyte abnormalities (leading to disorientation and seizures), metabolic alkalosis related to loss of stomach acid, and gastric ulcers. Frequent vomiting can also damage the esophagus which can then rupture (known as **Boerhaave syndrome**). However, as a general rule the medical complications associated with bulimia are generally not as severe as those seen in anorexia, and the mortality rate is significantly lower.

Frequent self-induced vomiting can lead to **esophageal ruptures** which is known as **Boerhaave syndrome**.

*Boer**H**aave syndrome = **B**een **H**eaving syndrome.*

Effective treatment for bulimia does exist, as **both medications and therapy** appear to be effective (with a combination of the two being superior to either alone). In particular, **CBT** and a form of psychotherapy known as **interpersonal therapy** are both associated with improvements in symptoms with a **moderate effect size**. SRIs are also helpful, with a **small effect size**. Of note, certain medications (like bupropion, a non-serotonergic antidepressant) must be absolutely avoided for patients with bulimia who are actively vomiting, as they may increase the risk of seizures.

On a mechanistic level, the presence of interpersonal rejection sensitivity should immediately remind you of **borderline personality disorder** and other cluster B personality disorders. Indeed, the comorbidity between these two disorders is incredibly high (over 50%), and people with bulimia share so many other features with borderline personality disorder (including impulsivity, chronic dysphoria, poor self-esteem, and extreme fear of abandonment) that it seems reasonable to suggest that in many cases bulimia can be thought of as following similar mechanisms as that condition. Interestingly, people with bulimia appear to have an exaggerated endogenous opioid response to food, which provides a clear mechanistic link to the underlying pathophysiology of borderline personality disorder.

Bulimia nervosa is highly comorbid with **borderline personality disorder**.

*Associate **B**ulimia with **B**orderline and other cluster **B** personality disorders!*

BINGE EATING DISORDER

Binge eating disorder is listed as a separate diagnosis in the DSM, but in practice it is similar in nearly every way to bulimia except that the bingeing episodes are *not* followed by compensatory purging behavior. However, the overall pattern of the disorder (including a strong association with cluster B personality disorders) is very similar to bulimia, and the treatments used are generally the same. Due to the lack of compensatory purging, people with binge eating disorder are often **quite overweight** (as compared to underweight in anorexia and normal weight in bulimia). Interestingly, binge eating disorder is equally prevalent in **men and women**, suggesting that purging as a specific compensatory behavior likely has a large learned component. Binge eating disorder has a better prognosis compared to bulimia, with 80% of people being in remission at 5 years. With all of this in mind, it is perhaps best to conceptualize binge eating disorder as a less severe variant of bulimia *without* compensatory behaviors (similar to how agoraphobia is seen as a more severe variant of panic disorder *with* compensatory behaviors). Because of this, we will lump binge eating disorder together with bulimia for the rest of this book.

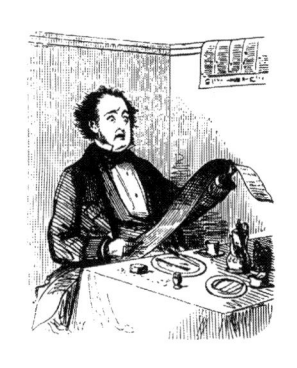

HOW TO DIAGNOSE EATING DISORDERS

When diagnosing eating disorders, keep in mind that patients will not always meet DSM criteria for either anorexia or bulimia. In fact, an eating disorder "not otherwise specified" is the most common diagnosis in this category! For this reason, don't get too hung up on exact criteria and instead focus on the overall pattern of eating.

Clinically, you can use the acronym **SCOFF** to screen for eating disorders. Answering "yes" to 2 or more of these questions is suggestive of an eating disorder:

"Do you make yourself **S**ick because you feel uncomfortably full?"
"Do you worry that you have lost **C**ontrol over how much you eat?"
"Have you recently lost more than **O**ne stone (14 lbs.) in a 3-month period?"
"Do you believe yourself to be **F**at when others say you are too thin?"
"Would you say that **F**ood dominates your life?"

Screening for eating disorders can be done in **just a few questions**.

SCOFF ("yes" to 2 or more is a positive screen):
*Feel **S**ick/uncomfortably full?*
*Lost **C**ontrol over eating?*
*Lost **O**ne stone of weight recently?*
*Feel **F**at when others say you are thin?*
*Feel that **F**ood dominates your life?*

While the SCOFF criteria can help to identify the presence of *an* eating disorder, they do not differentiate between anorexia and bulimia which is important to do given the differences in prognosis and treatment between them. Because the specific *behaviors* involved do not differentiate between anorexia and bulimia (as some people with anorexia purge while some people with bulimia restrict), it can be helpful to focus on the actual points of difference. Use the phrase **P**eanut **B**utter **I**ce **C**ream to tease apart the two disorders:

P is for Perceptions. Anorexia results from a **distorted self-perception** (as the person is actually *under*weight despite perceiving otherwise) while someone with bulimia or binge eating disorder who thinks they are fat may actually just have an accurate self-perception. For this reason, someone's body weight can be an easy way to distinguish between the different eating disorders, as people with anorexia must be underweight, people with bulimia are often a normal weight or slightly overweight, and people with binge eating disorder are generally overweight.

B is for Beliefs. People with anorexia and bulimia hold vastly different **fundamental beliefs about weight**. Someone with anorexia is more likely to believe that it is *wrong* to be fat. For someone with anorexia, being fat isn't just a matter of not looking attractive enough—it is a fundamental *error*, an aberration, a moral insult. In contrast, someone with bulimia does not necessarily feel distress about their weight due to an overactive error recognition system. Instead, beliefs about weight are related to their fear that being overweight will impair their ability to be loved and accepted by others.

IC is for Impulsivity vs Compulsivity. Finally, anorexia and bulimia differ in regards to the underlying **reasons for engaging in disordered eating**. Food-related behaviors in anorexia are highly *compulsive*, and people with anorexia often exert an incredibly **high degree of control** over their behavior. In contrast, food intake in bulimia is primarily *impulsive*, and people with this disorder often report a distinct **lack of control** over eating due to deficits in impulse control (as they are unable to resist the high level of **im**mediate **pos**itive reinforcement that foods, especially sweet or fatty foods like cake, are able to provide). While many people with bulimia will also engage in compulsive behaviors to lose weight, the purging would not be necessary if it were not for the impulse bingeing that starts off the chain reaction.

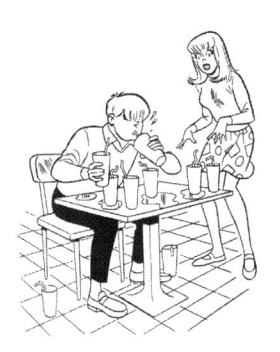

Anorexia and bulimia can be differentiated on the basis of **self-perceptions**, **beliefs about weight**, and **reasons for disordered eating**.

Peanut Butter Ice Cream:
*P*erceptions
*B*eliefs
*I*mpulsivity vs *C*ompulsivity

DIFFERENTIAL DIAGNOSIS OF EATING DISORDERS

Because the presence of disordered eating (including restriction, avoidance, bingeing, and purging) is fairly specific to eating disorders, misdiagnoses are rare. Nevertheless, it is important to be mindful of the way that other psychiatric syndromes can interact with appetite and eating patterns to avoid coming to the wrong diagnosis. Further, because both anorexia and bulimia share core mechanisms with other disorders (OCD and obsessive-compulsive personality disorder for anorexia and borderline personality disorder and addiction for bulimia), comorbidity is incredibly common, so make sure to be on the lookout for missed diagnoses.

NORMALCY

Desires to be thin or avoid overeating are not pathological. Indeed, restricting caloric intake to some degree would probably be beneficial for most people in industrialized countries where obesity is a bigger problem than hunger. In addition, many societies place a high degree of pressure on individuals (and women in particular) to meet unrealistic standards of beauty. Because of this, normalcy should always be on the differential for anyone with restricted food intake patterns, and no one should be diagnosed with an eating disorder on the basis of trying to lose weight alone.

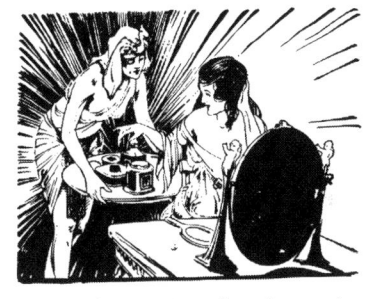

Instead, try to focus on the underlying process of each disorder (a distorted body image leading to compulsive behaviors in anorexia, and interpersonal rejection sensitivity combined with high impulsivity leading to bingeing and purging in bulimia) to make the call. Someone with disordered eating habits that are quickly corrected with simple education on what healthy eating involves is also unlikely to have either anorexia or bulimia, as by definition these disorders are characterized by specific cognitive distortions that prevent easy fixes.

BODY DYSMORPHIC DISORDER

It's easy to confuse anorexia and body dysmorphic disorder, as both involve an obsessive preoccupation with perceived bodily disfigurement leading to compulsive behaviors focused on appearance. In fact, some have argued that anorexia should be seen as a particular form of body dysmorphic disorder that is focused on weight rather than a specific body part. However, a few lines of evidence argue against the idea that anorexia is simply a form of body dysmorphic disorder, including differences in gender ratio (female-predominant in anorexia versus equal in body dysmorphic disorder) and treatment response (CBT and SRIs working for body dysmorphic disorder but not for anorexia). While the precise reasons are unclear, on a neurobiological level an obsessional preoccupation with *thinness* seems to differ enough from an obsessional preoccupation with *disfigurement* in specific parts of the body that the two warrant separate diagnoses.

OBSESSIVE-COMPULSIVE DISORDERS
As discussed previously, anorexia overlaps considerably with OCD to an extent that it is perhaps best understood within an obsessive-compulsive framework. The rate of comorbidity between anorexia and other obsessive-compulsive disorders is also quite high, suggesting a shared vulnerability between the two (even if anorexia ultimately has the most links to obsessive-compulsive *personality* disorder). Nevertheless, it is worthwhile to consider screening people with OCD and related disorders for anorexia and vice versa.

BORDERLINE PERSONALITY DISORDER
Patients with bulimia are 15 times more likely to show cluster B personality pathology than matched controls, and there are many overlapping symptoms between both. Therefore, careful assessment of personality disorders is needed for people with bulimia, with treatment considerations being revised to account for these disorders if they are present (such as making a referral to dialectical behavior therapy or other evidence-based treatments for borderline personality disorder when available).

ADDICTION
The impulsivity seen in bulimia appears to overlap with addiction, and some have argued that people with bulimia do in fact meet criteria for having an addictive disorder as they engage in repeated use of positive reinforcers (in this case, food) despite negative repercussions. Indeed, the neurobiology of bulimia resembles that of addiction, with increases in ΔFosB being observed in the nucleus accumbens. While the DSM doesn't officially recognize "food addiction" as a diagnosis, there is at least some merit to the idea as some of the same principles apply to both. In addition, the high impulsivity seen in bulimia likely predisposes to the development of other forms of addiction, making screening for substance use a good idea for these patients.

DEPRESSION
Depression has a complex relationship to anorexia. For one, appetite is often decreased in people suffering from depression (the **A** in SIGEC**A**PS) which can lead to large decreases in weight. However, patients with depression do not suffer from distorted body image and are not *actively* attempting to lose weight in the same way that people with anorexia are. To complicate matters further, the cognitive and neurovegetative symptoms of depression can be difficult to disentangle from the normal physiologic effects of starvation. However, some research has suggested that depressive symptoms in anorexia tend to resolve with restoration of regular eating habits. For this reason, antidepressants are generally indicated only when there is clear evidence of comorbid depression.

For bulimia, depressive symptoms should be clearly differentiated from chronic dysphoria related to borderline personality disorder. In cases where mood episodes are present, both SRIs and CBT have been shown to be effective at not only treating depression but also reducing the frequency of bingeing-purging episodes, and the combination of medications and psychotherapy is superior to either alone.

ANXIETY
People with both anorexia and bulimia often have severe anxiety related to weight gain and food intake. However, it's important to avoid diagnosing a separate anxiety disorder without clear evidence that this anxiety spreads into other domains outside of eating and weight. In addition, just having anxiety can lead to reduced appetite through activation of the "fight or flight" mode. This shouldn't be diagnosed as an eating disorder, as there is a clear upstream cause for the change in food intake.

AUTISM
While it is not a diagnostic requirement, people with autism often have restricted patterns of food intake (they are notoriously "picky eaters"). In contrast to anorexia, however, overall intake of calories is not compromised, and there is no evidence of distorted body image in these patients.

PUTTING IT ALL TOGETHER

For many people, eating (and its associated rituals such as having dinner with family, making a meal with friends, or experiencing a new type of food while traveling) are among the most delightful moments of life. If all eating disorders did was rob these moments of their joy, that would be bad enough. However, because eating disorders threaten not just the quality of life but even life itself, it is essential to stay vigilant for these conditions. Use the **SCOFF** mnemonic to screen for eating disorders, then use what you know about the underlying pattern of each disorder to figure out what mechanisms are at play. In **UNDER**-rexia, an **U**nderweight patient is abnormally **N**ervous about gaining weight, has **D**istorted perceptions about their weight, engages in **E**xercise or other weight-loss behaviors, and **R**estricts caloric. In **BOWL**-emia, **B**inges are followed by **O**ffsetting behaviors (purging) at least **W**eekly for 3 months in a way that is **L**inked to their self-esteem. Keep in mind that not everyone will fit perfectly into the precise patterns in the DSM, but don't let this deter you from finding the right forms of treatment for someone who has disordered patterns of eating.

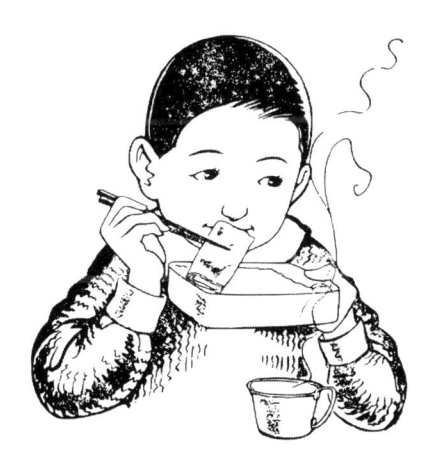

REVIEW QUESTIONS

1. A 14 y/o F begins following her friends into the bathroom after lunch to purge. She has done this every day for the past month but has never previously engaged in this behavior. She reports that she enjoys eating but worries that it will "make me fat and unpopular." She denies food avoidance, food restriction, or excessive exercise. She denies eating past the point that she feels full. When asked, she says that she believes herself to be "normal" weight but is engaging in these behaviors to avoid becoming fat. Her BMI is 20.2. What is the most likely diagnosis?
   A. Anorexia nervosa
   B. Bulimia nervosa
   C. Binge eating disorder
   D. More than one of the above
   E. None of the above

2. A 19 y/o F moves to New York to become a model. She lives with a roommate who is also a model who gives her advice on what foods to avoid, how frequently to exercise, and how to use diuretics and laxatives on days when there is a photo shoot to appear as thin as possible. She begins limiting her food intake to a single cucumber, a wedge of lettuce, and up to a dozen cups of green tea without sugar or milk per day. While she initially struggles with this diet, after a few weeks she finds that her hunger has gone away and that food no longer holds any appeal for her. Within several months, she has lost over 40 pounds. Her current BMI is 15.9. While initially she is able to find modeling contracts, recently she has been told that she looks "like you have cancer or something" and that she needs to gain weight. Despite being told this, she continues her attempts to lose weight. During a photo shoot the next day, she suddenly collapses and is rushed to the hospital. Vitals signs upon initial evaluation are HR 104, BP 98/60, RR 20, and T 94.9°F. She is confused and is oriented to person but not place, time, or situation. As she lacks capacity, a decision is made in consultation with the ethics department to initiate parenteral feeding given her risk of aspiration. On the fourth day of hospitalization, she suddenly develops psychomotor agitation, severe hypotension, and respiratory distress. An echocardiograph shows a left ventricular ejection fraction of 20%; however, electrocardiogram and cardiac markers are both normal. She is transferred to the intensive care unit in a state of cardiogenic shock. Which electrolyte is most implicated in the development of this outcome?
   A. Sodium
   B. Potassium
   C. Chloride
   D. Calcium
   E. Magnesium
   F. Phosphate

3. A 30 y/o M arrives for an initial consultation with a dietician. He recently suffered a heart attack and was found to have coronary artery disease, hyperlipidemia, and previously undiagnosed diabetes mellitus type 2. His BMI is 38.8. Upon initial evaluation, he reports having been overweight for as long as he can remember leading to frequent bullying and loneliness. He has attempted to lose weight at various times in his life but has been unable to continue these efforts for more than a few weeks at a time. His current diet consists primarily of prepackaged microwaveable food from the grocery store. Once or twice per week he will drive to the grocery store and pick up "all of my favorites," including ice cream, chips, and candy, and "ravenously devour" several grocery bags worth of food while watching television. He denies self-induced vomiting, use of laxatives, or exercise. He views himself as "hopelessly obese." Which of the following features of his case most argues *against* a diagnosis of bulimia nervosa?
    A. Current obesity
    B. Self-perception as being overweight
    C. Lack of purging
    D. Male gender
    E. Obesity beginning in childhood

4. A 38 y/o F sees her primary care doctor for an annual physical. Her doctor, who has known her since childhood, notices immediately that she appears thinner. Her current weight is 102 pounds, which has decreased from 128 pounds six months ago. On interview, she appears tired and sullen. When asked about the weight loss, she says that her appetite has "completely vanished" and that she only eats "when I feel like it, which is basically never." Her diet consists largely of granola bars, deli lunch meats, and "whatever else is around the house that I don't have to cook." She denies eating past the point of feeling uncomfortably full or any sense of having lost control over her eating habits. She does not exercise. She views herself as "thin." BMI is 17.0. She has stopped menstruating for the past three months, but multiple home urine pregnancy tests have been negative. Her mental status exam is notable for slowed movements, a restricted affect, absent prosody, and poor ability to concentrate. What is the most likely diagnosis?
    A. Anorexia nervosa
    B. Bulimia nervosa
    C. Binge eating disorder
    D. More than one of the above
    E. None of the above

1. **The best answer is E.** This girl does not suffer from an eating disorder, as her purging appears to be related to peer pressure rather than any cognitive or behavioral factors. Of note, she lacks a distorted body image and is not underweight, ruling out anorexia (answer A). While she engages in purging behaviors, she lacks impulsivity or a binge pattern to her food intake, ruling out bulimia and binge eating disorder (answers B and C).

2. **The best answer is F.** The diagnostic hallmark of refeeding syndrome is hypophosphatemia related to reinitiating feeding in someone who is chronically malnourished. While abnormalities in other electrolytes are often seen in cases of refeeding syndrome, it is most consistently associated with phosphate.

3. **The best answer is C.** This patient likely meets criteria for binge eating disorder which is related to bulimia nervosa but ultimately considered a separate diagnosis. While this patient engages in impulsive binges, he does not then compulsively purge as would be required for a diagnosis of bulimia. While people with binge eating disorder are often significantly overweight and those with bulimia are often a normal weight or just slightly overweight, this is a clinical observation and not part of the diagnostic criteria (answer A). His self-perception as being overweight is accurate in this case rather than representing a distorted body image as in anorexia (answer B). While bulimia is definitely more common in women compared to men, this is also not exclusionary (answer D). Finally, the fact that his obesity began in childhood is diagnostically irrelevant (answer E).

4. **The best answer is E.** While this patient has been restricting her diet recently, this appears to be secondary to a change in appetite rather than out of a desire to lose weight as would be seen in an eating disorder. She sees herself as thin, which argues against a diagnosis of anorexia (answer A), and does not engage in episodes of impulsive binge eating, which argues against a diagnosis of either bulimia or binge eating disorder (answers B and C). In this case, her change in appetite is possibly due to an episode of depression as evidenced by the findings on her mental status exam; however, a medical cause (such as hypothyroidism) cannot be ruled out at this time.

19 DEVELOPMENT

We now turn our attention to the process of **child development** which encompasses all of the physical and psychological changes that occur in the early stages of life, including infancy, childhood, and adolescence. Child development is an incredibly complex process that involves specific changes in physical attributes, motor skills, intellectual abilities, social interactions, and emotional range that occur at similar times in most people's lives. If all goes well, this core developmental process will ultimately create a physically, socially, intellectually, and emotionally mature adult.

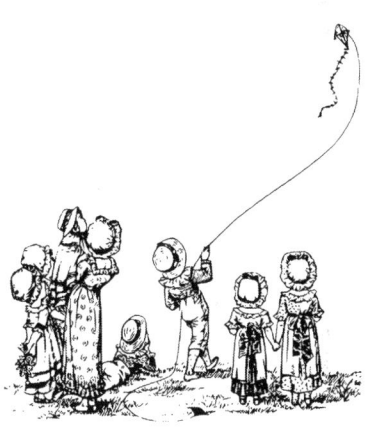

Many of the psychiatric disorders we have discussed so far can have their onset during development (including anxiety, eating disorders, and schizophrenia), and they will often present with different signs and symptoms and require distinct treatment considerations compared to cases beginning in adulthood. These variations are incredibly important and form the basis for the field of **child and adolescent psychiatry**. However, they are largely beyond the scope of this book.

Over the next few chapters, we will consider specific disorders of development that result in cognitive and behavioral impairment. These **neurodevelopmental disorders** include intellectual disability, autism, and attention deficit hyperactivity disorder (ADHD). To understand *disorders* of development, however, we must first know what is considered within the realm of *normal* development. For that reason, in this chapter we will begin with a discussion of normal child development before moving on to talk about various forms of intellectual disability (particularly those with neuropsychiatric manifestations). We will then turn our attention to autism and attention deficit hyperactivity disorder in the following two chapters.

NORMAL DEVELOPMENT

There is a **wide range of variability** in what is considered "normal" development, and different children progress through development at different rates. However, a few processes (primarily the development of specific motor, speech, and social skills) are considered vital for progressing towards full maturation. These are known as **developmental milestones**, and the typical expectation for children is that they will achieve these by a certain age. Failure to hit these milestones on time may be a sign of a medical condition that requires further investigation, so having a solid grasp of these milestones is essential for picking up on cases where there may be cause for concern.

INFANCY

Infancy is defined as the period between birth and when the child is able to walk or roughly the **first year of life**. Developmental milestones in infancy are primarily **motor skills** as speech has not yet developed. Infants should be able to **Lift their head** while laying prone on the ground at **2** months (notice how there are **2 brushstrokes** in the letter **L**). By **4** months, they should be able to **roll over** from laying on their back to their front (there are **4 letters** in both "roll" and "over"). At **si**x months they can **si**t upright, and by 9 months they should be able to both stand and crawl. Finally, at **w**one year of age, they should be able to **w**alk **w**ith some assistance.

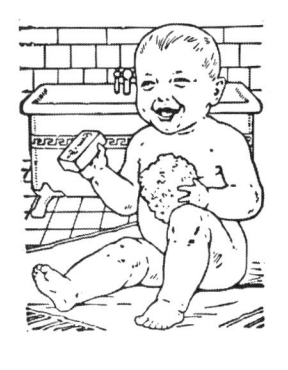

Speech is fairly limited before the age of 1. At **6** months, infants begin to **6**abble, and by 9 months they may say simple syllabic words like "mama" or "dada" (although not always used correctly). Finally, by age **w**one they should be able to use at least **w**one **w**ord **w**ith intention and follow **w**one step commands. While children do not develop full speech until after infancy, they are still social creatures. Infants demonstrate a preference for the sound of the human voice over other sounds immediately at birth. They will begin smiling in response to others by 4 months and laughing by 6 months. Between 6 and 12 months of age, infants can distinguish between different people and will form attachments to familiar caregivers such as parents or others living in the home. Infants often develop **stranger anxiety** around 6 months. This manifests as bouts of crying, becoming unusually quiet, or attempting to find their primary caregiver whenever they sense the presence of new or unfamiliar people. Stranger anxiety is a completely normal phase of social development and often subsides by 12 months (and almost always by the age of 2).

> **Infant milestones** primarily involve specific **motor and social** skills.
>
> Lift head at *2 months (**2 brushstrokes** in the letter **L**).*
> Roll over at *4 months (**4 letters** in both "roll" and "over").*
> Sit and **6**abble at six **(6)** months.
> **W**alk, say **w**one word, and follow **w**one-step commands at **w**one year.

EARLY CHILDHOOD

Early childhood is defined as the period between **1 and 3 years** of age. Children this age are called **toddlers** which underscores the primary importance of walking (or "toddling") and other motor and speech skills during these years.

Between the age of 1 and 2, toddlers go from knowing a single word to over **2** hundred words which they can put **2**-gether into **2** word sentences such as "Carry me!" or "Me go." About **2** out of every 4 words can be understood by strangers, and they should be able to follow a **2**-step command. Cube stacking is often used as a test of motor skills, and the number of cubes they can stack should be approximately equal to **their age times 3** (so a 2-year-old should be able to stack 6 cubes). They should also be able to copy a line (which is essentially a connection between **2** points). They can also feed themselves using a cup and spoon by the age of 2. Their motor abilities are generally well developed to the point that they can **run**. Socially, toddlers will often engage in **parallel play** rather than actively interacting with other children (recall that you need **2** lines to be in parallel). Toddlers also develop **separation anxiety** between 12 and 15 months of age. During this time, they will show a strong preference for known caregivers such as parents and will cry or tantrum when these caregivers leave. (Note that this is different than the *stranger* anxiety that is normal between 6 and 12 months of age. Stranger anxiety involves distress when new people are *introduced* whereas separation anxiety involves distress about when caregivers *leave*.) Separation anxiety is completely normal and often goes away by the age of 3.

Milestones at age **2** primarily involve **speech and motor** skills.

2-year-olds can:
*Say **2**-word sentences, with **2** of every 4 words understood by strangers.*
*Follow **2**-step commands.*
*Copy a **line** connecting **2** points.*
*Play in para**ll**el.*

By 3, speech has progressed to **3**-word sentences such as "I want milk," with **3** out of every 4 words understood by strangers. Toilet training occurs during this stage of development, and a 3-year-old should be able to exhibit both bowel and bladder control ("**pee at 3**"). A 3-year-old can also ride a **tri**cycle (though not yet a bicycle). Socially, a 3-year-old will begin to interact with other children their own age and will typically be able to name one or two people in particular as being friends.

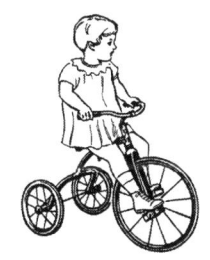

Milestones at age **3** primarily involve **speech and toileting**.

3-year-olds can:
*Say **3**-word sentences, with **3** of every 4 words understood by strangers.*
*Ride a **tri**cycle.*
*Show bowel and bladder control ("**pee at 3**").*

PRESCHOOL AGE

Years 4 and 5 are often called the **preschool age**. Children this age are generally independent enough to be left outside the immediate company of their parents and can socialize easily with others their own age, including engaging in **cooperative play**.

In terms of milestones, by age 4 speech should be mostly formed with **4** out of 4 words understood by strangers (although there may still be some small mistakes with complex grammar like saying, "I goed outside"). Motor skills include the ability to draw a **4**-pointed plus sign. By 5, all basic aspects of language should be present, and **5**peech should be fully comprehensible. They can also begin to perform more complex motor tasks including **5**kipping and tying their own **5**hoes. Children at this age enjoy both hearing and telling stories, and they can often begin **reading** (typically very simple books with lots of pictures). The ability to write begins around the age of 5 (note that there are **5** letters in the word **write**), often beginning with letters, numbers, and simple words (with fully formed sentences coming later).

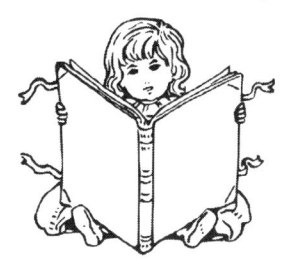

By age **5**, **complex motor skills** are possible, and **speech** should be **fully formed**.

5-year-olds can:
5peak fully.
5kip and tie their own 5hoes.
***Write** letters, numbers, and simple words (**5** letters in the word **write**).*

SCHOOL AGE

Ages 6 through 12 are when children begin going to school. Many basic motor and speech skills are already in place by this age (although a few more complex tasks such as being able to ride a bicycle will emerge during this time). Instead, developmental milestones tend to shift towards **social and cognitive** abilities. Children of school age tend to be rule oriented and respond to peer pressure. When interacting with others, they can be quite **conscience-driven** and will often rely on overly rigid notions of right and wrong. Cognitively, reading and writing abilities become more fully formed, and by the age of **8** children should be able to read a **8**ook independently.

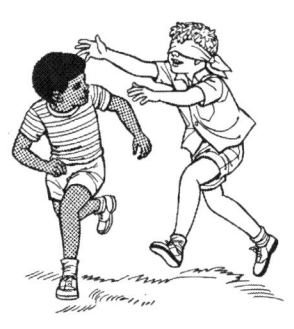

Following school age, development continues through adolescence and into adulthood. While there are additional developmental processes during this time such as puberty, **most cognitive, motor, and speech abilities are in place by age 12**.

By age **8**, children should be able to **read a book independently**.

An 8-year-old can read a 8ook.

ADOLESCENCE

Adolescence involves the process of maturation from childhood to adulthood. **Puberty** can begin during school age (most often at age 10 for girls and 12 for boys), but the most dramatic changes are typically not seen until age 13 and after. Puberty most directly involves maturation of the sexual organs, but this is also accompanied by the development of secondary sexual characteristics such as growth of body hair, changes in bone structure, and deepening of the voice.

Most adolescents are generally able to comprehend **abstract concepts** (rather than just concrete ones) and have fully developed reading comprehension. Socially, romantic feelings and exclusive relationships also emerge during this age. **Identity** is a key developmental concern during adolescence, and many teenagers will associate with various peer groups and "try on" different identities to see what fits. Contrary to what is commonly depicted in popular media, most adolescents **feel close to their parents**, although many also feel a need to separate from their parents and establish their own identity, especially in Western societies. There is often an increase in **risky behavior** that occurs during late adolescence and early adulthood, and many actions are done without taking the time to fully appreciate the possible consequences, leading to an increased rate of accidents, risky sexual behavior, and use of drugs. A number of psychiatric conditions can also begin to emerge during this time, including depression and eating disorders. The acronym **HEADSS** has been developed to assist in identifying common areas of stress or harm in adolescents. You can use this mnemonic in clinical settings to remember to assess the patient's **H**ome (who they live with), **E**ducation (how they are doing in school), **A**ctivities (what they do outside of school), **D**rugs, **S**exuality, and **S**uicide.

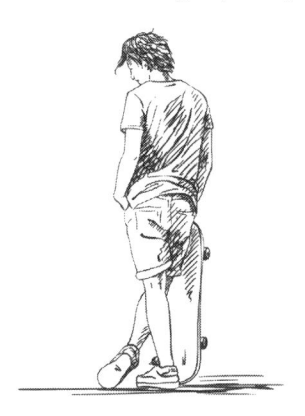

> Common sources of **stress or harm** in **adolescents** should be **routinely assessed**.
>
> *HEADSS:*
> *Home*
> *Education*
> *Activities*
> *Drugs*
> *Sexuality*
> *Suicide*

While all of the major physical changes of development are in place by the end of adolescence, a variety of cognitive, social, and emotional changes continue to occur throughout adulthood and even into older age. For this reason, development should be seen not as a task that is ever "completed" but rather as a continuing process of change that occurs over the entirety of a person's lifespan.

NEURODEVELOPMENTAL DISORDERS

Development is a complex process, and there are many places along the way for things to go awry. While the developmental milestones we have discussed are not hard and fast rules, a consistent **failure to meet milestones** should prompt an immediate medical work-up for possible underlying causes. Start by characterizing the nature of the deficits. Are they observed only in a **single area** (such as speech) or is there a **broad** failure to meet milestones in other domains like cognition and social skills as well? Is there a **sudden** slowing of development for a child who was previously developing without a problem, or has the child lagged behind their entire life? Is there any evidence that previously achieved milestones have been lost?

Abnormalities in development can occur for any number of reasons, including a wide range of genetic, environmental, infectious, anatomical, metabolic, nutritional, and immunologic diseases. However, most of these are well beyond the scope of this book. Instead, we will focus specifically on **neurodevelopmental disorders** (including intellectual disability, autism, and ADHD) which either are commonly evaluated by psychiatrists or are most likely to mimic other psychiatric syndromes. For the rest of this chapter, we will learn about intellectual disability and the various ways in which this can present, with a full discussion of autism and ADHD to come in the next two chapters.

INTELLECTUAL DISABILITY

An intellectual disability (previously referred to as mental retardation, although this term is now considered pejorative and should not be used clinically) involves **significant and persistent deficits in cognition** that result in a decreased ability to function independently on a day-to-day basis. Unlike most psychiatric syndromes, a diagnosis of an intellectual disability is not based upon the presence of specific signs or symptoms. Rather, it is based around the two things in its name: **assessments of intelligence** ("intellectual") and evidence of an **impaired ability to function independently** ("disability"). Intelligence is generally assessed using the intelligence quotient (IQ) which is a general measure of someone's abilities in multiple cognitive domains, including reading, math, vocabulary, memory, general knowledge, visual skills, verbal fluency, and reasoning. IQ tests are scored in such a way that the average person receives a score of 100, with a standard deviation of 15. This means that those who score **below 70** comprise the **lowest scoring 2.5% of the population**. This was chosen to be the cut-off under which someone is said to have an intellectual disability. However, it is not enough to simply score in the lowest 2.5% of the population; there must also be evidence of impaired functioning in daily living (such as difficulty in communication or an inability to care for one's self).

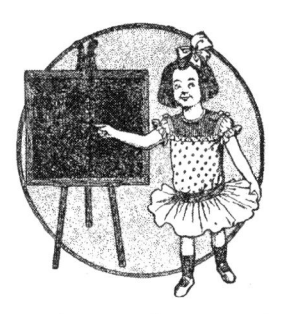

By definition, intellectual disability needs to be present during **early childhood** which distinguishes it from other disorders that similarly result in impaired cognition but only later in life (like dementia). For unknown reasons, **males** are affected by intellectual disability more often than females, with a gender ratio of 2 to 1.

While all cases of intellectual disability represent **lifelong conditions** with persistent deficits, the prognosis can vary widely from one case to the next. Some people with mild intellectual disability (with an IQ in the range of 50-69) will struggle in certain areas but can often complete school with some assistance, find jobs, and engage in meaningful relationships. Those with moderate intellectual disability (with an IQ in the range of 35-49) are often more impaired, with deficits in significantly more areas that necessitate assistance with even basic activities of daily living such as cooking or housework. However, they can often perform some tasks independently. Finally, those with severe intellectual disabilities may require assistance with every aspect of their lives, including feeding, bathing, and toileting. The majority of people (over 75%) with an intellectual disability have a mild form, with moderate and severe forms comprising the other 25%.

Intellectual disability is not a medical disease or a disorder, and there is no "cure." Management generally consists of various forms of **behavioral, occupational, physical, and/or speech therapy**. In almost all cases, an **individualized educational program** can help ensure that the patient is able to remain in school. Management can also involve training patients and/or caregivers to **enhance adaptive functioning**. For example, a child who has difficulty learning to use the toilet would be given specific trainings on this and provided with reinforcers when they do it correctly. In this way, the negative consequences of the intellectual disability are mitigated as much as possible, with the overall goal of increasing independence and autonomy.

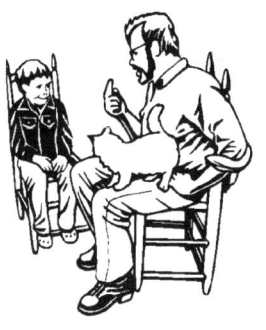

In over half of all cases of intellectual disability, no clear cause is found. This is known as an **idiopathic** or non-syndromic intellectual disability. In the other half of cases, however, an underlying medical cause can be identified, which is known as a **syndromic** intellectual disability. As a group, syndromic intellectual disabilities are often more severe than idiopathic cases (although this is not always the case).

For the remainder of this chapter, we will briefly cover some of the most common syndromic causes of intellectual disability. This is not intended to be a comprehensive list, as a full understanding of all forms of intellectual disability would require an entire book on its own. Nevertheless, this guide should serve as a high-yield starting point for recognizing some of the **most common causes** of syndromic intellectual disability as well as those with a **significant behavioral or psychiatric component**. (This information overlaps significantly with the field of pediatrics and may be beyond the scope of what is needed for some readers, so feel free to skip ahead to the next chapter if you don't think that it will apply to you!)

Jonathan Heldt

DOWN SYNDROME
Down syndrome is the **single most common genetic cause** of intellectual disability and occurs in around 0.1% all live births. It is caused by the presence of a third copy of chromosome 21 known as **trisomy 21**. (You can remember the association of Down syndrome with trisomy 21 by thinking of someone going out to hit the bars and **Down** some drinks on their **21st** birthday.) The likelihood of having a child with Down syndrome increases with maternal age, particularly above 35 years old.

Down syndrome is a **trisomy disorder** caused by a **third copy of chromosome 21**. It is the **most common genetic cause** of **intellectual disability**.

*Think of someone going out to hit the bars and **Down** some drinks on their **21st** birthday.*

Intellectual disability is the predominant clinical feature of Down syndrome, with significant delays in developmental milestones as a child and deficits in mental abilities even as an adult. A diagnosis of Down syndrome is based on genetic testing (either *in utero* or after birth) to look for the chromosomal abnormalities associated with the disorder. However, you can also often make a clinical diagnosis based upon certain signs. Physical exam often reveals a generally short stature and **distinctive facial features**, including flattening of the face, prominent eyelid folds, slanted eyes, a flat nose, and a large tongue relative to the small size of their mouth. People with Down syndrome often have additional medical comorbidities that are characteristic of the condition, including congenital heart disease and gastrointestinal abnormalities such as duodenal atresia.

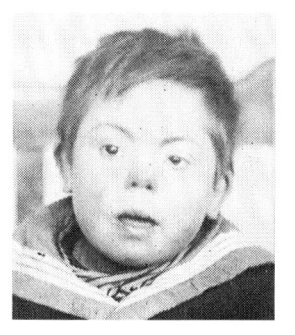

The prognosis for Down syndrome varies on the degree of intellectual disability present, with some people able to lead fairly independent lives and others being totally dependent upon others. However, people with Down syndrome have a significant risk of developing **Alzheimer's disease** later in life, with over half showing signs of further cognitive decline during their adult years.

FRAGILE X SYNDROME
Fragile X syndrome is the **second most common cause** of genetic intellectual disability after Down syndrome. In addition to cognitive deficits, people with fragile X syndrome often have additional neuropsychiatric symptoms, including social withdrawal, repetitive stereotyped behavior, and poor attention. Physical exam often reveals **X**-tra large testes (macro-orchidism), **X**-tra large jaws (macrognathism), and **X**-tra large ears (macrotia), all of which should be easy to associate with fragile **X** syndrome.

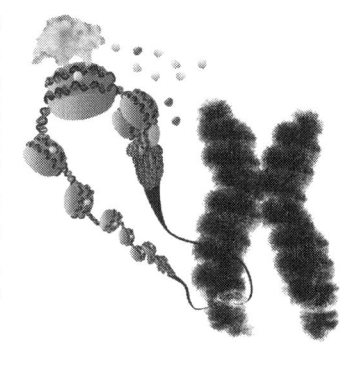

> **Fragile X syndrome** is a form of **genetic intellectual disability** characterized by **social withdrawal, repetitive behavior**, and **enlarged testes, jaws, and ears**.
>
> *Fragile **X** syndrome features **X**-tra large testes, jaws, and ears.*

    Fragile X syndrome is caused by an expansion of the trinucleotide repeat **CGG** on the X chromosome. While most people have less than 40 CGG repeats, someone with fragile X syndrome often has over 200. This increase in the number of CGG repeats results in suppression of a specific gene (known as FMR1) which produces a protein required for the development of interneuronal connections. Suppression of the FMR1 gene changes the shape of the X chromosome and causes it to appear "fragile" under a microscope, which gives the disorder its name. The poor connection between neurons is believed to underlie the intellectual deficits that individuals with this condition display. You can remember the association of the trinucleotide repeat **CGG** by associating it with **C**ongenitally **G**iant **G**onads.

> **Fragile X syndrome** is caused by **expansion of the trinucleotide repeat CGG** on the X chromosome.
>
> ***C**ongenitally **G**iant **G**onads are caused by a **CGG** repeat.*

FETAL ALCOHOL SYNDROME

Fetal alcohol syndrome is a common cause of intellectual disability that is related to **alcohol exposure *in utero***. The perinatal period is often complicated by low birth weights, preterm deliveries, and small stature. After birth, the extent of observed deficits depends largely on the amount of alcohol exposure, with some people having only mild symptoms and others experiencing profound disability. People with fetal alcohol syndrome often have problems with attention and behavior as well, leading to higher rates of **legal, academic, and social difficulties** compared to their peers. Many also suffer from problems with motor coordination. Individuals with fetal alcohol syndrome often have consistent physical characteristics that can help to guide a clinical diagnosis, including small eye openings, a smooth philtrum (the cleft between the nose and lips), and a thin upper lip. Like any form of intellectual disability, there is no cure for fetal alcohol syndrome, so the focus of medical intervention is largely on preventing prenatal alcohol exposure through public health education programs.

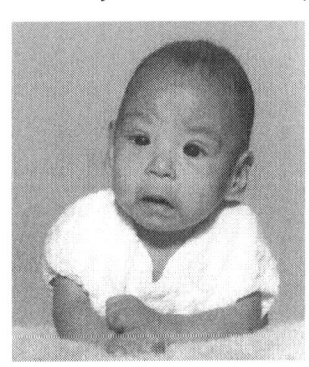

PRADER-WILLI SYNDROME

Prader-Willi syndrome is a genetic disorder that results in intellectual disability and specific neuropsychiatric signs including frequent tantrums, emotional lability, and self-injurious behavior such as scratching and skin picking. Physical examination can reveal a short stature and hypogonadism, with poor muscle tone sometimes being observed during infancy. However, by far the most specific symptom of Prader-Willi syndrome is a persistent state of **insatiable hunger** that is not relieved by eating. When permitted access to food, people with Prader-Willi syndrome can continue to eat for hours on end. This directly leads to various complications, both acute (like perforation of the stomach wall) and chronic (like obesity, insulin resistance, and type 2 diabetes mellitus). Because of the potential consequences of overeating, access to food must be strictly supervised at all times. Prader-Willi syndrome is caused by the deletion of a normally active **P**aternal allele on chromosome 15 (although it is still unclear how this deletion leads to the insatiable hunger that characterizes this syndrome). You can remember the association of **P-rader** Willi syndrome by remembering that it involves a **P**aternal gene deletion that results in "fridge **raider**" behavior.

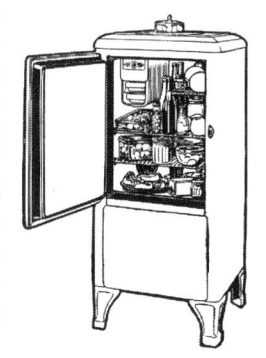

> **Prader-Willi syndrome** is a genetic disorder characterized by **insatiable hunger** along with intellectual disabilities, short stature, and hypogonadism.
>
> *P-rader Willi syndrome = Paternal gene deletion + "fridge raider."*

ANGELMAN SYNDROME

Angelman syndrome is similar to Prader-Willi syndrome in that both involve a deletion on chromosome 15. However, whereas in Prader-Willi syndrome the *paternal* gene is involved, in Angel**M**an syndrome the *Maternal* allele has been deleted. This results in a syndrome of **intellectual disability, speech impairment**, and **ataxia**. People with Angelman syndrome are often noted to have a **happy demeanor** and frequently laugh and smile in response to attention. There is also a characteristic facial appearance in many (but not all) cases. Angelman syndrome was initially known as "happy puppet syndrome" which captures the speech impairment, ataxia, and positive affect seen in this disorder. However, this term is considered pejorative and should not be used in a clinical setting. You can remember **Angel-M**an syndrome by thinking of someone who is **angel**ically happy due to a **M**aternal gene deletion.

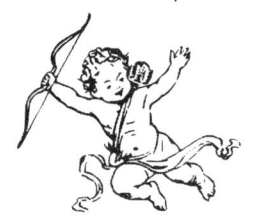

> **Angelman syndrome** is a genetic disorder characterized by a generally **happy demeanor**, intellectual disabilities, speech impairment, and ataxia.
>
> *Angel-Man syndrome = Angelically happy due to a Maternal gene deletion.*

DIGEORGE SYNDROME

DiGeorge syndrome (also known as velocardiofacial syndrome) is a genetic disorder caused by the deletion of a few dozen genes in the 22q11.2 region of chromosome 22. It is an **autosomal dominant** disease that varies widely in its presentation, with some having only a mild form of the syndrome and others being severely affected. DiGeorge syndrome causes abnormalities in multiple areas of physical development which you can remember using the convenient mnemonic **CATCH-22**: **C**ardiac malformations (such as tetralogy of Fallot), **A**bnormal facies, **T**hymic hypoplasia, **C**left palate, and **H**ypocalcemia related to gene deletion on chromosome **22**.

Like other aspects of the syndrome, the intellectual disability present is highly variable, with some having only mild cognitive deficits and others having severe disabilities. Interestingly, nearly a quarter of all individuals with DiGeorge syndrome go on to develop **schizophrenia** (a much higher incidence than seen in the general population). The exact mechanism linking DiGeorge syndrome to schizophrenia is unclear, but it remains an area of active research.

DiGeorge syndrome is a genetic condition resulting in **intellectual disability** and a variety of characteristic **anatomical and physiologic abnormalities**.

CATCH-22:
Cardiac malformations
Abnormal facies
Thymic hypoplasia
Cleft palate
Hypocalcemia
22nd chromosome

WILLIAMS SYNDROME

Williams syndrome is a genetic condition characterized by intellectual disability and an exceptionally **extroverted and outgoing personality**. People with Williams syndrome are often quite personable and will readily interact with strangers. (Interestingly, this appears to be related to hypoactivity of the amygdala in response to socially threatening stimuli such as disapproving faces, which is the *opposite* of what is seen in disorders like depression and PTSD.) Williams syndrome is generally associated with *mild* forms of intellectual disability, with reasoning and verbal abilities both being relatively spared. Physical exam tends to reveal a small head, a prominent mouth with widely spaced teeth, an elongated philtrum, and a flattened nasal bridge (sometimes known as **"elfin" features**). Unfortunately, people with Williams syndrome are vulnerable to a host of health problems including cardiac structural abnormalities (like aortic stenosis), gastrointestinal problems (such as frequent abdominal pain), and hypercalcemia. Life expectancy does not appear to be significantly impacted, however, and many people with Williams syndrome live into their 60s and beyond.

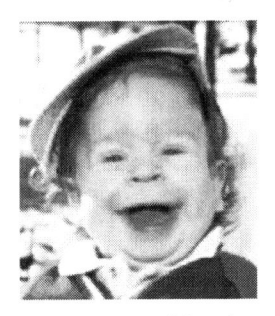

The cause of Williams syndrome is a genetic microdeletion on the long arm of chromosome 7 that leads to the loss of several genes. One of these genes produces the protein **elastin** which is found in structural connective tissue, and deletion of the elastin gene may account for some of the medical complications of Williams syndrome (including the cardiac structural abnormalities). If you picture a **7riendly person with el7in features**, you can remember the association of Williams syndrome with increased sociability and a microdeletion of chromosome **7**.

> **Williams syndrome** is a genetic cause of **mild intellectual disability** resulting in **increased sociability** and specific anatomical abnormalities.
>
> *Picture a **7riendly person** with **el7in features** a microdeletion on **chromosome 7**!*

CRI DU CHAT SYNDROME

Like Williams syndrome, cri du chat syndrome (French for "cat's cry") is caused by a genetic microdeletion, this time on the short arm of chromosome 5 (which you can remember by thinking that there are 5 letters in "kitty"). Unlike the overall mild intellectual disability found with Williams syndrome, cri du chat syndrome is associated with **severe intellectual disability**. People with cri du chat syndrome often have cardiac abnormalities (including ventricular and atrial septal defects) that may require surgical correction. **Self-injury** is sometimes seen, with hair pulling being particularly common. Diagnosis is based on the disorder's namesake cat-like mewing which is heard in patients as early as birth.

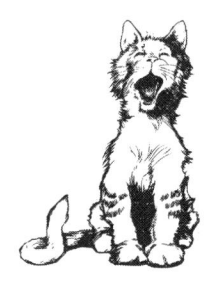

> **Cri du chat syndrome** is a genetic disorder resulting in **severe intellectual disability**, cardiac abnormalities, and a **characteristic cat-like cry** during infancy.
>
> *There are **5** letters in "**kitty**" (deletion on chromosome **5**).*

HOMOCYSTINURIA

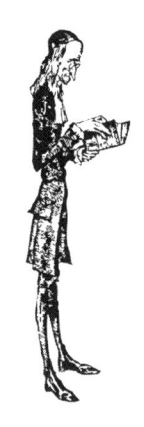

Homocystinuria is an **autosomal recessive metabolic disorder** where a deficiency of a specific enzyme (cystathionine beta synthase) results in accumulation of a toxic metabolite (homocysteine) not only in the urine but throughout the body as well. If untreated, elevated homocysteine can lead to developmental delays, intellectual disability, and neuropsychiatric symptoms resembling other disorders like ADHD. Physical manifestations of untreated homocystinuria include a **long thin body**, genu valgum (also known as "knock knees"), osteoporosis, and eye problems (including lens dislocation, retinal detachment, and myopia). Individuals with untreated homocystinuria are also at high risk for **thromboembolic events** such as heart attacks and stroke, and a significant number of people with this condition die before the age of 30 due to excess clotting. Because of this, your diagnostic suspicion for homocystinuria should be raised whenever you see a **young person with a history of thromboembolic events** (which are usually only found in older adults). Treatment involves high doses of **vitamin B₆** (pyridoxine) and/or a low-sulfur diet.

Homocystinuria can sometimes be confused for Marfan's syndrome, as both conditions feature a characteristic long and thin body habitus in addition to lens dislocation in the eyes. However, Marfan's syndrome does *not* feature intellectual disability and has a different pattern of lens dislocation with the lens moving *away* from the midline ("up and out"). In contrast, homocystinuria *does* feature intellectual disability, and the lens moves *towards* the midline ("down and in"). Focus on the "**in**" of homocyst**in**uria to remember the **in**tellectual disability, down-and-**in** lens dislocation, and thromboembolic **in**farction events seen in this condition.

> **Homocystinuria** is a genetic disorder resulting in **intellectual disability**, **lens dislocation**, **thromboembolic events**, and a **long thin body**.
>
> *Homocyst**in**uria causes **in**tellectual disability, down-and-**in** lens dislocation, thromboembolic **in**farction, and a long th**in** body.*

ADRENOLEUKODYSTROPHY

Adrenoleukodystrophy is an **X-linked genetic disorder** in which fatty acids cannot be metabolized, leading to their toxic build-up throughout the body. Deposition of fatty acids in the **brain** can result in not only intellectual disability but also hyperactivity, emotional lability, and disruptive behavior which can resemble disorders like ADHD. Other neurologic signs such as imbalance and seizures can be seen as well. The excess fatty acids also have a tendency to deposit in the **adrenal cortex** where they can cause adrenal insufficiency. (These two organs are captured in the name adrenoleukodystrophy, with "adreno" referring to *adrenal* insufficiency and "leuko" referring to the *white* matter of the brain.)

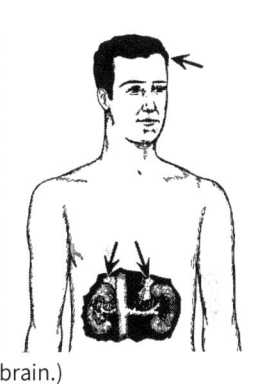

As an X-linked disorder, adrenoleukodystrophy is more common in **males**. The age of onset is variable, with some showing signs as early as 5 years while others are not diagnosed until adulthood. Adrenoleukodystrophy has a **variable prognosis**, with some people being completely asymptomatic, others having only adrenal problems, and still others being profoundly impaired both cognitively and physically. Treatment of the disorder involves hormone replacement to offset the adrenal insufficiency. Stem cell transplants can also be effective if used early enough in life, but given the high variability of the disorder, its use is controversial. Gene therapy is an emerging area of research which has shown some promise but needs further testing.

> **Adrenoleukodystrophy** is an X-linked genetic disorder resulting in **intellectual disability**, **behavioral problems**, and **adrenal insufficiency**.
>
> *Split the name apart: "**adreno**-" for **adrenal** and "**leuko**-" for **white** matter of the brain.*

RETT SYNDROME

Rett syndrome is an **X-linked genetic disorder** involving a **loss of developmental milestones**, including both motor and speech skills. Development proceeds normally until sometime between the ages of 1 and 4 when a sudden and profound backslide to previous developmental stages is seen. In addition to intellectual disability, Rett syndrome is characterized by specific movements including **hand-wringing**. A sudden decrease in **head circumference** can also be seen. Other conditions can co-occur, including an elevated risk of seizures, scoliosis, and sleeping problems.

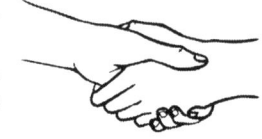

Rett syndrome is caused by mutations in the MECP2 gene on the X chromosome. The exact mechanism for how mutations in this gene lead to the characteristic signs and symptoms of the disorder are unknown. Unlike most X-linked disorders, the majority of people diagnosed with Rett syndrome are **girls**. This is because boys with this disorder generally die either *in utero* or shortly after birth due to a lack of an additional X chromosome containing a non-mutated form of the gene.

Rett syndrome is often **confused with autism** due to the fact that both begin around the same age (1 to 4 years old) and involve similar symptoms, including poor social skills, communication difficulties, and repetitive movements. In contrast to autism, however, Rett syndrome involves a **Rett**urn to stages of development that had previously been passed (in contrast to autism and other disorders where these milestones are never reached in the first place). Rett syndrome is also diagnosed primarily in girls (rather than the male predominance seen in autism) and features prominent motor symptoms (including gait abnormalities) that are not seen in autism.

Rett syndrome is an **X-linked genetic disorder** characterized by a sudden and dramatic **regression in development** to previous developmental stages.

*Rett syndrome involves a **Rett**urn to previous stages of development.*

LESCH-NYHAN SYNDROME

Lesch-Nyhan syndrome is an **X-linked recessive genetic disorder** that can cause severe intellectual disability. The diagnostic hallmark of Lesch-Nyhan syndrome is a pattern of **self-mutilating behaviors** (including frequent biting of the nails and lips) that appear around the age of 2. These behaviors are seen in almost all patients with the disorder. **Neurologic abnormalities** including poor muscle tone and inability to meet motor milestones are often seen as well.

As an X-linked condition, the majority of patients with the disorder are **male**. Lesch-Nyhan syndrome is caused by mutations in the gene coding for an enzyme known as hypoxanthine-guanine phosphoribosyltransferase (HGPRT). Deficiencies in this enzyme prevent cell breakdown products from being recycled back into DNA, so they are instead shuttled into a different metabolic pathway, resulting in increased **uric acid** production. Uric acid then deposits into various parts of the body, including joints (leading to inflammatory arthritis similar to gout) and the urinary tract (causing kidney stones and urinary tract infections).

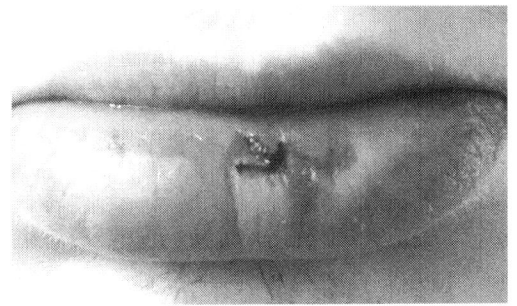

Lip biting in Lesch-Nyhan syndrome.

Lesch-Nyhan syndrome is an **X-linked recessive disease** that involves intellectual disability and characteristic **self-mutilating behaviors**.

*Le**X**-**Nyh**an is an **X**-linked disease that causes **Nyh**ilistic self-injurious behavior.*

SMITH–MAGENIS SYNDROME

Smith–Magenis syndrome is an **autosomal dominant genetic disorder** involving a microdeletion in the short arm of chromosome 17. It results in intellectual disability, hyperactivity, and a distinctive appearance (including short stature, a 'tented' upper lip, a depressed nasal bridge, a thick lower jaw, and a conjoined eyebrow in young adults). However, what is most diagnostic of the condition is a characteristic behavioral profile involving **severe self-injurious behavior** (including hand-biting, head-banging, skin-picking, insertion of foreign objects into bodily orifices, and pulling out fingernails and toenails) that is found in over 95% of people with the condition. A pattern of **stereotyped self-hugging** is also observed and may be pathognomonic for the condition. Sleep is often significantly disrupted owing to a disturbance of the circadian rhythm. Social interaction is often impaired as well, though people with Smith–Magenis syndrome still appear to desire the attention and affection of others. The characteristic combination of signs and symptoms in Smith–Magenis syndrome can be remembered using the mnemonic **SMITH** for **S**leep disturbances, **M**anual injuries (from biting of the hands and fingers), **I**ntellectual disability, a **T**hick lower jaw, and self-**H**ugging behaviors.

Smith–Magenis syndrome is a genetic disorder resulting in **intellectual disability**, **sleep disturbance**, and **severe self-injurious behaviors**.

SMITH:
Sleep disturbances
Manual injuries (from biting of the hands)
Intellectual disability
Thick lower jaw
Self-Hugging

CORNELIA DE LANGE SYNDROME
Cornelia de Lange syndrome is a **complex genetic disorder** that can be caused by mutations in various genes. It can **strongly resemble autism** in its neuropsychiatric presentation, as there is often poor social relatedness combined with a strong preference for structure and routine. Behavioral problems such as **aggression or self-injury** are often observed as well, and these appear to correlate directly with levels of pain or discomfort from related health conditions such as gastroesophageal reflux. Specific physical characteristics such as delayed growth, excessive hair, and small head circumference are often seen, while hearing loss is common (seen in 80% of people with the disorder). Cornelia de Lange syndrome can resemble Smith-Magenis syndrome in some ways as both involve a combination of intellectual disability and self-injurious behavior, but it can be identified by the *absence* of desire for attention from caregivers (whereas people with Smith-Magenis syndrome tend to show a desire for caregiver affection).

DIFFERENTIAL DIAGNOSIS OF INTELLECTUAL DISABILITY
Intellectual disabilities rarely tend to be confused with other psychiatric disorders due to their **onset in infancy or early childhood** (unlike the majority of mental disorders which begin in adolescence at the earliest). For this reason, *missed* diagnoses are more of a problem than *mis*diagnoses. While rates of psychiatric disorders are not necessarily *higher* in people with intellectual disability compared to the population as a whole, clinicians need to be vigilant not to assume that people with intellectual disability don't have other mental disorders as well. This is especially important when considering that people with intellectual disabilities often **underreport symptoms** due to difficulty communicating effectively. Because of this, care must be taken to investigate signs and symptoms when they occur, and a greater emphasis may need to be placed on objectively observed signs (such as the presence of psychomotor slowing, low appetite, and sleep disruption arguing for a diagnosis of depression) compared to subjectively reported symptoms.

NORMALCY
Like all of the syndromes we have talked about so far, intellectual disability occurs on a spectrum. However, what is unique to intellectual disability is the fact that this spectrum is **directly embedded into the definition of the condition**, with the lowest performing 2.5% of the population automatically given a diagnosis of an intellectual disability provided that they also have deficits in adaptive functioning as well. It is important not to overpathologize people who have intellectual disabilities, as many can lead healthy and full lives once familial and societal expectations have been adjusted (such as the idea that everyone must live independently, have a job, and get married). Indeed, there is as much of a danger from expecting too *little* from someone with an intellectual disability as there is from expecting too *much*, and clinicians working with people who have intellectual disabilities should keep an eye towards maximizing adaptive functioning wherever possible.

LEARNING DISABILITIES

Intellectual disabilities must be carefully distinguished from learning disabilities as they are **mutually exclusive diagnoses**. In contrast to intellectual disabilities (which affect functioning in *all* areas of life), learning disabilities are limited to **specific domains** such as reading (dyslexia), writing (dysgraphia), and math (dyscalculia). Therefore, diagnosing someone who has an intellectual disability with a comorbid learning disability is redundant, as their impairments in specific areas would likely stem from a *global* intellectual disability rather than representing a separate diagnosis in its own right.

People with learning disabilities differ from those with intellectual disabilities in that they are generally **able to bring their performance up to the level of their peers** by learning specific adaptive skills. In contrast, people with intellectual disabilities can show improvements in their adaptive functioning but are generally not able to catch up to their peers due to inherent limitations in their cognitive abilities.

COMMUNICATION DISORDERS

Communication disorders are a **large and heterogeneous group** of conditions that all share a core deficit in the ability to communicate effectively with others. They can range in severity from mildly impairing (such as stuttering) to profoundly disabling (such as the complete inability to hear or speak). Communication disorders are often comorbid with intellectual disabilities, although care should be taken to ensure that the signs and symptoms of the communication disorder aren't entirely accounted for by the intellectual disability itself.

AUTISM

Autism is both a missed diagnosis and misdiagnosis for intellectual disability, as they are often comorbid (indeed, as many as 70% of people with autism also meet criteria for an intellectual disability, which goes counter to media stereotypes of people with autism having genius-level intellect). However, it is also possible for intellectual disability to be misdiagnosed as autism (and vice versa) as both conditions present with failure to meet developmental milestones. The key is to focus on the nature of deficits. If all of the observed deficits fall within the domains of social communication and rigid adherence to structure (the "aloneness" and "sameness" discussed in the next chapter), then a separate diagnosis of intellectual disability is unnecessary. However, if the cognitive deficits exceed those domains and spill into other areas as well, a comorbid diagnosis of intellectual disability is likely warranted.

ATTENTION DEFICIT HYPERACTIVITY DISORDER

Similar to autism, ADHD can be confused for intellectual disability as they both have their onset in early childhood and can both cause impairment in academic and adaptive functioning. Just like with autism, the key is to determine whether the observed deficits are found entirely within the core domains of ADHD (inattention and hyperactivity) or whether they extend into other domains as well (such as learning, socialization, and intellect). Another clue is that treatment of ADHD using stimulants often results in dramatic improvement in symptoms whereas medications do not significantly improve the deficits seen in intellectual disability. In some cases, it is absolutely possible for someone to have both ADHD and an intellectual disability.

CEREBRAL PALSY

Cerebral palsy is a **highly heterogeneous condition** that involves poor coordination, muscle weakness, and/or spasticity resulting from damage to the central nervous system. This often results in pronounced **postural abnormalities** that often require the use of assistive devices such as wheelchairs or braces to enable movement. The potential causes of cerebral palsy are vast, although problems in pregnancy (such as pre-term birth and exposure to certain toxins or infections) account for a large proportion. Cerebral palsy is often accompanied by intellectual disability or learning disability, with up to half of all patients showing cognitive problems. However, it is important to point out that it should never be assumed that *all* patients with cerebral palsy are intellectually disabled! While cognitive deficits are common in patients with cerebral palsy, they are not universal, and care should be taken not to allow physical appearances to get in the way of promoting self-efficacy as much as possible.

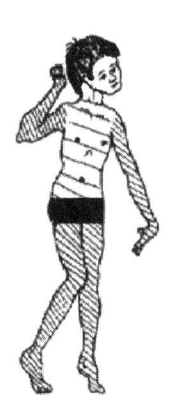

ADDICTION

People with intellectual disabilities have rates of addiction and substance abuse that are lower than the general population (likely reflecting decreased access to drugs). However, for the small subset of people with an intellectual disability who manage to get their hands on these substances, the risk of developing an addictive disorder is actually *higher* than average. Therefore, do not assume that people with intellectual disabilities are somehow "protected" from developing substance use disorders, especially those in the mild range of disability.

DEMENTIA

While both dementia and intellectual disability involve cognitive deficits, it is easy to tell them apart by focusing on two things: **onset and course**. By definition, intellectual disabilities begin early in life and follows a stable course while dementia occurs later (usually in one's 50s or 60s at the earliest) and is marked by progressive deterioration. It is possible for someone with an intellectual disability to develop dementia (in fact, many people born with Down syndrome later develop Alzheimer's disease as well).

SELF-HARM

Some forms of syndromic intellectual disabilities are characterized by frequent and repetitive self-injurious behavior. It is important to keep in mind that the nature of self-harm in intellectual disability differs significantly from both suicide as well as the non-suicidal self-injurious behavior seen in some cases of borderline personality disorder. Self-harm in intellectual disability appears to be related to **decreased pain perception** (as opposed to a desire to die in suicide and a way of regulating painful emotions in borderline personality disorder). In addition, people with intellectual disabilities can have difficulty communicating pain verbally and may engage in self-harm as a way of distracting themselves. Therefore, always be vigilant to consider that self-injury can be a sign of an unrecognized medical condition, especially if it is new or more severe than usual.

PUTTING IT ALL TOGETHER

An intellectual disability is ultimately quite simple to diagnose, as it requires only two things: **intelligence scores** in the lowest 2.5% of the population and evidence of **impaired adaptive functioning** as a result. Nevertheless, in practice (and on test questions) things quickly get more complicated. Much of this has to do with the fact that your ability to diagnose intellectual disabilities relies upon an understanding of what is encompassed by "normal" development. In addition, there are a large number of syndromic intellectual disabilities that each present with unique physical, cognitive, and behavioral features (making this probably the single densest chapter in the entire book). Unfortunately, there is no easy way around this, and a large amount of information will simply need to be memorized. As much as you can, study the **most specific features** of each disorder (such as an insatiable appetite in Prader-Willi syndrome, a loss of developmental milestones in Rett syndrome, and stereotyped self-hugging in Smith-Magenis syndrome) to identify syndromic cases when you see them.

Once an intellectual disability has been identified, switch your focus from the idea of finding a "cure" to instead trying to enhance adaptive functioning both on the part of the patient and their caregivers. There is danger both in having expectations that are *too high* as well as having expectations that are *too low*, and the treatment plan should be realistic about what can reasonably be achieved while never settling for anything less than as full and developed of a life as possible.

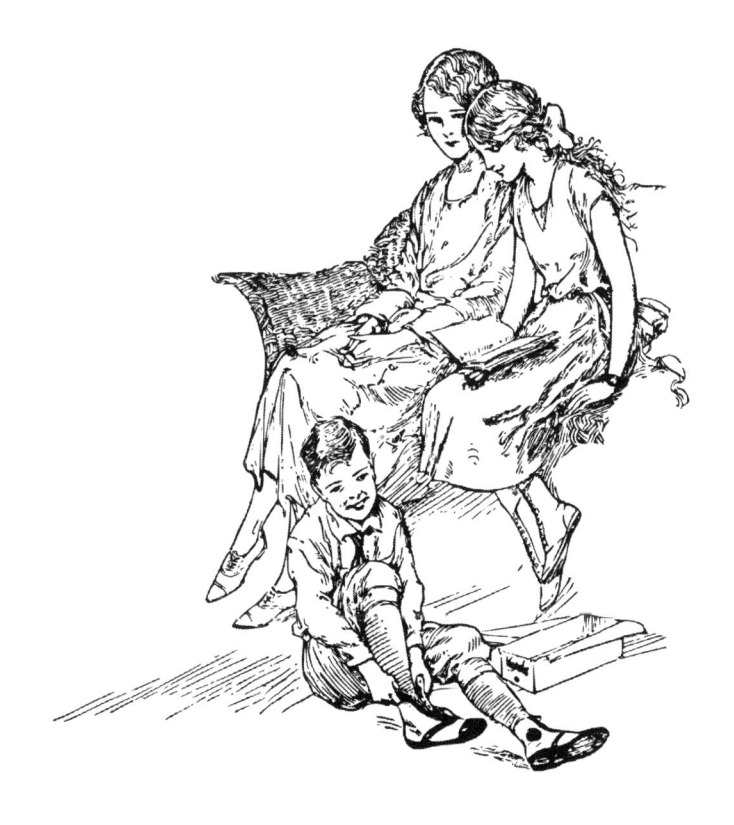

REVIEW QUESTIONS

1. A 2 y/o M is brought to the pediatrician's office by his parents on his birthday for an annual check-up. He is quiet with the pediatrician but will speak to his parents in short sentences consisting of no more than two or three words. He is able to walk independently but still wears diapers due to a lack of consistent control over both bowels and bladder. He continues to breastfeed but is able to eat solid foods as well. When around other children his same age, he does not spontaneously engage in conversation or do activities with them, preferring instead to play by himself. Which of the following findings is most concerning for abnormal development?
   A. Shyness around non-parent adults
   B. Inability to speak in sentences more than a couple of words
   C. Lack of bowel and bladder control
   D. Continued breastfeeding
   E. Playing by himself rather than with peers
   F. None of the above

2. A 5 y/o F is referred for formal testing after her pre-school teacher mentions that she seems "a little slow" compared to other children in her class. Her speech is generally understandable, although she makes occasional grammatical errors such as, "Your cookie is more bigger than my cookie." She is outgoing and social with other children in her class. Her parents are unaware if has difficulty with tying her own shoes as she wears shoes with Velcro straps. She can draw simple pictures but cannot yet write a complete sentence involving both a noun and a verb. She needs reminders from her parents at night to brush her teeth before going to bed. IQ testing reveals that she is in the 2nd percentile for children her age. What is the most likely diagnosis?
   A. An idiopathic intellectual disability
   B. A syndromic intellectual disability
   C. A communication disorder
   D. A learning disorder
   E. None of the above

3. A 2 y/o M is brought to the emergency department of a local hospital after he was found bleeding from his mouth. He was born at term after an uncomplicated pregnancy. However, at the age of 4 months he began appearing "limp" and was treated with physical therapy for generalized hypotonia. The boy's parents report that he is unable to walk and has been "essentially non-verbal" his entire life and communicates primarily with grunting noises. Over the past month he has begun aggressively biting his tongue and his lip. Immediately before coming to the hospital, he bit off the entirety of his lower lip, leading to severe bleeding. Physical examination reveals additional scarring on his thumb and fingers as seen in the following image:

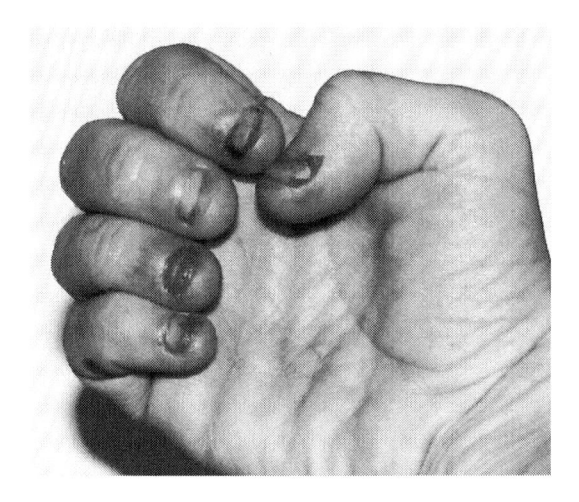

Which of the following is the most likely explanation for this patient's behavior?
   A. Nondisjunction of chromosomes resulting in additional copies
   B. Inability to metabolize fatty acids
   C. Deletion of a normally active maternal allele
   D. Overproduction of uric acid
   E. Exposure to toxic substances *in utero*

4. A 15 y/o M is seen by his ophthalmologist to evaluate a recent decrease in his visual acuity. He is otherwise healthy and eats a normal diet. He is 6'5" tall and appears to have longer than average limbs, fingers, and toes. While he is known to have severe nearsightedness resulting in use of corrective eyeglasses, in the past week he has noticed that his vision has become increasingly blurry. Ophthalmologic exam reveals a lens that is displaced away from the midline. Which of the following best describes this patient's level of intelligence?
   A. He is unlikely to have an intellectual disability (IQ 70 or above)
   B. He likely has a mild intellectual disability (IQ 50-69)
   C. He likely has a moderate intellectual disability (IQ 35-49)
   D. He likely has a severe intellectual disability (IQ below 35)
   E. It is impossible to tell whether he has an intellectual disability

1. **The best answer is F.** This 2-year-old child exhibits normal development in all domains mentioned in the question stem. While stranger anxiety is unusual past the age of 2, some degree of shyness around non-parent adults is completely normal (answer A). Speech at this age generally consists of two or three word sentences (answer B), while play is largely in parallel to, rather than directly with, other children (answer E). Bowel and bladder control are often not achieved until the age of 3 (answer C). Finally, stopping breastfeeding is not a developmental milestone (answer D).

2. **The best answer is E.** This patient has received scores on an IQ test that are in the range of intellectual disability (being in the lowest 2.5%). However, a diagnosis of intellectual disability is based not only on tests of intelligence but also on whether there are impairments in adaptive functioning as a result. Based on the case presentation, she is within normal limits on all developmental milestones described and shows no signs of significant impairment, effectively ruling out a diagnosis of either a syndromic or idiopathic intellectual disability at this time (answers A and B). It is possible that she will develop impairments in adaptive functioning in the future as the tasks expected of her become more complex, but at this time there is no basis for that diagnosis. Based on the description of her outgoing nature, she may have Williams syndrome, but it is probably more likely that this is simply within the range of normal personality. There is no evidence at this time that she has either a learning or a communication disorder (answers C and D).

3. **The best answer is D.** This boy likely has Lesch-Nyhan syndrome as evidenced by significant delays in various milestones (including motor and speech) as well as the presence of severe self-mutilating behaviors. While self-harm is seen in a variety of syndromic intellectual disabilities including Smith-Magenis syndrome and Cornelia de Lange syndrome, the early age of onset (2 years) and location of the injuries (lips and fingers) strongly suggest Lesch-Nyhan syndrome, which is associated with overproduction of uric acid. Nondisjunction of chromosomes results in trisomies like Down syndrome (answer A), inability to metabolize fatty acids suggests adrenoleukodystrophy (answer B), deletion of a normally active maternal allele suggests Angelman syndrome (answer C), and exposure to toxic substances *in utero* suggests fetal alcohol syndrome (answer E).

4. **The best answer is A.** This vignette describes a case of Marfan's syndrome. While commonly confused for homocystinuria due to a similar body habitus and the presence of lens dislocation, the pattern described in this case (including the outward dislocation of the lens and a lack of other medical history) contrasts with the "down and in" lens dislocation, presence of medical comorbidities, and requirement for a specialized low-sulfur diet seen with homocystinuria. While homocystinuria is associated with intellectual disability, intelligence in Marfan syndrome is often normal, so a lack of intellectual disability is the most likely scenario.

20 AUTISM

Autism is a neurodevelopmental disorder characterized by two things: **difficulties in social communication** and **restricted interests and activities**. Like intellectual disability, it is often diagnosed during **early childhood** based upon a failure to meet milestones on time (primarily those related to speech and language). Autism is referred to as a **spectrum disorder** due to the wide range in symptom severity and functional ability seen in this syndrome. Despite these variations, however, abnormalities in the two core domains must be present for *all* individuals diagnosed with this disorder, as these two traits (originally called an "**autistic aloneness**" and an "**insistence upon sameness**") have been associated with autism from the time it was first described in 1938. Unlike some of the other disorders we have talked about which come with their own long lists of diagnostic criteria, the criteria for autism are so simple that we can get them out of the way right off the bat: an **A**utism **S**pectrum **D**isorder is defined by an autistic **A**loneness and an insistence upon **S**ameness that are both present during early **D**evelopment! There is definitely more to say about each of those patterns, as we will discover in the next section.

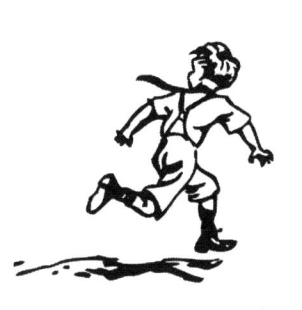

> **Autism** is defined by **impairments in social communication** as well as **restricted and repetitive interests and activities**.
>
> *Autism Spectrum Disorder (ASD):*
> *Autistic Aloneness*
> *Insistence upon Sameness*
> *Developmental onset*

SIGNS AND SYMPTOMS OF AUTISM

While "deficits in social communication" and "restricted interests and behaviors" capture most of what you need to know about diagnosing autism, there are some nuances here to be aware of. In addition, there are some other signs and symptoms that we'll discuss as well which are not part of the core diagnostic criteria but are still commonly seen in this disorder.

DEFICITS IN SOCIAL COMMUNICATION

Deficits in social communication can manifest in various ways, including **both verbal and non-verbal aspects of language** as well as difficulty understanding and following the **implicit rules of social interaction**.

Deficits in verbal language often manifest as **speech delays**, and failure to meet language milestones is the most common way that children with autism come to clinical attention. For some people with severe autism, speech can be entirely absent. However, speech delay is not *required* for a diagnosis of autism, and around half of people with autism (generally those with less severe forms) have overall normal speech abilities.

For these individuals, deficits in communication occur instead in other domains, including difficulty with understanding and using **non-verbal communication** such as body language and facial expressions. For example, most people understand that when someone points at something you should look at the object they are pointing to rather than looking at the finger itself. In contrast, someone with autism is more likely to misunderstand what is being communicated and will look at the pointing finger instead. People with autism are often **overly literal** and have difficulty understanding things like sarcasm that rely heavily on non-verbal aspects of communication including the context of the situation and the speaker's vocal intonations. Some people with autism have such difficulty recognizing facial expressions (even seemingly basic ones like "happy" or "sad") that they must be taught how to interpret these expressions explicitly. In this way, people with autism can sometimes come across as "robotic" in their interactions.

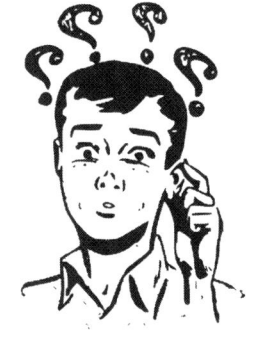

Deficits in social communication can also extend beyond language itself into the basic rules of social interaction. These rules are so intuitive and ingrained that most people follow them without even thinking about it. For example, most people know even from a very young age that when you meet someone you should say a greeting and introduce yourself by your name. Most people know that when you are talking with someone, it is polite to speak *sometimes*—not so much that you dominate the entire conversation but not so little that you come across as unengaged. Most people understand basic principles of social engagement such as **reciprocity** ("If you give me something, I should give you something back"), **turn-taking** ("I need to wait my turn in line"), and **sharing** ("If there is not enough for everyone, I should share"). In contrast, people with autism do not intuitively pick up on these rules and will often break them in subtle or not-so-subtle ways. They do not break these rules on purpose in order to be selfish; instead, they have difficulty understanding that they *should* behave this way to begin with. This lack of an intuitive understanding of the rules of social engagement often makes people with autism feel like "an anthropologist on Mars" trying to understand the laws of a society whose logic they cannot intuitively grasp. Despite their difficulties interacting with other people, people with autism often demonstrate a desire to be around others and often report loneliness or isolation when they lack meaningful friendships.

RESTRICTED INTERESTS AND ACTIVITIES
The other domain of autism involves **restricted or repetitive patterns of behavior, interests, and activities**. The phrase "insistence on sameness" captures the core pattern here very well, as people with autism often want, and will even demand of others, a strict adherence to specific routines and patterns such as wanting to eat the same food every day or needing to perform the same rituals before bed. Due to the difficulties in social communication that often co-occur, a child with autism may be unable to communicate their desires verbally and will instead act out, scream, or otherwise show distress when these patterns are interrupted.

Restrictions in interests and activities may also manifest through particular **fixations and fascinations** such as studying the schedules for every train at the local station or memorizing the weather patterns in certain parts of the world. This may also involve **stereotyped or repetitive movements** that do not necessarily make sense to an outside observer such as lining up objects in a specific order, flapping their hands in the air repeatedly, or spinning the wheels on a toy car for hours on end. For some individuals, this stereotyped behavior can even include self-harm such as repeatedly banging one's head against the wall (although the nature and purpose of this behavior differs significantly from that seen in borderline personality disorder and is more similar to the patterns of self-injury seen in people with certain forms of intellectual disability).

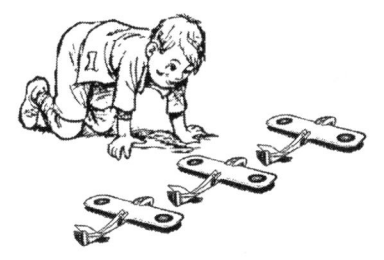

OTHER SIGNS AND SYMPTOMS
Many people with autism exhibit a variety of other signs and symptoms that, while common, are not required for a diagnosis of autism. First, **disturbances in sensory perception** are seen in up to 80% of patients with autism. These disturbances are often a combination of *hyper*sensitivity to certain stimuli (such as sounds or textures) and *hypo*sensitivity to other stimuli (such as pain or temperature). Second, a variety of **motor signs** are often seen in autism including poor coordination, low muscle tone, and unusual gait (such as walking on one's tip toes). While these signs are common (occurring in 60 to 80% of cases), they are also not required for a diagnosis of autism.

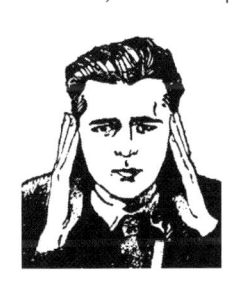

AUTISM ACROSS THE LIFESPAN

EPIDEMIOLOGY
The prevalence of autism varies significantly from study to study, ranging from 0.01% to 1.5% depending on the diagnostic standard used (reinforcing the idea that autism is a spectrum disorder that can encompass a wide range of symptoms and severities). However, it can generally be thought of as a **rare** disorder with a similar prevalence to schizophrenia or bipolar disorder. Notably, the prevalence of autism has increased over the past several decades. It is unclear why, but **changes in diagnostic patterns** (including more screening and increasing awareness of the disorder among both healthcare providers and families) appears to explain the majority of the increase.

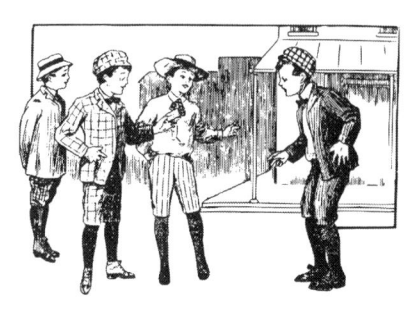

A significant gender gap exists with autism, as **boys** are diagnosed with autism more than 4 times as often as girls. Despite common misconceptions, there is no evidence that autism is linked to vaccines, and the endurance of this theory likely comes from the fact that the period of immunization occurs at the same age that symptoms of autism are first noticed (around **1 to 3 years old**).

PROGNOSIS
As a developmental disorder, autism does not occur in discrete episodes but rather has a **chronic and persistent course**. The functional prognosis for autism varies widely, as the disorder can present in forms ranging from mild impairments in social interaction to severe disability resulting in a complete lack of speech and total dependence upon caregivers for survival. Even without treatment, there appears to be a natural lessening of social deficits along with improvement in adaptive functioning over time as people with autism learn specific skills and ways of interacting with the world. However, some signs (such as restricted interests) are nearly always present.

TREATMENT
Treatment for autism involves **behavioral training** to teach specific adaptive skills (such as providing positive reinforcement to encourage the use of speech). In addition, **speech and language therapy** can also be helpful for teaching skills to overcome communication deficits, while interventions in the family and educational systems can improve functional skills and decrease stress on caregivers. While treatment earlier in life is associated with improved functional outcomes, the majority of individuals with autism remain dependent on others for support during adulthood (although people with high-functioning forms of autism are often be able to live, work, and maintain social relationships independently). At this time, **no medications** have been shown to be helpful for improving the core deficits seen in autism.

MECHANISMS OF AUTISM

Efforts to explain the causes of autism have been ongoing since the disorder was first described. While many of these theories have been discredited (such as an early attempt to link autism to "refrigerator mothers" who used emotionless parenting styles), there are some new explanations that are worth investigating.

A concept known as **hierarchical organization** suggests that, compared to those without the disorder, people with autism have a neurobiologically ingrained tendency to prioritize the *details* of what they see (the object's "local" properties) over the *overall meaning* (its "global" properties). Take a look at the following image:

```
SSSSSSSS        SSSSSSSS
SSSSSSSS        SSSSSSSS
SSSSSSSS        SSSSSSSS
SSSSSSSS        SSSSSSSS
SSSSSSSS        SSSSSSSS
SSSSSSSS        SSSSSSSS
SSSSSSSS        SSSSSSSS
SSSSSSSS        SSSSSSSS
SSSSSSSS        SSSSSSSS
SSSSSSSSSSSSSSSSSSSSSSSS
SSSSSSSSSSSSSSSSSSSSSSSS
SSSSSSSSSSSSSSSSSSSSSSSS
SSSSSSSSSSSSSSSSSSSSSSSS
SSSSSSSSSSSSSSSSSSSSSSSS
SSSSSSSS        SSSSSSSS
SSSSSSSS        SSSSSSSS
SSSSSSSS        SSSSSSSS
SSSSSSSS        SSSSSSSS
SSSSSSSS        SSSSSSSS
SSSSSSSS        SSSSSSSS
SSSSSSSS        SSSSSSSS
SSSSSSSS        SSSSSSSS
SSSSSSSS        SSSSSSSS
SSSSSSSS        SSSSSSSS
```

The *global* image is the shape of the letter **H**. However, the *local* image is many copies of the letter **S**. People *without* autism show a tendency to immediately interpret the shape as the letter H due to a preference for global processing over local processing. However, people *with* autism are more likely to say "the letter S" when asked to describe what the image is meant to communicate, reflecting their tendency to focus on the local details of something more than its global gist.

This tendency towards local detail-oriented processing over global meaning-related processing is observed in other ways as well, both beneficial and detrimental. Consider the image on the following page:

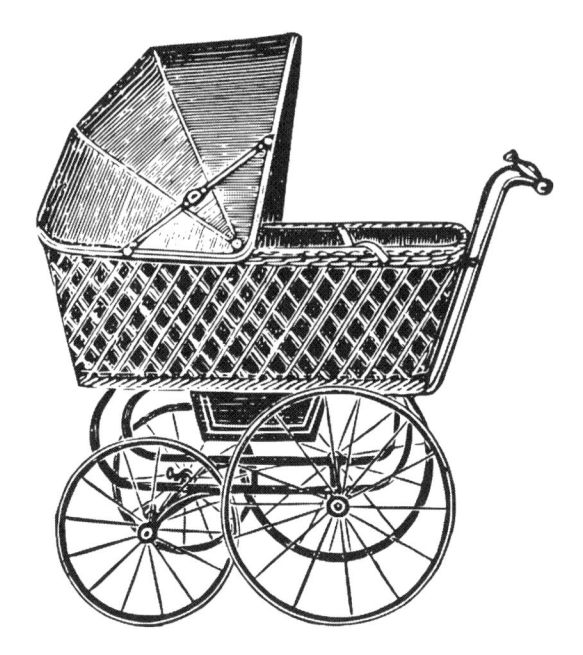

Now try to find this triangle ◣ in the image. For people with autism, the ability to break things down into their individual components makes this a relatively simple task that they can pull off with ease. For someone without autism, however, the tendency to focus on the *overall* message of the image (the shape of a baby carriage) makes it harder to perform this task. (For anyone curious, the location of the triangle in the baby carriage can be found by turning to the last page of this chapter.)

Differences in sensory processing are also apparent in optical illusions such as the following image:

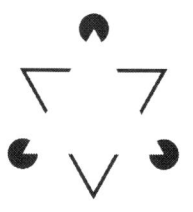

Because they tend to focus exclusively on the individual parts, it is difficult for someone with autism to get the overall "gist" of the image (the central white triangle), and studies have found that only around 10% of individuals with this disorder can "see" the illusion (in comparison with the majority of non-autistic people).

This lack of hierarchical organization explains why some individuals with autism show such proficiency with complex and detailed subjects such as mathematics or physics that people without autism often struggle with. However, it also explains the **deficits in verbal skills and use of language** that are core features of autism. For example, read the following sentence out loud:

His eyes filled with tears when he saw his mother's quilt riddled with tears.

Multiple studies have shown that people autism fail to differentiate between the pronunciation of each instance of the word "tear," as this relies upon an ability to quickly understand the overall meaning of the sentence (global processing) over the sound of each word in isolation (local processing).

These difficulties are compounded further when it comes to **non-verbal communication**, as this requires integration of multiple stimuli at the same time (including not only the words that are spoken but also the tone in which they are said, the context of the situation, and the speaker's body language and facial expressions). Because most people have a preference for global processing, integrating all of this information is a simple and automatic process. For someone with autism, however, the tendency to treat local details at the same level as global impressions proves impairing. Facial expressions are another area where the tendency to focus on details instead of the overall gist can produce difficulties. Consider these two expressions:

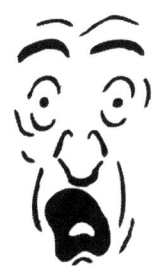

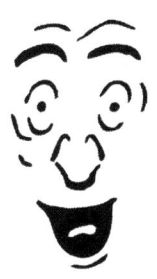

Most people are able to look at these images and immediately say that the one on the left represents a negative emotion like anger or fear while the one on the right is a more positive emotion like happiness or surprise. However, by breaking down the image into its individual components, one can see that the top of each face is in fact *exactly the same*, and only the contour of the mouth differs between them. By focusing too much on local details (the eyebrows, eyes, and nose being similar) rather than global gist, people with autism can struggle to accurately recognize facial expressions.

This innate preference for local over global processing also explains the **restricted interests and activities** seen in autism which often involve subjects that are better suited for local rather than global processing such as memorizing train schedules. Interestingly, relatives of patients with autism tend to be over-represented in fields like engineering, physics, and accounting that also reward detail orientation!

This preference for local over global processing is **not inherently a deficit or a disability**. Instead, this cognitive style confers specific advantages (like the ability to attend to minute details) while eliminating others (like the ability to communicate easily with others). It's important also to keep in mind that this processing style is *not* unchangeable, as people with autism can be taught (for example, using behavioral therapy) to overcome their instinctive tendency to get lost in the details and instead look at the overall meaning. In this way, the concept of hierarchical organization can help to assist in confirming a diagnosis of autism as well as explain why behavioral training is effective in managing the condition while medications, which cannot change processing style, are not.

DIAGNOSING AUTISM SPECTRUM DISORDERS

Diagnosis of an autism spectrum disorder is based upon both of the domains mentioned earlier (an autistic aloneness and an insistence upon sameness). Social communication deficits and restricted interests and activities must both be observed in **multiple settings** from **early childhood**. Abnormalities in behavior are often noticeable by the age of 2 and almost always by the age of 3 (even by people not formally trained in diagnosing autism). Diagnoses of children younger than 2 years should be given cautiously, as diagnosing too early or on the basis of minimal symptoms can lead to false positives (whereas diagnoses assigned later in life are more likely to be lasting and durable). However, that shouldn't deter you from referring these children for further evaluation and possibly even treatment, as earlier intervention is often associated with improved outcomes.

For many patients with autism, **speech delay** is the initial reason for a formal evaluation of autism. However, other causes for speech delay must be ruled out as well. Use the mnemonic **APHASIC** (meaning "unable to speak") to remember some common causes of speech delay in a child, including **A**utism, **P**hysical deficits such as apraxia (difficulty in generating motor impulses to produce speech) and dysarthria (the inability to form speech using vocal muscles), **H**earing impairment, **A**buse or neglect (which can also present with failure to meet milestones), **S**elective mutism (an anxiety disorder discussed in Chapter 9), **I**ntellectual disability, and **C**erebral palsy.

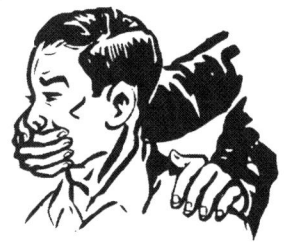

> **Speech delay** is the **most common initial symptom of autism** but can be a sign of other disorders as well.
>
> *APHASIC:*
> *Autism*
> *Physical deficits*
> *Hearing impairments*
> *Abuse or neglect*
> *Selective mutism*
> *Intellectual disability*
> *Cerebral palsy*

TYPES OF AUTISM

Historically, the DSM made a distinction between various types of autism. Individuals with high-functioning forms of autism were said to have **Asperger syndrome**, a milder version of the disorder which featured deficits in socialization and restricted interests and activities but lacked speech impairment or any comorbid intellectual disability. Another diagnosis known as "pervasive developmental disorder not otherwise specified" (sometimes called **atypical autism**) was given to individuals who exhibited multiple traits associated with the disorder but did not technically meet the core diagnostic criteria.

However, in the interest of bringing together all cases of autism under a single diagnostic banner (as well as no longer making reference to Dr. Hans Asperger who participated in euthanasia as part of a Nazi program), these distinctions were dropped in the DSM-5, and all of these cases would now be classified as an **autism spectrum disorder**. While there are no longer officially recognized subtypes of autism, there are still some clinical features that may be relevant which we will explore next.

SAVANTISM
Savantism refers to cognitive abilities in specific areas that are astoundingly over and above what is known to be in the realm of normal human ability. Individuals with savantism have **incredible cognitive capabilities**, often related to memory (like being able to memorize endless amounts of seemingly trivial information) or calculation (such as performing complex mathematical equations instantly in one's head). For example, someone might be able to tell you the day of the week and the weather for any specific date, even going back many years ("April 2, 1933 was a Sunday. It was cold, with frost in the morning and a dry wind in the afternoon").

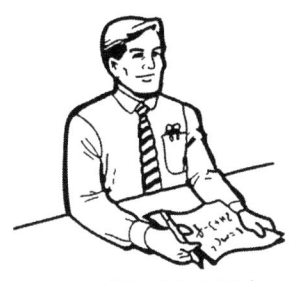

The relationship of savantism to autism is well characterized, with "islets of ability as well as deficits" having been described from the very first reported cases of the disorder. While over half of all savants have autistic traits, the reverse is not true, and the majority of people with autism are *not* savants. (Indeed, it is vastly more common for someone with autism to have an intellectual *disability* than to be a savant.) Nevertheless, the higher than average prevalence of savantism among people with autism suggests a link between the two conditions (likely related to superior local processing enabling seemingly superhuman mental feats). This serves as an important reminder that the features of autism are not inherently pathological and likely act as a double-edged sword in many areas.

PRAGMATIC LANGUAGE IMPAIRMENT
Someone who presents with deficits in social communication but does *not* have restricted interests or activities should not be diagnosed with autism, as impairments in *both* of these domains are required. However, these patients may still struggle as a result of social communication difficulties. To capture these patients, the DSM-5 introduced the concept of **pragmatic language impairment**, officially called "social (pragmatic) communication disorder." A diagnosis of pragmatic language impairment is mutually exclusive with a diagnosis of autism, with the presence or absence of restricted interests and behaviors being the deciding factor. Because it is such a new diagnosis, it is unclear how people diagnosed with this disorder will compare to those diagnosed with "textbook" autism.

DIFFERENTIAL DIAGNOSIS OF AUTISM SPECTRUM DISORDERS

As autism has become more prevalent, our understanding of how it relates to other disorders has deepened. For example, for a long time it was commonly assumed that people with autism did not become depressed, as the restricted affect seen in autism was seemingly incompatible with such a severe mood disorder. However, we now know that autism can be comorbid with nearly any psychiatric syndrome, making it important to be mindful of missed diagnoses with this condition.

NORMALCY

Neither of the two domains of autism (social communication deficits and restricted interests or activities) are inherently pathological, and decades of research shows that both of these traits are on the spectrum of normalcy. Because of this, avoid knee-jerk diagnoses of autism for anyone who has below-average social skills or above-average interest in their hobbies. Instead, look for evidence that these attributes are resulting in dysfunction. In severe cases, this is not hard to see. In less severe cases, however, the line may not be so clear. Review the advantages and disadvantages of diagnoses as outlined in Chapter 2 when making a decision about diagnosis. In some cases, the advantages (such as increased access to behavioral therapies or caregiving resources) may outweigh the downsides (including increased stigma and lowered expectations for families), but this decision should be made on an individual basis.

It is also worth mentioning that there is an ongoing debate over whether autism is a neurodevelopmental *disorder* in need of treatment or a neurologic *difference* that has been unnecessarily pathologized by the medical community. In fact, some people in the autism community advocate for the idea that autism is not a disorder at all and instead should be seen as a form of **neurodiversity** lying in the range of normalcy. As with all psychiatric syndromes, however, *at extremes the quantitative becomes qualitative*. For people with mild autistic traits, these differences can and should be celebrated as a distinct way of looking at the world. However, for people who have such a severe form of autism that they are completely unable to live independently or care for themselves, it is much harder to make the case that autism is simply a variant of normalcy. Nevertheless, it is an intriguing idea and an important reminder that autism should only be diagnosed if there is evidence of dysfunction (even if someone has behaviors or traits that are clearly "on the spectrum").

INTELLECTUAL DISABILITY

The relationship between autism and intellectual disability is complex. The two disorders are often comorbid, with around half of people with autism being intellectually disabled as well. (This even applies to savants as well, as they often have significant *dis*abilities even while having specific areas of extreme ability.) Diagnosing autism in the presence of intellectual disability can be a challenge, as intellectual disability itself can be associated with social dysfunction. Nevertheless, the social dysfunction must be **clearly out of proportion** to what would be expected purely from the intellectual disability alone. In addition, there must be evidence of restricted and repetitive interests or activities to make a clear diagnosis of autism.

PSYCHOSIS
The clinical features of schizophrenia and autism overlap in a few key ways which can lead to confusion. In particular, the prodrome of schizophrenia tends to involve very similar signs (such as social communication deficits and restrictions in affect) which can begin at the same early stage of life as autism. For this reason, it is possible that some people in the prodromal stage of schizophrenia will instead be diagnosed with autism, although these cases will eventually "declare themselves" at the time that clear psychotic symptoms emerge.

CLUSTER A PERSONALITY DISORDERS
Autism may at times be confused for a personality disorder, as both are chronic and enduring conditions. In fact, some studies have estimated that up to 50% of people with autism meet criteria for a personality disorder. Out of the three clusters, cluster A personality disorders are most likely to be misdiagnosed as autism due to several overlapping features including **social isolation** in schizoid personality disorder and **eccentric interests** in schizotypal personality disorder. It is notable that decreasing clinical interest in cluster A personality disorders has coincided with an increase in rates of autism, and it is possible that people who previously would have been diagnosed with a cluster A personality disorder would now receive a diagnosis of autism due to changes in diagnostic trends. However, as a rule the clinical features of autism tend to be noticeable by the age of 3 whereas those in cluster A personality disorders usually start in adolescence. In addition, people with autism do not necessarily lack a desire to engage in social relationships. Instead, they are often motivated to make friends but may come across as socially "clumsy" in their attempts to engage with others.

CLUSTER B PERSONALITY DISORDERS
At first glance, a diagnosis of autism seems unlikely to be confused with cluster B personality disorders given the wide range of affect associated with them (in contrast to the restricted affect seen in autism). However, both cluster B personality disorders and autism share similar **difficulties in mentalization** that can give the appearance of poor social skills. Don't confuse these two conditions! In cluster B personality disorders, difficulties in "reading" other people are more often related to *hyper*mentalization (or the tendency to get someone else's emotional state wrong by *overthinking* social cues) whereas in autism this appears to be connected to *hypo*mentalization as a result of engaging in local processing of facial expressions and social cues over global integration of contextual information.

CLUSTER C PERSONALITY DISORDERS
Out of all the cluster C personality disorders, obsessive-compulsive personality disorder is perhaps most likely to be misdiagnosed as autism as they share several features, including a preference for **rigid adherence to structure**. In differentiating between the two, evaluate whether the rigid patterns are the result of a desire for sameness (which would suggest autism) or an ego-syntonic hyper-conscientiousness (which would suggest obsessive-compulsive personality disorder). In addition, people with obsessive-compulsive personality disorder do not necessarily have any problems with social communication, so if these are present a diagnosis of autism is more likely.

ANXIETY DISORDERS
Individuals with autism appear to be at higher risk for anxiety, especially as they enter adolescence and become more aware of how their differences set them apart from their peers. Out of all the anxiety disorders, **social anxiety disorder** appears to have the most overlap with autism, and up to a third of adolescents with autism may meet criteria for social anxiety disorder. It is unclear how much of this co-occurrence has to do with the significant overlap in symptoms (as both autism and social anxiety involve difficulties in socializing) versus representing true comorbidity.

ATTENTION DEFICIT HYPERACTIVITY DISORDER
ADHD and autism should not be difficult to separate from each other, as ADHD primarily involves difficulties in the domains of inattention and hyperactivity and does not necessarily result in the "aloneness" and "sameness" that characterizes autism. However, diagnostic confusion can happen (largely due to the fact that both occur more often in boys and begin during early childhood).

OBSESSIVE-COMPULSIVE DISORDERS
Both autism and the obsessive-compulsive disorders feature the presence of rigid or compulsive behaviors. Of note, these behaviors are ego-dystonic in people with OCD (who are able to say *why* they are engaging in the behaviors even while they find them to be excessive or difficult to stop). In contrast, the restricted interests and behaviors of people with autism are **ego-syntonic**, and there is often an inability to describe the reasons for engaging in the behaviors (particularly in lower-functioning cases).

DEPRESSION
Depression is just as common in patients with autism as it is in the general population. However, due to the restricted emotional expression that many people with autism have, it can be difficult to assess this clearly. In particular, look for changes in the patient's baseline level of activity (such as less participation in hobbies or fewer attempts at social interaction) that may be related to depression.

EATING DISORDERS
Patterns of eating are often abnormal in people with autism, which is often noticeable from a very early age. Children with autism are often noted to be incredibly selective in what they eat (they are often described as "picky eaters"), with some preferring to eat a few foods exclusively. In general, there is a **normal amount of caloric intake** (even if the food choices are not diverse), and the thought patterns of autism lack the obsession with weight and body image seen in both anorexia and bulimia.

SLEEP DISORDERS
Similar to eating habits, sleeping patterns in people with autism are often quite dysregulated even from an early age. Specific sleep difficulties can include difficulty falling asleep, difficulty staying asleep, resistance to going to bed, and an out-of-sync circadian rhythm (such as staying up all night or sleeping all day). Sleep difficulties often persist across the lifespan. It is unclear why people with autism have abnormal sleep patterns, but when these occur they are generally considered to be a part of the syndrome itself (rather than necessitating a diagnosis of a separate sleep disorder).

PUTTING IT ALL TOGETHER

By virtue of its onset in early childhood and persistent deficits across the lifespan, autism can be among the most impairing of all psychiatric conditions. However, while there are severely disabled non-verbal people with autism, there is also no shortage of intellectually gifted individuals who may occasionally struggle with communication but nevertheless remain functional and independent in their daily life. This underscores the fact that autism is a **spectrum disorder**, so do not expect two people with the same diagnosis to necessarily have the same prognosis.

To remember the two core patterns of autism, think of **A**utism **S**pectrum **D**isorder as the "autistic **A**loneness" and "insistence upon **S**ameness" that occur during early **D**evelopment. The deficits in social communication can present as both language deficits as well as problems with understanding rules of social engagement. While **speech delay** is a common reason for initial presentation, not all cases of speech delay should be diagnosed as autism, so use the mnemonic **APHASIC** to remember other possible causes of delayed speech. Finally, keep in mind that on a mechanistic level autism appears to involve a preference for **local processing** over getting a global "gist," which can help to better identify cases of autism.

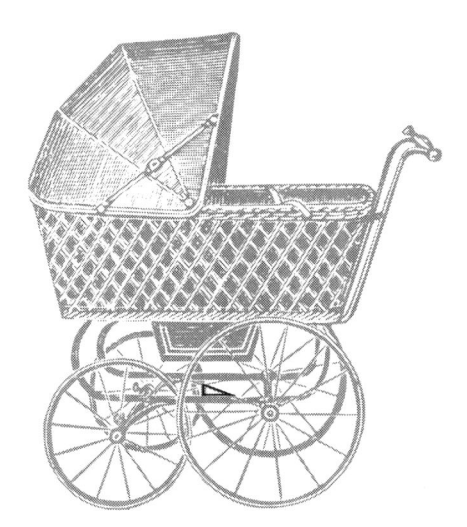

The location of the triangle from page 362.

REVIEW QUESTIONS

1. A 5 y/o M is brought into the pediatrician's office by his parents. They recently immigrated to the United States, and this is their first time visiting a doctor. Through a translator, the parents report that the boy does not speak in full sentences and communicates primarily by pointing at things and making loud noises. He spends the majority of his time playing with a set of marbles that was given to him by his grandparents one year ago. He will spend hours arranging these marbles in a specific order repeatedly, and if anyone moves or disturbs the marbles, he will scream and cry for up to an hour. He refuses to eat the majority of food placed in front of him and will only eat carrots, crackers, and a certain brand of cookie. His parents report that there were no problems with either pregnancy or childbirth. On exam, the boy does not respond to any questions that the pediatrician asks through the interpreter. Throughout the interview, his facial expression registers no change in emotion when approached by either his parents or any healthcare providers, and for the most part he appears indifferent to whether anyone else is in the room. Which of the following developmental milestones is this patient most likely to have missed?
   A. Babbling at 6 months
   B. Walking with assistance at 12 months
   C. Two-word sentences at 24 months
   D. Stacking 9 cubes at 36 months
   E. Parallel play at 2 months

2. (Continued from previous question.) The parents are informed of the diagnosis through the translator. They nod quietly in response and ask, "We came here so our son could have a better life. We want him to go to school and become successful. What can we do to ensure this?" What is the best response?
   A. "Your son will likely be very successful in life. He has been given abilities most of us don't have and will be able to memorize things perfectly."
   B. "The outlook for this condition is very good, and most cases resolve within a few years. However, it is possible that symptoms will return in the future."
   C. "As long as your son continues to take the medications he is prescribed, he will do just fine."
   D. "It is too early to say for sure, but it is likely that your son will struggle at least in some ways."
   E. "If your son had started treatment earlier, it may have been possible. But now it is out of the question: your son will not finish school."

3. A 16 y/o M is brought to a psychiatrist's office by his mother. His mother asks to speak with the psychiatrist separately. She says that the patient is "not normal" and requests a full evaluation. In particular, she says that he has "a lot of trouble reading people" and will often accuse his parents and others around him of being upset or angry at him when they are not doing anything out of the ordinary. She also says that he is "into some really weird things." She knows this because she has installed an internet monitoring device on his computer without his knowledge. She says that he is part of an online message board for people who believe that they are animal spirits inhabiting human bodies ("He thinks he's a platypus!"). Because of these interests and his difficulties interacting with others, he restricts his friendships to only two or three other students at school with whom he is very close. He is otherwise doing well at school, with mostly As and Bs. He has no medical conditions and saw a pediatrician yearly for check-ups throughout his life. On interview, the patient denies that there is anything wrong and that he wants to go home. He says flatly that he frequently fantasizes about running away so that he can "be with people who actually understand me." What is the most likely diagnosis?
    A. Autism spectrum disorder with intellectual disability
    B. Autism spectrum disorder without intellectual disability
    C. Intellectual disability without autism
    D. Pragmatic language impairment
    E. Rett syndrome
    F. None of the above

4. A 1 y/o F is brought by her parents to see a pediatrician. This is her first visit with a doctor. Upon entering the room, the pediatrician notices that the infant does not turn her head to look at him and makes no attempts to imitate his vocalizations. She does not attempt to speak or even babble. She instead largely points at objects that she is interested in. Her developmental milestones are otherwise intact. When taking a history from the family, they report that she is generally healthy other than an episode three months ago when she developed a high fever and cried inconsolably for several days. She experienced two seizures during this illness. They did not seek medical care at that time, and the fever resolved on its own within one week. Which of the following is the best next step?
    A. Inform the family of the diagnosis of autism and refer for speech and behavioral therapy
    B. Inform the family that autism is the most likely explanation but that the patient is too young to say with complete certainty
    C. Ask the parents to bring the patient back in one week after keeping a vocalization journal
    D. Refer the parents to an audiologist for evaluation
    E. Determine whether there are other children in the home

1. **The best answer is C.** This vignette describes a case of autism in a young boy as evidenced by deficits in social communication (including lack of speech and indifference to the presence of others) as well as restricted and repetitive activities (such as a rigid adherence to playing with the same toys in the same ways). Autism is most strongly associated with delays in speech-related milestones rather than motor milestones (answers B and D). However, these deficits in speech often do not begin until the age of 1 at the earliest, so deficits in babbling at 6 months are unlikely to be apparent without specifically looking for them (answer A). Parallel play at 2 years is not pathological and is consistent with a diagnosis of autism (answer E), although for this patient there was likely the absence of cooperative play at age 4.

2. **The best answer is D.** The clinical course of autism is characterized by chronic deficits in multiple domains rather than recurrent episodes of symptoms (answer B). However, the prognosis for the condition is also highly variable, making it too early to say for sure (although the lack of speech by age 5 is very concerning). While the prognosis for autism is improved with earlier initiation of treatment, most individuals still benefit from beginning treatment at the age of 5 (answer E). While some cases of autism include savantism, this is the exception rather than the rule, and most cases instead involve intellectual disability (answer A). Finally, medications play no role in improving outcomes in autism (answer C).

3. **The best answer is F.** While this patient's mother reports concerns in both the patient's social interaction and his interests, objectively there is little evidence of actual impairment in either of these domains, so it would not be appropriate to diagnose autism (answers And B). The fact that he has not been referred for evaluation prior to adolescence argues further against a diagnosis of autism. In addition, it is not clear that his difficulty with understanding the emotions of others is related to hypomentalization as would be seen in autism; if anything, he may engage in *hyper*mentalization by assuming that others have negative emotions that they may not have. He has an intact social support network which argues against pragmatic language impairment (answer D), and he is performing well as a student which argues against an intellectual disability (answer C). As a male, it is unlikely that he would have survived into adolescence with Rett syndrome (answer E).

4. **The best answer is E.** The patient has failed to meet her one-year language milestones which is cause for immediate concern. While autism is one possible explanation, there are many others that need to be ruled out as well (answers A and B). In this case, there is clear evidence of medical neglect as the family did not bring the child in for care despite a week-long fever with multiple seizures. As with all cases of suspected abuse or neglect, ensuring that the patient and other dependents in the home are safe is the highest priority, so it would not be appropriate to send the infant home with her parents at this time (answer C). While an auditory evaluation is likely necessary at some point to rule out hearing loss (especially in the context of an undiagnosed fever), it is not the highest priority at this time (answer D).

21 ADHD

Attention deficit hyperactivity disorder (ADHD) is a syndrome involving signs and symptoms in two domains: **inattention** and **hyperactivity**. (The diagnosis was previously called just "attention-deficit disorder," so you may hear "ADD" used instead of "ADHD" from time to time.) Like intellectual disability and autism, ADHD is considered to be a **neurodevelopmental disorder** that begins in childhood. However, unlike those conditions, ADHD does not present with failure to meet milestones. Instead, children with ADHD are most often brought to clinical attention due to **poor school performance**, **disruptive behavior**, or both.

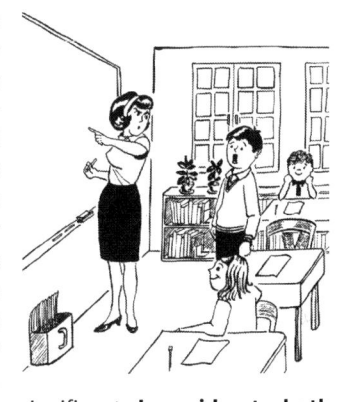

Diagnosing ADHD is tricky because there are significant **downsides to both undertreatment and overtreatment**. On one hand, children with untreated ADHD often have severe impairments in multiple areas of life as a direct consequence of this disorder including poor academic achievement, unstable peer relationships, and frequent run-ins with authority, some of which can have lasting consequences. For this reason, it seems cruel to deprive these children of the benefits of diagnosis (such as access to effective treatment). On the other hand, overdiagnosis of ADHD can also be impairing by inappropriately stigmatizing a child, communicating that there is something "wrong" with them, and taking away their sense of self-efficacy if they begin to believe that they are unable to do things without medications. There is also the risk of "medicalizing" structural problems (such as a child growing up in poverty who has trouble paying attention in school due to hunger, for whom a diagnosis of ADHD is missing the real problem). Because the risks of both overdiagnosis and underdiagnosis are so profound, taking the time to gain a good understanding about how to evaluate the signs and symptoms of ADHD across the lifespan is essential.

SIGNS AND SYMPTOMS OF ADHD

Let's look at each of the core symptom domains of ADHD in more detail.

INATTENTION

Inattention involves difficulties in focusing on a particular object or task over and above other stimuli. While most people have a train of thought that is able to stay on track for at least a few minutes at a time, in someone with ADHD **the train of thought is easily derailed**. This lack of ability to sustain attention leads to specific behavioral outcomes which are captured in the DSM-5 criteria for inattention in ADHD. You can remember these signs and symptoms using the mnemonic **DETAILS OFF** which will remind you that patients with ADHD often struggle with **D**etails of their work being sloppy, are **E**asily distracted ("Oh look a butterfly!"), tend to engage in **T**ask **A**voidance (especially if the task requires continuous attention), often appear to **I**gnore instructions, frequently **L**ose things, have trouble **S**ustaining attention on the same task, lack personal **O**rganization, are **F**orgetful when it comes to appointments or other responsibilities, and generally **F**ail to finish tasks once they have started. Of note, many people with ADHD still show good attention for subjects or tasks that they find intrinsically interesting, suggesting that it is not *impossible* for someone with ADHD to focus—it is just much harder for them than for most people.

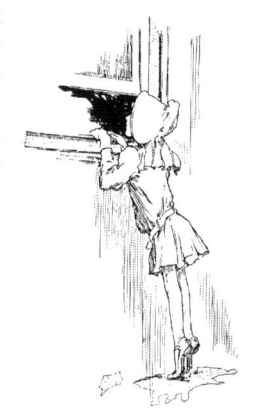

Inattention in ADHD is observable through a variety of **specific behaviors**.

DETAILS OFF:
Details sloppy
Easily distracted
Task Avoidance
Ignores instructions
Loses things
Sustained attention
Organization poor
Forgetful
Fails to finish tasks

HYPERACTIVITY

Hyperactivity involves a high level of energy that makes it difficult to sit still or to refrain from acting impulsively. The specific behaviors associated with hyperactivity in ADHD are captured in the mnemonic **HE RILED UP** which will remind you that patients with ADHD are **H**yperactive (often fidgeting and squirming in their seat), **E**nergetic (some describe them as "acting as if driven by a motor"), prone to **R**unning around or climbing even in situations where it is inappropriate (such as in the middle of class), predisposed to **I**nterrupting or intruding upon others' conversations, **L**oud (with difficulty doing activities quietly), **E**ffusive and talkative in their speech, intolerant of **D**elays or waiting, **U**nseated or up and about at times when they should stay in place, and inclined to **P**rematurely answer questions even before the person is done asking them. These behaviors can be a problem in the patient's home life, but they tend to become particularly pronounced when the child is placed in structured environments (like school) that rely upon a certain level of order and cooperation between the teacher and the students in class. Importantly, children with ADHD generally do not necessarily *intend* to be disruptive, but they find themselves unable to stop from acting impulsively (in contrast to the intentional behavior seen in conditions like oppositional defiant disorder).

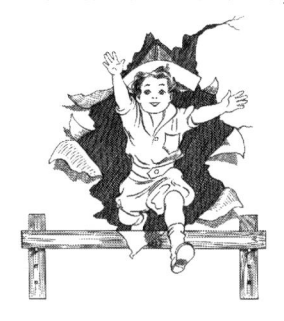

Hyperactivity in ADHD manifests through **unintentional disruptive behaviors**.

***HE RILED UP*:**
***H**yperactive*
***E**nergetic*
***R**unning around*
***I**nterrupts*
***L**oud*
***E**ffusive/talkative*
***D**elay intolerant*
***U**nseated/up and about*
***P**remature answers*

It's important to remember that neither of these symptoms are problematic in and of themselves. A certain level of inattention for tasks and subjects that we do not find interesting is completely normal, and hyperactivity is one of the perks of being a kid! However, when these traits become **persistent and inflexible**, a disorder can result. It's not a problem to be loud and hyperactive in places that can accommodate this (like a theme park), but it can be disruptive in places that cannot (like a funeral).

While the name "attention deficit hyperactivity disorder" suggests that both inattention and hyperactivity are required for a diagnosis (similar to how a diagnosis of autism requires both "aloneness" and "sameness"), the truth is that these two symptom domains do *not* always co-exist in the same patient. In fact, the most common form of ADHD involves inattention *without* hyperactivity! This brings up an important question: if these two symptom domains can occur in the absence of the other, why are they lumped together in the first place? There are two reasons. First, inattention and hyperactivity co-occur in the same person more often than would be predicted by chance. Second, both symptom domains appear to respond to the same kinds of treatment. Together, these facts likely suggest a **shared neurobiological mechanism** between inattention and hyperactivity.

ADHD ACROSS THE LIFESPAN

EPIDEMIOLOGY

ADHD affects approximately 10% of children and 5% of adults, making it a **common condition** with a high base rate in the population. The predominantly **inattentive subtype** is the most common, accounting for over two-thirds of all cases of ADHD (with the **combined subtype** making up around 20% and the **hyperactive subtype** accounting for the other 10%). ADHD subtypes tend to be **unstable over time**, and people may shift between them throughout their lives.

ADHD is more common in **males** compared to females, with a gender ratio of over 2 to 1. Males are more likely than girls to have the hyperactive subtype (which is reflected by the "he" in the HE RILED UP mnemonic). However, this may make ADHD in females more likely to be underdiagnosed.

ADHD is one of the **most heritable** psychiatric conditions, with studies showing that genes account for about 75% of the variance between different people. However, environmental factors are also believed to play a large role, with *in utero* tobacco exposure, maternal stress, premature delivery, low birth weight, poverty, and (weirdly enough) growing up in an English-speaking household all being risk factors for ADHD. Cultural factors are likely involved, as rates of diagnosis vary from country to country and even from place to place within the same country.

The signs and symptoms of ADHD **begin during childhood**, with an age of onset around 3 to 8 years. The age of diagnosis varies by how severe the symptoms are, with children who have severe symptoms often being diagnosed by the age of 5 while those who have only mild symptoms aren't diagnosed until 8 or even after. Despite some thought that there might be an "adult onset" version of ADHD occurring in people with no history of the disorder during childhood, evidence does not support this notion, as concurrent substance use appears to explain the vast majority of supposedly "adult onset" cases. This solidifies ADHD's status as a neurodevelopmental disorder which necessarily has its roots in childhood.

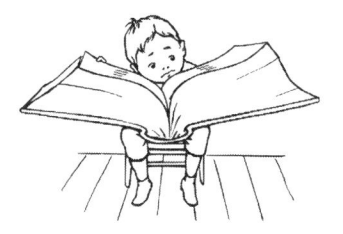

PROGNOSIS

Once symptoms appear, they are **chronic and enduring** (rather than episodic or fluctuating) which further helps to solidify ADHD's status as a neurodevelopmental disorder. Interestingly, the two domains of ADHD tend to follow different trajectories, as hyperactivity is often prominent during childhood but then slowly decreases with age whereas inattention tends to persist at roughly the same level throughout life.

On the whole, cases of ADHD tend to persist across the lifespan, and roughly two-thirds of people diagnosed with ADHD as children will continue to show signs of the condition as adults (either as a "full blown" disorder or in a subsyndromal form that falls short of diagnostic criteria but still remains impairing to some degree). However, this also means that up to one-third of children diagnosed with ADHD will show no signs of the disorder as adults, so the diagnosis should not be assumed to be lifelong in every case. For unknown reasons, cases of ADHD with a clear family history are most likely to "burn out" by adulthood while those with a stronger environmental component are more likely to persist into adulthood.

Untreated ADHD can have profoundly impairing effects both during childhood and later in life. School children with ADHD tend to have worse educational outcomes, greater stress in family and peer relationships, and increased rates of other psychiatric disorders (including anxiety and depression) compared to those without the disorder. For cases of ADHD that persist into adulthood, there is an association with poorer long-term outcomes in academic achievement, job performance, addictive behaviors, marital problems, unwanted pregnancies, and car accidents.

TREATMENT
Treatment of ADHD consists of **therapy, medications, or both**. The most commonly used therapies consist of behavioral management and training, including CBT and family therapy. In general, behavioral therapies for ADHD are associated with **medium effect sizes** in the range of 0.6 to 0.7. Like most psychotherapies, the beneficial effects of treatment last even after the treatment is discontinued.

Drug treatment of ADHD involves medications known as **stimulants**. Stimulants generally work by increasing the levels of the neurotransmitters **dopamine** and **norepinephrine** which results in improvement in both inattention and hyperactivity. The two most commonly used stimulants are methylphenidate (commonly known as Ritalin) and amphetamine salts (Adderall). As a class, stimulants are associated with a **very large effect size** above 1.0. In fact, stimulant medications are among the most effective treatments for any psychiatric syndrome, with over 70% of people treated with these medications showing significant improvement in the presenting symptoms. However, they are not without risk, including the possibility of growth restriction (although these children often "catch up" in height once the medication is stopped), appetite suppression, insomnia, and the potential for addiction and abuse at higher doses. Given these risks, behavioral therapies should generally be considered first, especially for those who are younger or only have mild symptoms.

A variety of **non-stimulant** medications (such as atomoxetine, guanfacine, and clonidine) are available as well. However, the effect size for non-stimulants is lower (around 0.5), making them comparable to behavioral therapies but without the benefit of long-lasting changes. Because of this, non-stimulants are generally only used in cases where medication is necessary but a stimulant cannot be used *or* to help increase the effect of a stimulant when additional improvement is needed.

MECHANISMS OF ADHD

While the precise mechanisms of ADHD are still unknown, one hypothesis suggests that the inattention and hyperactivity seen in the disorder are both related to abnormal signal processing in the central nervous system due to **excessive neuronal background noise**. To understand this, let's briefly review some neurophysiology. Neurons work by generating an electrical signal (an action potential) that then travels to specific other neurons to communicate a message. For example, if you were to accidentally hit your foot with a hammer, the neurons innervating your foot would send action potentials to the primary somatosensory cortex in your brain to register the sensation of pain. An action potential is meaningful because it represents a distinct **change from baseline**. However, this also means that the ability of a neuron to communicate information depends as much upon generating a signal when there *is* a stimulus as it does upon *not* generating a signal when there *isn't* a stimulus.

It is this process that appears to have broken down in ADHD, and studies have shown that neurons in the central nervous systems of people with this disorder are significantly more likely to generate signals even when not exposed to any stimuli. This creates a level of "background noise" that impairs the ability of these neurons to transmit information about *actual* stimuli to the brain, making it difficult for these individuals to focus on relevant stimuli. This is supported by studies showing that the "noisiness" of neuronal signals at baseline appears to correlate with the symptom severity of ADHD, supporting a direct link to the pathophysiology of the disorder.

To understand how a noisy baseline signal leads to inattention, imagine the mind as an old radio that receives radio waves via an antenna. The radio will stay on the same station (equivalent to sustaining attention) as long as it is receiving a clear signal. However, if the receiver loses the signal, it will assume that the station is off the air and attempt to switch over to another station with a clearer signal. For most people, this automatic switch from a station with a noisy degraded signal to another station with a clearer signal is helpful, as it prevents attention from being wasted on irrelevant or extraneous information. For people with ADHD, however, the signal is *always* noisy (like a busted radio that is constantly overloaded with static). This static interferes with the signal, causing the radio set to "think" that there is no meaningful information coming in. In response to this, the radio begins "searching" by constantly switching to different stations to find one with a cleaner signal. However, because the static is coming from the radio itself (not from the station that it is tuned to), a cleaner signal is never found, leading to an unending loop of attentional switches.

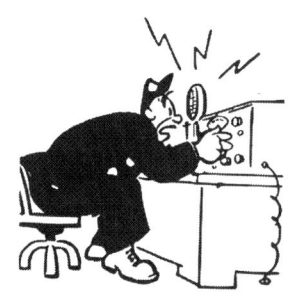

There are a variety of ways to compensate for the perpetual neuronal "noise" that people with ADHD experience. One is to boost levels of dopamine using stimulant medications, which causes a general **increase in the salience of information**. This allows incoming neuronal signals to stand out over the normal background "noise" (continuing the previous analogy, the radio is better able to hold onto this boosted signal, leading to less station switching). Salience can also be boosted by **novelty**, as new or exciting situations prompt the release of dopamine just like stimulants. Indeed, studies of brain metabolism in people with ADHD have shown that they have abnormally strong responses to new objects and environments. This could explain the disruptive and impulsive behaviors that people with ADHD engage in, as they help to generate novelty and thereby boost a signal that is noisy or degraded at baseline.

The images on the following page can help to illustrate the concepts we have discussed here, with the top image showing a signal with no noise (similar to someone without ADHD) and the middle image showing a signal with an increased level of background noise (representing someone with ADHD). The bottom image shows what happens when the background image is "boosted," demonstrating how stimulants and novelty (which both increase the underlying signal) can help to provide a clearer picture even when the signal is overlaid with noise.

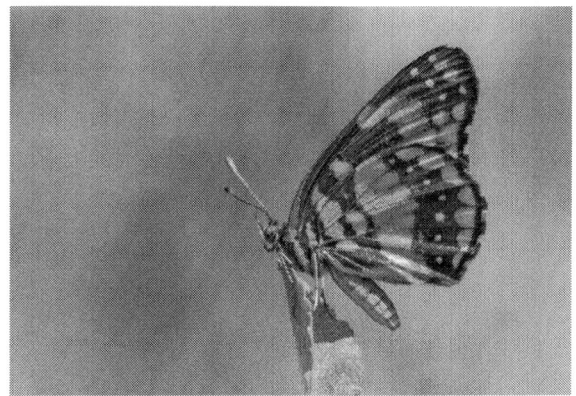

*Image of a butterfly **without static noise**.*

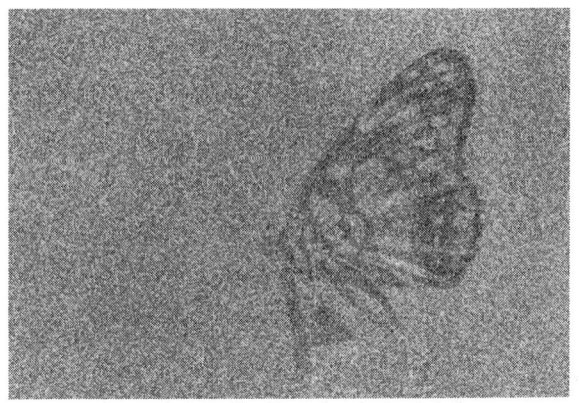

*Image of a butterfly **with static noise** to mimic the degraded signal of an individual with ADHD.*

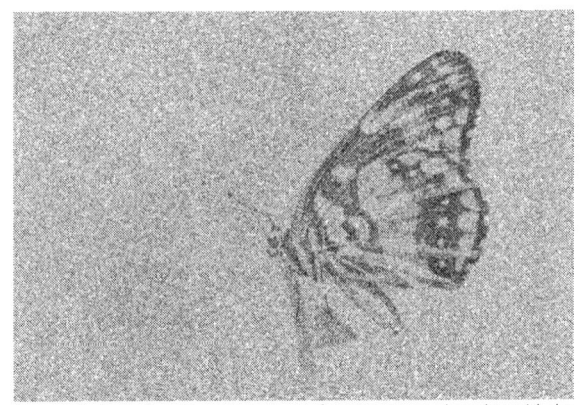

*Image of a butterfly with same amount of static noise as above but with the **underlying signal "boosted"** through enhanced contrast and brightness, leading to an increased ability to understand the image despite the noise.*

DIAGNOSING ADHD

On the face of it, the diagnostic criteria for ADHD don't appear to need a mnemonic, as the core patterns of the disorder are right there in the name: an "attention deficit" and "hyperactivity." However, there are a few nuances to pay attention to whenever you are diagnosing cases of ADHD.

ADHD should be considered a **diagnosis of exclusion**, as other medical, environmental, and social reasons for inattention and hyperactivity must be ruled out first. For example, a child who is stressed due to watching their parents fight every evening will likely have difficulty sleeping at night, leading to fatigue and difficulty staying awake during class. This may manifest as inattention, but it should not be automatically assumed to be ADHD. While this is a rather obvious example, more subtle forms may exist as well. For example, ADHD is diagnosed more frequently in the youngest children in each class (due to their earlier stage of cognitive development compared to their peers), illustrating how unconscious expectations play a large role in diagnosis as well.

To lower the risk of diagnosing a child with a disorder when the problem is actually in the environment, the DSM requires that signs of ADHD must be present in **at least two different settings** (such as at school *and* at home) before assigning the diagnosis. Nevertheless, as with any psychiatric syndrome, it is probably not possible to *completely* remove diagnostic subjectivity from the equation.

Putting this all together, you can use the mnemonic **FIDGETY** to remember the diagnostic criteria as listed in the DSM. The first half of the word will remind you that the core pattern of ADHD involves **F**unctionally impairing levels of either **I**nattention and/or behavioral **D**isinhibition. The second half of the word includes a few caveats to remember: that these symptoms must be **G**reater than expected (and not just the usual running around that is a completely normal part of growing up); that you need to **E**xclude other possible causes such as mood or anxiety disorders; that these patterns must be observed in **T**wo or more settings such as at school *and* at home; and finally that the patient must have been **Y**oung at the first onset of the disorder, with signs and symptoms first appearing before the age of 12 if not even earlier.

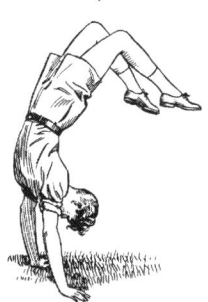

ADHD involves inattention and hyperactivity that is excessive, unrelated to other disorders, and has been observed in **multiple settings** from a **young age**.

FIDGETY:
Functionally impairing
Inattention
Disinhibition
Greater than normal
Exclude other disorders
Two or more settings
Young at onset (12 or less)

DIFFERENTIAL DIAGNOSIS OF ADHD

Over 70% of people with ADHD have at least one other comorbid psychiatric disorder. This includes not only externalizing disorders like oppositional defiant disorder and intermittent explosive disorder but also internalizing disorders like depression and anxiety. In addition, other neurodevelopmental disorders like intellectual disability and autism can be present as well. For this reason, it is important to evaluate for other psychiatric syndromes that can present with inattention and/or hyperactivity.

NORMALCY
ADHD is a **controversial diagnosis**. After all, isn't some degree of not wanting to sit quietly in school expected even downright *normal* during childhood? When thinking about ADHD, it is helpful to keep in mind that *at extremes the quantitative becomes qualitative*. Most children lie somewhere on a spectrum of severity in terms of inattention and hyperactivity. However, some children have inattention and hyperactivity that is *so* pronounced that it leaves little doubt that these characteristics impair their personal, social, and scholastic performance. In these cases, diagnosing ADHD is not difficult.

ADHD must also be separated out from the *normal* effects of *abnormal* circumstances. Because the symptoms of ADHD are so non-specific, it is important not to make a "knee-jerk" diagnosis when faced with a child who displays either inattention or hyperactivity and instead take a close look at the wide variety of factors that may be at play. To remember the various things that can frequently mimic ADHD, use the mnemonic **PAN LID NOISE**. (To link this phrase to ADHD, imagine an inattentive and hyperactive kid who is banging on pan lids and making lots of noise!)

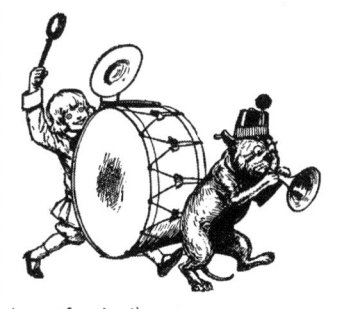

PAN is for Parenting, Abuse, and Neglect. Parenting styles can impact a child's behavior depending on what actions are rewarded or punished, and this can influence whether someone is diagnosed with ADHD. In more extreme cases, abuse and neglect can directly disrupt a child's ability to behave in accordance with what is expected of them (which can resemble the hyperactivity and impulsivity seen in ADHD).

LID is for Learning, Intellectual, and Developmental Disabilities. ADHD is a common cause of poor performance in school, but it is not the only one! Be mindful to screen for intellectual or learning disabilities as well. In contrast to a learning disability, academic impairment related to ADHD will improve with treatment. Learning disorders and ADHD can also co-occur, and in these cases both conditions must be treated separately (using educational techniques for learning disorders and behavioral management and/or stimulants for ADHD). ADHD should also be distinguished from autism and intellectual disabilities, both of which can closely mimic (or are often comorbid with) this condition. One way to do this is to remember that ADHD rarely presents with failure to reach specific developmental milestones (whereas this is a diagnostic hallmark of both autism and intellectual disability).

N is for Nutrition. Inadequate food can lead to persistent hunger that impairs one's ability to concentrate at school, making assessment of nutritional status an important part of the diagnostic process.

O is for Other conditions. Be on the lookout for any unusual signs or symptoms that could suggest an alternative medical or psychiatric explanation for the signs of ADHD. For example, a child who develops type 1 diabetes mellitus may begin to show signs of inattention, irritability, or hyperactivity when their blood sugar becomes abnormal. There will be other signs and symptoms of diabetes as well (such as excessive thirst or frequent urination), but these would only be picked up if the clinician is careful to take a full medical history.

I is for Intoxication. Use of certain substances can mimic symptoms of ADHD. The most common culprit is caffeine due to its easy availability. While caffeine can help keep people awake and potentially even improve concentration, it can also make people feel restless or hyperactive, especially when in situations that require them to sit still for long periods of time. Prescribed medications can impair cognition as well, with antihistamines (used for allergies) and anticonvulsants (used for seizures) being not uncommonly used in children.

S is for Sleep. Children who are unable to sleep at night will often have difficulty concentrating or even staying awake during the day, leading to persistent inattention and irritability that can resemble the symptoms of ADHD. For this reason, assessing the amount and quality of sleep for anyone presenting with ADHD-like symptoms is essential, and the presence of insomnia should lead to an investigation into possible causes of disrupted sleep (such as bullying or stress).

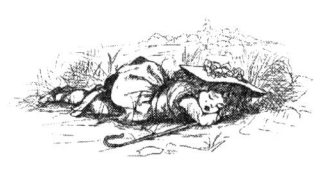

E is for Environment. Finally, please remember that the signs and symptoms of ADHD must be seen in **more than one environment**! Cases that are diagnosed based on only one environment likely suggest an outside factor that is specific to that place rather than to the child.

A variety of **medical and environmental factors** must be ruled out before assigning a diagnosis of **ADHD**.

PAN LID NOISE:
Parenting, Abuse, and Neglect
Learning, Intellectual, and Developmental disabilities
Nutrition
Other conditions
Intoxication
Sleep
Environment

EXTERNALIZING DISORDERS

ADHD and externalizing disorders are commonly confused, as both begin in childhood and feature the presence of frequent disruptive behaviors. Use the **PIRATES** framework to evaluate children brought in for evaluation of misbehavior. Increased levels of **A**ctivity is the surest sign of ADHD, as patients with ADHD display disruptive behaviors as the result of persistent hyperactivity. It is also crucial to evaluate **I**ntention, as patients with ADHD often do not *intend* to misbehave and will try to avoid annoying others, even if they find themselves unable to do so given their difficulty with sitting still. Children with ADHD will generally feel **R**emorse if they realize that they have upset others by cutting in line or interrupting them. Finally, **S**everity matters, as disruptive behaviors in patients with ADHD rarely rise to the level of flagrant disregard for the rights of others such as assault, bullying, or stealing that is seen in conditions like conduct disorder. In the real world, these lines are not always so clear cut, and many patients will have *both* ADHD and a comorbid externalizing disorder, making the drawing of lines difficult.

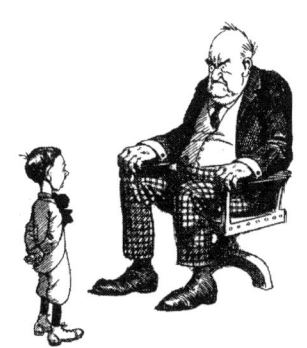

ABSENCE SEIZURES

An **absence seizure** (formerly called a "petit mal" seizure) is characterized by sudden episodes of altered consciousness. Someone experiencing an absence seizure can appear to be staring off blankly into space without paying attention to what is going on around them. While this can sometimes present with accompanying motor signs that make it obvious a seizure is occurring (like generalized body shaking), this is not always the case. For this reason, it is not uncommon for absence seizures to be initially misdiagnosed as ADHD. However, while children with absence seizures will experience inattentive staring episodes, they will generally show good attention when *not* having an seizure (unlike the *persistent* inattention seen in ADHD). Absence seizures can often be diagnosed clinically based on the history, although definitive diagnosis requires **electroencephalography** which will show a pattern of 3 Hz generalized "spike and wave" discharges that is practically pathognomonic for this disorder.

DEPRESSION

Given that depression and the inattentive subtype of ADHD can both present with difficulty concentrating, each should be on the differential for the other. However, the relationship between ADHD and depression goes deeper than that. For some people with untreated ADHD, chronic underachievement and difficulty meeting goals can result in a state of **demoralization** and **lack of motivation** that can strongly resemble depression. In addition, symptoms of ADHD can often prevent people from forming social relationships, with over 50% of children with ADHD reporting being lonely. To distinguish between these two diagnoses, focus on the presence of other symptoms of depression (the rest of **SIGECAPS**). In addition, in cases where someone's depressive symptoms stem entirely from the effects of ADHD, treatment of ADHD should itself improve depressive symptoms. In cases where these symptoms remain, consider making a separate diagnosis.

ADDICTION
The impulsivity seen in hyperactive or combined subtypes of ADHD can predispose people to developing addictions, and the rate of addictive disorders is significantly higher in people with ADHD than without. In addition, the medications used to treat ADHD can themselves be addictive (though typically only at much higher doses than those used therapeutically for ADHD), so be cautious if your patient begins asking for frequent or early refills. Finally, the effects of specific substances (either during intoxication or withdrawal) can easily mimic the inattention and hyperactivity seen in ADHD, so taking a careful substance history (and possibly obtaining a urine drug screen) can be diagnostically helpful.

ANXIETY
ADHD is frequently comorbid with anxiety in both children and adults. The anxiety present in the disorder is often (though not always) related to specific consequences of ADHD such as worrying about being into trouble with parents and teachers, not getting along well with peers, and doing poorly in school or at work. Treatment of ADHD will often result in decreased anxiety in these cases, though in cases where anxiety persists even after treatment, a separate diagnosis of an anxiety disorder (and treatment using CBT or SRIs) should be considered.

MANIA
The hyperactivity and impulsivity of ADHD can be mistaken for mania, although the timing of the two is completely different as these signs are *episodic* in mania and *chronic* in ADHD. Differences in the **age of onset** (childhood in ADHD and adolescence or early adulthood in bipolar disorder) can also differentiate between the two.

OBSESSIVE-COMPULSIVE DISORDERS
It may seem odd that ADHD and OCD would frequently be comorbid, as the impulsive disinhibited behavior seen in ADHD would seem to mix poorly with the compulsive risk-averse patterns seen in OCD. Indeed, studies of the neuropsychological profile of people with both ADHD and OCD have found that the inattention seen in people with OCD may be (at least in some cases) directly related to the obsessions themselves, which have become so frequent and intrusive that they make it difficult to concentrate on anything else. Because of this, consider whether inattentive symptoms in a patient with OCD can be attributed entirely to obsessive thoughts (in which case treatment of OCD should improve both) rather than to a separate diagnosis of ADHD.

TRAUMA
A history of abuse or neglect during early childhood is associated with an increased likelihood of developing ADHD. For this reason, it's important not to let the presence of hyperactivity and disruptive behaviors distract you from any trauma-related internalizing disorders that may be present as well (including not only "textbook" PTSD but also anxiety and depression as well). In fact, these internalizing disorders can often be even more impairing and distressing to the patient than the disruptive behaviors that may have brought them in for evaluation in the first place.

PERSONALITY DISORDERS

The disinhibition and impulsivity of cluster B personality disorders can strongly resemble ADHD, especially in those with a history of abuse or neglect. This association is strengthened further by the fact that these traits are chronic and enduring in both ADHD and personality disorders. In many cases, it is not always possible to tease out how much of the impulsivity present is related to ADHD versus a personality disorder, but the **function that the behavior has** can be a clue. People with ADHD tend to misbehave out of boredom or a need for stimulation, whereas people with cluster B personality disorders instead are often acting impulsively in order to escape from negative emotions or gain the approval of others.

PSYCHOSIS

Schizophrenia can present with impairments in attention that can resemble ADHD. The prodromal period is especially liable to misdiagnosis as the age range is roughly the same as ADHD while the dramatic positive symptoms of psychosis have yet to emerge. It is believed that disruptions of the salience network underlie both of these conditions, although in schizophrenia inattention is likely due to *too much* salience whereas in ADHD it is more likely related to *not enough* salience.

PUTTING IT ALL TOGETHER

ADHD is a neurodevelopmental disorder that begins in childhood and in many cases continues on into adulthood. Signs and symptoms of ADHD involve either inattention (as evidenced by the **DETAILS OFF** signs and symptoms) and/or hyperactivity (as evidenced by the **HE RILED UP** signs and symptoms). While symptoms of ADHD can be incredibly impairing, effective treatments are available, including both **behavioral therapy and medications**. The availability of treatment underscores the need to carefully screen for the condition, as untreated ADHD is associated with poor outcomes in various areas of life. When diagnosing ADHD, use the **FIDGETY** mnemonic to remember the core pattern of symptoms as well as important conditions to exclude. However, there are also significant downsides to diagnosing someone with ADHD, including a risk of overtreatment and stigma. Always rule out other factors that can mimic ADHD using the **PAN LID NOISE** mnemonic. Provided that these conditions are met, working with someone who has ADHD can be a very gratifying experience, as treatment often leads to improvements in functioning that are both immediate and dramatic.

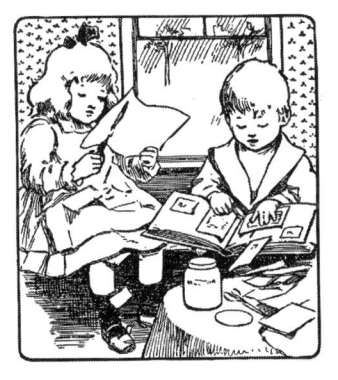

REVIEW QUESTIONS

1. A 6 y/o M is brought to the pediatrician's office by his mother. She says that he has developed "severe school anxiety" and throws tantrums every morning on the way to school. While at school, he is generally quiet and well-behaved. However, he has not done well on his assignments, and during a parent-teacher conference his mother was told that he often struggles to keep his focus on the subject at hand. He often has difficulty sitting with his parents long enough to work on homework at night, although he appears to have no difficulty sitting still to play video games for hours at a time on weekends. Pregnancy and delivery were both uncomplicated, and the patient has achieved all developmental milestones on time. He did well in preschool and is well liked by his classmates. Which of the following is *least* consistent with a diagnosis of ADHD as the primary explanation for this patient's behavior?
    A. Onset of symptoms at age 6
    B. Absence of hyperactivity at school
    C. Presence of inattention in multiple settings
    D. Being well-liked by his classmates
    E. Ability to focus on activities he finds enjoyable
    F. All of the above are consistent with a diagnosis of ADHD

2. (Continued from previous question.) The pediatrician places a referral for full neurocognitive testing. Results from the test are strongly suggestive of ADHD. At the next visit, the doctor discusses various treatment options and explains the risks and benefits of each. The mother says that she is hesitant about the idea of putting her child on medications. What is the most appropriate response?
    A. "That is entirely your choice. Medications are an option, but they are not the only one. Let's look into other possibilities."
    B. "Medications have been scientifically shown to be the single most effective treatment for ADHD, so we really should look at starting one right away."
    C. "A lot of parents have concerns about their children taking stimulants, but these tend to go away with time. Here is the number for a group of parents of children with ADHD who may be able to answer some more of your questions."
    D. "If you aren't interested in stimulants, there are a variety of non-stimulant options available that are just as effective. Your child really needs to be on some form of medication, though."
    E. "I agree. Children in this country are overmedicated, and even if you wanted to start a stimulant I wouldn't prescribe one."

3. A teacher requests a parent-teacher conference regarding a 9 y/o F in her class. During the conference, the teacher voices her concern that the girl frequently appears inattentive during class and has been turning in incomplete schoolwork for the past four weeks. The teacher notices several such episodes of "zoning out" throughout the day, each of which last around 5 seconds. Prior to this, the girl had been an "exceptional student" and was often seen reading at a level several years higher than her age. The girl is otherwise healthy with no history of trauma, drug exposure, or other medical conditions. The girl is referred to a child psychiatrist for further evaluation. The girl denies feelings of anxiety, depression, or irritability. However, she is concerned about her school performance and says, "I don't want to disappoint my parents." After a discussion with both the patient and her parents, a decision is made to start treatment with methylphenidate. At the follow-up visit two weeks later, her parents report no significant effect from the medication, so the dose is doubled. This only appears to increase the severity of her inattention. Which of the following best explains the patient's unusual reaction to methylphenidate?
    A. Some people are simply non-responsive to methylphenidate and need to be prescribed amphetamine salts instead
    B. The patient is having an allergic reaction to stimulants and should be prescribed a non-stimulant
    C. It was inappropriate for the psychiatrist to have prescribed medications for ADHD without attempting behavioral treatment first
    D. It was inappropriate for the psychiatrist to have prescribed medications for ADHD without completing a full work-up
    E. This is a normal and expected reaction to methylphenidate

4. A 14 y/o M is brought to a child psychiatrist along with a note from his teacher that reads "ADHD evaluation needed." He recently transitioned into high school where he has struggled both academically and socially. Prior to this, he went to a private school that strongly emphasized accommodating different learning styles. His learning style was determined to be "kinesthetic/tactile," and he was encouraged to build dioramas and art projects in place of taking written tests. He did very well at this school and showed good attention even for projects that he did not find interesting. He was born two months premature and spent four weeks in the neonatal intensive care unit but has otherwise been healthy during his life. Testing performed at age 5 showed a slightly above average IQ of 114, but he has not been retested since then. Both the patient's parents and the teachers at his new school confirm that he is well-behaved in class and shows no difficulty with waiting in line for his turn. As part of his evaluation, he is given a self-evaluation form to fill out. Despite taking an hour to look over the form, however, he hands it in blank with a look of embarrassment on his face. Which of the following is the most likely diagnosis at this time?
    A. Attention deficit hyperactivity disorder, inattentive type
    B. Attention deficit hyperactivity disorder, hyperactive type
    C. Attention deficit hyperactivity disorder, combined type
    D. An intellectual disability
    E. A learning disorder

1. **The best answer is F.** While other causes still need to be ruled out, the description of this patient's case is consistent with a diagnosis of ADHD. Cases of ADHD often begin between the ages of 3 to 8 (answer A). While both inattention and hyperactivity are found in the name, it is not necessary for both to be present for a diagnosis to given, so the absence of hyperactivity does not rule out ADHD in this case (answer B). The presence of symptoms in more than one setting is not only consistent with a diagnosis of ADHD, it is required (answer C). It is not uncommon for people with ADHD to be able to focus on activities they find intrinsically interesting or enjoyable (answer E). Finally, being well-liked by peers is not related to a diagnosis of ADHD (answer D).

2. **The best answer is A.** Medications are one of the primary treatment options for ADHD, but they are not the only option, as behavioral therapies have been shown to be effective for ADHD as well. While stimulants are the single most effective treatment, that does not mean that the mother should be pressured into starting one for her child (answer B). Non-stimulants are available as well, although it is incorrect to say that they are equally as effective as stimulants (answer D). Finally, it would not be appropriate either to defer a discussion about medications to non-professionals (answer C) or to refuse to prescribe stimulants for a clearly documented case of ADHD even if the mother desired it (answer E).

3. **The best answer is D.** This describes a case of absence seizures as evidenced by the fact that her inattention occurs in brief episodes lasting only a few seconds, which is highly characteristic of an absence seizure. It is also unusual, though not entirely outside the realm of possibility, for symptoms of ADHD to start suddenly in a girl who previously had no difficulties. Therefore, the psychiatrist should have established the nature of her inattention more clearly and ordered an electroencephalogram, which would show the 3 Hz "spike and wave" complexes associated with absence seizures. While it is true that some patients respond better to amphetamine salts than methylphenidate, a paradoxical worsening of inattention in response to a stimulant of any kind is highly unusual (answers A and E). This is not an allergic reaction to a stimulant, which would generally involve a rash, itching, swelling, or difficulty breathing (answer B). Finally, in most cases of ADHD it is reasonable to prescribe stimulants without first attempting behavioral therapy; however, in this case that would also have been ineffective as the underlying condition would remain undiagnosed (answer C).

4. **The best answer is E.** This patient likely suffers from a learning disorder such as dyslexia. While it is unusual for a learning disorder to suddenly "appear" during adolescence, the style of the patient's previous school likely allowed for difficulty reading to remain undetected for longer than usual. It is highly unusual for ADHD to spontaneously begin during adolescence or adulthood, and there are no reports of either inattention or hyperactivity (answers A, B, and C). In addition, an intellectual disability is absolutely ruled out by a lack of signs or symptoms beginning in early childhood (answer D).

22 DEMENTIA

In this chapter, we will shift our focus from disorders primarily seen in children to those seen in older adults. The process of aging (also known as **senescence**) is a normal part of human development. Unlike childhood development, there are no specific motor, speech, or cognitive milestones for adults to meet as they enter old age. Instead, aging is often accompanied by various *losses* in functioning that gradually increase over the years. Many of these changes (including some degree of memory loss) are considered to be completely within the realm of normalcy. However, there are also a variety of disorders associated with old age that cause distress and dysfunction not only for the patient themselves but also for their loved ones.

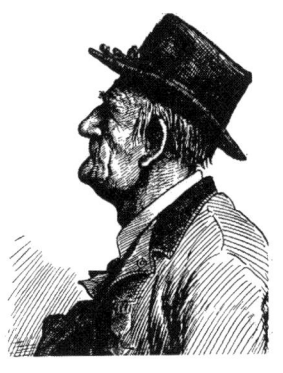

For the rest of this chapter, we will focus on a group of conditions known as **dementia** (formally called **major neurocognitive disorders** in the DSM-5). Dementia is a broad category of diseases characterized by a chronic and progressive **loss of memory and cognitive abilities**. Like the word "cancer," "dementia" does not refer to a single disorder but rather to many diseases that all share commonalities. The main forms of dementia are Alzheimer's disease, dementia with Lewy bodies, frontotemporal dementia, and vascular dementia. It is possible for multiple forms of dementia to be present at the same time, which is known as mixed dementia. For example, someone with loss of memory due to Alzheimer's disease may *also* have recurrent strokes that each reduce their cognitive abilities further. While we will spend the most time on Alzheimer's disease (as it is by far the most common type), we will also touch briefly on all forms of dementia with a specific focus on identifying the clinical signs and symptoms that are the most helpful in differentiating between each of these conditions. First, though, we will begin this chapter with a discussion of what is seen in normal aging, as this will help us identify when something is *ab*normal.

NORMAL AGING

Both **physical and psychological changes** are seen during the process of aging. Most organ systems in the body slow down or lose some degree of function, including the heart, lungs, liver, kidneys, bones, muscle, skin, and sensory organs. Sleep quality also declines, with increased nighttime awakenings and reduced restorative sleep.

The desire for **social interaction** is *not* significantly affected by aging, and social support remains important throughout the entire lifespan. While the *size* of one's social network often decreases due to deaths and other losses, the *quality* of each relationship often increases in response. Sudden changes in a patient's social patterns should prompt a further assessment for any physical or psychological barriers that could be present (such as social withdrawal due to depression). It is a myth that old people stop having sex, and many remain sexually active late into their lives.

Some degree of cognitive impairment is expected with aging. These losses in speed and flexibility occur primarily in the realm of **fluid intelligence**, which involves the ability to analyze and respond to *new* information. In contrast, **crystallized intelligence** (which is the result of well-practiced skills, abilities, and knowledge) is generally preserved and often even *increases* with old age. For example, a blacksmith with decades of experience would likely be able to make tools even in retirement due to preserved crystallized intelligence. However, if someone brought them a new computer to work on, they may have more difficulty with this (even if step-by-step instructions were available) due to reductions in fluid intelligence.

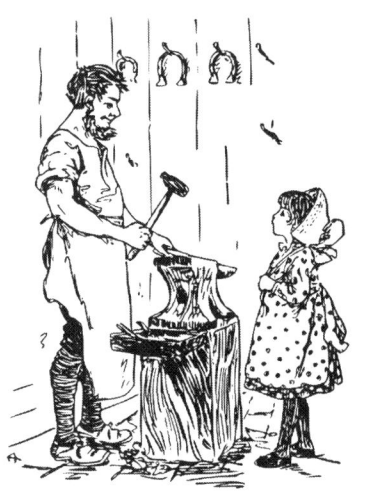

Acquisition of new memories and retention of old memories are both impaired. The type of memory most affected is **explicit memory** (also known as declarative memory) which involves consciously recalling specific facts or events ("Who was that person I ran into at the store yesterday?"). In contrast, **implicit memory** (or non-declarative memory) involving memories outside of one's conscious awareness ("Can you sing the melody of Happy Birthday?") remains intact throughout life.

There can also be deficits seen in some areas of language, including the ability to generate lists of words ("Tell me all the words beginning with the letter F that you can think of"). There can also be a small but noticeable loss of ability to speak and think abstractly, with a more **concrete thinking style** often seen in old age. In general, however, language and the ability to communicate meaningfully with others are *not* significantly impacted by normal aging.

Similar to knowing developmental milestones in childhood, understanding the cognitive domains that are or are not commonly affected during normal aging can assist in identifying when a patient's reported complaints are nothing to worry about versus being a sign of disease. You can remember the cognitive domains that are generally *preserved* during normal aging using the mnemonic **Crystal CLIR** which stands for **Cryst**allized intelligence, **C**oncrete reasoning, **L**anguage, **I**mplicit memory, and **R**ecognition of faces and situations. In contrast, the specific cognitive domains that are *impaired* during normal aging can be remembered using the mnemonic **Not so FAST** which stands for **F**lexibility, **A**bstraction, **S**peed, and **T**rain of thought (attention and concentration).

> **Crystallized intelligence, concrete reasoning, language, implicit memory,** and **recognition** are all preserved in **normal aging**.
>
> *Crystal CLIR:*
> **Crystal**lized intelligence
> **C**oncrete thinking
> **L**anguage
> **I**mplicit memory
> **R**ecognition

> **Normal aging** is accompanied by **decreases** in cognitive **flexibility**, **abstract** reasoning, processing **speed**, and **attention**.
>
> *Not so FAST:*
> **F**lexibility
> **A**bstraction
> **S**peed
> **T**rain of thought

When assessing for functional status, you may consider evaluating **activities of daily living** (ADLs) and **instrumental activities of daily living** (IADLs). ADLs are basic self-care tasks that a person needs to be able to do in order to survive. These can be remembered using the simple mnemonic **ABCDE**: **A**mbulating, **B**athing, **C**lothing, **D**efecating, and **E**ating. In contrast, IADLs are more complex tasks which are not as essential for survival but are still needed to live independently. IADLs can be remembered by packing each one into the acronym **IADLS** itself: **I**nteracting with other people, **A**ccounting (finances and bookkeeping), **D**omestic tasks (like cleaning and cooking), **L**eaving the house (driving, taking the bus, or otherwise getting around town), and **S**hopping for food and other necessities. Typically, the deficits seen in normal aging do *not* lead to functional impairment, and ADLs and IADLs give you a structured way of assessing this.

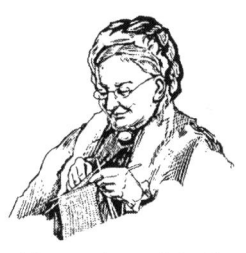

> **Activities of daily living** are a meaningful measurement of **functional status**.
>
> *ABCDE: **A**mbulating, **B**athing, **C**lothing, **D**efecating, and **E**ating.*
> *IADLS: **I**nteraction, **A**ccounting, **D**omestic tasks, **L**eaving the house, **S**hopping.*

SIGNS AND SYMPTOMS OF ALZHEIMER'S DISEASE

Dementia is characterized by cognitive deficits that are not only **unusual** but also result in **impairment** (in contrast to the memory loss seen in normal aging, which is both common and not disabling). **Alzheimer's disease** is the most common form of dementia and is considered to be the **prototypical neurocognitive disorder**, with other types of dementia often being compared and contrasted with it. For that reason, we will first learn about Alzheimer's disease in depth before moving on to other forms of dementia.

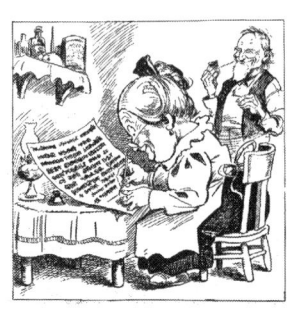

The signs and symptoms of Alzheimer's disease tend to come on **gradually** over months and years. (This helps to differentiate it from other forms of dementia, like those related to strokes, which instead occur in discrete episodes with plateaus in between.) The specific signs and symptoms involved can be remembered by thinking of two older grandparents who go by **MA 'N PA**:

M is for Memory. Memory losses in Alzheimer's disease a re more frequent and severe than those seen in normal aging. Whereas an older person may have *occasional* moments of forgetfulness (such as forgetting a specific word, where they placed an object, or why they walked into a room), someone with Alzheimer's disease is likely to forget these things on a regular basis and to a greater extent. **Short-term memory** (within the past several hours or days) is affected more severely than long-term memory, although in later stages of the illness long-term memory is impacted as well. **Explicit memory** is involved more often than implicit memory, although with time this distinction is also erased. Impaired **recognition of familiar faces** (such as close friends and family members) is a hallmark of severe Alzheimer's disease, as this tends to be intact in almost all healthy older adults.

A is for Awareness. The normal forgetfulness of aging is often accompanied by a distinct sense that information has been lost ("I can never remember where I put my keys!"). In contrast, people with Alzheimer's disease *lack* this awareness (they don't *know* that they don't know something). In later stages of the disease, the patient's level of **orientation** (their knowledge of who they are, where they are, what time it is, or why they are there) can be steadily lost as well.

N is for Neurocognitive deficits. To diagnose any form of dementia, the patient must have deficits in **multiple neurocognitive domains**, not just memory! Deficits in executive functioning, language, reasoning, and movement are all common. In formal clinical settings, **neuropsychological testing** can provide a structured assessment of all cognitive domains and highlight areas where the patient is struggling. If you are trying to assess based solely on the patient's presentation, look at their functional status as evidenced by their ability to care for their ADLs and IADLs. Often, one of the earliest signs of Alzheimer's disease is an **inability to plan and execute an idea**. For example, someone who is going fishing needs to have the ability to make a list of everything that they'll need to bring (executive functioning), fill out the fishing permit (language), use a map to find the lake (visuospatial), have the fine motor skills to put a piece of bait on the line (movement), and interpret what a sudden pull on the line means (recognition), among many other things. If there is impairment in any one of these domains, the trip will not work out. Because planning requires multiple cognitive abilities to be intact, an inability to plan can be a helpful indicator of which forms of cognition are impacted and to what extent.

P is for Psychiatric. Alzheimer's disease involves not only the *loss* of previous abilities but also the *presence* of new symptoms as well. Patients with Alzheimer's disease can show **mood changes** such as depression, irritability, and apathy. Around one-third of people with Alzheimer's disease develop **psychosis-like symptoms** including paranoia and delusions, with **delusional misidentification** (believing that a friend or family member is an impostor who has come to harm them) being a common pattern.

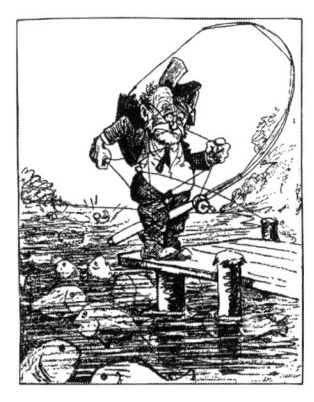

A is for Activity. The patient's level of activity in Alzheimer's disease is often both increased *and* decreased simultaneously, with **losses in complex behaviors** such as reading, writing, and socializing and **increases in purposeless behaviors** such as wandering and agitation. A particular pattern of behavior known as **sundowning** (a state of confused restlessness that is more prominent in the evening) is often observed. In some cases, the wandering and agitation can become so severe that patients need to be hospitalized or placed in long-term care to prevent them from injury or death (for example, if they are repeatedly trying to cross a busy street without using the crosswalk). As the disease progresses, patients lose their ability to perform IADLs which is then followed by ADLs. In final stages of the illness, many people with Alzheimer's disease are bed-bound and entirely dependent upon others for survival.

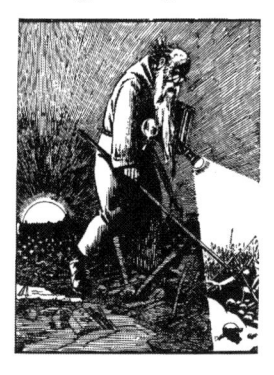

Alzheimer's disease involves not only the loss of cognitive abilities but also the presence of neuropsychiatric symptoms.

MA 'N PA:
Memory
Awareness
Neurocognitive deficits
Psychiatric
Activity

ALZHEIMER'S DISEASE ACROSS THE LIFESPAN

EPIDEMIOLOGY
Alzheimer's disease affects less than 1% of the total population at any given time, putting it on par with bipolar disorder or schizophrenia. While that would seem to make it a rare disorder and therefore more liable to overdiagnosis than underdiagnosis, in actual clinical practice you are going to be considering a diagnosis of dementia almost exclusively in patients who are **elderly**, a population where it is much more prevalent. While the chance of having Alzheimer's disease is around 3% at the age of 65, this risk **doubles every 5 years** after that, meaning that over 20% of people above the age of 80 and 50% of people above the age of 90 will develop this disease. However, younger age does not rule out this disorder entirely, as early-onset forms of Alzheimer's disease can begin in one's 50s or 60s. **Women** are affected more often than men, although this may have more to do with their longer lifespan than it does with any risk factors that are inherent to their gender.

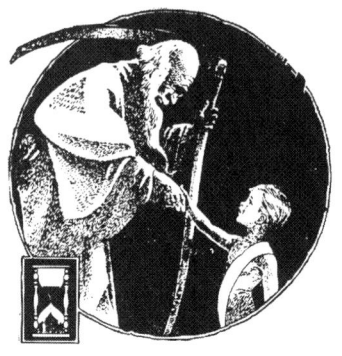

PROGNOSIS
Unfortunately, Alzheimer's disease is a **steadily progressive** condition, meaning that once it has begun it does not stop. For most patients with this disorder, additional deficits accumulate throughout the rest of their lifespan, leading to ongoing decreases in functional ability. People in early stages of Alzheimer's disease often require assistance with IADLs such as shopping or finances, while those in later stages of the disease can require assistance with even basic ADLs like eating and bathing. Incontinence of urine and stool is also seen in advanced stages of the disease and generally portends a poor prognosis, with a high risk of death within the next year. Alzheimer's disease is considered to be a **highly lethal** condition, as the risk of death is increased significantly compared to people the same age without the diagnosis. The average life expectancy from the time of diagnosis is around **5 years**, with death almost always occurring within 10 years. Alzheimer's disease is rarely the direct cause of death. Instead, the progressive functional decline leads to a lack of mobility which increases the risk of infection (which is the most common cause of death in Alzheimer's disease) as well as cardiovascular complications like clotting.

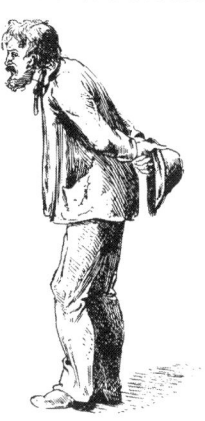

TREATMENT
Treatments for Alzheimer's disease are available. However, on the whole they are quite limited in their ability to make a meaningful impact on the condition. There is no medication or therapy that has been shown to halt or reverse the progression of Alzheimer's disease. Instead, the goal of treatment is limited to **symptom reduction** and **preservation** (not restoration) **of function**.

Psychotherapy (at least in the traditional sense) is not effective for people with Alzheimer's disease, as their cognitive deficits prevent them from meaningfully engaging in this type of treatment. In contrast, **behavioral interventions** are more effective and can improve quality of life in specific areas such as toileting abilities.

Most of the medications used to treat Alzheimer's disease are **cholinesterase inhibitors** which increase the amount of acetylcholine in the brain. (As we will see in the next section, destruction of acetylcholine-releasing neurons is a pathologic hallmark of Alzheimer's disease, and cholinesterase inhibitors help to temporarily offset this imbalance.) The only other antidementia drug is memantine which works as an **NMDA receptor antagonist**. Both cholinesterase inhibitors and memantine can be used to transiently improve symptoms of Alzheimer's disease, with a **small effect size** of around 0.2 to 0.3. However, the effect of these drugs tends to be **transient** and lasts only a few months before the normal course of the illness resumes. In addition, the primary metrics used to assess the effectiveness of these medications are the patient's scores on cognitive tests rather than their functional ability or quality of life (which are likely the more clinically relevant outcomes).

It is not uncommon for **antidepressants** and **antipsychotics** to be used for treating Alzheimer's disease, especially in cases where there are pronounced mood or behavioral features. There is some evidence that antipsychotics can reduce levels of agitation, though generally they have a very small effect size (around 0.1 to 0.2). However, antipsychotics have also been associated with an increased risk of mortality in elderly patients with dementia. Because of this, they should only be used after carefully weighing the possible benefits (a small chance of decreased agitation) against the known risks (increased mortality).

Because both therapy and medications are limited in their ability to treat this disease, the modality of treatment often shifts to **social and environmental interventions** instead. The first priority should be to protect the safety of the patient and those around them, such as removing the patient's driver's license to prevent accidents. Working with families and other caregivers during this process is also crucial. The specific goals of care should be made clear from the time of diagnosis, with education provided on whether the goals are reasonable ("I want my father to be able to continue living at home as long as possible") and when they are not ("I want my father to go back to working as an engineer again"). As the illness progresses, providing guidance with social interventions (such as arranging for residential care or conservatorship) can be invaluable. Finally, be mindful of **caregiver burnout**. Caring for people with Alzheimer's disease (especially in advanced stages of the disorder) can be physically, emotionally, and financially draining, so encouraging family members to engage in self-care and seek help when they need it can make a world of difference.

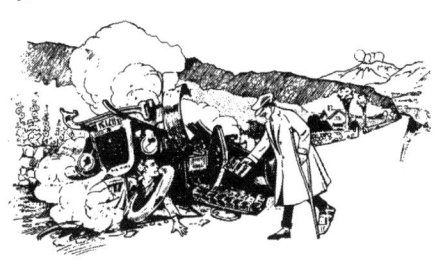

MECHANISMS OF ALZHEIMER'S DISEASE

In contrast to most psychiatric disorders, Alzheimer's disease features the presence of specific anatomic and physiologic findings, classifying it as a **pathology** rather than "just" a syndrome. Nowhere is this more apparent than when looking at the brains of patients with Alzheimer's disease during post-mortem autopsies, which often reveals widespread cortical atrophy as seen in this image:

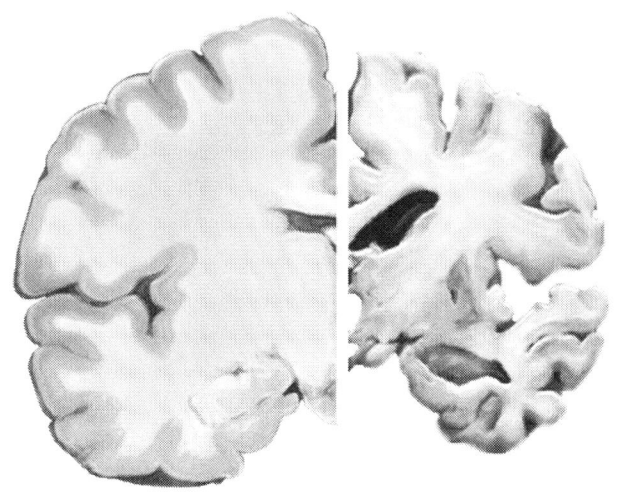

Normal brain   *Alzheimer's disease*

In particular, parts of the brain involved in releasing a neurotransmitter known as **acetylcholine** appear to be the most impacted, leading to a **loss of cholinergic neurons**. You can remember this association by thinking that **A**lzheimer's **D**isease is caused when **A**cetylcholine goes **D**own. This explains the symptomatic benefits seen with use of cholinesterase inhibitors, which increase the amount of acetylcholine that is active in the brain.

Alzheimer's disease is characterized by **loss of cholinergic neurons**.

Alzheimer's Disease is caused when Acetylcholine goes Down.

However, this explanation does not tell us *why* these nerve cells are dying in the first place. Research suggests that the neural destruction seen in Alzheimer's disease results from an inability of the brain to remove two types of **toxic waste products** known as senile plaques and neurofibrillary tangles.

Senile plaques consist of extracellular proteins known as **amyloid beta** that have clumped together. A certain amount of senile plaque is normal and likely accounts for the cognitive changes seen in normal aging. However, when too many amyloid beta proteins accumulate, they exert toxic effects in the brain by damaging nearby nerve cells. To prevent this toxicity from occurring, the brain produces a protein that is known as **apolipoprotein E** which functions as a "garbage truck" of sorts by clearing away amyloid beta and thereby preventing senile plaques from forming. However, some people have a gene variant known as **APOE4** that codes for a **poorly functioning** version of apolipoprotein E. The defective apolipoprotein E is unable to clear away amyloid beta which allows a high number of extracellular senile plaques to form. The number of senile plaques has been found to correlate with the severity of Alzheimer's disease, suggesting a clear relationship between these plaques and the cognitive deficits seen in this form of dementia. Because of this link, the APOE4 gene is the **largest risk factor** for developing Alzheimer's disease aside from age! Compared to those with no copies of the APOE4 gene, people with one copy have 3 times the risk of developing Alzheimer's disease while those with two copies have 15 times the risk.

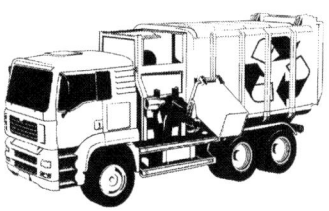

The **APOE4 gene** encodes a poorly functioning version of **apolipoprotein E** which allows **amyloid plaques** to build-up, increasing the risk of **Alzheimer's disease**.

APOE4 causes Amyloid Plaques in the Old and Elderly to form.

Neurofibrillary tangles, the second type of toxic waste product, also appear to be involved in Alzheimer's disease. Just as senile plaques are made up of amyloid beta proteins, these neurofibrillary tangles are made up of a protein called **tau**. Normally, tau is involved in stabilizing structures known as **microtubules** which make up the cytoskeleton on the inside of the cell. Microtubules act as tiny railroad tracks that transport nutrients and other molecules across the cell. However, if tau becomes damaged, the cell's ability to process nutrients is disrupted. These **misshapen tau proteins** then accumulate and form intracellular neurofibrillary tangles. Like senile plaques, the number of neurofibrillary tangles has been found to correlate with the severity of Alzheimer's disease.

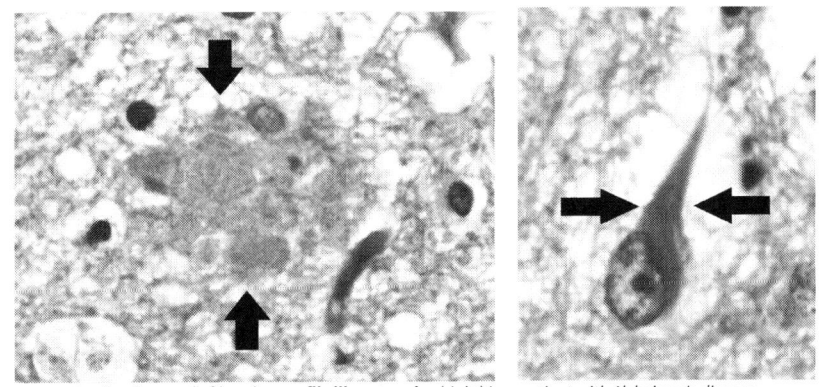

Senile plaques (left) and neurofibrillary tangles (right) in a patient with Alzheimer's disease.

Medications that target amyloid beta and tau are in the works, and it is possible that treatment of Alzheimer's disease in the future will look very different than it does now. For the time being, however, it is enough to know that the pathophysiology of Alzheimer's disease involves an **inability of the brain to take out the trash** (its extracellular senile plaques and intracellular neurofibrillary tangles specifically).

> **Senile plaques** and **neurofibrillary tangles** both contribute to **Alzheimer's disease**.
>
> *Alzheimer's disease neurons are SPeNT (Senile Plaques and Neurofibrillary Tangles).*

HOW TO DIAGNOSE DEMENTIA

Diagnosing dementia is a **two-step process**. First, you need to determine whether dementia is present or not. If it is, then you need to determine what *type* of dementia it is. While Alzheimer's disease is the most common form of dementia, it is not the only one, with other common causes being **dementia with Lewy bodies**, **frontotemporal dementia**, **vascular dementia**, or **mixed dementia** (with elements of more than one type). It is important to be keep non-Alzheimer's dementias on your differential, especially when it comes to treatment (as attempting to treat every type of dementia like Alzheimer's disease can be ineffective or even harmful).

Answering the first question ("Is dementia present?") can be accomplished using the diagnostic criteria in the DSM. The criteria for a major neurocognitive disorder are really quite simple and can be captured in the mnemonic **DIRE**: all you need is a clear **D**ecline in one or more cognitive domains leading to **I**mpairment and decreasing independence, provided that you have both **R**uled out delirium and **E**xcluded other psychiatric conditions such as depression as possible causes.

> **Dementia** involves a clear **cognitive and functional decline** that is not better accounted for by delirium, depression, or other disorders.
>
> *DIRE:*
> *Decline in cognition*
> *Impairment as a result*
> *Rule out delirium*
> *Exclude other psychiatric conditions*

A variety of clinical tests such as the Mini-Mental State Examination (MMSE) and Montreal Cognitive Assessment (MoCA) can be used as a standardized assessment of different cognitive domains. These tests provide a numerical score which is helpful not only for establishing the diagnosis but also for tracking progression over time. For example, the MoCA involves asking the patient to draw a clock from memory (among other things). The ability to successfully complete this task declines as dementia progresses, as seen in the following image:

Normal   ***Early*** *stages*   ***Late*** *stages*

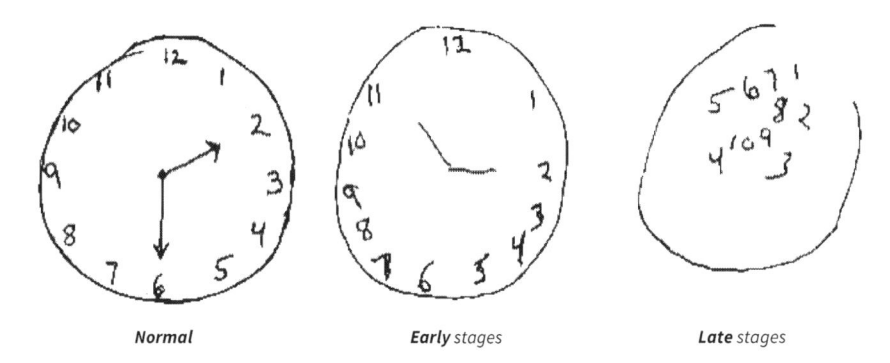

Once the diagnosis of dementia has been established, the second task is to differentiate between the different types of dementia. A clinical diagnosis can sometimes be determined through a psychiatric interview and physical examination, as each form of dementia is associated with specific clinical features that can help to differentiate between them. However, recognizing dementia subtypes on the basis of clinical findings alone produces inaccurate diagnoses around 25% of the time.

For this reason, it can be helpful to order neuroimaging for a definitive diagnosis. In particular, **functional neuroimaging** like positron emission tomography (PET) scans that reveal not only the *shape* of the brain but also its metabolic *activity* can be incredibly helpful. For example, the following brain scan shows the brain activity of a normal person compared to someone with Alzheimer's disease (with brighter colors indicating a higher amount of metabolic activity). An overall loss of brain volume is apparent as well. While the senile plaques and neurofibrillary tangles mentioned earlier would be apparent on brain biopsy, the invasive nature of this procedure (you're literally taking a chunk out of someone's brain) means that it is rarely performed while the patient is alive.

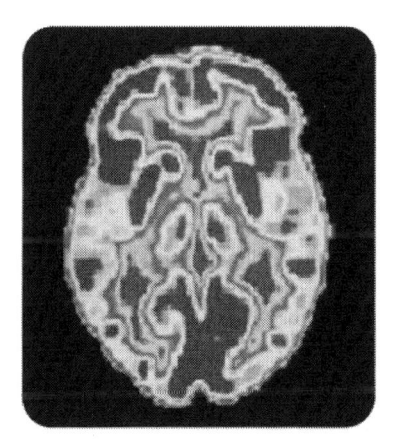

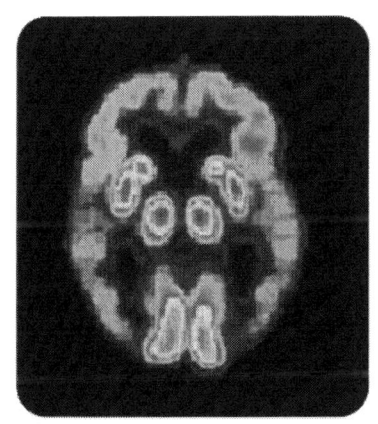

*Positron emission tomography (PET) scans of a **normal brain** (left) and **Alzheimer's disease** (right).*

With that established, we will now look at the various forms of dementia with a particular eye on how they differ from Alzheimer's disease.

EARLY-ONSET ALZHEIMER'S DISEASE
Early-onset Alzheimer's disease refers to cases beginning **before the age of 65**. Early-onset Alzheimer's disease is uncommon, accounting for less than 10% of all cases. In around a third of early-onset cases (or roughly 3% of the total population diagnosed with Alzheimer's disease) there is a clear familial pattern, with the disease inherited in an **autosomal dominant** fashion. Therefore, being below the age of 65 does not automatically rule out a diagnosis of Alzheimer's disease (especially if there is a positive family history).

VASCULAR DEMENTIA
Vascular dementia is the second most common type of dementia after Alzheimer's disease, accounting for around 20% of all cases. It is characterized by **repeated minor strokes** causing ischemic damage to brain tissue. Because strokes can affect different parts of the brain to various extents, vascular dementia is not associated with *specific* signs or symptoms. Instead, the clinical hallmark of vascular dementia is a series of **stepwise decreases in cognition**, with each drop in functional ability representing another ischemic event. (This stands in contrast to the steady and gradual decline seen in Alzheimer's disease.) From a treatment standpoint, cholinesterase inhibitors and memantine are used, although **addressing the underlying risk factors for stroke** (such as high blood pressure) is the most important goal.

DEMENTIA WITH LEWY BODIES
Dementia with Lewy bodies (DLB) is the third most common type of dementia after Alzheimer's disease and vascular dementia. It is characterized by the accumulation of **Lewy bodies** which are intracellular clumps of a protein known as **alpha-synuclein** that accumulate and cause neuronal damage (similar to how both senile plaques and neurofibrillary tangles damage neurons in Alzheimer's disease).

The hallmark symptom of dementia with Lewy bodies is **visual hallucinations** which are found in over 80% of all cases (even during early stages of the disease). These visual hallucinations commonly are vivid and well-formed, consisting of people or animals moving across one's field of vision ("I see a bunch of mice walking in a line across the floor"). To remember the hallmark symptom of dementia with **Lewy** bodies, think of these patients as having **visual hal-Lewy-cinations**.

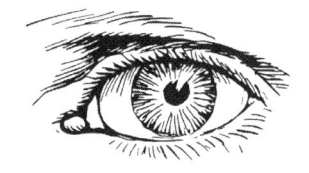

Dementia with Lewy bodies is characterized by **visual hallucinations**.

*Visual hal-**Lewy**-cinations are seen in dementia with **Lewy** bodies.*

Clinically, dementia with Lewy bodies can be differentiated from Alzheimer's disease by its **rapid cognitive decline** (with changes occurring in a matter of months instead of years) and **earlier onset** in life (with the incidence increasing after the age of 50 instead of 65). Dementia with Lewy bodies also differs from other types of dementia in that its progression is characterized by rapid **fluctuations in cognition** (with patients alternating between lucidity and confusion within the span of several hours) as well as **motor deficits** including muscle rigidity and difficulty walking. These motor deficits are pronounced enough that dementia with Lewy bodies is frequently misdiagnosed as Parkinson's disease (another condition involving both motor and cognitive deficits which will be discussed in more detail later in this chapter).

Like with Alzheimer's disease, treatment of dementia with Lewy bodies is symptomatic rather than curative and involves similar medications. Of note, people with this form of dementia are known to be **exquisitely sensitive to antipsychotics** with severe side effects such as confusion or catatonia occurring much more often in this population than others. For this reason, antipsychotics should be strictly avoided when treating dementia with Lewy bodies.

FRONTOTEMPORAL DEMENTIA
Frontotemporal dementia (FTD) is a form of dementia characterized by degeneration of the **frontal and temporal lobes** of the brain. In the majority of cases, this leads to a syndrome of **inappropriate and impulsive behavior** along with a decline in cognitive and social abilities. The overall pattern of frontotemporal dementia can be recalled using the mnemonic **OH DEAR**:

O is for Oral fixation. Frontotemporal dementia often involves a distinct pattern of **hyperorality**, with patients often trying to put things (particularly sweets and other carbohydrate-rich foods) into their mouths. This results in increased food intake, dietary changes (such as eating the same food over and over to the exclusion of all other foods), and even consumption of inedible objects in some cases.

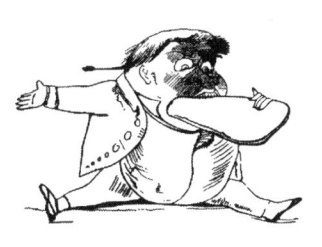

H is for Heartlessness. One of the earliest signs of frontotemporal dementia is impairment in social ability, with a **loss of sympathy and empathy** being the typical pattern observed. Patients often show a decreased interest in socializing and become oblivious to the emotions of other people. Unlike in psychopathy, this heartlessness is unintentional and is a distinct change from previous patterns of social interaction.

D is for Disinhibition. The frontal lobe is the part of the brain that says "no" to the baser instincts of the rest of the brain. When it becomes dysfunctional, it loses the ability to rein in these inappropriate impulses, leading to a pattern of disinhibited, socially inappropriate, and often pleasure-seeking behavior. In addition to the oral fixation noted early, behavior in frontotemporal dementia is often **hypersexual** (such as taking off clothes in public, grabbing body parts, or sexually propositioning others at extremely inappropriate times like at a work function).

E is for Executive dysfunction. While frontotemporal dementia features the same cognitive deficits seen in others forms of dementia, there are some nuances to take note of. The most affected cognitive domain in frontotemporal dementia is **executive dysfunction** resulting in inability to plan and execute complex ideas. In contrast, memory and visuospatial abilities are relatively preserved compared to Alzheimer's disease (although they are still involved to some extent).

A is for Apathy. When not engaging in impulsive, hyperoral, or hypersexual behavior, patients with frontotemporal dementia can often show a profound apathy that is also described as "listlessness" and "inertia." This emotionlessness can be disconcerting to family and friends, and in some cases it may be mistaken for depression.

R is for Ritualistic behavior. Finally, patients with frontotemporal dementia show a pattern of ritualistic, stereotyped, or compulsive behaviors. The specific behaviors involved can vary from simple movements such as pacing, tapping, or picking at one's skin to more involved actions such as hoarding food, cleaning the same spot over and over, or calling the same person repeatedly. Speech can also become restricted and stereotyped, such as repeating the same phrase or sound for minutes or hours on end.

> **Frontotemporal dementia** is characterized by a pattern of **disinhibited behavior** and **personality changes**.
>
> *OH DEAR:*
> *Oral fixation*
> *Heartlessness*
> *Disinhibition*
> *Executive dysfunction*
> *Apathy*
> *Ritualistic behavior*

In addition to these signs and symptoms, a variety of exam findings suggestive of upper motor neuron damage can be seen. These include **frontal release signs**, or a class of primitive reflexes that are normally seen only in very young infants whose frontal lobes have not yet fully developed.

Frontotemporal dementia is an uncommon cause of dementia and accounts for less than 10% of all cases. However, it tends to begin between the ages of 45 and 65, making it the second-most common cause of **early-onset** dementia. Like most forms of dementia, frontotemporal dementia is progressive, with a generally poor prognosis. Treatment is primarily symptomatic rather than curative. Given that there is no loss of cholinergic neurons (as occurs in Alzheimer's disease or dementia with Lewy bodies), cholinesterase inhibitors have little effect in frontotemporal dementia. Instead, pharmacologic management of frontotemporal dementia typically involves an **SRI** (as some evidence suggests that they are helpful for improving behavior), with atypical antipsychotics used as a last resort.

MIXED DEMENTIA

Mixed dementia occurs when multiple forms of dementia appear to be progressing at once. Most often, this involves the signs and symptoms of Alzheimer's disease combined with the stepwise progression of vascular dementia (as these are the two most common forms of dementia). However, because the term mixed dementia can encapsulate any combination of different neurocognitive disorders, there is a wide variety of other clinical presentations that can be seen as well.

MILD COGNITIVE IMPAIRMENT

Mild cognitive impairment (MCI) is a **halfway point** between normal aging and dementia where some level of cognitive deficit is present but it hasn't quite reached the level where it results in significant dysfunction. Cognitive deficits tend to be exclusively related to memory loss (with other cognitive functions generally remaining intact). In a way, mild cognitive impairment can be thought of as the **prodrome to dementia**, as people with the condition are up to 15 times more likely to develop Alzheimer's disease than those without any cognitive signs. Unfortunately, no medications or treatments have been shown to prevent the progression to dementia, so management of mild cognitive impairment largely involves educating both the patient and their family on what to expect and providing guidance on necessary steps.

"REVERSIBLE DEMENTIA"

A variety of non-psychiatric, non-neurologic conditions can cause cognitive symptoms which can strongly resemble dementia, including scoring poorly on tests like the MMSE or MoCA. These conditions are often referred to as **reversible dementias**, as treating the underlying condition can effectively restore cognitive function back to its previous state. You can remember the primary causes of reversible dementia using the mnemonic **DEMENTIA**:

D is for Drugs and drinking. A variety of prescription medications drugs can cause cognitive dulling, including benzodiazepines, anticonvulsants, antihypertensives, and anticholinergics. Look at the **timing** of symptom onset (especially if a new medication was started in the past few weeks or months) and consider discontinuing any new medications for a while to see if symptoms resolve.

Recreational substances can have profound effects on cognition as well. By far the substance most commonly linked to dementia-like symptoms is **alcohol**, as chronic use can lead to cognitive deficits that are indistinguishable from other cases of dementia (in fact, it is estimated that up to 10% of all cases of dementia are directly to alcohol use!). Unlike "textbook" dementia, these cases can often (though not always) be reversed with cessation of alcohol intake.

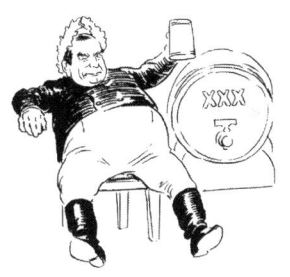

E is for Eyes and ears. Sensory impairments such as vision or hearing loss can easily mimic dementia, as not being able to see or hear can make a patient appear to be confused or experiencing memory loss. However, sensory impairments have also been found to correlate with an increased chance of developing *actual* dementia as well. Some evidence suggests that interventions such as updating an eyeglass prescription or providing hearing aids can help to modify this risk, so be mindful to screen for sensory impairments before diagnosing dementia.

M is for Metabolic. Conditions that alter metabolism (such as undiagnosed or poorly treated diabetes mellitus) can be major risk factors for cognitive impairment. In fact, diabetes is associated with an over 50% risk of developing any form of diabetes.

E is for Endocrine. While a variety of endocrine disorders can have neuropsychiatric symptoms, the one that most commonly resembles dementia is **hypothyroidism** due to its slow onset, profound cognitive deficits, and presence of apathy. Hypothyroidism is easily ruled out by ordering a thyroid stimulating hormone (TSH) test. If present, it is rapidly treatable using thyroid replacement.

N is for Nutrition. While malnutrition in general can itself be a risk factor for cognitive dulling, specific vitamin deficiencies have also been associated with cases of reversible dementia. In particular, a deficiency of **vitamin B$_{12}$** can lead to a syndrome of fatigue, confusion, irritability, and cognitive deficits that can easily be mistaken for dementia. A B$_{12}$ level can quickly rule this in or out.

T is for Tumors. Brain tumors or other space-occupying lesions can be associated with dementia-like symptoms. While the signs and symptoms can mimic dementia, there are often clues that something more is going on (such as the presence of specific neurologic deficits, a rapid progression, and/or cognitive problems in some domains but not others depending on where the lesion is located). When a tumor is suspected, head imaging is a good next step for evaluating further.

I is for Infection. Certain infections can cause a state of impaired cognition that can be hard to distinguish from dementia. For example, **HIV-associated neurocognitive disorders** can occur in cases of uncontrolled retroviral infection. Another example is **tertiary syphilis** (also known as neurosyphilis) which features the same insidious onset of profound cognitive symptoms that "normal" dementia does. Due to the relative rarity of syphilis in the age of antibiotics, testing for it as part of a routine dementia work-up is no longer indicated, but in particular cases (if there are signs of neurologic involvement such as ataxia or muscle weakness) it should be considered.

A is for Autoimmune. Some autoimmune diseases appear to have the potential to cause dementia-like symptoms. While there isn't enough evidence to justify ordering a "million dollar work-up" for *all* patients presenting with dementia-like symptoms, certain clues (such as a subacute onset of symptoms, a rapidly progressive course, or evidence of autoimmune signs in other organs) may raise your clinical suspicion.

Common causes of **reversible dementia** include **neurosyphilis, hypothyroidism, B$_{12}$ deficiency, substances, sensory impairment,** and **metabolic disease**.

DEMENTIA:
*D*rugs and drinking
*E*yes and ears
*M*etabolic
*E*ndocrine
*N*utrition
*T*umors
*I*nfection
*A*utoimmune

DIFFERENTIAL DIAGNOSIS OF DEMENTIA

Dementia lies at the boundary between a psychiatric syndrome and a neurologic disease. For this reason, the differential diagnosis for dementia must be **very broad** and encompass not only the psychiatric conditions we have discussed so far but also quite a few neurologic diseases that we haven't. While a full discussion of all relevant neurologic diseases is far outside the scope of this book, we will briefly make reference to some of the most common neurologic conditions that should be on your differential diagnosis for dementia.

NORMALCY

As discussed previously, a certain degree of cognitive decline and memory impairment is completely normal and expected with aging, especially in the domains covered by the **Not so FAST** mnemonic (including **F**lexibility, **A**bstraction, **S**peed, and a**T**tention). In contrast, if there are signs of deficits in areas that are normally **Crystal CLIR** (such as **Crystal**lized intelligence, **C**oncrete thinking, **L**anguage, **I**mplicit memory, and **R**ecognition) or if there is evidence of impairments in ADLs or IADLs, consider initiating a full evaluation for dementia.

PARKINSON'S DISEASE

Parkinson's disease is a neurodegenerative disorder caused by cell death in the **basal ganglia** which primarily affects **motor functioning** through the loss of dopamine-releasing neurons. This creates a state of motor dysfunction known as **Parkinsonism** that is characterized by a slowing of movements (bradykinesia), a resting tremor, muscle rigidity, and poor balance. A highly specific sign of Parkinson's disease is a **pill-rolling tremor** (so named because it looks like the patient is rubbing a pill between their index finger and thumb). A style of gait known as **festination** (which involves short shuffling steps, a forward-flexed posture, and a decrease in arm swing when walking) is also highly specific for Parkinson's disease. Many of the signs of Parkinson's disease (including the pill-rolling tremor and decreased arm swing) are notably **asymmetric** in nature and affect one side over the other, although they can sometimes become bilateral as the disease progresses.

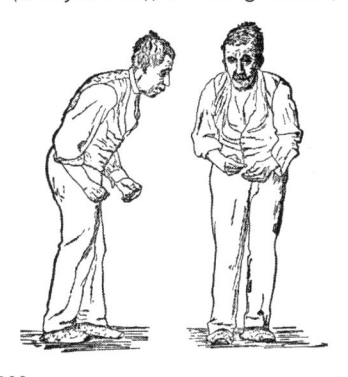

While motor signs are the most common clinical feature of Parkinson's disease, a significant minority of people with the condition experience profound cognitive and emotional deficits that can closely resemble dementia, particularly in later stages of the illness. People with Parkinson's disease are often described as having a **mask-like facial expression** that does not change or move, which is often accompanied by a slow and monotonous voice. Psychiatric symptoms (including depression, anxiety, paranoia, and visual hallucinations) are also common and can be even more impairing than the classic motor abnormalities. While medications are available to reverse many of the motor abnormalities of Parkinsonism, treatment of cognitive deficits remains symptom-driven rather than curative.

NORMAL PRESSURE HYDROCEPHALUS
Normal pressure hydrocephalus is a condition in which the cerebrospinal fluid-filled ventricles of the brain expand, raising intracranial pressure and causing dysfunction in nearby regions of the brain. Classically, patients with normal pressure hydrocephalus present with a characteristic **triad of dementia, incontinence, and gait instability**. Treatment involves neurosurgical placement of a shunt to drain the excess fluid, which effectively reverses symptoms of dementia in most patients.

> **Normal pressure hydrocephalus** is characterized by the clinical triad of **dementia, urinary incontinence**, and **gait instability**.
>
> *DIG = Dementia, Incontinence, and Gait.*

WERNICKE-KORSAKOFF SYNDROME
While chronic alcohol use can result in symptoms that are largely indistinguishable from cases of primary dementia, a specific condition known as Wernicke-Korsakoff syndrome warrants separate a discussion. Wernicke-Korsakoff syndrome is actually a combination of two conditions: **Wernicke encephalopathy** (confusion accompanied by an unsteady gait and difficulties with eye movement) and **Korsakoff syndrome** (profound *antero*grade amnesia, or an inability to form *new* memories). Due to the lack of ability to form new memories, people with Wernicke-Korsakoff syndrome often **confabulate** or make up information when asked questions ("What did you do for a living?" "I was... a sailor!" "Your wife says you were an accountant").

Wernicke-Korsakoff syndrome is caused by a deficiency of **thiamine** (or vitamin B$_1$) which is itself related to chronic alcohol use. On an anatomic level, Wernicke–Korsakoff syndrome is associated with damage to the **mammillary bodies**, a pair of structures in the brain that are involved in memory and recall. To remember these associations, think of a man who is so drunk that he begins inappropriately staring at a nearby statue's breasts (mammillary being Latin for "resembling a breast"). When someone asks him what he is doing, he responds by slurring the phrase, "I'm thorry, th1amine (I am in) a drunken thtupor." This story can help you make associations between alcohol, mammillary bodies, inappropriate behavior, and th**1**amine (or vitamin B$_1$) deficiency.

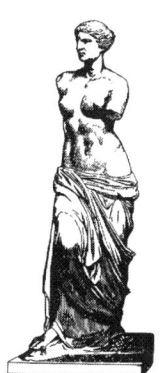

> **Wernicke-Korsakoff syndrome** is a syndrome of **confusion, gait imbalance**, and **amnesia** caused by **thiamine deficiency** related to **chronic alcohol use**. It is associated with damage to the **mammillary bodies**.
>
> *Think of a **drunk disinhibited** man looking at a statue's **mammillary bodies** and saying, "I'm thorry, **th1amine** a drunken sthupor."*

PRION DISEASE

Prion diseases are a group of **rapidly progressive neurodegenerative diseases** caused by the presence of abnormally folded proteins known as **prions**. These misshapen proteins develop the capability of inducing other proteins to misfold as well, setting off a chain reaction that leads to a rapid spread throughout the brain and other neural tissues. These misfolded proteins directly cause degeneration of nerve tissue, a process that quite literally punches holes in the brain and leads to a characteristic **spongiform** (or sponge-like) appearance under the microscope. On a clinical level, prion diseases present with profound memory loss, changes in behavior and personality, movement problems, and sensory deficits. While the highly variable presentation of the illness ensures that there are no pathognomonic signs or symptoms, cases of prion disease can often be recognized by their **rapid progression** involving multiple cognitive domains. Prion diseases are **uniformly fatal**, with almost all patients with the diagnosis dying within one year of symptom onset. The initial misfolded protein that starts the cascade can be acquired by being exposed to prions from other people (such as through cannibalism or brain surgery). In a minority of cases, prion disease is caused by a mutation in a gene known as PRNP.

TRAUMATIC BRAIN INJURY

Traumatic brain injury (TBI) is a catch-all term for the incredibly wide variety of medical abnormalities and cognitive deficits that can be seen following a physical injury to the head. Because the nature of physical injuries can vary so much in extent and severity (from something as minor as hitting one's head on a low doorway to as major as being in a coma for several weeks following a car crash), there is no single syndrome associated with traumatic brain injury. Instead, signs and symptoms following a traumatic brain injury can **mimic nearly every other psychiatric syndrome** including depression, anxiety, mania, psychosis, and OCD. **Memory loss** is the most common clinical findings, with up to 80% of all patients experiencing some form of memory loss following a head injury. Repeated injury to the head is even more closely associated with a dementia-like neurodegenerative process known as **chronic traumatic encephalopathy** (also called dementia pugilistica or "boxer's dementia"). Interestingly, chronic traumatic encephalopathy involves deposition of tau protein throughout the brain, a similar mechanism to Alzheimer's disease.

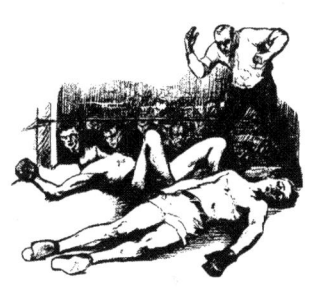

DELIRIUM

Dementia must be distinguished from delirium (discussed in Chapter 4) which is **transient** and **reversible** (unlike the chronic and progressive nature of dementia). By far the most reliable indicator of delirium is the **timing of symptoms**, as memory loss, disorientation, and other cognitive deficits tend to come on rapidly (often within a few days or weeks) compared to the insidious onset of dementia which occurs over several months or years. In addition, delirium often fluctuates from hour to hour which contrasts to dementia's persistent deficits. Delirium is caused by another medical condition (such as an infection), so the presence of any vital sign abnormalities or specific findings on physical exam should also raise your suspicion for delirium. It is entirely possible for someone to have both dementia and delirium (indeed, dementia is itself a significant risk factor for developing delirium), so in these cases look for a level of *increased* confusion that is an **acute change from baseline**.

DEPRESSION
Certain symptoms of depression (including fatigue, apathy, poor concentration, and reduced interest in activities) can strongly resemble dementia. If depression is severe enough, it can even cause patients to score poorly on tests like the MMSE or MoCA (although this is usually due to low motivation to complete the test rather than genuine cognitive deficits). This phenomenon is common enough that the term "**pseudodementia**" has been coined to describe these cases. It is imperative to distinguish between these two conditions, as depression is episodic and reversible while dementia is not. Depression can be differentiated from dementia by its more **rapid onset** (often over weeks rather than the months or years seen in dementia) and presence of specific **thought patterns** (like negative affective biases). In addition, someone who is having memory lapses as a result of being in a state of depression is more likely to say that they are *concerned by* these changes (as opposed to someone with dementia who generally lacks awareness that memory loss is occurring).

PSYCHOSIS
Paranoia, delusions, and hallucinations are often found in dementia, particularly in dementia with Lewy bodies or advanced stages of Alzheimer's disease. Differentiating between psychotic symptoms related to dementia and those that are a manifestation of schizophrenia can be aided by looking at the **age of onset** (as schizophrenia often begins earlier in life). However, this cannot be followed as a rule due to the fact that both *late-onset* schizophrenia and *early-onset* dementia exist. Further clues towards dementia rather than psychosis include a lack of prior psychiatric history, generally intact socio-occupational functioning prior to disease onset, and the presence of generalized deficits on cognitive testing.

INTELLECTUAL DISABILITY
The cognitive deficits seen in intellectual disability can mimic those in dementia is nearly every way. However, by definition intellectual disability **must be present from early childhood** whereas dementia begins later in life.

DISSOCIATION
Both dementia and dissociation involve memory loss. However, dissociative amnesia tends to involve retrograde amnesia about a specific (and often very stressful) time in the patient's life which generally reverses with time (the memory is later "recovered"). In contrast, memory loss in dementia is characterized by both retrograde *and* anterograde amnesia. The memory loss is also enduring, and in most cases these memories are not regained. Dissociation can further be distinguished from dementia in that people with dissociative amnesia generally show an **awareness** that they are afflicted by memory loss ("I can't remember anything from last summer") and will not show impairments in cognitive abilities, either in daily living or on formal testing.

SOMATIZATION AND MALINGERING

Memory loss can sometimes be the presenting complaint for someone who is somatizing or wants to feign an illness, as it is both entirely subjective and profoundly distressing. As with depression and dissociation, however, there is often **concern about memory loss** (which is highly unusual for dementia). In addition, when asked to complete cognitive tests, people who are malingering will often "overplay their hand" by trying to perform poorly on all parts of the test, including those that are so simple that even people with dementia would be able to do them ("Can you tell me your name?" "You know I can't do that, doc..."). Your clinical suspicion for somatization or malingering should be higher in cases where there is evidence for primary or secondary gain (such as someone presenting for a disability evaluation).

PUTTING IT ALL TOGETHER

Dementia is a tragic and disabling disease involving deficits in memory, cognition, awareness, and behavior. It is associated with a high disease burden not only for the patients themselves but also for their families and the societies in which they live. To avoid overdiagnosing the changes seen in normal aging as a pathological process, use the mnemonics **Crystal CLIR** and **Not so FAST** to remember which changes are expected and which are suggestive of disease. Once the presence of dementia has been established, use what you know about the specific signs and symptoms associated with each form of dementia (such as the **MA 'N PA** symptoms of Alzheimer's disease, the **stepwise progression** of vascular dementia, the **visual hal-Lewy-cinations** of dementia with Lewy bodies, and the **OH DEAR** symptoms of frontotemporal dementia) to determine the specific type you are working with.

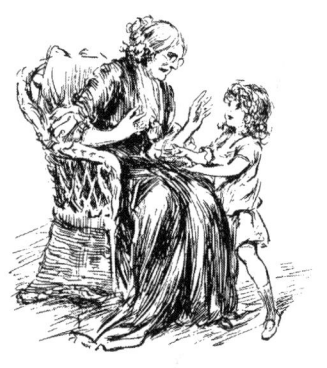

While current treatments are symptomatic rather than curative, diagnosing dementia still has the benefit of providing clarity to patients and their families on the nature of what they are experiencing as well as knowledge about what to expect in the future. Given the rate at which our knowledge about Alzheimer's disease and other forms is dementia is expanding, it is likely that in the future we will be able to do more to combat this progressive and lethal disease. In the meantime, do the best you can to maximize function for the patient and minimize burden for their caregivers.

REVIEW QUESTIONS

1. A 76 y/o F goes to her primary care provider for an annual visit. When asked about her memory, the patient says that she has occasional episodes of entering a room and not being able to remember why she entered. She also has noticed that she will often not be able to recall the name of a friend that she encountered earlier that same day. She has called the police two times in the past month to report an intruder after not recognizing that the person entering her house was her home care nurse. While she used to be able to sit and read the Bible for hours on end, she finds that now she has trouble keeping track of what she is reading for more than 30 minutes at a time. Which of the following features is most concerning for a diagnosis of dementia?
   A. Being unable to remember why she entered a room
   B. Being unable to recall the name of a friend whom she saw the same day
   C. Being unable to recognize her home care nurse
   D. Being unable to focus on reading for more than 30 minutes at a time
   E. None of the above are concerning for dementia

2. (Continued from previous question.) The primary care provider performs a MoCA (a cognitive screening test with a normal score of 25 and above), and the patient scores 19/30. Observed deficits include delayed recall, executive functioning, and abstraction. The patient denies use of alcohol, cigarettes, or any other drugs ("I've been a churchgoer all my life."). She denies visual hallucinations. According to her home care nurse, she has not had any changes in her eating or speaking habits. The nurse describes the patient as having experienced a "progressive decline" rather than one characterized by sudden decreases in cognitive and functional abilities. Physical exam, including a complete neurologic exam, is generally normal. Her blood pressure is 128/78, and she has never had a stroke. Which of the following diagnoses can be given with certainty at this time?
   A. Alzheimer's disease
   B. Frontotemporal dementia
   C. Dementia with Lewy bodies
   D. Vascular dementia
   E. Mixed dementia
   F. None of the above

3. (Continued from previous question.) On the way to her next appointment, the patient is involved in a motor vehicle accident for which she is at fault. She is admitted to the hospital for a broken femur. Which of the following could have prevented this outcome had it been done at the first visit?
   A. Prescribing a cholinesterase inhibitor
   B. Ordering positron emission tomography
   C. Inquiring about the presence of osteoporosis
   D. Performing a test of auditory and visual acuity
   E. None of the above

4. (Continued from previous question.) The patient is discharged from the hospital. Over the next 2 years, she experiences progressive loss of cognitive ability and soon is dependent upon others for all activities of daily living including eating and bathing. She is admitted to the hospital for pneumonia and dies several days later. Which of the following findings is *least* likely to be seen on a post-mortem autopsy?
    A. Widespread cortical atrophy
    B. Selective loss of cholinergic neurons
    C. Spongiform appearance of brain tissues under the microscope
    D. Intracellular neurofibrillary tangles
    E. Extracellular senile plaques
    F. All of these are likely to be observed

5. A 66 y/o M is brought to see his primary care provider by his daughter who is concerned about him. According to his daughter, the patient experienced the death of his wife 6 months ago and since then has had a "major decline" in his ability to function. His daughter now feels the need to stop by his house at least once per day to ensure that there are meals available for him to eat "or else he would probably just starve." He scores a 14/30 on the MoCA, with points lost primarily for several tasks which he declines to attempt ("That sounds like a lot of work. What's the point of all this? I want to go home."). When asked about his memory, he says, "Yeah I forget things all the time. Phone numbers, names, dates—they're all gone." He reports difficulty sleeping at night and says that sometimes he hears the voice of his wife "calling out my name." Which of the following most strongly argues *against* a diagnosis of Alzheimer's disease for this patient?
    A. Age of onset of symptoms
    B. Presence of auditory hallucinations
    C. Recent death of his wife
    D. Awareness of memory loss
    E. Score on the MoCA

1. **The best answer is C.** Normal aging is accompanied by a variety of cognitive changes, including deficits in short-term memory (answer A), declarative memory (answer B), and attention (answer D). However, recognition of familiar faces is often spared. Therefore, changes in one's ability to recognize faces and objects is concerning and should be accompanied by a thorough evaluation.

2. **The best answer is F.** While this patient is likely suffering from some form of dementia, the specific subtype remains unclear. The lack of changes in oral habits argues against frontotemporal dementia (answer B), the absence of visual hallucinations argues against dementia with Lewy bodies (answer C), and the lack of a stepwise progression argues against vascular dementia (answer D). This makes Alzheimer's disease the most likely diagnosis. However, it is important to keep in mind that Alzheimer's disease is *not* a diagnosis of exclusion and that diagnoses of dementia subtypes based only on clinical examination are incorrect 25% of the time. Therefore, it is not possible to diagnose Alzheimer's disease with any degree of certainty in the absence of further testing (answer A).

3. **The best answer is E.** Patients with a clinical suspicion for dementia should not be permitted to drive or operate complex machinery that could potentially put their own lives or the lives of others at risk. Medication treatments for dementia have only a mild benefit at best and would not necessarily prevent accidents (answer A). Aiding the diagnosis through neuroimaging (answer B) or ruling out sensory impairments (answer D) could have been helpful but would also not have necessarily prevented this outcome. Finally, assessing for osteoporosis would not have prevented the proximal cause of the broken femur—the accident itself (answer C). This outcome could have been prevented by removing her license and arranging alternate transportation.

4. **The best answer is C.** A spongiform appearance is seen in prion diseases. However, the fact that the patient lived for 2 years following her initial diagnosis strongly argues against prion diseases being the cause of her cognitive decline. Instead, the clinical picture suggests that Alzheimer's disease is the most likely explanation. Widespread cortical atrophy, selective loss of cholinergic neurons, intracellular neurofibrillary tangles, and extracellular senile plaques (answers A, B, D, and E) are all likely to be observed in a patient with Alzheimer's disease.

5. **The best answer is D.** This patient's recent decline in function appears to be most consistent with a diagnosis of depression, which can resemble dementia in elderly patients (including scoring poorly on cognitive tests). Awareness of memory loss strongly argues against a diagnosis of dementia, as people in all but the earliest stages of dementia often lack an awareness that their cognition is decreasing. His age is consistent with a diagnosis of Alzheimer's disease (answer A). Psychotic symptoms can occur in dementia, including auditory hallucinations and delusional misidentifications (answer B). The recent death of his wife can be consistent with a diagnosis of Alzheimer's disease, especially if she was previously taking care of his activities of daily living (answer C). His score on the MoCA is abnormal, although this appears to be due to low motivation (answer E).

23 SLEEP

Sleep needs no introduction. Every person on earth has had the experience of being asleep, with most people spending up to a third of their lives in this state. However, for the purposes of clarity, let's take time to introduce some definitions. Sleep is a temporary state of **decreased consciousness** characterized by reduced wakefulness, inhibition of most incoming sensory information, and lowered muscle activity. Sleep allows the body to regenerate its energy and restore muscle tissues used during the day. On a cognitive level, sleep promotes memory formation by consolidating recently learned information.

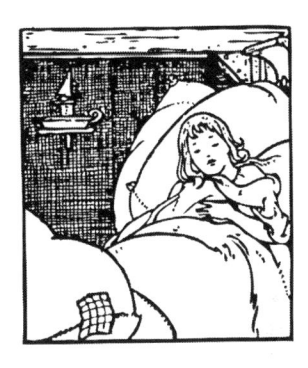

Most people understand on an intuitive level that sleep is incredibly important for maintaining not just physical health but mental health as well. However, while the fact that there *is* a relationship between sleep and mental health is obvious, the exact nature of the relationship is not quite so simple. While psychiatric disorders are often associated with changes in the amount and quality of sleep, it is not always clear whether the disruption in sleep *preceded* the mental distress or is an *aftereffect* of it. For example, international travel across multiple time zones is a well-known trigger for manic episodes, suggesting that dysregulation of sleep itself may prompt a sudden change in mood. However, the reverse can also be true, as depression itself is known to induce changes in one's sleep cycle but only *after* someone has already started exhibiting symptoms of depression. It is likely that the interactions between sleep and mental health is a **two-way street** where each impacts the other in a reciprocal manner. Because understanding sleep is central to maintaining mental health, we will spend our final full chapter discussing sleep physiology, insomnia, and other disorders related to sleep.

SLEEP PHYSIOLOGY

The daily cycle of alternating between periods of sleep and wakefulness is known as the **circadian rhythm**. This cycle is regulated by the hormone **melatonin**, which is secreted at night by the pineal gland in response to low light in the environment. Melatonin decreases wakefulness and promotes sleep induction. Secretion of melatonin stops in the morning, at which time the hormone **cortisol** (which forms part of the HPA axis) is at its peak. This daily alternation between melatonin and cortisol correlates with the subjective feelings of being "awake" or "sleepy" throughout a 24-hour period. You can remember the function of both of these hormones by thinking that mela-**turn**-**in** makes you want to **turn in** for the night. In contrast, corti-**sol** is released during the daytime in response to **sol**-ar rays.

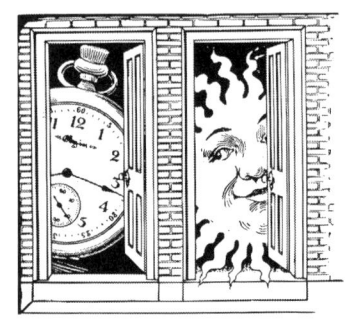

> The **circadian rhythm** is the result of a **daily alternation** between **melatonin**, which promotes sleep, and **cortisol**, which promotes wakefulness.
>
> Mela-**turn**-**in** makes you want to **turn in** for the night.
> Corti-**sol** is released in response to **sol**-ar rays.

Sleep itself is a **dynamic process** that ebbs and flows throughout the night even if we are not necessarily conscious of this. Sleep generally occurs in **sleep cycles** that last 90 minutes on average (meaning that most people will have 4-6 sleep cycles in a single night). Sleep cycles involve a regular progression through various stages of sleep as seen in the following figure:

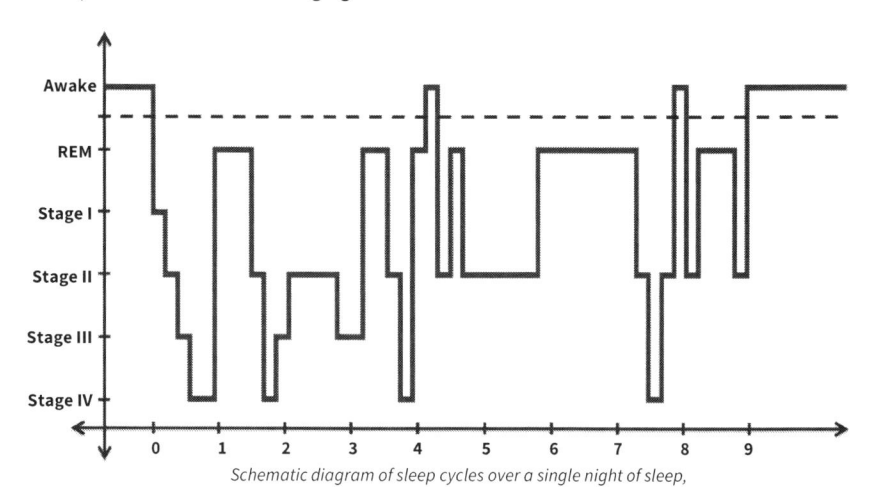

Schematic diagram of sleep cycles over a single night of sleep, with hours of sleep on the x-axis and stage of sleep on the y-axis.

Each stage of sleep is characterized not only by specific signs (mostly involving levels of muscle activity) but also by a specific pattern of electrical activity in the brain which can be seen using an electroencephalogram (EEG). A sleep cycle proceeds in a fairly regular order from lighter phases of sleep (stages I and II) down towards deeper phases of sleep (stages III and IV) which are associated with slower and less frequent activity on EEG. The order of the sleep cycle can be memorized using the mnemonic **BATS Drink Red Blood**:

B is for Beta waves. Beta waves are the patterns of electrical brain activity that occurs during waking consciousness.

A is for Alpha waves. On average, people take 15 minutes to fall asleep from the time they go to bed. Between wakefulness and sleep is an **in-between state** where one feels drowsy but remains conscious. This state is characterized by alpha waves on EEG, which reflects slowed brain activity compared to wakefulness.

T is for Theta waves. Theta waves mark the time when someone crosses over from wakefulness into stage I sleep. Stage I sleep is also known as **light sleep**, as someone is *just barely* asleep and is easily arousable by various stimuli (such as the sound of the television in the other room). In general muscle tone is reduced, although sudden muscle twitches known as hypnic jerks can occur.

S is for Spindles and K complexes. Stage II sleep is characterized by the absence of consciousness and a further decrease in muscle tone. On EEG, this appears in the form of specific forms of electrical activity known as sleep spindles and K complexes.

D is for Delta waves. The presence of low frequency **de**lta waves characterizes **de**ep sleep. This is the **most restorative** phase of sleep both physically and mentally. In this state, someone becomes unaware of all but the most intrusive external stimuli. For example, outside traffic noise or the sound of a television are typically blocked out, although louder noises (like the sound of an alarm clock going off) may break someone out of this stage of sleep.

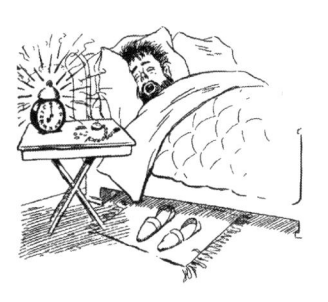

The **deepest stages of sleep** are characterized by **delta waves** on EEG.

*Slow frequency **de**lta waves indicate **de**ep sleep.*

R is for Rapid eye movement. Rapid eye movement (REM) sleep is a paradoxical stage of sleep in which the brain's level of activity is *increased* to levels similar to wakefulness but one's consciousness as a whole feels most deeply asleep. The name REM sleep comes from the fact that the eyes are noted to move rapidly during this time even though the eyelids remain closed. Consistent with the high levels of brain activity observed during this stage, REM sleep is when the most dramatic **dreaming**

occurs. (Dreaming can occur during non-REM sleep as well, but it tends to be less vivid and is less likely to be remembered compared to dreams occurring in REM sleep). REM sleep is also characterized by **muscle paralysis**, with no movement of voluntary muscles occurring during this stage.

> **Vivid dreaming** most often occurs during **REM** sleep.
>
> *You're more likely to **REM**ember your d**REM**s during **REM** sleep.*

B is for Back again. Following REM, the brain moves backwards through previous stages of sleep to begin another cycle (or, if they have had enough sleep, to wake up).

Sleep cycles between REM and non-REM phases several times per night. While sleep progresses through its various stages in a specific order (as captured in the **BATS Drink Red Blood** mnemonic), this progression tends to become more erratic and less consistent as the night goes on, with less deep sleep and more REM sleep occurring in each cycle. After enough time, the person spontaneously wakes up. Someone waking up from a lighter stage of sleep often feels more well rested than if they had woken up directly from deeper sleep. At this point, the amount of melatonin secretion is minimal while levels of cortisol are near the highest levels for the day, creating a sensation of alertness and wakefulness to prepare for the day ahead.

> The **sleep cycle** proceeds in a generally consistent order, with each stage characterized by different **clinical and electroencephalographic findings**.
>
> **BATS D**rink **R**ed **B**lood:
> **B**eta waves (awake)
> **A**lpha waves (drowsy)
> **T**heta waves (Stage I sleep)
> **S**pindles and K complexes (Stage II sleep)
> **D**elta waves (Stage III and IV sleep)
> **R**EM sleep
> **B**ack again

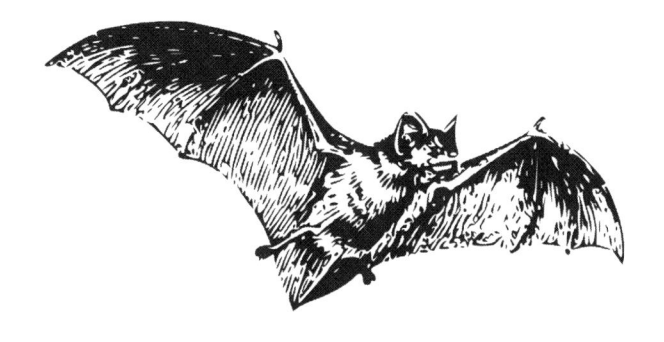

INSOMNIA

Sleep is critical for health, with most experts recommending at least 7 to 8 hours of sleep per night for most adults. Lack of sleep is associated with various physical and mental consequences, including increased risks of obesity, hypertension, heart disease, diabetes, and infection. Because of the consequences of inadequate sleep, anything that threatens someone's ability to consistently get enough sleep can be cause for concern. These impairments in sleep are known as **sleep disorders**. By far the most common form of sleep disorder is **insomnia** which is defined as any form of difficulty sleeping. However, there are other conditions that lead to a reduced quality of sleep or to episodes of falling asleep at inappropriate times which can be equally impairing (these will be discussed later in this chapter).

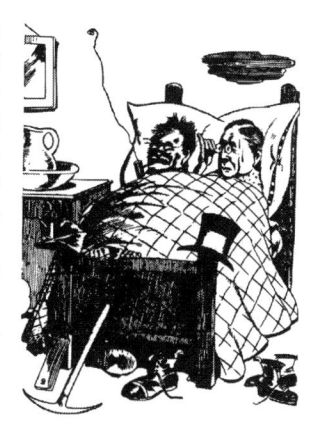

Insomnia can involve difficulty sleeping in multiple ways, including trouble falling asleep, frequent awakenings throughout the night, or waking up long before desired. Insomnia is not inherently pathological, and occasional nights of bad sleep are completely normal. However, if the inability to sleep continues for too long or becomes severe, it can be the source of significant stress and dysfunction. On a symptomatic level, people with chronic insomnia often struggle with fatigue, poor mood, irritability, and inattention throughout the day. These symptoms are often accompanied by some level of distress about their lack of sleep.

Insomnia can occur as a result of a variety of factors, including stress, lifestyle, drugs, medical conditions, and psychiatric comorbidity. However, it can also occur on its own without a clear etiology, sometimes called idiopathic or "primary" insomnia. Insomnia is **common**, with around 30% of the population reporting problems with sleep on at least an occasional basis. For this reason, insomnia should not be considered a disorder until it becomes frequent and severe. The majority of cases are *secondary*, with insomnia being attributed to upstream factors like lifestyle, drugs, or other disorders. Once these have been excluded, the prevalence of *primary* insomnia falls to around 5% of the general population.

Age and **gender** are the largest risk factors for insomnia, with older adults and women both being at higher risk compared to the rest of the population. The presence of a comorbid psychiatric disorder is also a major risk factor, with studies showing that around 40% of all people with recurrent insomnia meet criteria for at least one mental disorder (compared to only 15% of people without sleep complaints). Of these, **depression** is the most common, although anxiety is a close second.

As a general rule, insomnia tends to be **persistent**, although it may come and go in an episodic fashion across one's lifespan. Chronic insomnia is associated with worse outcomes in nearly all areas of one's life, including physical health, mental well-being, pain perception, and levels of social support. Physical and cognitive performance decreases as well, with people who miss even one night of sleep driving just as badly (if not worse) than someone who is under the influence of alcohol. In fact, people who are chronically sleep deprived have a rate of accidents that is up to 4.5 times higher than the average. All of these together predict a greatly increased **risk of mortality**, with severe insomnia (sleeping less than 4 hours a night) being associated with a 15% higher mortality rate.

Treatment of insomnia involves therapy, medications, or both. The first-line treatment should be a variant of CBT known as **cognitive behavioral therapy for insomnia** (CBTi). CBTi involves practicing good **sleep hygiene** combined with addressing and correcting any dysfunctional beliefs that may be contributing to sleep-relaxed anxiety ("If I don't get enough sleep tonight, I'm going to have a terrible day tomorrow and everything will be ruined!"). CBTi has been associated with significant reductions in both *subjective* sleep-related distress (with a **large effect size** as high as 1.0) as well as *objective* improvements in the amount and quality of sleep (albeit with a smaller effect size around 0.1 to 0.3). In addition, the beneficial effects of CBTi tend to persist even after treatment has ended.

Medications used to treat insomnia are known as **hypnotics** and consist of a wide variety of drugs with different mechanisms of action, including antihistamines, benzodiazepines, and "Z-drugs" like zolpidem (Ambien). While the efficacy of these drugs varies depending on the class, as a whole their effects tend to be limited to the time in which they are taken, and people tend to develop **tolerance** to their sedative effects after only a few nights of regular use. Finally, hypnotics can cause daytime sedation and poor balance, leading to an increased risk of falls (especially in the elderly). For this reason, hypnotic drugs should generally be recommended only after other interventions (such as CBTi) have been tried, and even then only for as short a period of time as possible.

SECONDARY CAUSES OF INSOMNIA

The prognosis of insomnia varies considerably depending on whether it is primary or secondary. Some causes of secondary insomnia (such as obstructive sleep apnea) will resolve immediately with treatment while others (like restless leg syndrome) are more difficult to treat. Therefore, appropriate diagnosis and treatment of insomnia rests upon looking at the most common underlying causes of insomnia. Because the range of possible causes is so wide, it can be helpful to have a systematic way of evaluating someone who presents with complaints about sleep. You can use the mnemonic **SOUR DREAMS** to remember those factors that commonly contribute to insomnia:

S is for Stress. Stress is well known to make both falling and staying asleep more difficult, so someone who comes in saying that they are not sleeping well should be asked about particular circumstances in their life that may be a source of stress.

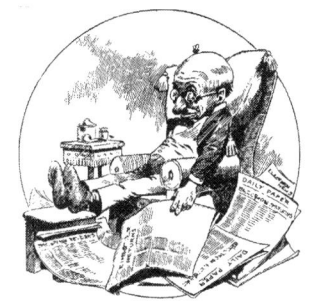

O is for Obstructive sleep apnea. Obstructive sleep apnea (OSA) is a condition in which people suffer from brief but recurrent episodes of apnea (or pauses in breathing) throughout the night. This occurs as a result of **anatomical blockage of the airways** due to both the muscle relaxation that occurs during sleep as well as the recumbent position that most people sleep in. These hypoxic episodes lead to transient "micro-awakenings" that occur throughout the night and prevent the person from entering into deep sleep, resulting in sleep that is not restorative. This leads to **persistent daytime fatigue** and other symptoms such as headaches. While intuitively it would seem like the poor quality sleep associated with obstructive sleep apnea would make people *more* able to fall asleep at night, studies have shown that as many as half of all people with obstructive sleep apnea still struggle with bedtime insomnia.

It's important to ask about obstructive sleep apnea for anyone presenting with chronic fatigue, as patients are not always aware that they are waking up frequently at night. You can use the mnemonic **STOP BANG** to remember the specific factors that are predictive of obstructive sleep apnea, including **S**noring loudly, feeling **T**ired all the time, apneic episodes that have been directly **O**bserved by someone else, high blood **P**ressure, high **B**ody mass index, older **A**ge, a large **N**eck circumference, and male **G**ender. Sleep apnea is a major threat to health, as untreated sleep apnea is associated with a higher risk of heart attack and stroke. Treatment for obstructive sleep apnea involves using a **continuous positive airway pressure** (CPAP) machine that provides a steady stream of air to keep the airway from getting compressed.

> Risk factors for **obstructive sleep apnea** include **snoring, fatigue, hypertension, obesity, older age**, a **large neck**, and **male** gender.
>
> *STOP BANG:*
> *Snoring*
> *Tired all the time*
> *Observed apnea*
> *High blood Pressure*
> *High Body mass index*
> *Older Age*
> *Large Neck circumference*
> *Male Gender*

U is for Urination. Frequent urination at nighttime (known as **nocturia**) can cause chronic sleep deprivation, which is especially common in the elderly. Treatment of underlying causes can provide significant improvements in sleep quality.

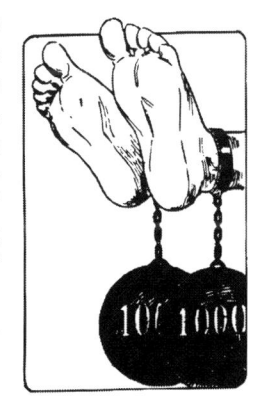

R is for Restless legs. Restless legs syndrome (RLS) is a condition in which a person experiences recurrent feelings of internal energy or restlessness while trying to sleep. This restlessness is temporarily alleviated by moving one's legs, leading to frequent leg movements at bedtime. This can often impair both the length and quality of sleep, leading to symptoms of sleep deprivation. Around half of all cases of restless legs syndrome are idiopathic, with genetics playing a large role. However, it can also occur as the result of other medical or psychiatric conditions. The most common culprit is **iron deficiency** (seen in 20% of all cases), although other disorders like renal failure, diabetes, and Parkinson's disease can play a role as well. In these cases, treatment of the underlying condition (such as giving iron supplementation) takes priority. For idiopathic cases, no curative treatments are available. Instead, a variety of symptomatic treatments can help to improve sleep duration and quality of life. Medications that boost dopamine (such as pramipexole) are often effective. However, their benefits must be balanced against the potential downsides including a risk of rebound symptoms (where restlessness becomes even more severe than it initially was when the drug is stopped).

D is for Drugs. A wide variety of prescription and recreational drugs can interfere with sleep. The most common culprit by far is **caffeine**, which is widely available and consumed by the majority of the population. People tend to underestimate the amount of caffeine that they drink, so ask your patients with insomnia to keep track of their intake so they can tell whether their insomnia is likely related to caffeine intake. Another common culprit is **alcohol**. While it can initially help to induce sleep through its sedative effects, it often leads to a poor quality of sleep or even nighttime awakenings several hours later when a mild state of withdrawal occurs.

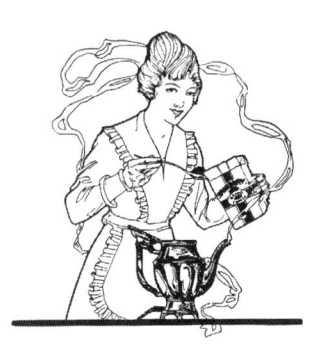

R is for Routine. Asking about the patient's daytime and nighttime routine can help to reveal particular habits that may be contributing to difficulty falling asleep, including frequent naps, exercising too close to bed, or exposure to bright lights at night (which can suppress melatonin secretion and throw off one's circadian rhythm). Having a bedtime routine like making a cup of decaffeinated tea or going to bed at the same time each night can help to improve sleep quantity and quality.

E is for Environment. Sleeping should be done in a space that is quiet, peaceful, and cool. The bed should be used only for sleeping and sex, as other activities (including eating, watching television, or using the phone) can undo the association of your bed as being a place where you go to sleep.

A is for Anxiety. Anxiety is associated with difficulty both falling and staying asleep, so assessing for the presence of anxiety disorders is critical. Often, anxiety about not getting enough sleep can itself perpetuate a cycle of sleeplessness. In addition, someone may have anxiety about falling asleep if they have frequent nightmares (as can occur in PTSD) or experience night terrors or sleep paralysis.

M is for Mood. Mood disorders such as depression and bipolar disorder have disruptions in sleep as core clinical features (remember **S**IGECAPS and DIG FA**ST**!). Depression is often associated with impaired ability to fall asleep at night and early morning awakenings, while mania presents with decreased *need* for sleep.

S is for Subjective. A number of people report a feeling that they aren't getting enough sleep, but a sleep study then reveals that their sleep patterns are adequate. Always consider the possibility that the amount of sleep that someone gets may be greater than they sense, and if this appears to be the case, consider educating on ways of reducing sleep-related anxiety.

> **Insomnia** can be **idiopathic** but is more likely **secondary** to a number of other **medical and psychological factors**.
>
> *SOUR DREAMS*:
> **S**tress
> **O**bstructive sleep apnea
> **U**rination
> **R**estless legs
> **D**rugs
> **R**outine
> **E**nvironment
> **A**nxiety
> **M**ood
> **S**ubjective

MECHANISMS OF PRIMARY INSOMNIA

Mechanistically, cases of insomnia that are not attributable to any secondary causes often involve overactivation of the **HPA axis**, as the severity of insomnia appears to correlate with measurable differences in levels of corticotropin-releasing factor and cortisol. This overactive HPA axis leads to a state of persistent **hyperarousal** during the day. On a cognitive level, this hyperarousal manifests as anxious thoughts about particular life stresses. These thoughts begin to persist at night, which interferes with the ability to fall asleep and worsens one's quality of sleep. After a few nights of bad sleep, the focus of worry often shifts to include not only whatever someone was stressed about in the first place but also the detrimental effect of poor sleep itself. This results in **hypervigilance about falling asleep**, leading to an increase in anxiety around bedtime which only *further* prevents someone from entering the state of relaxation necessary for sleep and creating a vicious cycle. The involvement of the HPA axis appears to explain the common comorbidity of insomnia with both depression and anxiety disorders, as they all likely share a common mechanism. It also explains the effectiveness of CBT in breaking the cycle of insomnia, as anxious thought patterns about sleep are replaced by healthier thought processes and habits.

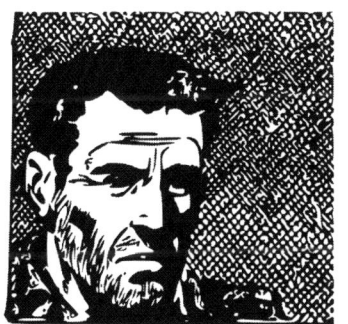

OTHER SLEEP DISORDERS

In addition to insomnia, there are a variety of other sleep disorders that you should be aware of. While a full discussion of sleep disorders would take an entire book on its own, this section can serve as a brief introduction to each major type of sleep disorder to help you recognize them when they occur clinically.

CIRCADIAN RHYTHM DISORDERS

People who are not able to consistently follow a set daily schedule (such as those who work night shifts or travel across time zones) are at risk for circadian rhythm disorders. These disorders are characterized by excessive sleepiness during the daytime (when they should be awake) and involuntary wakefulness at night (when they should be asleep). Providing education on sleep hygiene (such as avoidance of naps and caffeine prior to sleep) can be an initial first step. For those with excessive difficulty *falling asleep* at night, **melatonin supplements** can be incredibly helpful. For those with difficulty *staying awake* during the day, exposure to bright lights can be effective, as can the medication **modafinil** which helps to promote wakefulness.

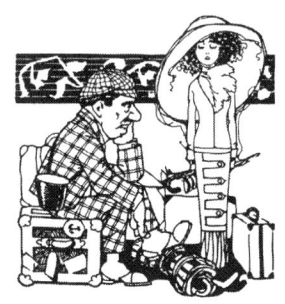

SLEEPWALKING

Sleepwalking (also called somnambulism) is when an individual performs activities as if they are awake despite being in a state of deep sleep. This most commonly involves walking around, although other activities (such as going to the bathroom, cooking, and even driving) have been reported. Sleepwalking is a type of **parasomnia**, a category of sleep disorders characterized by abnormal movements or behaviors during sleep. Parasomnias like **SL**eepwalking occurs during **SL**ow-wave sleep when muscles are not paralyzed (like they are during REM sleep). Most cases of sleepwalking are idiopathic, with no clear cause ever being found. However, in some cases they may be related to use of Z-drugs like zolpidem.

REM SLEEP BEHAVIOR DISORDER

REM sleep behavior disorder is characterized by **abnormal movements during REM sleep**. Recall that REM is the stage of sleep when dreaming is most vivid but one's muscles are paralyzed. For someone with REM sleep behavior disorder, however, a **lack of muscle paralysis during REM sleep** leads to their acting out their dreams. This can be very disruptive to others sharing the bed, and people with REM sleep behavior disorder can sometimes even unintentionally injure themselves or their partners if they are experiencing a particularly violent dream. Compared to sleepwalking, REM sleep behavior disorder is more often related to another disorder (such as Parkinson's disease or dementia with Lewy bodies) than it is idiopathic.

NIGHTMARE DISORDER

Nightmares are **unpleasant or terrifying dreams** that occur during REM sleep. Most people have nightmares from time to time, but a minority of people are afflicted by nightmares that are frequent or severe enough to qualify as a disorder. People with nightmare disorder are more likely to have a history of trauma. If treatment is desired, **stress reduction techniques** such as mindfulness can help, as can the medication **prazosin** which has been shown to reduce the frequency and severity of nightmares.

SLEEP TERRORS
Sleep terrors (also called night terrors) differ from nightmares in that they occur during **non-REM sleep**. As is typical of dreams during non-REM sleep, the person its typically **unable to remember** what they were dreaming about. However, upon awakening they are clearly distressed, often crying out or sitting upright with eyes wide open. Physiologic signs can resemble a panic attack, with tachycardia and hyperventilation being common. Sleep terrors are most common during **childhood**, and the vast majority of cases do not persist into adulthood (with less than 1% of adults experiencing sleep terrors on a regular basis). For this reason, **reassurance** is typically sufficient for children who suffer from sleep terrors (as well as their parents).

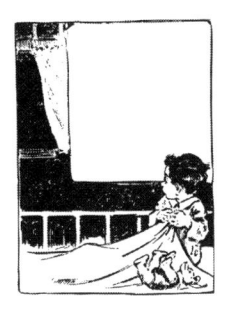

SLEEP PARALYSIS
Capping off the trio of conditions involving terrifying experiences while asleep is sleep paralysis. Sleep paralysis occurs when someone wakes up from REM sleep and gains consciousness of the world but remains **unable to move**. This sensation is often accompanied by a feeling of **fear or panic**. In addition, many people report a distinct sensation of being watched and can even hallucinate a malevolent figure in the room. Episodes of sleep paralysis can be highly disturbing, especially if they are so regular or severe that someone develops anxiety about going to bed. Up to half of all adults have experienced at least one episode of sleep paralysis, although less than 5% experience them on a regular basis. Education on the nature of sleep paralysis and teaching of relaxation techniques can often be treatment enough, although in more severe cases CBT or medications (typically SRIs) can been used.

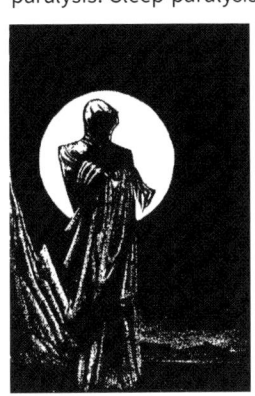

NARCOLEPSY
Narcolepsy is a neurological disorder characterized by **excessive daytime sleepiness** that in some cases leads to people having episodes where they suddenly fall asleep without intending to. While these sudden "sleep attacks" are the most dramatic and memorable symptom, there are a variety of clinical features found in narcolepsy that can inform your diagnosis. The mnemonic **CHAP** will help you remember these:

C is for Cataplexy. Cataplexy refers to **sudden episodes of muscle paralysis** during wakefulness. This can span the range from more subtle signs (such as slight weakness in one's limbs) all the way up to more dramatic events (such as collapsing on the ground due to a complete loss of muscle tone). Cataplexy is often triggered by strong emotional states, but it can occur "out of the blue" as well. Cataplexy is likely related to activation of the same state of muscle paralysis seen in REM sleep but *without* the accompanying loss of consciousness (it is only **half of the REM sleep state**). Cataplexy is unique to narcolepsy, making it a **very specific sign**. Of note, cataplexy should be differentiated from cata*lepsy* which is associated with catatonia. You can remember this by thinking that cata**psy** is found in **psy**chiatric conditions whereas catap**lexy** is related to the bedroom (as you use a bed for both sleep and s**exy** time).

> **Cataplexy**, or sudden episodes of **muscle paralysis during wakefulness**, is a core feature of **narcolepsy**.
>
> *Catale**psy** is found in **psy**chiatric conditions while catap**lexy** is related to narcolepsy (use a bed for both **sleep** and s**exy** time).*

H is for Hypnagogic and hypnopompic hallucinations. The term **hypnagogic** refers to the transition from wakefulness to sleep, while **hypnopompic** refers to the transition from sleep to wakefulness. People with narcolepsy are known to experience vivid hallucinations during both transition. This imagery can range from random lights or "speckles" all the way to fully formed images of people and places. In contrast to the hallucinations seen in dreaming, it is rare for hypnagogic or hypnopompic hallucinations to involve any sort of story or narrative. You can remember the difference between hypnagogic and hypnopompic hallucinations by thinking that hypno-**grog**-ic hallucinations occur when you are **grog**-gy, while hypno-**pump**-ic hallucinations occur when you need to **pump** yourself up in the morning.

> **Hypnagogic and hypnopompic hallucinations** are sensory experiences that occur during the **transition between sleep and wakefulness**.
>
> *Hypno-**grog**-ic is when you are **grog**-gy at night, while hypno-**pump**-ic is when you need to **pump** yourself up in the morning.*

A is for sleep Attacks. Sudden episodes of sleep are perhaps the most dramatic and well-known sign of narcolepsy. These "sleep attacks" (which are distinct from the "dream attacks" seen in dissociative episodes) typically last only a few seconds or minutes, but due to their unpredictable nature they can be incredibly distressing and impairing. Not all people with narcolepsy experience such sudden "attacks" of sleep, with some people primarily experiencing **excessive daytime sleepiness** (even when they get adequate sleep).

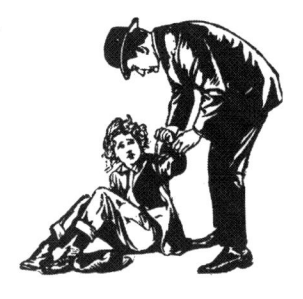

P is for sleep Paralysis. Sleep paralysis is common in narcolepsy and, like cataplexy, represents a manifestation of the tendency these patients have towards experiencing **only half of the REM sleep state** (muscle paralysis without the sleepiness), only this time occurring at night instead of during the day (as occurs during cataplexy).

> **Narcolepsy** is characterized by the tetrad of **cataplexy, hypnagogic and hypnopompic hallucinations, sleep attacks,** and **sleep paralysis**.
>
> **CHAP:**
> **C**ataplexy
> **H**ypnagogic and hypnopompic hallucinations
> Sleep **A**ttacks
> Sleep **P**aralysis

While diagnosing narcolepsy is easy when someone has *all four* of these clinical features, not everyone with narcolepsy does. In cases where the diagnosis is less clear, **sleep studies** can help to detect the specific abnormalities (such as rapid transitions between wakefulness and REM sleep) that characterize narcolepsy.

Narcolepsy is a **rare diagnosis**, affecting less than 0.1% of the population (although it may be underdiagnosed, especially in people who do not have all four of the characteristic symptoms). It tends to have its onset during **adolescence and early adulthood**, with **men and women** being affected equally. Treatment is symptomatic rather than curative. Sodium oxybate (better known by its street name gamma-hydroxybutyric acid or **GHB**) is effective at reducing the severity of multiple symptoms of narcolepsy, including excessive daytime sleepiness, episodes of cataplexy, and altered sleep architecture. In addition, the wakefulness-enhancing drug **modafinil** appears to be effective at reducing daytime sleepiness and sleep attacks but does not significantly affect episodes of cataplexy. Careful maintenance of sleep hygiene and avoidance of sleep-impairing substances such as caffeine and alcohol are crucial as well. **Behavioral and lifestyle changes** such as scheduling naps and exercise sessions can be beneficial as well.

PUTTING IT ALL TOGETHER

Sleep is a vital part of life that is essential not only for *living* but for living *well*. In the field of psychiatry, impaired sleep has been associated with nearly all forms of mental illness in a bidirectional fashion (with disturbances in sleep increasing the risk for developing a mental disorder as well as mental disorders themselves increasing the risk of impaired sleep). Because of the close relationship of sleep to mental health, you should consider assessing sleep patterns as part of **every psychiatric evaluation**.

Understanding the physiology of normal sleep can help with identifying the exact stages in the process where things have gone awry. Use **BATS D**rink **R**ed **B**lood to remind yourself of the stages of sleep. From there, evaluate where in the process the dysfunction is occurring, then use the **SOUR DREAMS** mnemonic to evaluate for common causes of insomnia dysfunction. Once these have been ruled out, consider a referral to CBTi or another evidence-based form of therapy, with medications used sparingly if at all.

REVIEW QUESTIONS

1. A 29 y/o F awakens suddenly at 2:53 in the morning and experiences an "electrical sensation" running down her entire body from head to toe. She has a distinct sense that someone has broken into her house and is standing in the doorway, but she finds that she is unable to roll over in bed to look and know for sure. She feels her heart begin beating loudly in her ears and feels short of breath. A few seconds later she is able to turn over and sees that there is no one in the doorway. Which of the following best describes this episode?
    A. Nightmare
    B. Hypnagogic hallucination
    C. Cataplexy
    D. Sleep paralysis
    E. Sleep terror
    F. None of the above

2. (Continued from previous question.) Which of the following statements is true about this condition?
    A. Taking prazosin regularly will help to prevent these episodes
    B. It is likely to recur frequently once it has started
    C. It is common in children but rare in adults
    D. It is less likely to occur while taking medications to treat depression
    E. None of these statements are true

3. A 25 y/o M sees her primary care provider complaining of insomnia. He says that for the past 2 months he has had severe difficulty falling asleep and will often feel the need to move his legs for up to 2 hours before finally falling asleep. He says, "I just can't seem to get comfortable. It's like I just drank coffee except I don't drink anything." Asking about additional sources of caffeine, including chocolate and tea, confirms the absence of caffeine intake. He also denies drinking alcohol or using other psychoactive substances. He denies having specific thoughts going through his head while falling asleep, saying, "I'm not worried about anything. I mean, since this started I have begun to get worried about *it*, but otherwise my life is going fine." He denies daytime fatigue, saying, "I only get 5 or 6 hours which is enough to function, although I'd like to get more." Which of the following is the best next step?
    A. Prescribe an antidepressant
    B. Prescribe a hypnotic
    C. Refer for a sleep study
    D. Refer to a specialist in cognitive behavioral therapy for insomnia
    E. Order laboratory tests

4. A 13 y/o F is brought to see a neurologist for recurrent "fainting spells" that she has been experiencing for the past two months. She reports feeling "super tired all day, every day" and often falls asleep during class. She has been sent to the principal's office several times who has encouraged her to "go to bed earlier and stop drinking so much coffee at night." At a surprise birthday party that her family arranged for her over the weekend, she suddenly collapsed several seconds after the guests yelled, "Surprise!" She denies losing consciousness at that time and has full memory of the event. However, she also has experienced other episodes when she will fall down for several minutes and wake up with no memory of the experience. She recently has begun waking up from nightmares but finds herself unable to move. She denies hearing or seeing things as she is falling asleep. She otherwise has no medical or psychiatric history. Which of the following is the most appropriate statement for the neurologist to make at this time?

    A. "This is likely a dissociative disorder. You need to see a psychiatrist who can help you with this more than I can."
    B. "This sounds like narcolepsy, but without the presence of hypnagogic hallucinations we cannot diagnose it as such."
    C. "Your principal is right: you need to get more sleep and drink less coffee in the evenings."
    D. "I can see what you are trying to do here, but there are better ways of getting out of class than this."
    E. "I wish I could do more to help, but this is a completely untreatable condition."
    F. None of the above would be appropriate statements to make

1. **The best answer is D.** This vignette describes a case of sleep paralysis which involves becoming conscious while in a state of muscle paralysis related to REM sleep. Panic-like psychological and physiologic symptoms as well as a feeling that someone or something else is present in the room are common. Nightmares also occur during REM sleep, but the hallucinated objects and paralysis do not persist after awakening (answer A). Hypnagogic hallucinations refer to seeing or hearing things while falling asleep, not while waking up from sleep (answer B). Cataplexy is a state of sudden muscle paralysis during daytime *wakefulness*, not sleep (answer C). Sleep terrors occur during deep sleep and are not accompanied by muscle paralysis (answer E).

2. **The best answer is D.** Antidepressants like SRIs are sometimes used to treat recurrent sleep paralysis, so someone taking them to treat depression is likely to experience these episodes less often. Sleep paralysis is rarely recurrent, although for a minority of people they can be (answer B). Prazosin helps reduce the frequency and severity of nightmares, not sleep paralysis (answer A). Sleep terrors are common in children but rare in adults (answer C).

3. **The best answer is E.** This vignette describes a case of restless legs syndrome. Restless legs syndrome can be idiopathic, but in many cases it is related to a medical condition. Of these, iron deficiency is the most common, so this should be ruled out immediately. If no cause is found, drugs that increase dopamine such as pramipexole can be used. Antidepressants have not been shown to help in cases of restless legs syndrome (answer A). Prescribing a hypnotic, ordering a sleep study, or referring to a specialist in CBT for insomnia may be helpful but should not be done before the most obvious underlying causes are ruled out first (answers B, C, and D).

4. **The best answer is F.** This describes a case of narcolepsy involving cataplexy, sleep attacks, and sleep paralysis. While hypnagogic hallucinations are also found commonly in narcolepsy, most cases of narcolepsy do not involve all four symptoms (answer B). Narcolepsy is a treatable condition (answer E) but requires more than just telling someone to get more sleep and drink less caffeine (answer C). Narcolepsy should be differentiated from dissociation which involves "dream attacks" rather than the "sleep attacks" (answer A). Diagnosing malingering is inappropriate as this clinical case matches what is known about the phenomenology of narcolepsy almost exactly (answer D).

24 FINAL REVIEW

Hey, you made it! *Congratulations*. Learning about an entire field of medicine over a few hundred pages is no easy task, so kudos to you for your hard work and determination. While **psychiatric diagnosis is neither simple nor easy**, hopefully you have gained some of the skills and knowledge required to approach this task with a clear mind. Psychiatric diagnosis is a **powerful tool**, but like any tool it must be used responsibly to avoid being unintentionally turned into a weapon. Despite the inherent shortcomings of the process, we cannot sidestep diagnosis entirely as it remains the cornerstone of our ability to bring understanding and hope to the people struggling with these syndromes.

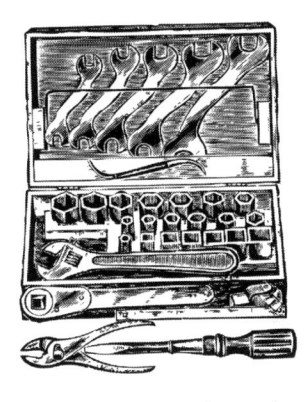

To avoid the downsides of diagnosis, remember to *always keep normalcy on the differential*, as sadness is not depression, happiness is not mania, hearing voices is not schizophrenia, worrying is not an anxiety disorder, being orderly is not OCD, experiencing trauma is not PTSD, having emotions is not a personality disorder, and so on. Keep this crucial distinction in mind as you prepare to help a world of people who need your knowledge, guidance, and compassion more than ever.

While each chapter so far has made references to topics in other chapters, these final review questions are intended to supercharge your learning by helping you draw additional comparisons between the various disorders we have studied. This will also help to **consolidate the information** that you have learned so far and better prepare you for real-world clinical situations where patients can come in with **any possible problem** (rather than just the one from the chapter you happened to be studying at the time).

Good luck!

FINAL REVIEW QUESTIONS

1. A 28 y/o F brings her 1-month-old baby girl to her pediatrician's office for a well-child check. She has been raising the baby alone after her boyfriend left upon discovering that the girl had Down syndrome. Examination of the baby reveals that she is at the 4th percentile in weight for her age. Upon entering the room, the pediatrician notices that the baby is crying and that the mother is wearing large amounts of makeup. The mother says, "Thank you doctor for seeing my baby. She's a tiny little girl now, but she's going to grow up to be a star. She's already singing right now, and it's beautiful, beautiful, absolutely booty-full." When the pediatrician tries to pick up the infant for examination, her mother pulls her back suddenly, yelling, "Oh no you don't! She's mine! If you think you're getting rich off me and my baby, you're dead wrong!" The baby continues crying throughout this exchange. What is the next best step?
   A. Prescribe an antipsychotic
   B. Prescribe a mood stabilizer
   C. Prescribe an antidepressant
   D. Arrange for transfer to the hospital
   E. Provide reassurance and conclude the appointment

2. A 7 y/o M is brought to see a child psychiatrist by his mother for "problems at school." Pregnancy, birth, and early childhood were non-eventful, and he met all developmental milestones on time. However, halfway through the school year, the patient began having difficulty sitting still. He previously was completing his schoolwork without any problem, but he suddenly started showing no interest in school. His mother is concerned because he appears to have forgotten things that he has previously learned, including the alphabet and how to do arithmetic. He lives with both of his parents and an older sister. There is no history of medical or psychiatric problems in the family. Which of the following is the most likely diagnosis?
   A. Attention deficit hyperactivity disorder, inattentive type
   B. Attention deficit hyperactivity disorder, hyperactive type
   C. Attention deficit hyperactivity disorder, combined type
   D. Rett syndrome
   E. Disruptive mood dysregulation disorder
   F. Oppositional defiant disorder
   G. Autism spectrum disorder
   H. None of the above

3. (Continued from previous question.) The patient is referred for neuropsychiatric testing. Five days after the initial evaluation, he experiences a tonic-clonic seizure lasting for approximately one minute. He is sent by ambulance to the emergency department. Vitals signs are HR 108, BP 84/58, RR 22, and T 100.7°F. Laboratory studies show severe hyponatremia. An MRI of the brain is conducted which reveals white matter changes in the posterior periventricular area. Physical examination of his mouth shows the following:

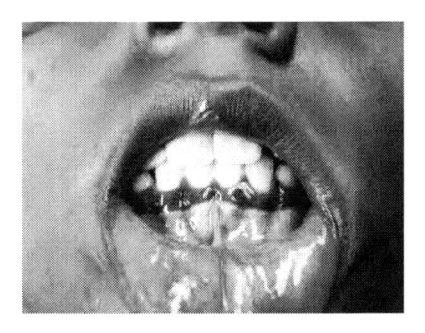

Which of the following is true of this condition?
- A. It is untreatable
- B. It is equally common in males and female
- C. It was previously known as Asperger's syndrome
- D. Some people with this condition are completely asymptomatic
- E. It tends to respond to stimulant medications
- F. None of the above are true

4. A 25 y/o M comes to a psychiatrist's office for an initial evaluation for difficulty sleeping. He says that he has always been "a bit of an introvert" but has generally been successful in his life. He graduated from college with a degree in geological engineering several years ago and has a well-paying job. He is currently single but has dated in the past. He has never seen a psychiatrist or taken psychotropic medications prior to this visit but did see a therapist for two months around the time of his parents' divorce at the age of 12. His primary concerns today are trouble sleeping, daytime fatigue, and difficulty concentrating at work. He often cannot fall asleep for several hours and has been averaging only 4 hours of sleep per night. Once he falls asleep, he is generally able to sleep through the rest of the night. He has noticed these symptoms for the past 3 months over which time they have been slowly getting worse. He denies any major stresses or changes in his life. His mood is generally "good" and he finds that he still enjoys his favorite activities such as going mountain biking (although he does not do it as often due to fatigue). He denies feelings of hopelessness or thoughts of suicide. He feels that sometimes he is moving more slowly but is unsure (he looks confused when asked the question). Which of the following is the most likely diagnosis?
    - A. Unipolar depression
    - B. Bipolar depression
    - C. Dysthymia
    - D. Adjustment disorder
    - E. Generalized anxiety disorder
    - F. None of the above

5. An 18 y/o F with a history of the hyperactive subtype of ADHD undergoes extensive neuropsychiatric testing which reveals very high levels of impulsivity (in the 92nd percentile for adults her age) and very low levels of compulsive behavior. Which of the following behaviors is she *least* likely to engage in?
   A. Eating lots of food in a single sitting and then vomiting them up
   B. Using a razor to make superficial cuts on her wrist following a break-up
   C. Pulling out small patches of hair from her head until it bleeds
   D. Going to a friend's party to drink despite having had her driver's license revoked after a DUI one month ago
   E. Throwing a plate against the wall during an argument with her parents

6. A 20 y/o M is brought to the psychiatrist's office by his mother who says that she "doesn't know what to do with him anymore." On interview, the patient declines to speak with the psychiatrist because "he will steal my energy," so the mother provides the majority of the history. Per the mother, the patient rarely showers or changes clothing until his parents tell him to. He worked at a local fast food restaurant until he was fired for coming into work "looking like he lost a fight with a homeless person." He now spends most of his free time on various online message boards. He previously did very well in school and graduated with straight As. However, he declined several scholarships at prestigious colleges. When asked why, he says, "Colleges are like banks for your mind, and I want to keep mine stuffed under the bed." The psychiatrist tries again to ask him questions, and this time he responds. He says he prefers not to shower because it "replaces my internal aura with something more artificial." He denies feeling depressed or anxious. He has no trouble sleeping and says he does not hear voices. He wants nothing from the psychiatrist at this time, describing himself as "happy." When asked if he has friends, he says, "Mostly people online who also enjoy the wonders of the jade stone arts." His mental status exam is unremarkable except for an affect that is sometimes inappropriate to the topic at hand. After finishing the session, the psychiatrist asks to speak with the patient's mother separately. She begins crying and says, "I want answers. My brother is schizophrenic. Will my son be too?" Which of the following is the most appropriate response?
   A. "Your son has schizophrenia. Let's talk about treatment."
   B. "Your son does not have schizophrenia, but he may develop it later."
   C. "I can say definitively that your son will not develop schizophrenia."
   D. "Your son won't develop schizophrenia, but he has a related condition known as schizoid personality disorder."
   E. "These beliefs may come across as being related to schizophrenia, but they are caused by something called paranoid personality disorder."
   F. "Your son is completely normal. I'd like to see you alone next time."

7. A 15 y/o F is hospitalized after a second suicide attempt. While speaking with the patient's parents, the psychiatrist says, "We need to work together to come up with a comprehensive plan, as the next few years won't be easy. Your daughter's condition has the highest chance of death of any psychiatric condition, so we really need all hands on deck." What is the patient's most likely diagnosis?

A. Major depressive disorder
B. Bipolar disorder
C. Schizophrenia
D. Panic disorder
E. Obsessive-compulsive disorder
F. Post-traumatic stress disorder
G. Factitious disorder
H. Borderline personality disorder
I. Anorexia nervosa
J. Bulimia nervosa

8. A 53 y/o M is seen for the first time by a neurologist specializing in memory loss. He says that he worked in construction for many years and recently found out that he was exposed to "some kind of toxic chemical, I don't remember the name but apparently it's pretty bad" on a regular basis. He believes that exposure to this chemical is related to some "annoying brain problems" he has been having and desires a full evaluation. He has contacted other people that he worked with in the past who are planning on filing a class action lawsuit against their previous employer. In regards to specific complaints, the patient says that his ability to remember letters and numbers has "basically evaporated" in the past 5 years. While he is able to read, he says that he cannot recall phone numbers, addresses, or other pieces of information that involve combinations of letters and numbers. When asked to spell his own name, he says, "That's one of those things, I can't do it anymore." His MoCA score today is 5/30 (normal range of 25 and above). When asked about his driving, he says, "That I can do—driving, going to the store, putting on my shoes—that's all fine." Which of the following would be the best next step?
    A. Writing a report that suggests the patient is suffering from a severe neurocognitive disorder
    B. Conducting a thorough physical and neurologic examination
    C. Ordering a CT scan of the brain
    D. Telling the patient to "stop lying and get out of my office"
    E. Taking a non-confrontational approach and politely reassuring the patient that there is nothing wrong with him

9. An 18 y/o F is admitted to the hospital after telling her therapist that she is "hearing voices telling me to kill myself." She began hearing these voices 2 weeks ago and describes them as originating from inside her head. She has been hospitalized over 10 times since the age of 14 and has multiple diagnoses in her chart, including depression, bipolar II disorder, an unspecified anxiety disorder, PTSD, and irritable bowel syndrome. At her most recent hospitalization, she was told by a frustrated nurse, "Don't come back here until you are really sick like the other people here!" after which she became incredibly agitated. During rounds with her team on the morning after admission, she describes feeling depressed "for as long as I can remember" and denies periods of normal or balanced mood. She says that she feels unloved by her mother at home and desires to go to a residential treatment program after discharge. When told by the social worker

that her insurance doesn't cover this, her affect rapidly darkens and she tells the social worker, "The voices say you're stupid and worthless." Which of the following is true of this patient's condition?
   A. She is unusually young for a female to develop this condition
   B. It is a rare diagnosis that bridges psychotic and mood disorders
   C. It responds well to a combination of antidepressants and antipsychotics
   D. It is a lifelong condition, and her symptoms will continue to worsen over the next several decades
   E. It is correlated with a history of abuse

10. An 18 y/o M is brought to the hospital by his parents who found him making cuts to his wrist while sitting in his room. A picture of his injuries is seen below:

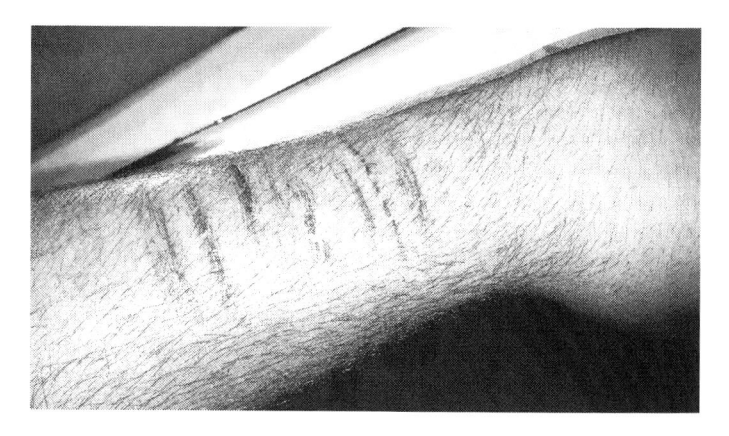

The injuries are determined by the triage nurse to be non-life-threatening, and given that it is a busy Saturday night in the emergency department, he ends up waiting to be evaluated by a physician for over 8 hours. When seen by the physician, he complains of bilateral headache, nausea, and dizziness beginning one hour ago. Vitals signs are HR 74, BP 120/76, RR 16, and T 98.2°F. He appears somewhat lethargic and is slurring his words. However, there are no other abnormalities on physical exam. He continues to report suicidal ideation, so a plan is made to admit him to the psychiatric unit. On the unit, he tells one of the nurses that he is having severe pain in his right upper abdomen. At this time he is alert and oriented to person only. A rapid response is called, and he is quickly transferred to the intensive care unit where he is diagnosed as being in fulminant hepatic failure. Which of the following could have prevented this outcome?
   A. Being seen by the physician within one hour of arriving at the hospital
   B. Taking a complete substance history including the time of last drink
   C. Having a high index of suspicion for occult overdoses
   D. Ensuring that the patient had access to adequate hydration while waiting in the emergency department
   E. Nothing could have prevented this outcome

11. (Continued from previous question.) The patient is determined to need an urgent liver transplant to survive. However, his mental status continues to fluctuate, and he is unable to answer questions about his condition other than saying his name and "it hurts" repeatedly. Which of the following is the best next step?
    A. Ask the patient if he understands the risks and benefits of the procedure
    B. Ask the parents what they would like to do based on their own beliefs
    C. Call the outpatient psychiatrist to determine the psychiatric diagnosis
    D. Cancel plans for transplantation
    E. None of the above

12. A 20 y/o F nursing student with no prior medical or psychiatric history is attending a learning session on how to perform an intradermal injection. She is paired with another student to practice inserting a needle into each other's skin. Her partner follows the instructions including proper sterile technique and begins to insert the needle as seen below:

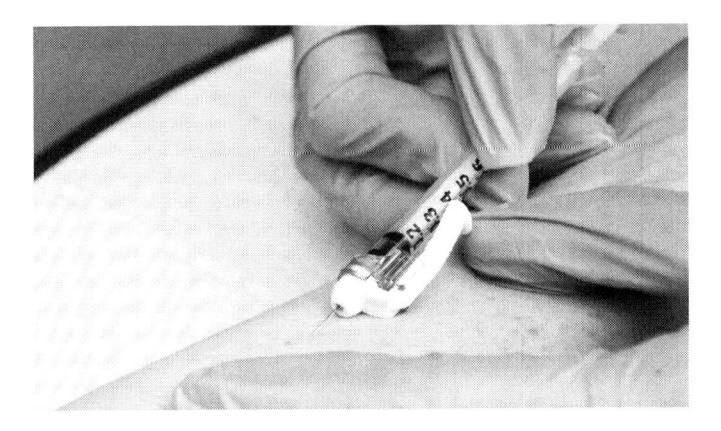

    Upon insertion of the needle, the girl suddenly feels faint. Her heart begins racing and she feels lightheaded. She experiences a distinct sense that the world is not real, and she feels that she is controlling herself in the same way she would control a puppet or doll. She begins screaming, and an ambulance is called. Which of the following is the most likely diagnosis?
    A. Acute stress disorder
    B. Post-traumatic stress disorder
    C. Obsessive-compulsive disorder
    D. Panic disorder
    E. Dissociative amnesia
    F. Depersonalization-derealization disorder
    G. None of the above

13. A 31 y/o F makes an appointment to see her primary care provider to discuss her weight. She has been mildly obese for much of her life. However, over the past 6 months she has gained 25 pounds. She acknowledges eating too much, including a strong preference for fatty and carbohydrate-rich foods like snack cakes. She

denies episodes of binge eating, saying, "Recently I eat this way all the time." She notes that her increase in food intake coincided with her boyfriend of 11 years breaking off their engagement. She has felt "pretty down" since then, but then says, "But that's life, you know? Life is a shit sandwich sometimes." She denies a persistent depressed mood, saying, "When I see friends I still have a good time, but on an average day I feel like crap." She is worried about the effect that her recent weight gain will have on her ability to find a new romantic partner, saying, "Who wants to date a whale?" She has cried frequently over the past few weeks, often in response to a friend making a comment that she perceives as making fun of her weight ("He said my cookies were 'almost too good'! What's *that* supposed to mean?"). She then asks for a prescription for Adderall, saying, "It's supposed to help you lose weight, right? And I could use the energy boost. I feel like I'm spending all day in bed." Which of the following is the best response?
- A. "Based on what you're telling me, an antidepressant will likely help even more than Adderall."
- B. "Medications won't do anything to help you. The only thing that will help is a type of therapy known as dialectical behavior therapy."
- C. "This sounds like you have social anxiety. Let me refer you to someone who can do cognitive behavioral therapy."
- D. "It's not uncommon for people with bulimia to get depressed, but we need to focus on treating the bulimia first."
- E. "Adderall sounds like a good option for you. I'll write you a script."
- F. None of the above

14. A 9 y/o F comes to school wearing a turtleneck sweater. It is the end of August, with temperatures outside approaching 100°F. An observant lunch lady pulls the girl aside to ask her if she isn't too warm and wouldn't prefer to take her sweater off. However, the girl resists this suggestion, so she is sent to the nurse's office. The nurse conducts a full physical examination and observes the findings below:

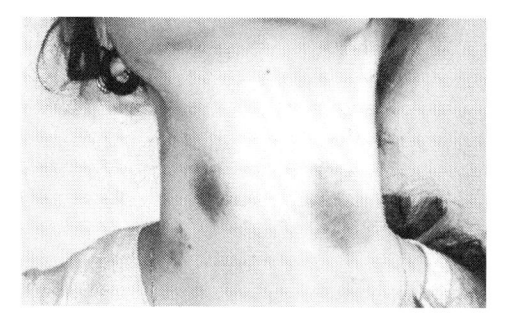

The girl refuses to answer any of the nurse's questions. Later, when the girl's father comes to pick her up, the nurse asks about her neck. The father replies, "It's nothing. She plays a lot. She probably just fell." When the nurse continues to ask him questions, he says, "Look, I told you it's nothing. She was clumsy this morning and clocked herself while getting out of bed. Can I go now?" Which of the following conditions is this girl most likely to have at this time?

A. Social anxiety disorder
B. Post-traumatic stress disorder
C. Oppositional defiant disorder
D. Borderline personality disorder
E. Dissociative identity disorder

15. (Continued from previous question.) The girl is referred to a child and adolescent psychiatrist whom she sees at least twice yearly for the next decade. At the age of 18, she is working at a local daycare and going to school in the evenings to study early childhood education. However, she often finds herself unable to fully concentrate on either her job or her studies. She suffers from muscle tension and is unable to relax even when at home on the weekends or around friends. She frequently worries about how she will do at school and frequently visualizes her boss firing her. These thoughts often come to her head as she goes to bed, leading to frequent nights of poor sleep with resultant daytime fatigue. Which of these conditions is she *least* likely to develop over her lifetime?
    A. Anxiety about most things most of the time
    B. Episodes of depressed mood
    C. Persistent depressed mood
    D. Nightmares more often than average
    E. Flirtatious attention-seeking behaviors which come across as shallow

16. A 21 y/o M is pulled over for driving 40 miles per hour above the speed limit. He greets the police officer with a smile and says, "Hiya fuckface! How about you quit being such a do-gooder choad and let me go?" The officer arrests him. Urine toxicology reveals the presence of opioids, cannabis, amphetamines, and alcohol. Seven days later, he is seen by a psychiatrist. Chart review reveals that the patient has been arrested under similar circumstances on one previous occasion. There is no history of violent crime or interactions with the legal system prior to the age of 20. However, he was hospitalized at age 19 after a suicide attempt. The patient has spent most of the previous week pacing around his room and talking endlessly to neighbors in adjacent cells. On multiple occasions, he has disrobed and begun to masturbate before being stopped by guards. When this happens he becomes very upset and punches the walls of the cell. On interview, the patient describes himself as "the magnificent Mr. Miyagi" and asks the psychiatrist to observe his "karate judo moves." He says that he plans to "synthesize all martial arts into a single discipline" that he will teach to school children "so that no one will ever be afraid again." He laughs frequently during the interview and attempts to leave several times before being asked to sit back down by the guard. Which of the following is the most likely primary diagnosis?
    A. Narcissistic personality disorder
    B. Psychopathic antisocial personality disorder
    C. Non-psychopathic antisocial personality disorder
    D. Schizophrenia
    E. Bipolar I disorder
    F. Multiple substance use disorders
    G. Attention deficit hyperactivity disorder

17. An 8 y/o M is admitted to the hospital while on vacation with his family for severe abdominal pain and vomiting. While staying at an all-inclusive resort, the patient unlocked his door and walked to the all-you-can-eat buffet where he proceeded to eat until he began crying and vomiting. He speaks slowly and is unable to understand most questions asked of him, though his parents say that this is his baseline behavior. A picture of the patient taken before the incident is below:

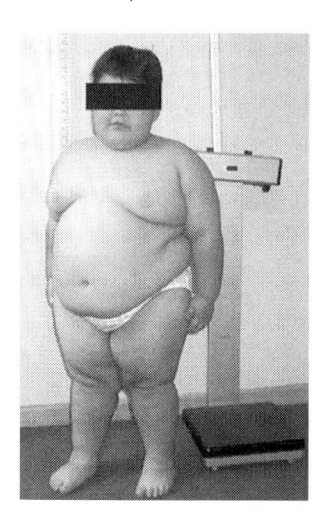

The patient subsequently undergoes an exploratory laparotomy which reveals gastric rupture and necrosis. Which of the following diagnoses most likely explains this patient's behavior?
A. Binge eating disorder
B. Bulimia nervosa
C. Down syndrome
D. Prader-Willi syndrome
E. Angelman syndrome
F. William syndrome
G. None of the above

18. A 58 y/o F comes into the psychiatrist's office complaining of depression after realizing "what a complete and utter failure my life has been." She voices a desire to both engage in psychotherapy and start taking medications for depression. She denies an episodic pattern to her depression and instead says that she has been "constantly depressed" for several decades. She denies changes in sleep, appetite, or energy levels. She denies having close friends, saying, "My whole world has been at home." She lives with her husband who previously worked as a car salesman. However, they are now living on disability payments since her husband hurt his back while working in the garage (although she says, "Sometimes I wonder if he's really as hurt as he says he is."). Financially, they frequently struggle to make ends meet, but he has refused to discuss the possibility of her returning to work to bring in additional income. Earlier in life, she was accepted into law school but declined the offer after her husband

disapproved of her going to school. He has recently begun to bring additional sexual partners into their bedroom so that they can have threesomes ("and sometimes foursomes," she says sheepishly). When asked if she enjoys these sexual encounters, she says, "No! I hate them. I want him to look at me the way he looks at these random strangers he brings home." She has never told him of her dislike of these sexual encounters and says that she "plays along" to make him happy. During times when he is away, she feels "a physical pain deep down in my body" that only goes away when he returns. The patient is provided with a referral for a psychotherapist who takes her insurance. However, she then asks for "at least 5 referrals" as "I want to make sure that my husband is okay with them." Which of the following is true of this patient's condition?
   A. It is unlikely to change
   B. It is likely to resolve on its own without treatment
   C. It is likely to resolve with use of an antidepressant
   D. It is known to respond well to cognitive behavioral therapy
   E. It is likely related to dysregulation of the sympathetic nervous system

19. A 56 y/o M comes to a psychiatric clinic with his wife. He is observed to walk very slowly and requires assistance from his wife when turning to walk through the clinic door. When asked how the clinic can help, the wife immediately breaks down crying and says, "He doesn't love me anymore." As his wife is crying, the patient shows no change in affect and continues to stare straight ahead. His wife soon stops crying and composes herself. She then says, "Things haven't been the same for the past year. I don't think he loves me anymore. He doesn't say more than a few words each day. But he also doesn't let me go anywhere. If I leave him for even a few minutes to go to the store, he'll call me on my phone and ask where I am. He doesn't do anything for himself. I cook for him, and if I don't remind him he won't shower or change his clothes." The patient was started on an antidepressant by his primary care provider three months ago. When asked if he is depressed, he flatly answers, "No." When asked if he has any concerns, he again answers, "No." His voice is notable for a complete absence of prosody. A resting tremor is noted in his left hand but not his right. A MoCA is performed, and the patient scores an 18/30 with significant deficits in executive functioning and delayed recall. There are no abnormalities in cranial nerve function. Which of the following is the most likely diagnosis at this time?
   A. Alzheimer's disease
   B. Early-onset Alzheimer's disease
   C. Frontotemporal dementia
   D. Dementia with Lewy bodies
   E. Vascular dementia
   F. Mixed dementia
   G. Parkinson's disease
   H. Prion disease
   I. None of the above

20. A 6 y/o M is brought to see his pediatrician after he begins refusing dinner. He spends dinnertime arranging his food in such a way that no different foods are touching each other. If someone tries to get him to eat, he screams and runs away from the table. He now refuses to eat any foods that are not individually wrapped. While there is no evidence of either weight loss or weight gain, the patient's mother is concerned about the effect that eating only pre-packaged foods will have on his health. She says that this behavior started after he was gifted a children's book on microbiology by his grandmother. Since then, he has spent several hours each day reading about different forms of bacteria on the internet. When the pediatrician asks him why he does this, he says, "Bacteria friends!" When asked what the consequences of eating bacteria would be, he cannot think of any. He makes poor eye contact with the pediatrician and often looks around the room. Which of the following is the most likely explanation for his behavior?
    A. Obsessive-compulsive disorder
    B. Obsessive-compulsive personality disorder
    C. Autism spectrum disorder
    D. Intellectual disability
    E. Anorexia nervosa
    F. None of the above

21. A 14 y/o F is brought to see a doctor by her parents who say that she is "out of control" the past 3 days. Per their report, she has been incredibly irritable and has frequently yelled not only at her parents but also her friends, classmates, and teachers at school. They say that "a lot of the time what she says makes no sense" and play a video they took of her arguing with a friend and accusing her of being "a witch with broom booms." At times, she has needed to be restrained by others out of fear that she may attack someone else. She also sometimes has "fits of crying" that do not appear to be related to any specific events or circumstances. They also note that she has stopped sleeping regularly and returned home this morning at 6:00 appearing as if she had been outside wandering all night. There is no prior medical or psychiatric history, and the patient was previously doing very well in school. There are no recent psychosocial stressors that the parents are aware of, although they note that the patient appeared to have "the flu" about one week ago. On exam, the patient herself is entirely mute but will direct her eyes to the person asking her questions. She makes a repetitive chewing-like motion with her lips. There are beads of sweat on her brow, and she appears to have urinated on herself. Which of the following is most likely to result in a change in behavior?
    A. Gentle reassurance that the behavior is normal
    B. Starting an antidepressant
    C. Starting a mood stabilizer
    D. Starting an antipsychotic
    E. Referring to cognitive behavioral therapy
    F. Referring to dialectical behavior therapy
    G. Surgical intervention

22. A 44 y/o M with a history of binge eating disorder in remission for the past year comes in to see his psychiatrist for a follow-up visit. Despite no longer engaging in episodes of binge eating, the patient remains overweight with a BMI of 34.9. He describes feeling tired all of the time. While he often falls asleep during the day, he frequently has difficulty falling asleep at night and asks to be started on a medication to help with sleep. All of the following should be part of his initial evaluation *except*:
    A. A substance intake history
    B. A sleep study
    C. A physical examination
    D. A review of systems
    E. Taking vital signs
    F. All of these should be part of his initial assessment

23. (Continued from previous question.) His psychiatrist starts him on zolpidem. At the next visit one month later, the patient has gained 10 pounds. He says that he still is not binge eating but often wakes up in the morning to find food stains on his shirt and empty cartons of food that he does not remember eating in his trash can. He lives alone. What is the most likely explanation for this behavior?
    A. The patient has returned to binge eating but does not remember them
    B. The patient has returned to binge eating but does not want to tell his doctor
    C. The patient is experiencing an idiopathic parasomnia
    D. The patient is experiencing a substance-induced parasomnia
    E. None of the above

24. A 45 y/o M with Down syndrome is brought to see his primary care provider by a sister who acts as his caretaker. His sister reports that over the past year she has noticed that he does not appear to recognize her anymore. He has also had several episodes of wetting the bed over the past few months which he normally does not do. He also previously enjoyed painting but has not engaged in this activity recently, even with her direct prompting. She says, "Over the past month in particular, he has seemed to be more irritable than usual, which isn't the sweet boy I've known my whole life." His vital signs and recent labs are all within normal limits. Which of the following is the most appropriate response?
    A. "This is typical behavior for someone with Down syndrome. How long have you been his caretaker?"
    B. "His lack of painting is likely a sign of depression. He can't do therapy so we should start an antidepressant."
    C. "This is likely the result of a urinary tract infection. We should take him to the hospital for further evaluation."
    D. "I'm concerned about this, but we need to perform cognitive testing before we can be certain of a cause."
    E. "I know this can be hard to hear, but what you're telling me suggests that your brother's condition will likely continue to get worse."

25. A 39 y/o M is brought to the hospital by ambulance after he collapsed at work. He was in the middle of cleaning out his desk after being fired from his job for repeatedly looking at pornography on his company computer. He did not appear to lose consciousness when he fell as his co-workers reported that his eyes remained open. However, he has not responded to any questions asked of him. He appears to be unable to walk and needs to be lifted by the paramedics into the ambulance. When interviewed by the emergency medicine physician, he still does not respond to questions asked of him. All vital signs are within normal limits. A complete physical exam reveals no abnormalities. He does not respond to requests to cooperate with a neurologic exam. A CT of the head is ordered and shows no evidence of pathology. A psychiatric consultation is ordered. The patient continues to not respond to questions, although he is noted to become tearful when the psychiatrist asks him, "What happened at work today?" Chart review reveals that he was admitted to the psychiatric hospital once five years ago for transient suicidal ideation that resolved within one day of admission. Which of the following is the most likely diagnosis at this time?
    A. Catatonia
    B. Selective mutism
    C. Hypochondriasis
    D. Conversion disorder
    E. Somatic symptom disorder
    F. Factitious disorder
    G. Malingering
    H. None of the above

26. (Continued from previous question.) The patient's wife arrives and asks to know more about this condition. Which of the following statements could be made?
    A. "This condition has a good prognosis, and he will likely be back to normal by the time he leaves the hospital."
    B. "It's not really up to us. He'll get better when he decides to get better."
    C. "Based on what we know, we are quite certain about his diagnosis."
    D. "Once he is discharged, he will likely need to see a neurologist for the rest of his life."
    E. None of the above

27. A 33 y/o F is seen by her psychiatrist for a yearly follow-up visit. She has a history of treatment-resistant depression that was treated with electroconvulsive therapy three years ago. Since then, she has been generally euthymic. At today's visit, however, she says that she is "not good." She reports that over the past month she has felt herself "slide back into the abyss" and has begun to feel hopeless about her future and believes that she will never find a full-time job or have a stable relationship. She works as a freelance journalist and has begun staying up until late at night to write more articles because "the more you write, the more likely you are to get picked up." She has also joined a dating website and has started to go on "a lot of dates, I try for one a day but last week I met three guys on a single day." In spite of these efforts, she has not yet found a steady job or a stable relationship, and she now feels like "it's probably pointless

to keep trying." She feels that she has "brought this on myself" and that she should have "gone to podiatry school like my parents wanted." She feels anxious and restless most of the day and reports only sleeping 2 or 3 hours most nights. She denies use of caffeine, alcohol, or other substances. Which of the following is the most likely diagnosis given her current symptoms?
- A. Major depressive disorder
- B. Bipolar disorder
- C. Schizoaffective disorder, depressive type
- D. Schizoaffective disorder, bipolar type
- E. Dysthymia
- F. Cyclothymia
- G. Borderline personality disorder
- H. None of the above

28. A 29 y/o F is brought to the psychiatrist's office by her sister. She has a history of schizophrenia beginning at age 25 resulting in two hospitalizations, the last being over one year ago. Her psychotic symptoms are currently well controlled on risperidone at night. However, her sister is concerned because she "appears depressed." Her sister reports that the patient used to love playing the violin but has stopped playing entirely in the past several years. On interview, the patient reports feeling lonely and isolated. She denies a history of major depressive episodes prior to the age of 25. She denies thoughts of hopelessness, guilt, or suicide. She sleeps several hours per night and eats three full meals per day. Her affect is dysthymic with a restricted range. What is the most likely diagnosis?
    - A. Schizophrenia
    - B. Schizoaffective disorder, depressive type
    - C. Major depressive disorder
    - D. Major depressive disorder with psychotic features
    - E. Both schizophrenia and major depressive disorder

29. A 24 y/o M who works in food delivery comes to the county clinic requesting an evaluation. He says that over the past year he has developed a distinct sensation that he cannot feel his own body. He reports feeling "hollow like a kick drum" on a daily basis and describes a sensation that "my skin is just covering a sack of meat." He describes being socially isolated due to intense anxiety regarding social encounters. When he does attempt to make contact with old friends, he feels "dead inside, even though I try to smile so that the other person doesn't feel all awkward and weird." This sensation tends to come and go over a period of weeks, but recently it has lasted for a month straight. The patient reports a history of childhood abuse at the age of 8 by his older stepbrother ("I think that's probably where I actually died, now this feeling is just confirmation"). He says, "I realize that these thoughts are strange, and that's why I'm here." He suffers from chronic feelings of depression and reports thoughts of suicide most days. He denies compulsive behaviors, auditory hallucinations, or feelings that others are out to harm him. Which of the following diagnoses best accounts for this patient's presentation?

A. Schizophrenia
B. Schizoaffective disorder
C. Social anxiety disorder
D. Primarily obsessional obsessive-compulsive disorder
E. Depersonalization-derealization disorder
F. Schizotypal personality disorder
G. Schizoid personality disorder
H. None of the above

30. A 28 y/o F comes to a psychiatrist's office for an evaluation. She reports a history of "depression and bipolar" going back for "as long as I can remember." After taking a thorough history, the psychiatrist diagnoses her with major depressive disorder, borderline personality disorder, opioid use disorder, social anxiety disorder, binge eating disorder, and post-traumatic stress disorder. Which of these conditions should be the initial focus of treatment?
    A. Major depressive disorder
    B. Borderline personality disorder
    C. Opioid use disorder
    D. Social anxiety disorder
    E. Post-traumatic stress disorder
    F. All of these conditions should be treated concurrently

31. A 29 y/o M is brought to the hospital by his sister after he stopped returning her phone calls for three days. When she arrived, she found him sitting motionless on the bed in a pool of dark yellow urine. The trash at his home was empty, and the refrigerator is completely empty except for moldy bread and a few pieces of rotten fruit. He normally works a full-time job. However, upon calling a co-worker, his sister finds out that the patient has not been seen at work for over one week. On interview, he is entirely mute and responds to questions by making small nods or shakes of the head. His affect is flat. The psychiatrist is unable to assess his mood, thought content, thought process, perception, insight, or judgment. When finishing the interview, the consulting psychiatrist offers to shake his hand. The patient raises his hand in response to the psychiatrist's offered hand but does not actually make contact with it. When the psychiatrist puts her hand down, the patient's hand remains in the air as seen below:

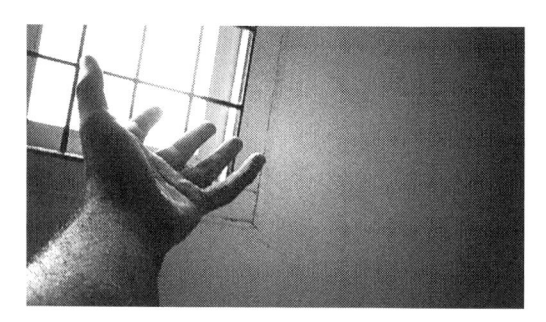

Which of the following is the most likely diagnosis?

A. Major depressive disorder
B. Bipolar disorder
C. Schizophrenia
D. Conversion disorder
E. Factitious disorder
F. Malingering
G. None of the above

32. A 50 y/o M is brought in to the psychiatrist's office by his wife after he was fired from his job as an accountant. He says that he has been "unjustly let go" and plans to hire a lawyer. When asked why he was fired, he says that he discovered that his boss was "bilking our customers" by transferring "black money" and engaging in tax evasion. His wife looks upset when he starts talking, saying, "This again! He never stops talking about this, and I'm sick of it!" She threatens to divorce him if he ever brings this up again, to which he responds, "I'm going to take those bastards down if it's the last thing I do." His wife throws her hands up and walks out of the room, saying, "There's something wrong with him. He's never been like this before. I can't take it anymore." When asked, the patient denies auditory hallucinations, visual hallucinations, or suicidal ideation. He describes his mood as "good," and he averages 7 hours of sleep per night. His thought process is linear and logical. Despite losing his job, he has been able to support himself, saying that he is a "big saver." However, he is planning on using up most of his savings to hire a lawyer. What is the most likely diagnosis?
    A. Schizophrenia
    B. Delusional disorder
    C. Paranoid personality disorder
    D. Depression with psychotic features
    E. Bipolar disorder with psychotic features
    F. None of the above

33. A 42 y/o F is playing basketball with a friend when she suddenly experiences a sensation that her heart is beating incredibly fast in her ears along with shortness of breath and dizziness. She feels incredibly scared that something bad is going to happen and tells her friend who drives her to the closest hospital. By the time they arrive in the hospital 15 minutes later, her symptoms have resolved, and she decides not to go in to avoid having to pay for the medical expenses. One year later, she experiences the same symptoms while having sex with her husband. This time the symptoms last over 30 minutes, so she calls an ambulance. Again the symptoms resolve by the time she reaches the emergency room, so no work-up is performed and she is immediately discharged with a referral to see her primary care provider. In the next few days, she experiences episodes of palpitations lasting no more than a few seconds each. They are so brief that she is unsure if she is merely imagining them. She experiences life as less enjoyable, as she is constantly worried about whether her palpitations will return. She avoids having sex or playing sports, and she is considering whether or not she feels that she can continue driving ("What if this happened while I was on the freeway?"). Which of the following is the most likely diagnosis?

A. Panic attacks
   B. Panic disorder
   C. Generalized anxiety disorder
   D. Somatic symptom disorder
   E. Hypochondriasis
   F. None of the above

34. (Continued from previous question.) Which of the following regions of the brain is most likely initially involved in recognizing the sensation of her heart beating rapidly in her ears?
   A. The insula
   B. The anterior cingulate cortex
   C. The orbitofrontal cortex
   D. The medial prefrontal cortex
   E. The hippocampus
   F. None of the above

35. A 74 y/o M is brought to see a psychiatrist by his wife for "delusions." The patient recently has begun to become more paranoid and has rejected food and water from his wife on several occasions, saying, "Don't try to poison me." Over the past week, he has been seen arguing with houseplants and empty tables. The patient's wife says that he seems to "come and go" mentally, as sometimes he seems completely confused and disoriented while at other times he is "the same old Jim." She denies any prior psychiatric history or substance use that she is aware of. He is diagnosed with late-onset schizophrenia and prescribed risperidone, an antipsychotic. At the follow-up visit one week later, the patient's wife says that he's "completely worse" and now "walks like a statue." His confusion has also become persistent rather than transient over the past week, and he has forgotten the names of people around him. One morning, his wife became scared that he had died in his sleep when it took several minutes to awaken him in the morning. The patient is oriented to person and place only. His MoCA score is 20/30. Which of the following is the best next step?
   A. Discontinue risperidone
   B. Continue risperidone at its current dose
   C. Increase the dose of risperidone
   D. Add a cholinesterase inhibitor
   E. None of the above

36. A 51 y/o M Army veteran makes an appointment to see a psychiatrist. On interview, he says that he is suffering from "bad, bad PTSD" from his time in the military and requests an evaluation to see if he is entitled to benefits as a result. Which of the following would be the best question to ask if the interviewer is concerned about malingering?
    A. "Tell me about what you are experiencing."
    B. "What was the nature of the traumatic event?"
    C. "Do you find yourself avoiding places that remind you of the trauma?"
    D. "Do you find yourself easily startled?"
    E. "Do you experience frequent nightmares?"
    F. "How long has this been going on?"

37. A 15 y/o M is brought to the hospital after he engaged in self-injurious behavior. On interview, he denies thoughts of suicide or any desire to die. Which of the following patterns of self-injurious behavior would be most consistent with a diagnosis of autism?
    A. Cutting his abdomen with a kitchen knife with the stated purpose of "destroying the evil within"
    B. Hitting himself in the head repeatedly and not giving a verbal response when asked why he is doing this
    C. Banging his head against a wall while repeatedly yelling "I'm stupid, I'm bad, I'm stupid, I'm bad" after hitting his sister during an argument
    D. Making repeated superficial cuts to his wrists after being told that he is "ugly and worthless" by an ex-girlfriend
    E. Using bleach to wash his hands after touching a bathroom door handle
    F. Injecting himself with a syringe containing water mixed with his own feces and then calling 911
    G. None of the above

38. A 56 y/o M is arrested while following a young girl on her way home from school. When he attempted to grab her by the arm on several occasions, she screamed. A neighbor heard her cry and called the police. When the police arrived, he opened his coat and exposed his naked body to them. When interviewed by the detective assigned to the case, the patient acknowledges that his actions were wrong but expresses no remorse for them. The patient's wife arrives. She reports that over the past year he has had multiple incidents, including being fired from his work as an office supplies salesman after he continued to take inventory home with him despite multiple reprimands. Since he has been home, she has noticed him eating out of the garbage can on several occasions. She denies any prior psychiatric history or interactions with the legal system. Which of the following regions of his brain is most likely to demonstrate pathology?
    A. The amygdala
    B. The temporal lobe
    C. The anterior cingulate cortex
    D. The endogenous opioid system
    E. The pituitary gland

39. A 59 y/o F makes an appointment with a therapist to address feelings of depression and loneliness. She reports a history of depression beginning in her teenage years but has not been in any form of treatment for over 20 years. She says that she regularly went to therapy in her 20s and 30s for "anger towards myself and my family." She has tried various medications for depression, none of which had any positive effects. While she says that she's not the "burning ball of rage" that she was in her youth, she is still "angry at my family for betraying me, at my friends for abandoning me, and at God for letting this all happen." Her depression is described as "this dull feeling, like I'm an empty shell of a person without a purpose." She denies changes in appetite or weight. She suffers from regular periods of insomnia but generally gets 6 or 7 hours of sleep per night. She has had three marriages, the longest of which lasted 3 years. She describes being in "constant pain" from a variety of medical symptoms for which she has not found a diagnosis. Her current list of specialists includes a rheumatologist and a gastroenterologist. Which of the following is true of this patient's condition?
    A. It is likely to respond to electroconvulsive therapy
    B. Psychotherapy is unlikely to help unless it is paired with medications
    C. Medication treatment should consist of more than one drug at a time
    D. Cognitive behavioral therapy is the most helpful form of therapy
    E. It has a high suicide rate

40. A 19 y/o M comes to see a psychiatrist requesting to be "put on antidepressants so I don't do anything bad." He tells the psychiatrist that since graduating from high school last year he has started to regularly see mental imagery of young girls. He finds this imagery incredibly disturbing and says, "It doesn't even make sense! I'm not attracted to children!" Recently he has begun hearing voices whispering, "Touch them!" when he sees a young girl. He also has begun only showering at the gym, as when he showers at home he constantly worries that there is a naked girl standing behind him. When told that this is impossible, he replies, "Well yes, *duh*, I know that. But it's still terrifying as hell." He has done extensive reading online about the dulling effects that antidepressants have on sex drive and says, "I need to start one right away at the highest dose. If I don't start one, I don't know what I would do. I've thought about killing myself. It would be better than molesting a child!" He denies spending time engaging in behavior related to these thoughts "unless if you count doing everything I can to not be anywhere near a school or daycare." Which of the following interventions is most likely to reduce his distress over the long-term?
    A. Prescribing a serotonin reuptake inhibitor
    B. Prescribing an antipsychotic
    C. Prescribing both a serotonin reuptake inhibitor and an antipsychotic
    D. Asking him to imagine being near young girls during a therapy session
    E. Asking him to look up pictures of young girls on the internet
    F. None of the above

41. A 16 y/o M comes with his mother to a family therapy session. He is slightly overweight for his age. His mother is concerned because he has started refusing to eat dinner for the past two weeks. When asked, he says, "I don't know, I'm not

hungry. And my stomach hurts a lot." His mother responds, "Maybe it's because of all that crap you're eating!" Turning to the therapist, she says, "Did I tell you he ate both tubs of ice cream I brought home for the school social? They weren't even in the house 24 hours and then I see them in the trash!" He yells, "Mom, shut up!" The therapist asks to speak with the patient and his mother separately. When speaking with the therapist alone, the mother says, "Recently I saw him sneaking into my bathroom and looking through my medicine cabinet. Now all my laxatives are missing." When interviewed alone, the patient denies self-induced vomiting. He says, "I told you. My stomach just hurts a lot so I don't want to eat." The therapist notices the following marks on the patient's right hand:

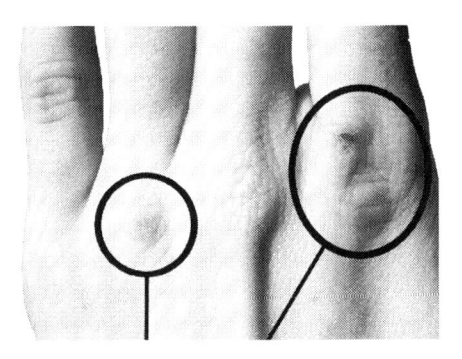

Which of the following is the most likely cause of his decreased food intake?
A. Oppositional defiant disorder
B. Bulimia nervosa
C. Binge eating disorder
D. Anorexia nervosa
E. Depression
F. Somatic symptom disorder
G. None of the above

42. A 40 y/o M is seen by his primary care doctor for an annual physical. He is found to be in good health with the exception of mildly elevated cholesterol levels. He is in a long-term relationship and has two children. He works as a salesman at a local sporting goods store. There is no history of legal trouble. During the interview, the doctor asks about substance use. He reports use of alcohol on a weekly basis when with friends and cocaine around 2 or 3 times per year. He denies a history of depression but reports difficulty falling asleep for an hour around once per week. Family history is positive for alcohol abuse in his father who died from liver failure in his 50s. Which of the following is the most likely diagnosis?
A. Major depressive disorder
B. A substance-induced mood disorder
C. Alcohol addiction
D. Cocaine addiction
E. Addiction to both alcohol and cocaine
F. Idiopathic (primary) insomnia
G. None of the above

43. (Continued from previous question.) One month later, the patient is brought to the hospital on a Saturday night by ambulance at around 2:00 in the morning. He was at a night club when a fire broke out and spread rapidly. He evacuated within several minutes, but after leaving the building he began coughing continuously and reporting shortness of breath, palpitations, and extreme dizziness. He stated, "I feel like I'm going to die" several times on the way to the hospital. Upon arriving at the hospital, he is very agitated and talks continuously. Laboratory tests show a positive urine toxicology screen for cocaine and an elevated blood alcohol level. Which of the following is the most likely diagnosis at this time?
    A. Alcohol and cocaine use disorders
    B. Post-traumatic stress disorder
    C. Acute stress disorder
    D. Substance-induced psychotic disorder
    E. Panic attack
    F. Panic disorder
    G. None of the above

44. A 35 y/o F makes an appointment with a psychiatrist. She was encouraged to seek treatment by her sister who recently started an antidepressant that "worked wonders" for her. The patient initially went to see her primary care provider for this prescription but was told that she was "not depressed" based on the results of a screening she did and that she would not be prescribed an antidepressant. When asked, the patient reports that her mood has been "incredibly low" for the past 3 months. She does not enjoy activities as she usually does and feels that "things will never get better." She spends most of her day thinking about past mistakes and wondering what she has done to bring this upon herself. She feels tired and has headaches most of the day, although she notes that she is sleeping 7 hours per night. She denies difficulty concentrating, changes in appetite, or thoughts of suicide. Her mental status exam is notable for a dysthymic affect with a restricted range and lack of prosody in her voice. No psychomotor retardation is noted. She denies use of alcohol or other substances. She reports a clear episodic pattern to her mood with multiple prior episodes of depression beginning in her early 20s which each last around 9 months. She denies major life stressors either now or with past episodes. She asks, "I'm really hoping to get started on something, as things have been bad for me recently." She is not interested in therapy at this time. Which of the following is the most appropriate response?
    A. "You definitely meet criteria for major depressive disorder. Let's talk about different treatment options."
    B. "Your primary care provider is right: you don't actually meet criteria for major depressive disorder, so there is no role for treatment right now."
    C. "You technically have adjustment disorder. I know you're not keen on therapy, but it's really the best treatment for what you have."
    D. "I'm worried that you have bipolar disorder, so antidepressants are more likely to harm than help in your case."
    E. "You have what is known as dysthymia. Let's start an antidepressant."
    F. None of the above

45. A 30 y/o M is brought to the hospital by his wife who reports that he has been "acting bizarrely" for the past week, including telling others that he is "covered in all-seeing eyes" and that he is being followed by "the eye holders" who want to capture and enslave him for his abilities. He has no prior psychiatric or medical history and works at an art gallery downtown. He reports that for the past year he has been smoking cannabis around 2 times per week "to enhance my artistic abilities." When using cannabis, he finds that colors are "brighter," and recently colors have started to "talk to me and tell me how they would like be used in a painting." During the interview, a nurse enters and tells the patient that he will need to change into a hospital gown. He immediately becomes furious and yells, "Shows don't wear clothes!" and begins pounding on the walls of the room. Security is called, and the patient is given an intramuscular antipsychotic. He is hospitalized for four weeks and then referred to a psychiatrist for long-term follow-up. Six months after his initial presentation, he has remained abstinent from cannabis. However, he continues to state that "the walls talk to me" and that he is being watched. Which of the following are the most accurate diagnoses at the time of admission and discharge, respectively?
    A. Brief psychotic disorder and schizophreniform disorder
    B. Cannabis use disorder and schizophrenia
    C. Substance-induced psychotic disorder and schizophrenia
    D. Substance-induced mood disorder and bipolar disorder
    E. Schizophrenia at both admission and discharge
    F. None of the above

46. A 28 y/o M is brought to the hospital after he attempted to rob a bank using a firearm. Security camera footage shows him repeatedly threatening a teller with the gun before accidentally dropping it, at which point the gun fires a bullet into his foot, as seen below:

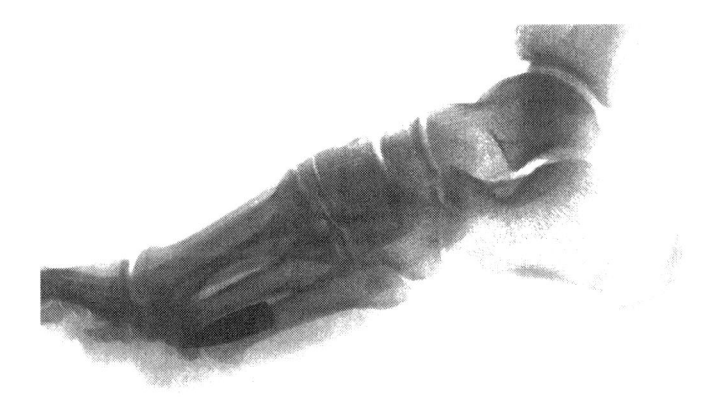

The patient is taken to the operating room for surgical repair. Upon awakening from anesthesia, he appears startled and attempts to find ways of leaving the hospital. However, police officers have been stationed outside of his room to

place him under arrest as soon as he is medically stabile. The on-call psychiatrist is asked to evaluate his condition and determine whether he needs psychiatric hospitalization. On interview, the patient expresses remorse for his actions but says that he "had no choice." He says that he needed to rob the bank to pay people who will "kill me without a second thought if I don't get them their money." However, he refuses to identify these individuals. The patient claims to have no prior medical, psychiatric, or criminal record which is confirmed both by the police outside and later by the patient's wife. His mental status exam is generally within normal limits with the exception of an anxious affect and an exaggerated startle response. His speech, thought content, thought process, perceptions, and cognition are otherwise intact. Which of the following is the most likely diagnosis?
    A. A psychotic disorder
    B. A psychopathic disorder
    C. An externalizing disorder
    D. An addictive disorder
    E. A neurodevelopmental disorder

47. A 20 y/o F is brought to the hospital by her college roommate saying that she is "acting completely crazy." The patient is incredibly hostile and attempts to bite the nurse bringing in her food tray. The on-call psychiatrist is consulted but is unable to interview the patient, as she is sedated from the intramuscular medications that were administered after the attempted attack. The psychiatrist instead speaks with the patient's roommate who has lived with her for the past two years. On interview, the roommate describes that she is "a totally different person" from time to time. She says further that the patient has "like three or four different personalities—sometimes she's super fun and outgoing, but other times she's really moody and hostile." She says that she has looked into switching roommates on multiple occasions, but due to a housing shortage on campus she has not been able to. Which of the following questions would best discriminate between dissociative identity disorder and bipolar disorder for this patient?
    A. "How long do each of these personalities last?"
    B. "Is she ever seemingly both happy and sad at the same time?"
    C. "Has she ever become so moody that she has attempted suicide?"
    D. "Do you know if your roommate drinks alcohol, smokes marijuana, or uses any other substances on a regular basis?"
    E. "Do you know what medications your roommate takes?"
    F. None of the above

48. An 81 y/o M is seen by his primary care provider. During the pre-visit assessment, the patient registers a high score on the PHQ-9, a depression screening tool. During the interview, the patient indicates that he has been drinking half a bottle of wine each night for the past 5 years. When asked, the patient indicates that he has felt depressed for several years. He denies a history of depression prior to the age of 75 but says that "after my wife died, it's like the floor fell out from under me." He is unaware of whether he began drinking before his mood symptoms appeared or if his mood worsened after he began drinking. The patient also

indicates that he has difficulty sleeping through the night and often wakes up feeling "very awake and anxious" around 3:00 in the morning. He is generally unable to return to sleep, leaving him feeling tired most of the next day. As part of routine screening for older adults, the primary care provider administers a screening test for dementia on which the patient scores below the cut-off for normal cognition. Which of the following is the best next step for management at this time?
- A. Prescribe a cholinesterase inhibitor to enhance memory
- B. Prescribe fluoxetine, an antidepressant that is highly energizing, to be taken in the morning
- C. Prescribe trazodone, an antidepressant that is highly sedating, to be taken at night
- D. Prescribe a benzodiazepine to help with sleep
- E. Prescribe naltrexone to reduce the pleasurable effects of drinking
- F. Refer to cognitive behavioral therapy for depression
- G. Refer to cognitive behavioral therapy for insomnia
- H. Refer to a substance rehabilitation program
- I. Assess the patient's readiness to change his pattern of drinking
- J. Instruct the patient that his driver's license will need to be revoked

49. (Continued from previous question.) The patient is very concerned after being told that his driver's license will be revoked, saying, "I can't survive without my car. How will I get around? I need to get my license back. I don't care about anything else. That's my highest priority." Which of the following is the next best step in management?
    - A. Prescribe a cholinesterase inhibitor to enhance memory
    - B. Prescribe fluoxetine, an antidepressant that is highly energizing, to be taken in the morning
    - C. Prescribe trazodone, an antidepressant that is highly sedating, to be taken at night
    - D. Prescribe a benzodiazepine to help with sleep
    - E. Prescribe naltrexone to reduce the pleasurable effects of drinking
    - F. Refer to cognitive behavioral therapy for depression
    - G. Refer to cognitive behavioral therapy for insomnia
    - H. Refer to a substance rehabilitation program
    - I. Assess the patient's readiness to change his pattern of drinking

50. A 31 y/o M makes an appointment with a psychiatrist but asks to be seen on the ground floor of the building rather than in the psychiatrist's usual office on the third story. On interview, the patient thanks the psychiatrist for meeting him on the ground floor, saying, "I don't do elevators." The patient denies a history of panic-like responses around elevators. Instead, he says, "I just don't trust things like that, you know? So many ways for things to go badly in an elevator." He reports similar fears of vehicles and cooking appliances. He is currently living in his parents' house as he has been unable to find a job, saying, "I want to do something meaningful with my life, but I'm pretty sure I'll screw it up if I'm actually given something important to do." He desires a romantic relationship as

well but is fearful that any girl is "only going to break my heart." He describes a constant sensation of being "on edge" and says that he has never been able to relax, even when on vacation or spending time with friends. He says that this is a big part of the reason that he feels socially isolated, as he was "always harassing my friends about whether we should buy plane tickets now or wait until they come down in price later or whether we should take that trip to San Francisco if a big earthquake is probably going to hit soon." Which of the following biological markers is most likely to show abnormalities in this patient?
- A. Levels of serotonin in the brain
- B. Metabolism of the frontal and temporal lobes
- C. Release of cortisol from the adrenal glands
- D. Reactivity of the amygdala to fear-inducing stimuli
- E. Resting signal-generating activity in the retinas
- F. Receptivity of the insula to afferent nerve signals

51. A 30 y/o M is brought to the police station after he was found attempting to break into the headquarters of the Central Intelligence Agency. He reports that he is being followed by North Korean spies and needs to enter the building to "gather splintelligence" so that he can fight back. He describes himself as "the only thing standing between this country and all-out nuclear war" and demands to be let go. He reports having "radio implants" in his ears that allow him to listen in on the North Korean spies who "constantly talk about me." He becomes incredibly irritable when told that he cannot leave, yelling, "You bastards don't get it! I'm the key! Just put me in the lock and you'll see!" He lacks identification of any kind, and he appears disheveled and unkempt. Which of the following features definitively rules *out* a diagnosis of bipolar disorder with psychotic features in this case?
    - A. His disheveled and unkempt appearance
    - B. His use of the word "splintelligence"
    - C. His rhyme between "key" and "see"
    - D. His belief that he is the only one who can save the world
    - E. His belief that he is being followed by spies
    - F. His irritability when he is blocked from his goals
    - G. His belief that he can listen in on North Korean spy communications
    - H. None of the above

52. A 66 y/o F is diagnosed with multiple myeloma after experiencing several months of bone pain in her spine and ribs. She is started on chemotherapy but still experiences significant pain, so her oncologist prescribes her oxycodone (an opioid). While this is initially effective at managing her pain, she now finds that she is "sneaking" additional doses throughout the day to achieve the same level of pain control. She often experiences a great deal of pain getting out of bed in the morning and will often take an additional pill within 5 minutes of waking up. She feels very guilty about this and has taken to hiding her prescriptions from her daughter who normally helps with her medical care. Her oncologist notices that she has been requesting early refills from the pharmacy and calls her in for an appointment. Which of the following is the best next step at this time?
    A. Increase the dose of oxycodone
    B. Maintain the same dose of oxycodone
    C. Decrease the dose of oxycodone
    D. Discontinue oxycodone
    E. Refer to an addiction medicine clinic
    F. More than one of the above

53. A 41 y/o M sees his psychiatrist for an evaluation. He has previously been diagnosed with depression and is taking both fluoxetine (an antidepressant) and clonazepam (a benzodiazepine) prescribed by his primary medical doctor. Given the risks of long-term benzodiazepine use, his psychiatrist discontinues clonazepam. At a follow-up appointment one month later, the patient reports persistent irritability, restlessness, insomnia, palpitations, and anxiety about most things for the past month. He denies recent stressors or an episodic pattern to his anxiety. Which of the following is the most likely diagnosis?
    A. Generalized anxiety disorder
    B. Panic disorder
    C. Social anxiety disorder
    D. Anxiety related to major depressive disorder
    E. None of the above

1. **The best answer is D.** This mother is likely suffering from postpartum psychosis as evidenced by her grandiose thought patterns and erratic behavior. Postpartum psychosis often begins during the first two weeks following delivery and is considered to be a psychiatric emergency warranting immediate hospitalization and treatment to protect both the mother and the child. Postpartum psychosis is not a normal reaction to childbirth (answer E), and while medications will likely be needed for treatment (answers A, B, and C), the immediate priority is to ensure that both the patient and the child are in a safe and monitored environment. *(Chapter 6—How to Diagnose Bipolar Disorders)*

2. **The best answer is H.** This boy is presenting with symptoms of inattention and hyperactivity that suggest a diagnosis of ADHD. However, it is very unusual for ADHD to present with sudden onset or with the loss of previously learned cognitive abilities like doing math (answers A, B, and C). Rett syndrome does present with a loss of developmental milestones but is diagnosed almost exclusively in girls (answer D). This patient has shown no behavior that is consistent with an externalizing disorder (answers E and F) or the deficits in social communication and restricted interests seen in autism (answer G). Therefore, the best answer is none of the above. *(Chapter 21—ADHD Across the Lifespan)*

3. **The best answer is D.** The presence of seizures, hyponatremia, white matter changes on MRI, and hyperpigmentation of the oral mucosa are highly suggestive of adrenoleukodystrophy, a condition that can sometimes be mistaken for ADHD due to the presence of similar clinical features. Adrenoleukodystrophy is a highly variable condition, with some people being completely asymptomatic and others having very severe symptoms. It is an X-linked genetic disorder that is more common in males (answer B). It is treatable, though not curable (answer A). Unlike ADHD, it does not respond to stimulants (answer E). Asperger's syndrome was used to describe high-functioning cases of autism (answer C). *(Chapter 19—Intellectual Disability)*

4. **The best answer is F.** While this patient shows some signs of depression (including sleep changes, fatigue, poor concentration, and possibly psychomotor slowing), it is notable that all of these symptoms are consistent with the effects of sleep deprivation. In addition, the two most sensitive symptoms of depression (depressed mood and anhedonia) are both absent. For this reason, a diagnosis of either unipolar or bipolar depression is unlikely (answers A and B). While dysthymia can similarly present with subsyndromal depressive symptoms, the lack of cognitive features such as hopelessness or low self-esteem both argue against this disorder (answer C). Adjustment disorder could be a reasonable diagnosis, but there is no major recent change or stressor (answer D). Generalized anxiety disorder can similarly present with difficulty sleeping, but there should be evidence of excessive worrying in multiple areas of life (answer E). In the absence of any other information, a primary sleep disorder such as idiopathic insomnia could be entertained, although other causes of poor sleep such as obstructive sleep apnea should be ruled out as well. *(Chapter 23—Insomnia)*

Memorable Psychiatry

5. **The best answer is C.** Trichotillomania is considered to be a compulsive behavior that is similar to obsessive-compulsive disorder in nature. In contrast, the other behaviors listed are generally more impulsive in nature, including binge eating (answer A), self-injurious behavior (answer B), addiction (answer D), and externalization (answer E), which would all be more common in someone with high impulsivity. *(Chapter 10—How to Diagnose Obsessive-Compulsive Disorders)*

6. **The best answer is B.** This patient shows signs of having unusual beliefs and makes odd associations between thoughts and ideas. However, he does not show signs of psychosis as evidenced by a lack of delusions, auditory hallucinations, and disorganized behavior or speech which together argue against a diagnosis of schizophrenia at this time (answer A). The most likely diagnosis is schizotypal personality disorder which is considered to be on a similar spectrum to schizophrenia, as people with the disorder are at higher risk of developing it (answer C). The presence of these unusual beliefs as well as a desire for social companionship both argue against schizoid personality disorder (answer D). While there is an element of paranoia to some of what he says, someone with paranoid personality disorder would likely be more mistrustful and wouldn't have the same degree of odd beliefs present (answer E). Finally, it is worth considering whether the patient has a disorder at all as he appears generally satisfied with his life; however, the fact that he has been fired from jobs and appears to not be living up to his potential due to his beliefs argues against complete normalcy (answer F). *(Chapter 14—Cluster A Personality Disorders)*

7. **The best answer is I.** Anorexia nervosa has the highest mortality rate of any single psychiatric condition at 20%. *(Chapter 18—Anorexia Nervosa)*

8. **The best answer is B.** There are many signs that point to malingering in this case, including a presentation that does not match known causes of memory loss, reported deficits that are severely out of proportion to what is normally seen in similar cases, the possibility of financial gain from having a more severe illness, and resistance to considering other consequences of having the disorder such as one's license being taken away. However, even in cases where there is a high degree of suspicion for malingering, it remains a diagnosis of exclusion. Therefore, it would be inappropriate to respond as if the patient were definitively malingering until a complete work-up had been completed (answers D and E). However, ordering a CT scan is likely unnecessary at this time and risks exposing the patient to unnecessary ionizing radiation (remember to "Do no harm") (answer C). Finally, diagnosing a neurocognitive disorder should not be done until there is additional evidence of a primary neurologic cause, especially with such a high chance of malingering in this case (answer A). *(Chapter 13—How to Diagnose Somatoform Disorders, Chapter 22—Differential Diagnosis of Dementia)*

9. **The best answer is E.** This case describes a typical presentation of psychotic symptoms in a patient with borderline personality disorder as evidenced by the presence of affective instability, hostility, chronic dysphoria (rather than episodic depression), somatoform complaints, and dysfunction beginning in adolescence.

There is possibly an element of factitious disorder as well, as the patient may be fabricating psychotic symptoms to appear more ill and therefore warrant hospitalization. Cases of borderline personality disorder are more common in people with a history of abuse. While she would be unusually young to develop schizophrenia, the phenomenology of her auditory hallucinations is inconsistent with primary psychosis (answer A). Schizoaffective disorder is a rare diagnosis that bridges psychotic and mood disorders, but it is unlikely to be the diagnosis here (answer B). Depression with psychotic features responds well to a combination of antidepressants and antipsychotics, but the non-episodic pattern of her mood symptoms argues against this diagnosis (answer C). Finally, while some degree of dysfunction related to borderline personality disorder is likely to persist across the lifespan, it is generally considered to have a good prognosis after early adulthood with a gradual lessening of symptoms (answer D). *(Chapter 7—Differential Diagnosis of Psychotic Disorders, Chapter 15—Differential Diagnosis of Borderline Personality)*

10. **The best answer is C.** This vignette describes a case of acetaminophen poisoning in a patient with suicidal ideation. Acetaminophen is often used for intentional overdoses due to its easy availability as an over-the-counter drug. Cases of acetaminophen poisoning are not always immediately obvious, as signs and symptoms are often not seen for up to 72 hours after ingestion. That is why it is essential to have a high index of suspicion for occult overdoses in patients presenting with suicidal ideation. It is tempting to think that alcohol withdrawal could account for his symptoms, especially considering that alcohol can cause liver damage and a withdrawal state that begins in the same time period (24 to 72 hours after ingestion). However, it is rare for alcohol withdrawal to cause fulminant hepatic failure, especially in a young patient (answer B). Being seen by the physician within one hour of arriving at the hospital would not have made a difference here as the physician did not screen for this (answer A), although having seen a different physician may have. Adequate hydration is unrelated to treatment for acetaminophen overdose (answer D). *(Chapter 4—Suicide)*

11. **The best answer is E.** For major medical and surgical interventions like a liver transplantation, a capacity evaluation is warranted. However, it is clear from the vignette that this patient is not able to meaningfully communicate, so it is already impossible to determine his level of capacity (answer A). In cases where a patient lacks capacity, the next step is to locate a surrogate decision maker, which in this case would likely be the parents. However, the parents should be asked to make a decision as the *patient* would have, not based on their own belief systems (answer B). Determining the psychiatric diagnosis is not a priority in an emergent situation like this (answer C). A liver transplantation is often required for survival, and canceling it on the basis of the patient lacking capacity would be grossly unethical (answer D). *(Chapter 4—Delirium)*

12. **The best answer is G.** This patient is experiencing a panic attack in response to a specific stimulus. However, a single panic attack is insufficient for a diagnosis of panic disorder, as panic disorder involves sudden, unexpected, repeated panic

attacks that give rise to dysfunction in one's life (answer D). It is more likely that this girl has a specific phobia of needles. She would not be diagnosed with a traumatic disorder as the stimulus was not a life-threatening or extremely violent event (answers A or B). While she experienced distinct sensations of both depersonalization and derealization, the fact that these have only occurred in the setting of a panic attack rules out depersonalization-derealization disorder, as the dissociative symptoms must be severe and persistent (answer F). There is no evidence of either obsessions or compulsions (answer C), nor is there evidence of amnesia at this time (answer E). *(Chapter 9—How to Diagnose Anxiety Disorders, Chapter 12—How to Diagnose Dissociative Disorders)*

13. **The best answer is A.** This patient has many features consistent with a diagnosis of atypical depression, including the presence of depressed mood with preserved mood reactivity, high interpersonal rejection sensitivity, hypersomnia, and hyperphagia. She is also in her early 30s which is around the average age of onset for episodic depression. Therefore, the best treatment at this time would be an antidepressant and/or psychotherapy. A stimulant would likely only help with symptoms rather than treating the underlying cause (answer E). While atypical depression has many features that overlap with borderline personality disorder, the later age of onset and lack of other features of the disorder argue against that diagnosis (answer B). The interpersonal rejection sensitivity seen in atypical depression can also resemble social anxiety, but the presence of additional features such as hyperphagia and hypersomnia are unaccounted for by a diagnosis of only social anxiety disorder (answer C). Finally, bulimia is ruled out by the lack of binge eating episodes which are a prerequisite for this diagnosis (answer D). *(Chapter 5—How to Diagnose Depressive Disorders)*

14. **The best answer is A.** This is a case of probable child abuse as evidenced by the appearance of bruising in an unexposed area that is unlikely to be injured on accident as well as the father's denial and inconsistent responses. The effect of trauma on children is different compared to adults, with children under the age of 10 being very unlikely to develop the same signs and symptoms of PTSD that are seen in adults (answer B). Instead, the most common immediate response to childhood trauma is an internalizing disorder such as social anxiety disorder. The fact that anxiety disorders generally begin during childhood and are the single most common form of psychiatric condition (giving them a high base rate in the general population) also argue for social anxiety disorder being the most likely diagnosis (although it's important to keep in mind that it is very possible that, despite her exposure to abuse, she has not developed any form of psychiatric pathology). Externalizing disorders are associated with neglect more than abuse and are more common in boys than girls (answer C). Borderline personality disorder and dissociative identity disorder are both associated with a history of trauma as a child. However, these disorders do not tend to develop until adolescence or young adulthood, making them unlikely to be present at this time (answers D and E). *(Chapter 11—PTSD Across The Lifespan)*

15. **The best answer is E.** The symptoms described in this case, including muscle tension, restlessness, fatigue, insomnia, and inattention, are consistent with overactivation of the HPA axis which is commonly seen in people who have experienced childhood abuse. Abnormalities of the HPA axis are seen in a variety of psychiatric disorders, all of which this patient is at increased risk for including generalized anxiety disorder (answer A), depression (answer B), dysthymia (answer C), and nightmare disorder (answer D). In contrast, histrionic personality disorder does not have this same association with an abnormal HPA axis and is notably the only cluster B personality disorder that does not have an association with a history of abuse. *(Chapter 9—Signs and Symptoms of Anxiety, Chapter 14—Cluster B Personality Disorders)*

16. **The best answer is E.** This case describes a patient with classic symptoms of mania including increased goal-directed activity, distractibility, impulsivity, grandiosity, and talkativeness. In addition, a previous suicide attempt suggests a history of depression which is commonly seen in people with bipolar I disorder. This case is complicated by the presence of substance abuse, and it is possible that his initial presenting symptoms were at least partially related to substance use. However, the persistence of these symptoms long after the effects of these drugs would have worn off argues against substance use disorders being a primary (rather than secondary) cause of his condition (answer F). While there are narcissistic elements to his goals, it is unclear that these would persist in the absence of this mood episode, so narcissistic personality disorder should not be diagnosed at this time (answer A). While there is a high degree of recklessness to his behavior that could endanger others, this does not appear to be his primary goal; in combination with a lack of previous violent crimes, this argues against antisocial personality disorder (answers B and C). Hyperactivity must be demonstrated outside of a current mood episode for a diagnosis of ADHD (answer G). Finally, while he has grandiose delusions and some degree of disorganized behavior, he lacks other symptoms of a primary psychotic disorder like schizophrenia (answer D). *(Chapter 6—Differential Diagnosis of Bipolar Disorders, Chapter 8—Differential Diagnosis of Addictive Disorders)*

17. **The best answer is D.** This describes a case of Prader-Willi syndrome, a genetic condition characterized by an insatiable sense of hunger that leads to excessive food intake. In severe cases, this behavior can directly lead to gastric rupture and necrosis, as occurred here. Prader-Willi syndrome is caused by the deletion of a normally active paternal allele. Angelman syndrome is caused by a similar deletion of a *maternal* allele but presents with completely different symptoms (answer E). The early onset of symptoms and the co-occurrence of receptive and expressive language deficits both argue against binge eating disorder or bulimia, and it is rare for binges related to an eating disorder to be so excessive that they cause gastric perforation (answers A and B). Neither Down syndrome nor William syndrome are related to excessive food intake (answers C and F). *(Chapter 19—Intellectual Disability)*

18. **The best answer is A.** This describes a case of dependent personality disorder as evidenced by her extremely deferential nature towards her husband in multiple areas of life which directly results in distress and dysfunction. Dependent personality disorder involves an extreme and inflexible level of agreeableness, which is a core personality trait that may not change over time (answer B) even with use of medications or psychotherapy (answers C and D). There is no evidence that dependent personality disorder is related to dysregulation of the sympathetic nervous system (answer E). *(Chapter 14—Cluster C Personality Disorders)*

19. **The best answer is G.** This patient presents with several changes in personality, cognition, and level of functioning that are immediately concerning for some form of dementia. However, the presence of specific neurologic findings including an abnormal gait, a flat affect (the highly characteristic "mask-like" face), absent prosody, and a unilateral resting tremor all strongly suggest Parkinson's disease over and above other causes of dementia (answers A through F and H). *(Chapter 22—Differential Diagnosis of Dementia)*

20. **The best answer is C.** Rigid behaviors can be seen in a variety of psychiatric conditions, including OCD, obsessive-compulsive personality disorder, autism, and anorexia. In this case, the patient's rigid behavior involves limited food preferences occurring in the context of restricted interests in microbiology and bacteria. There is also evidence of poor language structure, minimal eye contact, and abnormal social interactions with the pediatrician, all of which together argue for a diagnosis of autism. While it would be unusual for OCD to start so young, it is not unheard of. However, the patient does not report any obsessional thoughts that directly lead to his behaviors which makes OCD less likely (although his verbal deficits it is hard to say with certainty). In addition, the belief appears to be ego-syntonic rather than ego-dystonic (answer A). Obsessive-compulsive personality disorder would result in rigid behaviors done because it is more moral or ethically correct (answer B). There is no evidence that the patient is avoiding food due to a distorted body image, and his caloric intake appears to remain the same (answer E). Finally, there is no evidence of intellectual disability, as the patient's deficient grammar is more likely explained by a diagnosis of autism (answer D). *(Chapter 20—Signs and Symptoms of Autism)*

21. **The best answer is G.** This patient is presenting with externalizing behaviors and psychotic symptoms that have begun in the past 3 days. While this sudden onset is itself unusual, there are a variety of signs and symptoms that are highly concerning for a medical etiology of her condition, including a recent flu-like illness, the presence of tardive dyskinesia in a patient who has no prior psychiatric history, and signs of autonomic dysfunction including sweating and urinating on herself. This combination is highly suggestive of anti-NMDA receptor encephalitis, a condition that can strongly mimic cases of primary psychosis. In some cases, the condition is associated with ovarian teratomas in which case surgical removal of the tumor will result in rapid improvement of symptoms. While it is not yet certain that she has an ovarian teratoma, compared to the

other treatment options (all of which have virtually zero chance of working) surgical intervention is the *most* likely to result in a change in her behavior even if we cannot yet say that it will definitively do so. Remember to consider anti-NMDA receptor encephalitis when a young patient presents with sudden onset of psychotic symptoms with no prior psychiatric history, especially when features of autonomic or neurologic dysfunction are present. *(Chapter 7—Differential Diagnosis of Psychotic Disorders)*

22. **The best answer is F.** A substance history, physical exam, and review of systems should be part of every psychiatric evaluation (answers A, C, and D). A substance history in particular can elucidate patterns of caffeine and/or alcohol intake that could be interfering with a normal sleep schedule. Vital signs are not required for every psychiatric evaluation. However, in the context of someone with an eating disorder and possible obstructive sleep apnea, they can help to diagnose comorbid conditions (such as hypertension) that may be related to the problem (answer E). A sleep study is not required at every psychiatric evaluation, but for someone who is obese, male, and complains of feeling tired all the time, the clinical suspicion is high enough to warrant one (answer B). *(Chapter 3—The Psychiatric Interview, Chapter 23—Insomnia)*

23. **The best answer is D.** Parasomnias (including "sleep-eating") are a known side effect of Z-drugs like zolpidem, and the emergence of this behavior soon after starting this medication strongly argues for a substance-induced parasomnia. While most parasomnias are idiopathic, the timing argues against that in this case (answer C). It is possible that the patient has experienced a recurrence of binge eating disorder, but in the context of the behavior only happening at night this is less likely (answers A and B). *(Chapter 23—Other Sleep Disorders)*

24. **The best answer is E.** It can be difficult to detect cases of dementia in someone with an existing intellectual disability due to the presence of cognitive deficits at baseline. However, it can usually be detected based on reports of changes in personality and ability to do things that one normally could (in this case, things like recognizing his sister or painting pictures). Over half of people with Down syndrome will develop Alzheimer's disease during their lifetime. As with all cases of Alzheimer's disease, the onset of the disorder portends a poor prognosis. While not engaging in one's usual hobbies can be a sign of depression, in the context of other signs such as urinary incontinence it is less likely (answer B). An infection could account for the incontinence, but it is unlikely to have persisted for several months without other signs of infection (answer C). Cognitive testing is helpful for diagnosing cases of dementia in an otherwise healthy population, but for someone with an intellectual disability it is unlikely to be revealing (answer D). Finally, dismissing a caregiver's observations is completely unwarranted and risks ignoring the most important source of information available (answer A). *(Chapter 19—Intellectual Disability, Chapter 22—Alzheimer's Disease Across the Lifespan)*

25. **The best answer is D.** This patient is showing signs of multiple neurologic deficits (including mutism and bilateral extremity weakness) following a major psychosocial stressor, which is strongly suggestive of conversion disorder. In addition, thus far all objective tests of neurologic disease are negative, further supporting the diagnosis. The patient's mutism could be related to catatonia, but in the absence of other signs such as muscular rigidity, waxy flexibility, or negativism, this is less likely (answer A). Selective mutism is an extreme variant of social anxiety disorder and is typically chronic rather than sudden onset (answer B). Both hypochondriasis and somatic symptom disorder present with concern about *symptoms* rather than neurologic *signs* (answers C and E). Finally, there is no evidence that the patient is intentionally fabricating these deficits as would be seen in factitious disorder and malingering, although these cannot be ruled out for sure (answers F and G). *(Chapter 13—How to Diagnose Somatoform Disorders)*

26. **The best answer is A.** Conversion disorder is a diagnosis with a relatively good prognosis, with most patients showing resolution of their neurologic deficits by the time of discharge (although a quarter will have a recurrence within one year). However, because conversion disorder is a diagnosis of exclusion, it should never be given to anyone with absolute certainty, as a medical or neurologic cause is eventually found in up to a third of all cases (answer C). Long-term care will likely involve a psychiatrist, not a neurologist (answer D). Finally, it is inappropriate to assume that the patient is fabricating his condition or to imply that to others (answer B). *(Chapter 13—How to Diagnose Somatoform Disorders)*

27. **The best answer is B.** This patient is experiencing a mixed state. While she endorses depressive symptoms including guilt, hopelessness, and depressed mood, she also reports symptoms of mania including increased goal-directed activity and a lack of need for sleep. This combination of both depressive and manic symptoms simultaneously should be re-diagnosed as bipolar disorder rather than continuing her previous diagnosis of unipolar depression (answer A). There is no evidence of psychotic symptoms, ruling out schizoaffective disorder (answers C and D). A mixed state is a very high-risk time and rules out subsyndromal disorders such as dysthymia and cyclothymia (answers E and F). Finally, there is no evidence of affective lability or a strong interpersonal aspect to her current presentation, arguing against borderline personality disorder (answer G). *(Chapter 6—How to Diagnose Bipolar Disorders)*

28. **The best answer is A.** While this patient reports depressive symptoms including anhedonia, all of them overlap with the standard symptoms of schizophrenia, making a separate diagnosis of major depressive disorder (with or without psychotic features) unnecessary (answers C, D, and E). There is no history of depressive symptoms prior to the onset of schizophrenia, making the depressive type of schizoaffective disorder an unlikely diagnosis (answer B). *(Chapter 7—Differential Diagnosis of Psychotic Disorders)*

29. **The best answer is E.** This patient is describing chronic and severe feelings of depersonalization which along with a history of trauma best fit a diagnosis of

Jonathan Heldt

depersonalization-derealization disorder. While the patient's reported beliefs may sound odd to most people, they are notably ego-dystonic as he recognizes that they sound strange, which argues against a diagnosis of a primary psychotic disorder (answers A and B) or schizotypal personality disorder (answer F). A recurrent ego-dystonic belief brings to mind OCD, although there is no pattern of overactive error recognition to his beliefs (answer D). While the patient reports some degree of social anxiety, his symptoms are pronounced enough that they extend far beyond "just" social anxiety disorder (answer C). While the patient avoids others, he appears to desire companionship on some level as evidenced by the fact that he continues to reach out to old friends (answer G). *(Chapter 12—How to Diagnose Dissociative Disorders)*

30. **The best answer is C.** People with borderline personality disorder often have multiple psychiatric comorbidities. This makes prioritizing an essential part of treatment for these patients as it is generally not possible to meaningfully engage in treatment for all of these disorders at the same time (answer F). As a general rule of thumb, treatment of borderline personality disorder should take priority over other conditions such as depression, anxiety disorders, and PTSD (answers A, D, and E), as leaving borderline personality disorder unaddressed tends to worsen treatment outcomes for the other disorders. The primary exceptions to this are active substance use, severe mania, and a severe eating disorder all of which either represent a more immediate threat to health or would interfere with their ability to be treated for their other disorders (answer B). Out of these, this patient only has a current opioid use disorder, so this should be addressed first. *(Chapter 15—Borderline Personality Across the Lifespan)*

31. **The best answer is B.** This patient is exhibiting classic signs of catatonia including mutism, echopraxia, and catalepsy. While no additional history is available, in any given population bipolar disorder is the most common cause of catatonia and accounts for over half of all cases, with depression and schizophrenia accounting for a third and 15%, respectively (answers A and C). While there are some neurologic deficits observed including mutism, it is not clear that the patient is suffering from conversion disorder, and the presence of signs specific to catatonia argues for this as the better explanation (answer D). Both factitious disorder and malingering are diagnoses of exclusion and should not be diagnosed in the presence of clear signs of another disorder (answers E and F). *(Chapter 4—Catatonia)*

32. **The best answer is F.** This patient lacks evidence of significant pathology on mental status exam. The lack of auditory hallucinations or disorganized thought process makes schizophrenia unlikely (answer A), while his intact mood and sleep patterns argue against a diagnosis of a mood disorder (answers D and E). His wife's comment that "he has never been like this before" strongly suggest against a diagnosis of paranoid personality disorder which is characterized by a life-long pattern of paranoia resulting in dysfunction (answer C). This leaves delusional disorder (answer B) as the most likely diagnosis. However, while the patient is experiencing occupational dysfunction as a result of his belief, it is not clear that

his belief is a delusion, as it is notably non-bizarre and cannot be assumed to be false. In fact, there have been cases similar to this where whistleblowers have been accused of being psychiatrically ill when attempting to call attention to unfair practices. While it is certainly possible that this patient's beliefs are false, there is insufficient evidence to diagnose a delusional disorder at this time. *(Chapter 7—How to Diagnose Psychotic Disorders)*

33. **The best answer is F.** This vignette describes a case of an arrhythmia (in this case, supraventricular tachycardia) whose symptoms strongly resemble those of a panic attack. It is notable that at no point in this vignette does the patient receive a medical work-up for her symptoms. If she had, her doctors may have discovered specific abnormalities on electrocardiogram that would have alerted them to the presence of an arrhythmia. This reinforces the fact that panic attacks are a diagnosis of exclusion, as a medical cause for the symptoms must be ruled out (answers A and B). The patient's symptoms of anxiety are episodic rather than persistent, ruling out generalized anxiety disorder (answer C). While she shows concern about her symptoms, this is a normal and reasonable response to her experiences (answers D and E). *(Chapter 9—Differential Diagnosis of Anxiety Disorders)*

34. **The best answer is A.** Palpitations, or the sense that one can hear their own heartbeat, is a form of interoception which is largely processed in the insula. While hyperactive signaling in the insula is believed to underlie psychiatric disorders related to somatization, interoception is ultimately a helpful function (in this case, it has allowed this person to recognize that there is a problem and seek medical help). The anterior cingulate cortex is involved in *interpreting* an interoceptive signal as representing an error, not in *recognizing* it initially (answer B). The orbitofrontal cortex is most implicated in mood disorders while the medial prefrontal cortex and hippocampus are implicated in PTSD (answers C, D, and E). *(Chapter 13—Mechanisms of Somatization)*

35. **The best answer is A.** This patient is most likely suffering from dementia with Lewy bodies as evidenced by the fluctuating pattern of his cognitive impairments, his sensitivity to antipsychotic medications, and his likely visual hallucinations as he has been observed talking to unseen objects. Antipsychotics should generally be avoided for people with dementia with Lewy bodies, so continuing or increasing the dose of risperidone would not be appropriate (answers B and C). Simply adding a cholinesterase inhibitor without stopping risperidone would also not resolve the problem (answer D). *(Chapter 22—How to Diagnose Dementia)*

36. **The best answer is A.** When concerned about malingering, the best approach is to use open-ended questions whenever possible. Asking questions about specific symptoms may inadvertently provide information on what symptoms are most salient to the interviewer (answers B, C, D, and E). Asking about the duration of symptoms does not necessarily do this, but in general closed-ended questions are less preferable than open-ended ones (answer F). *(Chapter 3—The Psychiatric Interview, Chapter 11—Differential Diagnosis of Trauma-Related Disorders)*

37. **The best answer is B.** While non-suicidal self-injurious behavior is most often associated with borderline personality disorder, it is found across many different psychiatric conditions and is not specific to any one disorder. People with autism or intellectual disabilities will often engage in self-injurious behavior without a discernable purpose, especially in cases where the patient is non-verbal. Cutting one's abdomen in response to a bizarre delusion is more consistent with schizophrenia (answer A), punishing one's self after impulsive misbehavior is more consistent with an externalizing disorder (answer C), making superficial cuts after an interpersonal rejection is more consistent with borderline personality disorder (answer D), using bleach to calm a contamination obsession is more consistent with OCD (answer E), and intentionally inducing an illness is more consistent with factitious disorder (answer F). *(Chapter 20—Signs and Symptoms of Autism)*

38. **The best answer is B.** This patient has likely developed frontotemporal dementia as evidenced by his disinhibited sexual behavior, change in eating habits, and poor impulse control. The onset of symptoms in his late 50s is also highly suggestive of this disease. As the name implies, frontotemporal dementia is associated with hypometabolism in both the frontal and temporal lobes of the brain. Abnormal emotional processing in the amygdala is associated with psychopathic traits. However, despite his recent remorseless antisocial behavior, the lack of any prior history strongly argues against this diagnosis (answer A). The anterior cingulate cortex is involved in processing error recognition in OCD and somatization and would not be expected to be involved here (answer C). The endogenous opioid system is likely dysregulated in borderline personality disorder and other cluster B disorders, not frontotemporal dementia (answer D). Finally, the pituitary gland is part of the HPA axis which is implicated in a variety of internalizing disorders; it is also unlikely to be involved in this case (answer E). *(Chapter 22—How to Diagnose Dementia)*

39. **The best answer is E.** This vignette describes a case of borderline personality disorder in an older adult as evidenced by the presence of chronic dysphoria, persistent anger, relationship dysfunction, likely somatization, and a poor sense of identity. While she denies the dramatic symptoms of borderline personality disorder such as self-harm, impulsivity, and psychosis-like symptoms, this is consistent with the idea that these symptoms often remit with age while these other symptoms tend to remain. Borderline personality disorder is associated with a high suicide rate on par with mood disorders like depression and bipolar disorder. While ECT is an effective treatment for treatment-refractory depression, there is no evidence that it is helpful for chronic dysphoria related to borderline personality disorder (answer A). Medications should play a limited role in treating borderline personality disorder due to a lack of efficacy (answers B and C). There is little evidence supporting the use of CBT in borderline personality disorder (answer D). Instead, other forms of therapy such as dialectical behavior therapy and mentalization-based treatment have the most evidence. *(Chapter 15—Borderline Personality Across the Lifespan)*

40. **The best answer is D.** This vignette describes a case of OCD as evidenced by this patient's recurrent, distressing, and intrusive ego-dystonic thoughts about wanting to molest young girls. Exposure and response prevention is the gold standard of treatment. In cases like this where exposure to the feared stimulus is immoral or illegal, asking the patient to imagine scenarios during therapy allows them to be exposed to situations that cannot be experienced through traditional exposure and response prevention. While antidepressants are also effective at treating OCD, they are less effective than exposure and response prevention, so they should not be the first-line treatment if only one can be pursued (answer A). Despite the presence of psychotic-sounding symptoms including auditory hallucinations, these thoughts are notably ego-dystonic and are recognized as coming from within the patient's own mind, making them more consistent with OCD than with any kind of psychotic disorder that would warrant use of an antipsychotic (answers B and C). Asking the patient to do an illegal and immoral activity is not appropriate (answer E). *(Chapter 10—OCD Across the Lifespan)*

41. **The best answer is B.** This patient's food intake appears to follow the pattern of bulimia, including binge eating episodes and purging with the use of laxatives. While bulimia is uncommon in males, it is not unheard of. It is likely that he is self-inducing vomiting as well given the lacerations on his knuckles which can be caused by the skin brushing against the teeth when activating the gag reflex (sometimes known as Russell's sign). If the patient were not engaging in purging efforts, he would instead likely be diagnosed with binge eating disorder (answer C). As he is overweight, it is impossible to determine whether he suffers from anorexia which relies upon the presence of a distorted body image (answer D). While it is possible that the patient's stomach pain is related to either a somatoform disorder (answer F) or a medical condition (answer G), the presence of both bingeing and purging behaviors provides a better explanation. If the pain persists after these behaviors have stopped, then these disorders should be considered. While decreased food intake can often be seen in depression, there is not enough additional evidence of this disorder for it to be diagnosed (answer E). Finally, arguing with one's parents as a teenager is not evidence of oppositional defiant disorder (answer A). *(Chapter 18—Bulimia Nervosa)*

42. **The best answer is G.** Based on the vignette, there is no evidence of psychiatric pathology in this patient. While he admits to use of alcohol, this appears to be culturally normal (answers C and E). While cocaine use is illegal, he does not appear to have suffered significant personal consequences as a result of use, and having negative repercussions is a required component for diagnosing addiction (answer D). He denies depression or any mood symptoms (answers A and B). Finally, while he reports difficulty sleeping once per week, this is also common in the general population and should not be diagnosed as pathological (answer F). *(Chapter 2—Normal Versus Abnormal, Chapter 8—Signs and Symptoms of Addiction, Chapter 23—Insomnia)*

43. **The best answer is G.** As before, there is no evidence of psychiatric pathology in this case, as the patient's reaction to a life-threatening situation is completely within the realm of normalcy, ruling out both acute stress disorder and PTSD (answers B and C). While he reports symptoms consistent with a panic attack, these same symptoms could also be accounted for by smoke inhalation (answers E and F). While he was using substances at the time of the incident, they do not appear to have directly resulted in negative repercussions, as he would have been exposed to this event whether he was using substances or not (answer A). Finally, there is no evidence of psychotic symptoms at this time (answer D). *(Chapter 2—Normal Versus Abnormal, Chapter 8—Signs and Symptoms of Addiction, Chapter 11—Differential Diagnosis of Trauma-Related Disorders)*

44. **The best answer is A.** This case illustrates the pitfalls of relying too strictly on diagnostic criteria when approaching patient care. While this patient technically does not meet DSM-5 criteria for major depressive disorder (she has only 4 symptoms instead of the required 5), she fits the pattern of depression in every other way. She should therefore be offered treatment in the form that she desires, as not offering treatment based on a rigid reliance upon diagnostic criteria is confusing the criteria for the actual disorder and is akin to mistaking the map of an area for the terrain itself (answer B). It may be tempting to diagnose a different disorder that also features subsyndromal symptoms of depression such as adjustment disorder or dysthymia, but the lack of a major life stressor rules out the former (answer C) while the clearly episodic nature of symptoms lasting less than 2 years rules out the latter (answer E). While we cannot say for sure that the patient does *not* have bipolar disorder, there is no evidence of it at this time (answer D). *(Chapter 2—The Algorithmic Approach to Diagnosis, Chapter 5—How to Diagnose Depressive Disorders)*

45. **The best answer is C.** At the time of initial presentation, this patient is best classified as having a substance-induced psychotic disorder related to cannabis, as diagnostically it is impossible to tell whether he has a primary psychotic disorder until he has been abstinent from cannabis and other substances long enough for their effects to have worn off. However, after six months it is clear that his psychotic symptoms have remained even in the absence of cannabis use, so a diagnosis of schizophrenia is more appropriate. It would not be appropriate to diagnose a primary psychotic disorder at the time of admission in the context of using a substance that can induce psychosis in some people who take it (answers A and E). While the patient is experiencing negative repercussions as a result of cannabis use, he was able to stop his use of the substance. Only if he had been unable to quit using cannabis despite having experienced negative repercussions would cannabis addiction be diagnosed (answer B). Finally, the symptoms described in this case are more consistent with a psychotic disorder than a mood disorder (answer D). *(Chapter 7—Differential Diagnosis of Psychotic Disorders, Chapter 8—Signs and Symptoms of Addiction)*

46. **The best answer is D.** This patient presents to the hospital after attempting to engage in instrumental violence. Instrumental violence is more often associated with psychopathy than an externalizing disorder, which is instead characterized by reactive violence in response to negative emotions (answer C). However, the patient's stated remorse and his lack of psychiatric or legal history prior to this incident strongly argue against psychopathy (answer B). It is notable that the patient's mental status exam is almost entirely normal which strongly argues against a psychotic disorder (answer A). There is no evidence of either autism or intellectual disability for this patient. While ADHD is also a neurodevelopmental disorder, misbehavior associated with this condition is generally impulsive rather than instrumental as was the case here (answer E). Therefore, the most likely explanation is that what the patient is saying is true, which may be related to an addictive disorder such as gambling disorder. Addictive disorders should be considered whenever there is no evidence of overt pathology on the mental status exam. *(Chapter 8—How to Diagnose Addictive Disorders)*

47. **The best answer is A.** The mood states seen in bipolar disorder can sometimes be so extreme that it appears to others that one's core personality has changed to a completely different person. A key differentiating factor is the frequency at which these changes occur, as the mood states seen in bipolar disorder tend to last for weeks or months while the identity states in dissociative identity disorder can change in a matter of minutes, hours, or days. Suicide is found in both bipolar disorder and dissociative identity disorder and does not reliably distinguish between them (answer C). Features of both happiness and sadness at the same time can either represent a mixed state due to bipolar disorder or the extreme affective instability seen in many cases of borderline personality disorder, which is frequently comorbid with dissociative identity disorder (answer B). While knowing the substance history is incredibly helpful for assessment, it would not distinguish between bipolar disorder and dissociative identity disorder in this case (answer D). Finally, because both bipolar disorder and dissociative identity disorder are frequently misdiagnosed and improperly treated, it would be unwise to rely too strongly on the medication history for differentiating between these two conditions (answer E). *(Chapter 12—Differential Diagnosis of Dissociative Disorders)*

48. **The best answer is J.** This is a complicated case of an elderly man with multiple problems including cognition deficits, depression, alcohol abuse, and insomnia, so deciding on a treatment strategy should involve prioritizing these various conditions. As with any case, the highest priority should be given to keeping both the patient and others safe. In this case, that will involve revoking the patient's license to drive, as this has the greatest potential to result in immediate harm to either the patient or others. *(Chapter 22—Alzheimer's Disease Across the Lifespan)*

49. **The best answer is I.** Once the immediate threat to safety is addressed, deciding which of the patient's conditions to prioritize becomes more challenging. In looking at the patient's complaints, it becomes clear that all of them may be related at least in some way to alcohol. Alcohol use can exacerbate depression or even cause it entirely by itself; it can directly cause cognitive deficits which often resolve with alcohol cessation; and it can often disrupt sleep significantly which can directly cause the kinds of nighttime awakenings that the patient is experiencing. For this reason, addressing the patient's alcohol use should take priority over treatment of dementia (answer A), treatment of depression (answers B, C, and F), or treatment of insomnia (answers C, D, and G). To treat his alcohol addiction, a variety of treatment options are available, including medications like naltrexone and referrals to substance rehabilitation programs. However, neither of these interventions will be effective if the patient is not committed to change (answers E and H). Therefore, assessing the patient's current readiness to change as directed by the principles of motivational interviewing is the best next step for managing this patient's concerns. *(Chapter 8—Addiction Across the Lifespan)*

50. **The best answer is C.** This vignette describes a stereotypical case of generalized anxiety disorder as evidenced by persistent worries in multiple domains of his life directly leading to impairment. Generalized anxiety disorder is most correlated with dysregulation of the HPA axis which manifests through abnormalities in the release of cortisol from the adrenal glands. Abnormal metabolism in the frontal and temporal lobes is associated with frontotemporal dementia (answer B), hyperreactivity of the amygdala is seen in PTSD (answer D), high resting neuronal activity in the retina has been demonstrated in ADHD (answer E), and high receptivity of the insula to afferent signals is seen in somatization (answer F). No conditions have been reliably associated with abnormal serotonin levels in the brain (answer A). *(Chapter 9—How to Diagnose Anxiety Disorders)*

51. **The best answer is H.** Bipolar disorder with psychotic features shares many signs and symptoms with primary psychotic disorders such as schizophrenia, with a lack of self-care (answer A), grandiose delusions (answer D), paranoid delusions (answer E), and auditory hallucinations (answer G) being found commonly in both conditions. This makes distinguishing between the two a clinical challenge. Some signs and symptoms are more often associated with one of these conditions than the other, such as disorganized speech (answers B and C) being more common in schizophrenia while irritability when blocked from reaching one's goals is more consistent with bipolar disorder (answer F). However, none of these are absolutely diagnostic of either condition, and it is impossible to definitively rule out bipolar disorder based on the information provided. Knowing how the patient has functioned across his lifespan would be much more helpful, with preserved functioning in between episodes being highly characteristic of bipolar disorder while a progressive decline in functioning is much more consistent with schizophrenia. *(Chapter 6—How to Diagnose Bipolar Disorders, Chapter 7—Signs and Symptoms of Schizophrenia)*

52. **The best answer is A.** This patient has poorly controlled pain related to a severe medical condition that warrants additional treatment, such as increasing the analgesic dose or switching to another drug that offers better coverage. Maintaining, reducing, or discontinuing her current level of pain management would not be appropriate (answers B, C, and D). While some of the features of this case (including a pattern of escalating use and feelings of guilt related to substance use) are found in addictive disorders as well, they can also be seen as a result of physiologic tolerance and societal stigma. In addition, there is no evidence that this patient is using opioids for their positively reinforcing effects. Rather, she appears to use them appropriately to remove pain (a negative reinforcement). Therefore, referring to an addiction medicine clinic would not be appropriate as she is not suffering from an addiction (answer E). You could consider using non-pharmacologic pain reduction techniques such as mindfulness meditation in addition to pain medications for greater effect. *(Chapter 8—Differential Diagnosis of Addictive Disorders)*

53. **The best answer is E.** This patient is experiencing the effects of benzodiazepine withdrawal which is characterized by both psychological and physiologic arousal that can manifest in feelings of severe anxiety. In this context, it would be inappropriate to diagnose a new anxiety disorder (answers A, B, and C) or to attribute his anxiety to his depressive disorder (answer D). This is a common clinical scenario when lowering the dose of or discontinuing a benzodiazepine, and patients should be counseled on what to expect prior to beginning this process. Slowly tapering the dose of the benzodiazepine can also help to reduce the chances of a severe withdrawal state, although it cannot always be avoided entirely. *(Chapter 8—Psychoactive Substances, Chapter 9—Differential Diagnosis of Anxiety Disorders)*

RECOMMENDED READING

The following articles are intended to provide those who are interested with directions for further reading on many of the subjects we have discussed so far. This list is not meant to be a comprehensive catalog of references for the information in this book. For any questions about the sources of specific data, please contact the author at **memorablepsych@gmail.com**.

CHAPTER 2 | DIAGNOSIS
- Prince et al. "No health without mental health." Lancet. 2007 Sep 8;370(9590):859-77.
- Kindler KS. "Explanatory models for psychiatric illness." Am J Psychiatry. 2008;165:695-702
- Rosenhan. "On being sane in insane places." Science. 1973;179:250-258
- Croskerry. "The importance of cognitive errors in diagnosis and strategies to minimize them." Acad Med. 2003 Aug;78(8):775-80.
- Crumlish et al. "How psychiatrists think." Advances in Psychiatric Treatment. 2009;15(1):72-79.
- Aboraya et al. "The Reliability of Psychiatric Diagnosis Revisited: The Clinician's Guide to Improve the Reliability of Psychiatric Diagnosis." Psychiatry (Edgmont). 2006 Jan;3(1):41-50.

CHAPTER 3 | EVALUATION
- Warner. "Clinicians' guide to evaluating diagnostic and screening tests in psychiatry." Advances in Psychiatric Treatment. 2004;10:446–454.
- McGough et al. "Estimating the Size of Treatment Effects: Moving Beyond P Values." Psychiatry (Edgmont). 2009 Oct;6(10):21–29.
- Pewsner et al. "Ruling a diagnosis in or out with 'SpPIn' and 'SnNOut': a note of caution." BMJ. 2004;329(7459):209-213.
- Grimes et al. "Refining clinical diagnosis with likelihood ratios." Lancet. 2005 Apr 23-29;365(9469):1500-5.

CHAPTER 4 | PSYCHIATRIC EMERGENCIES
- Hawton et al. "Suicide." Lancet. 2009 Apr 18;373(9672):1372-81.
- Harris et al. "Suicide as an outcome for mental disorders. A meta-analysis." Br J Psychiatry. 1997;170:205-228.
- Skegg. "Self-harm." Lancet. 2005 Oct 22-28;366(9495):1471-83.
- Klonsky. "The functions of deliberate self-injury: a review of the evidence." Clin Psychol Rev. 2007 Mar;27(2):226-39.
- Elbogen et al. "The intricate link between violence and mental disorder: results from the National Epidemiologic Survey on Alcohol and Related Conditions." Arch Gen Psychiatry. 2009 Feb;66(2):152-61.
- Petit. "Management of the Acutely Violent Patient." Psychiatric Clinics;28(3):701-711.
- Legano et al. "Child abuse and neglect." Curr Probl Pediatr Adolesc Health Care. 2009 Feb;39(2):31.e1-26.

- Christian et al. "The evaluation of suspected child physical abuse." Pediatrics. 2015 May;135(5):e1337-54.
- Inouye. "Delirium in older persons." N Engl J Med. 2006;354:1157-1165.
- Appelbaum. "Assessment of patients' competence to consent to treatment." N Engl J Med. 2007;357:1834-1840.
- Bhati et al. "Clinical Manifestations, Diagnosis, and Empirical Treatments for Catatonia." Psychiatry (Edgmont). 2007;4(3):46-52.

CHAPTER 5 | DEPRESSION
- Kendler. "The Phenomenology of Major Depression and the Representativeness and Nature of DSM Criteria." Am J Psychiatry 2016 Aug 1;173(8):771-80.
- Burcusa et al. "Risk for Recurrence in Depression." Clinical psychology review. 2007;27(8):959-985.
- Paykel et al. "Life events and depression. A controlled study." Arch Gen Psychiatry. 1969 Dec;21(6):753-60.
- Harmer et al. "Why do antidepressants take so long to work? A cognitive neuropsychological model of antidepressant drug action." Br J Psychiatry 2009; 195:102-108.
- Nelson et al. "Childhood maltreatment and characteristics of adult depression: meta-analysis." Br J Psychiatry. 2017 Feb;210(2):96-104.
- Cipriani et al. "Comparative efficacy and acceptability of 21 antidepressant drugs for the acute treatment of adults with major depressive disorder: a systematic review and network meta-analysis." Lancet 2018 Apr 7;391(10128):1357-1366.
- Bostwick et al. "Recognizing mimics of depression: The '8 Ds'." Current Psychiatry. 2012 Jun;11(6):30-36.

CHAPTER 6 | BIPOLAR DISORDER
- Kendler. "The clinical features of mania and their representation in modern diagnostic criteria." Psychol Med. 2017 Apr;47(6):1013-1029.
- Ghouse et al. "Overdiagnosis of Bipolar Disorder: A Critical Analysis of the Literature." The Scientific World Journal. 2013;2013:297087.
- Joffe et al. "A prospective, longitudinal study of percentage of time spent ill in patients with bipolar I or bipolar II disorders." Bipolar Disord. 2004 Feb;6(1):62-6.
- Cuellar et al. "Distinctions between bipolar and unipolar depression." Clinical psychology review. 2005;25(3):307-339.
- Geddes et al "Treatment of bipolar disorder". Lancet. 2013;381(9878):10.1016/S0140-6736(13)60857-0.
- Cipriani et al. "Comparative efficacy and acceptability of antimanic drugs in acute mania: a multiple-treatments meta-analysis." Lancet. 2011; 378:1306-1315
- Nusslock et al. "Elevated reward-related neural activation as a unique biological marker of bipolar disorder: assessment and treatment implications." Behav Res Ther. 2014 Nov;62:74-87.
- Paris et al. "Borderline personality disorder and bipolar disorder: what is the difference and why does it matter?" J Nerv Ment Dis. 2015 Jan;203(1):3-7.

CHAPTER 7 | SCHIZOPHRENIA
- Picchioni et al. "Schizophrenia." British Medical Journal. 2007;335(7610):91-95.
- Kendler. "Phenomenology of Schizophrenia and the Representativeness of Modern Diagnostic Criteria." JAMA Psychiatry. 2016 Oct 1;73(10):1082-1092.
- Fusar-Poli et al. "The psychosis high-risk state: a comprehensive state-of-the-art review." JAMA Psychiatry. 2013;70:107-120.
- Kapur. "Psychosis as a state of aberrant salience: a framework linking biology, phenomenology, and pharmacology in schizophrenia." Am J Psychiatry. 2003;160:13-23.
- Emsley et al. "The nature of relapse in schizophrenia." BMC Psychiatry. 2013;13:50.
- Schwartz et al. "Congruence of diagnoses 2 years after a first-admission diagnosis of psychosis." Arch Gen Psychiatry. 2000 Jun;57(6):593-600.
- Kendler. "Psychosis within vs outside of major mood episodes: a key prognostic and diagnostic criterion." JAMA Psychiatry. 2013 Dec;70(12):1263-4.
- Leucht et al. "Comparative efficacy and tolerability of 15 antipsychotic drugs in schizophrenia: a multiple treatments meta-analysis." Lancet. 2013;382:951-962.
- Resnick et al. "Faking it: How to detect malingered psychosis." Current Psychiatry. 2005 Nov;4(11):12-25.

CHAPTER 8 | ADDICTION
- Lüscher et al. "The mechanistic classification of addictive drugs." PLoS Med. 2006 Nov;3(11):e437.
- Koston et al. "Management of drug and alcohol withdrawal." N Engl J Med. 2003; 348:1786-1795.
- Nestler et al." DeltaFosB: a sustained molecular switch for addiction." Proc Natl Acad Sci U S A. 2001 Sep 25;98(20):11042-6.
- Lopez-Quintero et al. "Probability and predictors of remission from lifetime nicotine, alcohol, cannabis, or cocaine dependence: Results from the National Epidemiologic Survey on Alcohol and Related Conditions" Addiction. 2011 March;106(3):657–669.
- Berlin et al. "Understanding the Differences Between Impulsivity and Compulsivity." Psychiatric Times. 2008 Jul;25(8):58-61.
- Olsen. "Natural Rewards, Neuroplasticity, and Non-Drug Addictions. Neuropharmacology." 2011;61(7):1109-1122.
- Grant et al. "Introduction to Behavioral Addictions." The American journal of drug and alcohol abuse. 2010;36(5):233-241.

CHAPTER 9 | ANXIETY
- Craske et al. "Anxiety." Lancet. 2016 Dec 17;388(10063):3048-3059.
- Bystritsky et al. "Current Diagnosis and Treatment of Anxiety Disorders." Pharmacy and Therapeutics. 2013;38(1):30-57.
- Steimer. "The biology of fear- and anxiety-related behaviors." Dialogues in Clinical Neuroscience. 2002;4(3):231-249.
- Faravelli et al. "Childhood stressful events, HPA axis and anxiety disorders." World Journal of Psychiatry. 2012;2(1):13-25.

- Zorn et al. "Cortisol stress reactivity across psychiatric disorders: A systematic review and meta-analysis." Psychoneuroendocrinology. 2017 Mar;77:25-36.
- Stein et al. "Social anxiety disorder." Lancet. 2008 Mar 29;371(9618):1115-25.
- Roy-Byrne et al. "Panic disorder." Lancet. 2006; 368:1023-1032.
- Aronson et al. "Phenomenology of panic attacks: a descriptive study of panic disorder patients' self-reports." J Clin Psychiatry. 1988 Jan;49(1):8-13.
- Bystritsky et al. "Acute responses of anxiety disorder patients after a natural disaster." Depress Anxiety. 2000;11(1):43-4.

CHAPTER 10 | OCD
- Abramowitz et al. "Obsessive-compulsive disorder." Lancet. 2009; 374:491-499.
- Hollander. "Obsessive-compulsive disorder and spectrum across the life span." Int J Psychiatry Clin Pract. 2005;9(2):79-86.
- Huey et al. "A psychological and neuroanatomical model of obsessive-compulsive disorder." J Neuropsychiatry Clin Neurosci. 2008 Fall;20(4):390-408.
- Bjornsson et al. "Body dysmorphic disorder." Dialogues Clin Neurosci. 2010;12(2):221-32.
- Scarella et al. "The Relationship of Hypochondriasis to Anxiety, Depressive, and Somatoform Disorders." Psychosomatics. 2016;57(2):200-207.
- Leckman. "Phenomenology of tics and natural history of tic disorders." Brain Dev. 2003 Dec;25 Suppl 1:S24-8.
- Woods et al. "Diagnosis, Evaluation, and Management of Trichotillomania." The Psychiatric clinics of North America. 2014;37(3):301-317.

CHAPTER 11 | PTSD
- Bisson et al. "Post-traumatic stress disorder." The BMJ. 2015;351:h6161.
- Ehlers et al. "A cognitive model of posttraumatic stress disorder." Behav Res Therapy 2000;38:319-345.
- Brewin et al. "Meta-analysis of risk factors for posttraumatic stress disorder in trauma-exposed adults." J Consult Clin Psychol. 2000 Oct;68(5):748-66.
- Santiago et al. "A Systematic Review of PTSD Prevalence and Trajectories in DSM-5 Defined Trauma Exposed Populations: Intentional and Non-Intentional Traumatic Events." PLoS ONE. 2013;8(4):e59236.
- Creamer et al. "The relationship between acute stress disorder and posttraumatic stress disorder in severely injured trauma survivors." Behav Res Ther. 2004 Mar;42(3):315-28.
- Sullivan et al. "Pharmacotherapy in post-traumatic stress disorder: evidence from randomized controlled trials." Curr Opin Investig Drugs. 2009 Jan;10(1):35-45.
- Flory et al. "Comorbidity between post-traumatic stress disorder and major depressive disorder: alternative explanations and treatment considerations." Dialogues in Clinical Neuroscience. 2015;17(2):141-150.

CHAPTER 12 | DISSOCIATION
- Lynn et al. "Dissociation and Dissociative Disorders Challenging Conventional Wisdom." Current Directions in Psychological Science. 2012 Jan;21(1):48-53.

- Lyssenko et al. "Dissociation in Psychiatric Disorders: A Meta-Analysis of Studies Using the Dissociative Experiences Scale." Am J Psychiatry. 2018 Jan 1;175(1):37-46.
- van der Kloet et al. "Fragmented Sleep, Fragmented Mind: The Role of Sleep in Dissociative Symptoms." Perspect Psychol Sci. 2012 Mar;7(2):159-75.
- Simeon et al. "Feeling unreal: a depersonalization disorder update of 117 cases." J Clin Psychiatry. 2003 Sep;64(9):990-7.
- Brand et al. "A review of dissociative disorders treatment studies." J Nerv Ment Dis. 2009 Sep;197(9):646-54.
- Brand et al. "Dispelling myths about dissociative identity disorder treatment: an empirically based approach." Psychiatry. 2014 Summer;77(2):169-89.

CHAPTER 13 | SOMATIZATION
- Fink. "Physical complaints and symptoms of somatizing patients." J Psychosom Res. 1992 Feb;36(2):125-36.
- Smith. "The course of somatization and its effects on utilization of health care resources." Psychosomatics. 1994 May-Jun;35(3):263-7.
- olde Hartman et al. "Medically unexplained symptoms, somatisation disorder and hypochondriasis: course and prognosis. A systematic review." J Psychosom Res. 2009 May;66(5):363-77.
- Boeckle et al. "Neural correlates of somatoform disorders from a meta-analytic perspective on neuroimaging studies." Neuroimage Clin. 2016 Apr 10;11:606-13.
- Harvey et al. "Conversion disorder: towards a neurobiological understanding." Neuropsychiatric Disease and Treatment. 2006;2(1):13-20.
- Eastwood et al. "Management of factitious disorders: a systematic review." Psychother Psychosom. 2008;77:209-218.
- Lebourgeois. "Malingering: Key Points in Assessment." Psychiatric Times. 2007 Apri;24(4).
- Mellers. "The approach to patients with 'non-epileptic seizures.'" Postgraduate Medical Journal. 2005;81(958):498-504.

CHAPTER 14 | PERSONALITY
- Tyrer et al. "Classification, assessment, prevalence, and effect of personality disorder." Lancet. 2015 Feb 21;385(9969):717-26.
- Newton-Howes et al. "Personality disorder across the life course." Lancet. 2015 Feb 21;385(9969):727-34.
- Bateman et al. "Treatment of personality disorder." Lancet. 2015 Feb 21;385(9969):735-43.
- Trull et al. "Dimensional models of personality: the five-factor model and the DSM-5." Dialogues in Clinical Neuroscience. 2013;15(2):135-146.
- Lynam et al. "Using the Five-Factor Model to Represent the DSM-IV Personality Disorders: An Expert Consensus Approach." Journal of Abnormal Psychology. 2001;110(3):401-412.
- Esterberg et al. "A Personality Disorders: Schizotypal, Schizoid and Paranoid Personality Disorders in Childhood and Adolescence." Journal of psychopathology and behavioral assessment. 2010;32(4):515-528.

- Caligor et al. "Narcissistic personality disorder: diagnostic and clinical challenges." Am J Psychiatry. 2015 May;172(5):415-22.
- Disney. "Dependent personality disorder: a critical review." Clin Psychol Rev. 2013 Dec;33(8):1184-96.
- Mancebo et al. "Obsessive compulsive personality disorder and obsessive compulsive disorder: clinical characteristics, diagnostic difficulties, and treatment." Ann Clin Psychiatry. 2005 Oct-Dec;17(4):197-204.
- Weinbrecht et al. "Avoidant Personality Disorder: a Current Review." Curr Psychiatry Rep. 2016 Mar;18(3):29. doi: 10.1007/s11920-016-0665-6.
- Bierer et al. "Abuse and neglect in childhood: relationship to personality disorder diagnoses." CNS Spectr. 2003 Oct;8(10):737-54.

CHAPTER 15 | BORDERLINE
- Leichsenring et al. "Borderline personality disorder." Lancet. 2011; 377:74-84.
- Paris. "Why Psychiatrists are Reluctant to Diagnose: Borderline Personality Disorder." Psychiatry (Edgmont). 2007;4(1):35-39.
- Zanarini et al. "Fluidity of the Subsyndromal Phenomenology of Borderline Personality Disorder Over 16 Years of Prospective Follow-Up" Am J Psychiatry. 2016 Jul 1;173(7):688-94.
- Gunderson et al. "Ten-Year Course of Borderline Personality Disorder: Psychopathology and Function From the Collaborative Longitudinal Personality Disorders Study." Archives of general psychiatry. 2011;68(8):827-837.
- Stanley et al. "The Interpersonal Dimension of Borderline Personality Disorder: Toward a Neuropeptide Model." The American Journal of Psychiatry. 2010;167(1):24-39.
- Fonagy et al. "Borderline personality disorder, mentalization, and the neurobiology of attachment." Infant Ment Health J. 2011 Jan;32(1):47-69.
- Lieb et al. "Pharmacotherapy for borderline personality disorder: Cochrane systematic review of randomised trials." Br J Psychiatry. 2010 Jan;196(1):4-12.
- Chapman. "Dialectical Behavior Therapy: Current Indications and Unique Elements." Psychiatry (Edgmont). 2006;3(9):62-68.

CHAPTER 16 | ANTISOCIAL
- Jenson et al. "Externalizing Disorders in Children and Adolescents: Behavioral Excess and Behavioral Deficits." Oxford Handbook of School Psychology. 2011.
- Zoccolillo et al. "The outcome of childhood conduct disorder: implications for defining adult personality disorder and conduct disorder." Psychol Med. 1992 Nov;22(4):971-86.
- Guttmann-Steinmetz et al. "Attachment and Externalizing Disorders: A Developmental Psychopathology Perspective." J Am Acad Child & Adolescent Psychiatry;45(4):440-451.
- Bronsard et al. "The Prevalence of Mental Disorders Among Children and Adolescents in the Child Welfare System: A Systematic Review and Meta-Analysis." Medicine. 2016;95(7):e2622.
- Sala et al. "Phenomenology, longitudinal course and outcome of children and adolescents with bipolar spectrum disorders." Child and adolescent psychiatric clinics of North America. 2009;18(2):273-vii.

- Grant et al. "Choosing a treatment for disruptive, impulse-control, and conduct disorders." Current Psychiatry. 2015 Jan;14(1):28-36.

CHAPTER 17 | PSYCHOPATHY
- Gregory et al. "The antisocial brain: psychopathy matters." Arch Gen Psychiatry. 2012 Sep;69(9):962-72.
- Ogloff. "Psychopathy/antisocial personality disorder conundrum." Aust N Z J Psychiatry. 2006 Jun-Jul;40(6-7):519-28.
- Gregory et al. "Punishment and psychopathy: a case-control functional MRI investigation of reinforcement learning in violent antisocial personality disordered men." Lancet Psychiatry. 2015 Feb;2(2):153-60.

CHAPTER 18 | EATING DISORDERS
- Treasure et al. "Eating disorders." Lancet. 2010;375:583-93.
- Yager et al. "Anorexia nervosa." N Engl J Med. 2005;353:1481-1488.
- Eddy et al. "Diagnostic crossover in anorexia nervosa and bulimia nervosa: implications for DSM-V." Am J Psychiatry. 2008 Feb;165(2):245-50.
- Hadad et al. "Addicted to Palatable Foods: Comparing the Neurobiology of Bulimia Nervosa to that of Drug Addiction." Psychopharmacology. 2014;231(9):1897-1912.
- Morgan et al. "The SCOFF questionnaire: a new screening tool for eating disorders." Western Journal of Medicine. 2000;172(3):164-165.

CHAPTER 19 | DEVELOPMENT
- McLaughlin. "Speech and Language Delay in Children." American Family Physician. 2011 May;83(10):1183-88.
- Noritz et al. "Motor delays: early identification and evaluation." Pediatrics. 2013 Jun;131(6):e2016-27.
- Daily et al. "Identification and evaluation of mental retardation." Am Fam Physician. 2000 Feb 15;61(4):1059-67,1070.
- Kendall et al. "Intellectual disability and psychiatric comorbidity: Challenges and clinical issues." Psychiatric Times. 2015 May;32(5).

CHAPTER 20 | AUTISM
- Levy et al. "Autism." Lancet. 2009;374(9701):1627-1638.
- Kanner. "Autistic disturbances of affective contact." Acta Paedopsychiatr. 1968;35(4):100-36.
- Constantino et al. "Diagnosis of autism spectrum disorder: reconciling the syndrome, its diverse origins, and variation in expression." Lancet Neurol. 2016 Mar;15(3):279-91.
- Grodberg et al. "The Autism Mental Status Exam: Sensitivity and Specificity Using DSM-5 Criteria for Autism Spectrum Disorder in Verbally Fluent Adults." Journal of autism and developmental disorders. 2014;44(3):609-614.
- Landa et al. "Developmental Trajectories in Children With and Without Autism Spectrum Disorders: The First 3 Years." Child development. 2013;84(2):429-442.
- Rajendran et al. "Cognitive Theories of Autism." Developmental Review. 2007 Jun;27(2):224-260.

CHAPTER 21 | ADHD
- Cherkasova et al. "Developmental course of attention deficit hyperactivity disorder and its predictors." J Can Acad Child Adolesc Psychiatry. 2013 Feb;22(1):47-54.
- Elder. "The importance of relative standards in ADHD diagnoses: evidence based on exact birth dates." J Health Econ. 2010 Sep;29(5):641-56.
- Bubl et al. "Elevated background noise in adult attention deficit hyperactivity disorder is associated with inattention." PLoS One. 2015 Feb 18;10(2):e0118271.
- Faraone. "Using Meta-analysis to Compare the Efficacy of Medications for Attention-Deficit/Hyperactivity Disorder in Youths." P&T. 2009 Dec;34(12):678-94.
- Fabiano et al. "A meta-analysis of behavioral treatments for attention-deficit/hyperactivity disorder." Clin Psychol Rev. 2009 Mar;29(2):129-40.

CHAPTER 22 | DEMENTIA
- Harada et al. "Normal Cognitive Aging." Clinics in geriatric medicine. 2013;29(4):737-752.
- Burns et al. "Dementia." BMJ. 2009 Feb 5;338:b75.
- Blennow. "Alzheimer's disease." Lancet. 2006 Jul 29;368(9533):387-403.
- Carlesimo et al. "Memory deficits in Alzheimer's patients: a comprehensive review." Neuropsychol Rev. 1992 Jun;3(2):119-69.
- Velayudhan et al. "Review of brief cognitive tests for patients with suspected dementia." International Psychogeriatrics / Ipa. 2014;26(8):1247-1262.
- Mortimer et al. "Neuroimaging in dementia: a practical guide." Pract Neurol. 2013 Apr;13(2):92-103.
- Sabbagh et al. "Increasing Precision of Clinical Diagnosis of Alzheimer's Disease Using a Combined Algorithm Incorporating Clinical and Novel Biomarker Data." Neurol Ther. 2017 Jul;6(Suppl 1):83-95.
- McKeith et al. "Diagnosis and management of dementia with Lewy bodies." Neurology. 2005;12:1863-1872.
- Warren et al. "Frontotemporal dementia." The BMJ. 2013;347:f4827.
- Jorge. "Neuropsychiatric consequences of traumatic brain injury: a review of recent findings." Curr Opin Psychiatry. 2005 May;18(3):289-99.

CHAPTER 23 | SLEEP
- Roth. "Insomnia: Definition, Prevalence, Etiology, and Consequences." Journal of Clinical Sleep Medicine. 2007;3(5 Suppl):S7-S10.
- Irish et al. "The Role of Sleep Hygiene in Promoting Public Health: A Review of Empirical Evidence." Sleep medicine reviews. 2015;22:23-36.
- Abad et al. "Diagnosis and treatment of sleep disorders: a brief review for clinicians." Dialogues in Clinical Neuroscience. 2003;5(4):371-388.
- Williams et al. "Cognitive behavioral treatment of insomnia." Chest. 2013 Feb 1;143(2):554-565.
- Edinger et al. "Subtyping primary insomnia: is sleep state misperception a distinct clinical entity?" Sleep Med Rev. 2003 Jun;7(3):203-14.

ATTRIBUTIONS

The fonts **Oswald** and Source Sans Pro were used for the cover and inside text, respectively. They were accessed from Google Fonts under an open-source license.

All images displayed in this book are under the public domain, with the following exceptions. Use of this content does not suggest that the content's original creator(s) endorse this book or its author in any way.

COVER AND BACK
- Cover and back design by Stephen Sauer (SingleFinDesign.com).
- Images and icons designed by Freepik.

CHAPTER 2 | DIAGNOSIS
- "A patient consulting his friendly doctor." Credit: Wellcome Images (Creative Commons Attribution 4.0 International license).
- "Nosebleed aid." Credit: TenarAiuola (Creative Commons Attribution-Share Alike 3.0 Unported license).

CHAPTER 3 | EVALUATION
- "Doctor talking with pregnant woman." Credit: P.S.Art-Design-Studio (Shutterstock.com).

CHAPTER 4 | PSYCHIATRIC EMERGENCIES
- "An alcoholic man with delirium." Credit: Wellcome Images (Creative Commons Attribution 4.0 International license).
- "Catatonic grimacing." Credit: Owald Bumke. *Lehrbuch der Geisteskrankheiten, 2nd ed.* 1924. (Believed to be in public domain as copyright for photographs and pictures published in Germany expire fifty years after their first publication.)
- "Croquis fait a Murcie." Credit: Davillier, Jean Charles, barón, 1823-1883 (Creative Commons Attribution 2.0 Generic license).

CHAPTER 8 | ADDICTION
- "Cookie jar." Credit: LHF Graphics (Shutterstock.com).
- "Hand sanitizer pump dispenser." Credit: Zern Liew (Shutterstock.com).
- "Injecting drugs." Credit: KUCO (Shutterstock.com).
- "S'mores." Credit: pimlena (Shutterstock.com).

CHAPTER 9 | ANXIETY
- "Scary clown." Credit: Danny PiG (Creative Commons Attribution 2.0 Generic license).
- "Stuffed bird with Mom leg." Credit: Daniel Hatton (Creative Commons Attribution-NonCommercial-NoDerivs 2.0 Generic license).

CHAPTER 10 | OCD
- "Man putting toilet paper up to his mouth." Credit: txking (Shutterstock.com).

- "OCD Letter Blocks." Credit: amenclinicsphotos ac (Creative Commons Attribution-ShareAlike 2.0 Generic license).

CHAPTER 13 | SOMATIZATION
- "Male torso, revealing internal organs and system." Credit: Wellcome Images (Creative Commons Attribution 4.0 International license).

CHAPTER 14 | PERSONALITY
- "Drawing of a bride with bridesmaids." Credit: pixy.org/4477409 (Creative Commons Attribution-NonCommercial-NoDerivatives 4.0 International license).

CHAPTER 19 | DEVELOPMENT
- "Sketch of skateboarder." Credit: Olga Tropinina (Shutterstock.com).
- "Boy with Down syndrome." Credit: Wellcome Images (Creative Commons Attribution 4.0 International license).
- "Silencing of the FMR1 Gene in Fragile X Mental Retardation Syndrome." Credit: Dr. Marian L. Miller (Journal-Cover-Art.com) (Creative Commons Attribution-Share Alike 3.0 Unported license).
- "Baby with fetal alcohol syndrome." Credit: Teresa Kellerman (Creative Commons Attribution-Share Alike 3.0 Unported license).
- "Distinctive facial appearance of person with Williams syndrome." Credit: E. A. Nikitina, A. V. Medvedeva, G. A. Zakharov, and E. V. Savvateeva-Popova, 2014 Park-media Ltd (Creative Commons Attribution 3.0 Unported license).
- "Dermatophagia." Credit: 6th Happiness (Creative Commons Attribution 3.0 Unported license).
- "Cerebral palsy forms." Credit: Δρ. Χαράλαμπος Γκούβας (Harrygouvas) (Creative Commons Attribution-Share Alike 3.0 Unported license).

CHAPTER 22 | DEMENTIA
- "The progressive deterioration of pattern processing ability in a subject as they progress from mild cognitive impairment (MCI) to severe Alzheimer's disease (AD)." Credit: Mattson M (Creative Commons Attribution 3.0 Unported license).

CHAPTER 24 | FINAL REVIEW
- "Intradermal injection." Credit: British Columbia Institute of Technology (Creative Commons Attribution 4.0 International license).
- "Love bite." Credit: Janek B. (Creative Commons Attribution-Share Alike 3.0 Unported license).
- "8 year-old patient with Prader-Willi syndrome." Credit: Fanny Cortés M1, M. Angélica Alliende R1,a, Andrés Barrios R1,2, Bianca Curotto L1,b, Lorena Santa María V1,c, Ximena Barraza O3, Ledia Troncoso A2, Cecilia Mellado S4,6, Rosa Pardo V (Creative Commons Attribution 4.0 International license).
- "Dare to reach out your hand into the darkness, to pull another hand into the light." Credit: Sundaram Ramaswamy (Creative Commons Attribution 2.0 Generic license).
- "X-ray of a foot, showing a bullet." Credit: Wellcome Images (Creative Commons Attribution 4.0 International license).

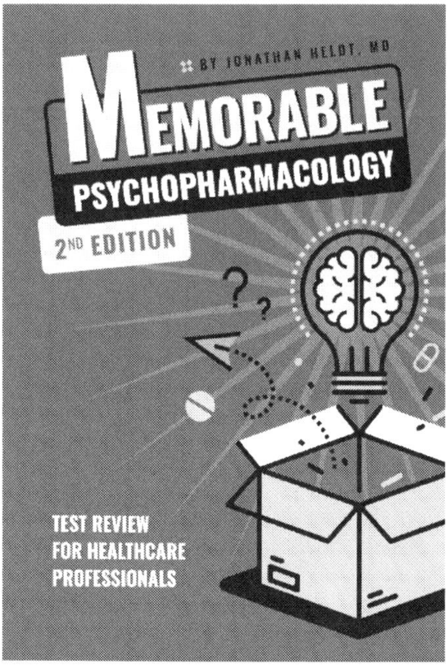
BY JONATHAN HELDT, MD
MEMORABLE
PSYCHOPHARMACOLOGY
2ND EDITION
TEST REVIEW
FOR HEALTHCARE
PROFESSIONALS

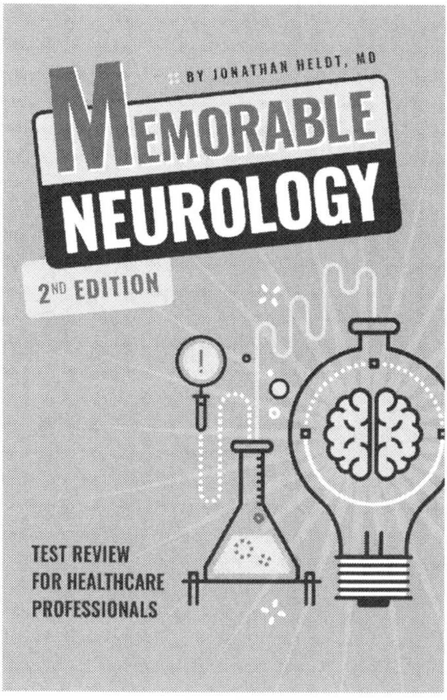
BY JONATHAN HELDT, MD
MEMORABLE
NEUROLOGY
2ND EDITION
TEST REVIEW
FOR HEALTHCARE
PROFESSIONALS

INTERESTED IN LEARNING MORE?

Get *Memorable Psychopharmacology* and *Memorable Neurology*,
both available now from the same author!

Memorable Psychopharmacology

Now that you have the information needed to approach psychiatric diagnosis, take your learning to the next step by understanding the evidence behind the treatment of these disorders! *Memorable Psychopharmacology* uses a conversational tone, catchy mnemonics, visual aids, and practice questions to ensure that you not only learn the material but retain it far into the future. For anyone preparing to meet the mental health needs of their patients, *Memorable Psychopharmacology* is an indispensable review.

Memorable Neurology

The nervous system can be a scary place to explore without a guide! *Memorable Neurology* gives you the tools you need to understand the structure, function, and potential dysfunction of the most complex organ system in the body. *Memorable Neurology* combines a solid foundation in neuroanatomy with a focus on clinical diseases to give you a leg up in the field of neurology. A generous helpful of mnemonics, visuals, and practice questions makes learning the material simple, straightforward, and enjoyable.

BOTH AVAILABLE NOW ON AMAZON.COM!

ABOUT THE AUTHOR

Jonathan Heldt is currently on faculty at the UCLA Semel Institute for Neuroscience & Human Behavior. He completed his Bachelor's degree in Biochemistry at Pacific Union College, his medical degree at the Loma Linda University School of Medicine, and his residency at the UCLA Psychiatry Residency Training Program. He is interested in both mental health and medical education and hopes that this book will inspire these interests in others. He has no conflicts of interest to disclose.

For questions, comments, and updates, please visit **memorablepsych.com** *or email* **memorablepsych@gmail.com**.

Memorable Psychiatry by Jonathan Heldt

Diagnosis and Evaluation

Psychiatric Interview

CHAMPION'S PSYCH EVAL

Chief Cx	**P**rescriptions
How to Help	**S**ubstances
Add'l Info	**Y**outh
Medical Hx	**C**ollateral
Psych Hx	**H**ousing
Ideation	**E**mployment
Orientation	**V**ictimization
Navigation	**A**ncestry
Social Support	**L**egal

Mental Status Exam

A Beautiful **M**ental **S**tatus **A**lways **P**leases **C**ustomers, **P**rovided **O**f **C**ourse **I**t's **J**ustified

- **A**ppearance
- **B**ehavior
- **M**otor
- **S**peech
- **A**ffect and mood
- **P**erception
- **O**rientation
- **C**ognition
- **I**nsight
- **J**udgment
- **T**hought **P**rocess
- **T**hought **C**ontent

Major Diagnostic Categories

A MAP TO MIND SPACE

Addiction	**M**edical
Mood	**I**ntoxicants
Anxiety	**N**ormalcy
Psychosis	**D**elirium
Trauma	**S**omatoform
OCD	**P**ersonality
	ADHD/autism
	Cognitive
	Eating

Psychiatric Emergencies

Suicide Tx

DIOS MIO
- **D**etainment
- **I**npatient
- **O**bservation
- **S**harps
- **M**edical clearance
- **I**njuries
- **O**ccult overdoses

Delirium Dx/Tx

Where THE F AM I
- **Where** (disor.)
- **T**hought disorg.
- **H**allucinations
- **E**nergy changes
- **F**luctuating
- **A**cute
- **M**edical causes
- **I**ntoxicants

Capacity

U R SAFE
- **U**nderlying cause
- **R**eorientation
- **S**leep
- **A**ntipsychotics
- **F**amily/friends
- **E**nvironment

CURBSIDE
- **C**ommunicate
- **U**nderstand
- **R**isks &
- **B**enefits
- **S**ituation
- **I**mpact
- **D**ecide
- **E**xplain

Catatonia Sx

LIMP MEN
- **L**ethargy (stupor)
- **I**mmobility
- **M**utism
- **P**ositioning
- **M**otor abnormalities
- **E**cholalia/echopraxia
- **N**egativism

Homelessness Tx

A TRIP HOME
- **A**ddiction
- **T**raumatization
- **R**ehabilitation
- **I**mmunization
- **P**sychiatric services
- **H**ousing
- **O**utreach
- **M**ultidisciplinary
- **E**ssentials

Mood Disorders

Mood Assessment

Reactive PLANETS
- **R**eactivity
- **P**olarity
- **L**ability
- **A**ttributability
- **N**ormality
- **E**pisodicity
- **T**reatment responsivity
- **S**everity

Depression Dx

SIGECAPS
- **S**leep
- **I**nterest/enjoyment
- **G**uilt/hopelessness
- **E**nergy
- **C**oncentration
- **A**ppetite
- **P**sychomotor ret.
- **S**uicide

5/9 "2 blue weeks"

Dysthymia Dx

HE'S 2 SAD
- **H**opelessness
- **E**nergy
- **S**elf-esteem
- **2**+ years
- **S**leep
- **A**ppetite
- **D**ecision-making

Bipolar Disorder Dx

Mania = **DIG FAST**
- **D**istractibility
- **I**mpulsivity
- **G**randiosity
- **F**light of ideas
- **A**ctivity ↑
- **S**leep (↓ need for)
- **T**alkativeness

3-4/7 "1 fun week"

Hypomania
DIG FAST (but lesser, not impairing)

Mixed Episode
↓ mood + ↑ activity

Psychosis

Schizophrenia Dx

HD BS Network
- **H**allucinations (auditory)
- **D**elusions (paranoid)
- **B**ehavior (disorganized)
- **S**peech (disorganized)
- **N**egative symptoms

2-4-6-ophrenia
2 symptoms for at least 6 months

Positive and Negative Sx

The 5 A's of Negative Sx
- **A**ffect
- **A**mbivalence
- **A**logia
- **A**nhedonia
- **A**sociality

Positive sx = Present = s**P**ecific
Negative sx = Not present = se**N**sitive

Malingered Psychosis

Vague AWD LIARS
- **V**ague
- **A**ssociated **W**ith **D**elusions
- **L**aterality
- **I**nside
- **A**ble to resist
- **R**educing strategies
- **S**econdary gain

Addiction

Psychoactive Substances

CAN HIS DOG Behave?
- **C**annabis
- **A**lcohol
- **N**icotine
- **H**allucinogens
- **I**nhalants
- **S**timulants
- **D**epressants
- **O**pioids
- **G**ambling
- **Beh**avioral

Addiction Dx

The 3 Reapers
Repeated use of **R**einforcers (positive) despite negative **R**epercussions
- or -

Time 2 CUT DOWN PAL
- **Time** spent
- **2**+ symptoms
- **C**ravings
- **U**nable to cut down
- **T**olerance
- **D**angerous use
- **O**thers affected
- **W**ithdrawal
- **N**eglecting roles
- **P**roblems resulting
- **A**ctivities given up
- **L**arger amounts or for longer

Complete Substance Hx

TRAPPED
- **T**reatment history
- **R**oute of administration
- **A**mount used
- **P**attern of use
- **P**rior abstinence
- **E**ffects of use
- **D**uration of use

Memorable Psychiatry by Jonathan Heldt

Anxiety

Anxiety Assessment

ONSTAGE
- **O**bsessive
- **N**ormalcy
- **S**omatization
- **T**rauma
- **A**ttributable
- **G**eneralized
- **E**pisodic

Generalized Anxiety Dx

EGADS! I'm MISERA-ble!
- **E**xcessive
- **G**eneralized
- **A**nxiety
- **D**aily
- **S**ix or more months

- **M**uscle tension
- **I**rritability
- **S**leep
- **E**nergy
- **R**estlessness
- **A**ttention
- (3+ sx)

Panic Dx

Attacks = STUDENTS Fear C's
- **S**weating
- **T**rembling
- **U**nsteadiness
- **D**issociation
- **E**levated heart rate
- **N**ausea
- **T**ingling
- **S**hortness of breath

- **F**ear of dying, etc.
- **C**hest pain
- **C**hills
- **C**hoking

Disorder = SURPrise
- **S**udden **U**nexpected **R**ecurrent **P**anic

OCD

Obsessions

I MURDER?
- **I**ntrusive
- **M**ind-based
- **U**nwanted
- **R**esistant
- **D**istressing
- **E**go-dystonic
- **R**ecurrent

Compulsions

Calm-pulsions help to **calm** obsessive thoughts

Body Dysmorphic Dx

Fix ME DOC!
- **Fix**ation on flaw
- **M**edical care-seeking
- **E**go-syntonic
- **D**isabling
- **O**bsessive thoughts
- **C**ompulsive behaviors

OCD Spectrum

Icks: **T**ic, **trich**otillomania, **sick** (hypochondriasis), body dysmor**phic**

Hypo-**conned**-riasis = patient believes doctor is being **conned** by normal signs & lab findings

TIC = **T**ransient **I**rresistible **C**ontraction

Two-rette syndrome = **Two** forms (motor + vocal)

PTSD, Dissociation, and Somatization

PTSD Dx/Tx

TRAUMA
- **T**raumatic event
- **R**e-experiencing
- **A**rousal
- **U**nable to function
- **M**onth or more
- **A**voidance

Post Traumatic Stress?
Prazosin/**T**herapy/**S**erotonin

Dissociation Sx

DDREAMS
- **D**epersonalization
- **D**erealization
- **R**etrograde amnesia
- **E**rrors of commission
- **A**bsorption
- **M**otor automaticity
- **S**uggestibility

Somatization Tx

I Do CARE
- **I**nterface
- "**D**o no harm"
- **C**BT
- **A**ntidepressants
- **R**egular visits
- **E**mpathy

Somatic Sx D/o Dx

SOME ATTIC
- **S**ymptoms
- **O**ne or more
- **M**edically unexpl.
- **E**xcessive
- **A**nxiety
- **T**hinking about
- **T**ime and energy
- **I**mpaired/distressed
- **C**hronic

Conversion Dx

CAN'T-version
- **C**linically unexplained
- **A**bnormality
- **N**eurologic
- **T**rigger (sometimes)
- Can't: genuinely unable

Malingering/Factitious
- **MAL**ingering **Al**ways **Leaves**, **FAC**titious **A**lways **C**omes back

Personality Disorders

Personality Clusters

At a party...
Cluster A will **PaSS**:
Paranoid, **S**chizoid, and **S**chizotypal

Cluster B will get **BAHN**ed:
Borderline, **A**ntisocial, **H**istrionic, and **N**arcissistic

Cluster C will make party **D**ead **O**n **A**rrival: **D**ependent **O**bsessive-compulsive **A**voidant

Borderline Dx/Tx

I DESPAIR
- **I**dentity
- **D**ysphoria/emptiness
- **E**motional instability
- **S**uicide/self-harm
- **P**sychotic/dissociative
- **A**nger
- **I**mpulsivity
- **R**elationships

DELAPSE
- **D**iagnose
- **E**ducate
- **L**ife outside of tx
- **A**void meds
- **P**rioritize
- **S**afety plan
- **E**xpect change

Antisocial Dx

ACID LIAR
- **A**dult (18+)
- **C**riminality
- **I**mpulsivity
- **D**isregard for safety
- **L**ying
- **I**rresponsibility
- **A**ggression
- **R**emorselessness

Psychopathy, Eating Disorders, and ADHD

Psychopathy Sx

BDSM
- **B**oldness
- **D**isinhibition
- **S**hallowness
- **M**eanness

Eating D/o Screen

SCOFF (2+)
- **S**ick/uncomfortably full
- **C**ontrol over eating lost
- **O**ne stone of weight loss
- **F**eel fat when thin
- **F**ood dominates life

Anorexia Dx

UNDER-rexia
- **U**nderweight
- **N**ervous about wt gain
- **D**istorted perception
- **E**xercise, purging, etc.
- **R**estricting intake

Bulimia Dx

BOWL-imia
- **B**ingeing
- **O**ffsetting (purging)
- **W**eekly >3 mo
- **L**inked to self-esteem

Autism Dx

ASD
- **A**loneness
- **S**ameness
- **D**evelopmental onset

ADHD and Dementia

ADHD (Inattentive) Sx

DETAILS OFF
- **D**etails sloppy
- **E**asily distracted
- **T**ask **A**voidance
- **I**gnores instructions
- **L**oses things
- **S**ustained attention poor
- **O**rganization poor
- **F**orgetful
- **F**ails to finish tasks

ADHD (Hyperactive) Sx

HE RILED UP
- **H**yperactive
- **E**nergetic
- **R**unning around
- **I**nterrupts
- **L**oud
- **E**ffusive/talkative
- **D**elay intolerant
- **U**nseated/up and about
- **P**remature answers

ADHD Dx

FIDGETY
- **F**unctionally impairing
- **I**nattention
- **D**isinhibition
- **G**reater than normal
- **E**xclude other disorders
- **T**wo or more settings
- **Y**oung at onset (≤12)

Dementia Dx

DIRE
- **D**ecline in cognition
- **I**mpairment
- **R**ule out delirium
- **E**xclude psych d/o's

Alzheimer's Sx

MA 'N PA
- **M**emory
- **A**wareness
- **N**eurocognitive deficits
- **P**sychiatric
- **A**ctivity

Made in United States
Orlando, FL
04 January 2025